BASIC PHARMACOKINETICS
AND PHARMACODYNAMICS

BASIC PHARMACOKINETICS AND PHARMACODYNAMICS

An Integrated Textbook and Computer Simulations

Second Edition

Edited by

SARA E. ROSENBAUM

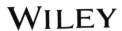

For general information on our other products and services or for technical support, please contact our Customer Care Department within the United States at (800) 762-2974, outside the United States at (317) 572-3993 or fax (317) 572-4002.

Wiley also publishes its books in a variety of electronic formats. Some content that appears in print may not be available in electronic formats. For more information about Wiley products, visit our web site at www.wiley.com.

Library of Congress Cataloging-in-Publication Data:

Names: Rosenbaum, Sara (Sara E.), author, editor.
Title: Basic pharmacokinetics and pharmacodynamics : an integrated textbook and computer simulations / edited by Sara E. Rosenbaum.
Description: Second edition. | Hoboken, New Jersey : John Wiley & Sons, Inc., [2017] | Includes bibliographical references and index.
Identifiers: LCCN 2016031846 (print) | LCCN 2016034126 (ebook) | ISBN 9781119143154 (pbk.) | ISBN 9781119143161 (pdf) | ISBN 9781119143185 (epub)
Subjects: | MESH: Pharmacokinetics | Pharmacological Phenomena | Computer Simulation
Classification: LCC RM301.5 (print) | LCC RM301.5 (ebook) | NLM QV 38 | DDC 615/.7–dc23
LC record available at https://lccn.loc.gov/2016031846

Printed and bound by CPI Group (UK) Ltd, Croydon, CR0 4YY

C9781119143154_310524

To Steve, Molly and Lucy

CONTENTS

5   **Drug Elimination and Clearance**   **99**

Sara E. Rosenbaum

6   **Compartmental Models in Pharmacokinetics**   **145**

Sara E. Rosenbaum

18 Introduction to Physiologically Based Pharmacokinetic Modeling   367

Sara E. Rosenbaum

19 Introduction to Pharmacodynamic Models and Integrated Pharmacokinetic–Pharmacodynamic Models   391

Drs. Diane Mould and Paul Hutson

20 Semimechanistic Pharmacokinetic–Pharmacodynamic Models   413
Drs. Diane Mould and Paul Hutson

Appendix A   Review of Exponents and Logarithms   469
Sara E. Rosenbaum

Appendix B   Rates of Processes   **479**

Sara E. Rosenbaum

Appendix C   Creation of Excel Worksheets for Pharmacokinetic Analysis   **489**

Sara E. Rosenbaum

**Appendix D   Derivation of Equations for Multiple Intravenous Bolus
Injections**   **505**

Sara E. Rosenbaum

PREFACE

The goal of the second edition of Basic Pharmacokinetics and Pharmacodynamics is to update and strengthen existing chapters of the book and to add additional chapters in response to recent trends in the application of pharmacokinetics and pharmacodynamics in clinical practice and pharmaceutical research.

Notable areas of update and expansion include both the text and the interactive computer models associated with drug transporters and hepatic clearance. Additionally, the chapters on drug absorption/bioavailability and pharmacodynamics have been updated, expanded and strengthened to reflect the importance of these topics and the need to cover the material both comprehensively and in a manner compatible with their present application. I felt that these areas would be most effectively strengthened by experts in each of the fields. To this end, I am delighted that Dr. Steven Sutton, who has had extensive experience as a researcher in the pharmaceutical industry and as an educator at the College of Pharmacy, University of New England, agreed to take over Chapters 3 and 9 that cover drug absorption and bioavailability. I am also delighted that Drs. Diane Mould and Paul Hutson agreed to revamp and expand the chapters on pharmacodynamics (Chapters 19 and 20). Dr. Mould of Projections Research Inc is a well-known pharmacokinetic and pharmacodynamic modeler, who has extensive experience in the application of pharmacodynamic models. Dr. Hutson from University of Wisconsin, School of Pharmacy, is similarly experienced and was able to provide an academic perspective to the overhaul of this material.

Owing to the increasing prominence of personalized and precision medicine, it has become important that clinical pharmacists and researchers in pharmaceutical fields have a basic knowledge of pharmacogenomics. Dr. Daniel Brazeau, an experienced educator and researcher in this area from the College of Pharmacy, University of New England, graciously agreed to write an introductory chapter on pharmacogenetics for the second edition. In response to the increasing use and diverse application of physiologically based pharmacokinetic (PBPK) modeling that has occurred over the last 15 years, it has become essential for modern students of pharmacokinetics to have a foundation in this topic. Chapter 18 introduces PBPK models and describes how they are built and applied. The third new chapter in the second edition presents the predictive models used to evaluate drug–drug interaction (DDI) risk using *in vitro* data. These models are used increasingly by pharmaceutical companies and drug regulators to try to reduce the large health risks and costs posed by DDIs. While not all readers of the book will need to apply these models professionally, an understanding of this topic will allow students to better understand and appreciate the mechanism, characteristics, and varied outcome of DDIs. Finally, in order to provide interested students with a foundation to this latter chapter, the second edition includes an appendix on basic enzyme kinetics and the mathematical basis of the predictive models. My colleague at the College of Pharmacy, Dr. Roberta King, an expert in drug metabolism, collaborated in the preparation of this material. Each of the new chapters is supported by new interactive computer models.

It is hoped that the second edition of this textbook provides a comprehensive and thorough presentation of all essential topics in the contemporary application of pharmacokinetics and pharmacodynamics. While not all chapters will be necessary for the immediate needs of all audiences, collectively the book should serve as a valuable reference for the future.

I would like to thank the many scientists who generously gave of their time and provided me with information and input in many areas. I would especially like to thank Dr. Karthik Venkatakrishnan for his valuable input on the chapter on predictive models for DDIs. I would also like to thank and recognize the wonderful work of Pragati Nahar who prepared the custom color figures in the book, including the figure used on the cover. I would also like to thank many undergraduate and graduate students at URI who helped in a variety of ways especially Jamie Chung who provided valuable support for the preparation of the materials, and Benjamin Barlock and Rohitash Jamwal for their input in the creation of the simulation models. Finally, I would like to thank Jonathan Rose at Wiley for his patience, understanding, and responsiveness in the preparation of this edition.

CONTRIBUTORS

Daniel Brazeau   Daniel Brazeau is a Research Associate Professor at the University of New England. He holds joint appointments in the Department of Pharmaceutical Sciences in the College of Pharmacy and Department of Biomedical Sciences in the College of Osteopathic Medicine. Dr. Brazeau is a Director of UNE's Genomics Core, a research training core providing the expertise, technologies and most importantly, training support for faculty and students. He received his B.S. and M.S. in Biology from the University of Toledo and earned his Ph.D. in Biological Sciences (1989) from the University at Buffalo. After completing postdoctoral training in population genetics at the University of Houston, he was a Research Assistant Professor in the Department of Zoology at the University of Florida and Director of the University of Florida's Genetic Analysis Laboratory in the Interdisciplinary Research Center for Biotechnology. For 10 years prior to joining UNE, he was a Research Associate Professor in the Department of Pharmaceutical Sciences at the University at Buffalo and Director of the University at Buffalo's Pharmaceutical Genetics Laboratory. Dr. Brazeau's research interests involve the areas of population molecular genetics and genomics. He teaches courses in molecular genetics methodologies and a required course in pharmacogenomics for graduate and pharmacy professional students. Dr. Brazeau is also a participating scientist in the National Science Foundation's Geneticist-Educator Network Alliances (GENA) working with high school science teachers to incorporate genetics into the classroom.

Paul Hutson   Paul Hutson, whose baccalaureate and master's degrees are in biochemistry and chemistry, respectively, completed an oncology/pharmacokinetics fellowship at St. Jude Children's Research Hospital in Memphis. He was a Faculty Member at the University of Illinois for 5 years before moving to the University of Wisconsin School of Pharmacy in Madison in 1988. He now practices pharmacy with the oncology and palliative care group at the UW Hospital and Clinics and is an Associate Member of the UW Carbone Cancer Center. His three course offerings at the School of Pharmacy are Clinical Pharmacokinetics, Pediatric Pharmacotherapy, and Dietary Supplements, and he supervises an Advanced Pharmacy Practice Experience (APPE) in basic pharmacometrics. Dr. Hutson provides pharmacometric modeling services to the pharmaceutical industry and to University of Wisconsin—Madison investigators through its CTSA-funded Institute for Clinical and Translational Research.

Roberta S. King Roberta S. King is an Associate Professor at the University of Rhode Island, College of Pharmacy. Her research expertise is in metabolism and enzymology focusing on individual variation in activity of the drug-metabolizing enzymes. She teaches Drug Metabolism and Structure-based Drug Design.

Dr. Mould Dr. Mould obtained her bachelors degree at Stevens Institute of Technology in 1984 in Chemistry and Chemical Biology. She received her Ph.D. in Pharmaceutics and Pharmaceutical Chemistry at The Ohio State University (OSU) in 1989. She spent 26 years as a pharmacokineticist in industry where she specialized in population pharmacokinetic/pharmacodynamic modeling and was an Associate Research Professor at Georgetown University. She has conducted population PK/PD analyses of hematopoietic agents, monoclonal antibodies, anticancer and antiviral agents, antipsychotic, cardiovascular, and sedative/hypnotic agents. Dr Mould is involved in clinical trial simulation and optimal study design in drug development. She was a member of the Scientific Advisory Group for Phar-Sight, where she assisted in development of clinical trial simulation software.

Currently, Dr Mould is President of Projections Research Inc., a consulting company offering pharmacokinetic and pharmacometric services. She is also the founder of iDose LLC, a company that develops systems to individualize doses of drugs that are difficult to manage. She has published 62 peer-reviewed articles, 16 book chapters, made 97 national and international presentations, and presented six podium sessions on advanced modeling and simulation approaches. Dr Mould has authored 97 posters at both national and international meetings. She is an Adjunct Professor at the University of Rhode Island (URI), OSU, and the University of Florida, and teaches an annual class on disease progression modeling at the National Institutes of Health. Dr Mould taught nine courses (OSU, URI, and SUNY Buffalo) on specialized aspects of population pharmacokinetic and dynamic modeling. She is a member of the editorial board for Journal of Pharmacokinetics and Pharmacodynamics, Clinical Pharmacology and Therapeutics, and Clinical Pharmacology and Therapeutics Pharmacometrics and Systems Pharmacology. Dr. Mould is a member of the Board of Regents for the American College of Clinical Pharmacology and is a Chairman of the Publications committee for this organization. She is a Fellow of the American College of Clinical Pharmacology and the American Association of Pharmaceutical Sciences.

Steven C. Sutton Steven (Steev) C. Sutton, B.S. Pharmacy, Ph.D., University of New England, Portland, Maine Dr. Sutton is an Associate Professor and Chair of Pharmaceutics, College of Pharmacy, University of New England in Portland, Maine. He received his B.S. in Pharmacy from Massachusetts College of Pharmacy and a Ph.D. in Pharmaceutical Sciences from the State University of New York at Buffalo, New York. Dr Sutton began his career in the pharmaceutical industry working for CIBA-Geigy in Ardsley, NY (now Novartis), for INTERx in Lawrence, KS (then a part of Merck), and for Pfizer in Groton, CT, before embarking in a second career—that of academia—at the University of New England College of Pharmacy in Portland in 2009. Dr. Sutton founded the AAPS Oral Absorption Focus Group and in 2003, he became a Fellow of the AAPS. His research interests include predicting active pharmaceutical ingredient concentration–time profile in human after oral administration from chemical structure, modeling, and simulation of oral absorption of low permeability and/or low aqueous soluble compounds, *in vitro—in vivo* correlation of orally

administered controlled release dosage forms, species differences in gastrointestinal (GI) physiology, and transport of nanoparticles across the GI epithelium. Dr. Sutton has authored or coauthored over 120 book chapters, abstracts of work in progress, invited presentations, and patents.

1

INTRODUCTION TO PHARMACOKINETICS AND PHARMACODYNAMICS

Sara E. Rosenbaum

Objectives

The material in this chapter will enable the reader to:

1. Define pharmacodynamics and pharmacokinetics
2. Understand the processes that control the dose–response relationship
3. Gain a general appreciation of how mathematical expressions in pharmacodynamics and pharmacokinetics can be used for the rational determination of optimum dosing regimens

Basic Pharmacokinetics and Pharmacodynamics: An Integrated Textbook and Computer Simulations,
Second Edition. Edited by Sara E. Rosenbaum.
© 2017 John Wiley & Sons, Inc. Published 2017 by John Wiley & Sons, Inc.

1.1 INTRODUCTION: DRUGS AND DOSES

Drugs may be defined as chemicals that alter physiological or biochemical processes in the body in a manner that makes them useful in the treatment, prevention, or cure of diseases. Based on this definition, any useful drug must affect body physiology or biochemistry. By extension, any useful drug must, if used inappropriately, possess the ability to do harm. Drug action begins with administration of the drug (input) and concludes with the biological response (output, which can be a beneficial and/or an adverse effect). The inputs (dose, frequency of administration, and route of administration) must be selected carefully to optimize the onset, intensity, and duration of therapeutic effects for a particular disease condition. At the same time, the inputs selected must minimize any harmful effects of drugs.

The design of optimum dosing regimens requires a complete understanding of the processes and steps that translate the input into the output. It also requires an understanding of how the input–output relationship may be influenced by individual patient characteristics that may exist at the very beginning of therapy, as well as conditions that may arise during the course of drug therapy. These will include the age and weight of the patient, the presence of other diseases, genetic factors, concurrent medications, and changes in the disease being treated over time.

The material presented in this book will address and explain why, as shown in Table 1.1, there is such tremendous variability in the value of drug doses and dosing frequencies among therapeutic drugs. Additionally, it will address why different routes of administration are used for different drugs and different indications (Table 1.1).

The steps between drug input and the emergence of the response can be broken down into two phases: pharmacokinetic and pharmacodynamic. The *pharmacokinetic phase* encompasses all the events between the administration of a dose and the achievement of drug concentrations throughout the body. The *pharmacodynamic phase* encompasses all the events between the arrival of the drug at its site of action and the onset, magnitude, and duration of the biological response (Figure 1.1). The rational design of optimum dosing regimens must be based on a thorough understanding of these two phases and will, ideally, include the development of one or more mathematical expressions for the relationship between dose and the time course of drug response.

Optimum drug administration is important not only for ensuring good patient outcomes in clinical practice, but also in the design of clinical trials during drug development. The

TABLE 1.1 Examples of Common Daily Doses and Dosing Intervals

Drug	Daily Dose (mg)	Dose Frequency (h)	Route
Calcium carbonate	3000	2	Oral
Ibuprofen	1600	6	Oral
Vancomycin (for MRSA[a])	2000	12	Intravenous
Amoxicillin	750	8	Oral
Vancomycin (for pseudomembranous colitis)	1000	6	Oral
Atenolol	100	24	Oral
Fluoxetine	20	24	Oral
Ramipril	10	12	Oral
Digoxin	0.250	24	Oral
Chloroquine	300	Weekly	Oral

[a]Methicillin-resistant *Staphylococcus aureus*.

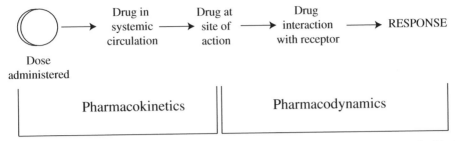

FIGURE 1.1   The two phases of drug action. The pharmacokinetic phase is concerned with the relationship between the value of the dose administered and the value of the drug concentrations achieved in the body; the pharmacodynamic phase is concerned with the relationship between drug concentrations at the site of action and the onset, intensity, and duration of drug response.

cost of drug research and development is enormous, so it is critical that all drug candidates selected for human trials are evaluated in the most efficient, cost-effective manner possible.

The application of pharmacokinetic and pharmacodynamic principles to this process has been shown to enhance the selection of optimum doses and optimum designs of phase II clinical trials.

1.2 INTRODUCTION TO PHARMACODYNAMICS

Pharmaco- comes from the Greek word for "drug," *pharmackon*, and *dynamics* means "of or relating to variation of intensity." *Pharmacodynamics (PD) is the study of the magnitude of drug response. In particular, it is the study of the onset, intensity, and duration of drug response and how these are related to the concentration of a drug at its site of action.* An overview of some basic drug terminology and the drug response–concentration relationship is provided below.

1.2.1 Drug Effects at the Site of Action

Note that although some references and textbooks distinguish the terms drug *effect* and drug *response*, this distinction has not been adopted universally. In this book, *effect* and *response* are used interchangeably.

1.2.1.1 Interaction of a Drug with Its Receptor
Drug response is initiated by a chemical interaction between a drug and a special binding site on a macromolecule in a tissue. This macromolecule is known as a drug *receptor.* The drug–receptor interaction results in a conformational change in the receptor, which results in the generation of a stimulus that ultimately leads to a biochemical or physiological response (Figure 1.2). Most receptors (over 95%) are proteins; however, other types of receptors exist such as the DNA receptors of the alkylating agents used in cancer chemotherapy. The drug–receptor interaction involves chemical bonding, which is usually reversible in nature and can be expressed using the law of mass action (Figure 1.2). Thus, at the site of action, the drug binds to its receptor and equilibrium is established between the bound and the unbound drug. As the drug is eliminated from the body and removed from its site of action, it dissociates from the receptor, which is left unchanged, and the response dissipates.

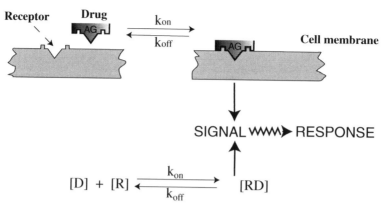

FIGURE 1.2 Drug–receptor interaction. Here, AG signifies a drug agonist, [D] is the free drug concentration (not bound to the receptor), R is the concentration of free receptors, [RD] is the concentration of the drug–receptor complex, and k_{on} and k_{off} are the rate constants for the forward and backward processes, respectively.

In contrast, a few drugs form *irreversible* covalent bonds with their receptors. For example, aspirin inhibits platelet aggregation by inhibiting the formation of thromboxane in the platelets. It accomplishes this by binding covalently to and blocking the catalytic activity of cyclooxygenase, the enzyme that produces thromboxane. The effect of a single dose of aspirin will persist long after the drug has been removed from its site of action and will continue until new cyclooxygenase molecules are synthesized, which can then resume the production of thromboxane. Other examples of drugs that bind irreversibly to their receptors include the alkylating agents mentioned above and proton pump inhibitors, such as omeprazole, which block the secretion of gastric acid by binding irreversibly to the H^+, K^+-ATPase pumps of parietal cells.

The drug–receptor interaction is highly dependent on the chemical structure of both the drug and the receptor and, therefore, small changes in the structure of the drug can reduce or destroy activity. For example, the drug–receptor interaction can distinguish between the R- and S-isomers of drugs that have chiral carbon atoms. Usually, one isomer is much more active than the other. The S-isomer of warfarin, for example, is two to five times more active than the R-isomer. The development and promotion of S-omeprazole (Nexium) is based on the premise that the S-isomer has the higher affinity for the binding site and thus offers therapeutic advantages over preparations containing racemic mixtures (equal quantities of each isomer) of omeprazole, such as Prilosec and its generic equivalents.

Receptors are assumed to exist for all active endogenous compounds (*natural ligands*) such as neurotransmitters and hormones. The interaction between natural ligands and their receptors controls and/or regulates physiological and biochemical processes in the body. In most cases, drugs mimic or antagonize the actions of endogenous ligands by interacting with their cognate receptors. For example, epinephrine is a natural ligand that interacts with β_2-adrenergic receptors in bronchial smooth muscle to bring about bronchial dilation. Albuterol, a drug, also interacts with this receptor to produce bronchial dilation. Acetylcholine transmits signals through a synapse by interacting with its nicotinic receptor found on postsynaptic neuronal membranes. This interaction, which is mimicked by the drug nicotine, results in the production of a response called an action potential.

It should be noted that there are a few drugs that do not act on receptors but that exert their action by bringing about *physicochemical changes* in the body. For example, conventional antacids, such as calcium carbonate, act as buffers to reduce acidity in the stomach and polyethylene glycol, an osmotic laxative, acts by preventing the absorption of water in the large intestine.

1.2.1.2 Postreceptor Events

Drugs almost always bring about some type of change in the *intracellular environment* of cells, but the lipophilic cell membrane presents a physical barrier to most drugs and endogenous ligands. As a result, most receptors are located on the cell membrane itself. The stimulus generated from the interaction of the drug with the membrane bound receptor has to be relayed to the inside of the cell. The relaying of the initial stimulus, known as *coupling* or *signal transduction*, often involves a cascade of different steps during which the initial signal may be amplified or diminished. Some important transduction mechanisms are summarized below (see Figure 1.3).

1. Interaction of a drug with a receptor can lead directly to the opening or closing of an *ion channel* that lies across a cell membrane. In this case, the signal is relayed by changes in the ion concentration within the cell. For example, the interaction of acetylcholine with its nicotinic receptor results in the opening of an ion channel allowing Na^+ to move into the cell thus, initiating the production of an action potential.

2. Signal transduction for a large number of drugs involves the *activation of a G-protein* (guanine nucleotide-binding protein). The drug–receptor interaction on the membrane triggers the activation of a G-protein on the cytoplasmic side of the membrane, which then initiates a series of events that culminate in the biological response. Activated G-protein can produce a variety of effects, including stimulation or inhibition of enzymes, and the opening or closing of ion channels. These events usually result in changes in the concentration of an intracellular compound known as the

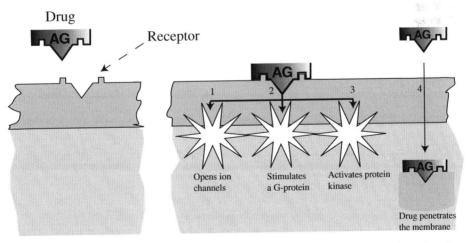

FIGURE 1.3 Diagrammatic representations of how a drug receptor interaction brings about intracellular events. The intracellular relay of the initial signal resulting from the interaction of a drug with a membrane-bound receptor can be accomplished in one of three ways: (1) the direct opening of ion channels; (2) the activation of a G-protein that may lead to the activation of another enzyme or to a modulation of an ion channel; (3) the activation of protein kinase. Alternatively, (4), some drugs are able to penetrate membranes and directly activate intracellular receptors.

second messenger. Examples of second messengers include cyclic adensine-3′,5′-monophosphate (cAMP), calcium, and phosphoinositides. The second messengers then relay the response further through a series of complex steps. For example, the interaction of catecholamines such as norepinephrine with certain β-receptor sub-types involves G-protein activation. This then stimulates adenylate cyclase to convert adenosine triphosphate to cAMP, which acts as the second messenger. Subsequent events include the stimulation of specific protein kinases, activation of calcium channels, and modification of cellular proteins. Other examples of G-protein–coupled receptors are the action of acetylcholine on its muscarinic receptors and the action of serotonin on its 5-HT receptors.

3. The interaction of a drug with its receptor can also result in the stimulation of a receptor-associated enzyme, tyrosine kinase. The activated tyrosine kinase phosphorylates key macromolecules, which are often a part of the receptor itself, to relay the signal. Insulin and peptide growth factors, for example, use this form of signal transduction.

Some drugs are lipophilic enough to penetrate the cell membrane, while others may be transported across the cell membrane by uptake transporters. Drugs that are able to enter a cell can interact directly with intracellular receptors. Examples of drugs that act on intracellular receptors include many steroids such as glucocorticoid steroids, sex hormones, and thyroid hormones. The HMG-CoA reductase inhibitors (commonly known as *statins*) and metformin also act within the cell (hepatocyte) and both are dependent on uptake transporters to deliver them to the intracellular space and their site of action.

1.2.2   Agonists, Antagonists, and Concentration–Response Relationships

A drug that mimics the endogenous receptor ligand to activate the receptor is referred to as an *agonist*. The typical relationship between the drug effect and the agonist concentration at the receptor site is shown in Figure 1.4a. Note that as the concentration of the drug increases, the effect increases. At *low concentrations, there is a linear relationship between concentration and effect* (i.e., the response is proportional to the concentration). At higher drug

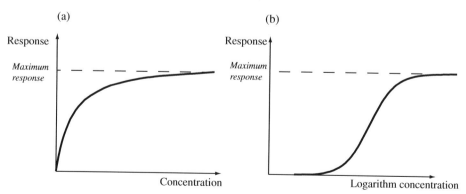

FIGURE 1.4   Plots of response versus drug concentration: (a) on a linear scale and (b) on a semilogarithmic scale.

concentrations, increases in concentration bring about much smaller changes in effect (the *law of limited returns*). Eventually, at very high concentrations, the effect achieves a maximum value and then remains constant and independent of concentration. In this area of the curve, increases in concentration will not result in further increases in response. This relationship is observed because response is generated by a saturable, capacity-limited process. For example, the response may be limited by the number of receptors that a tissue contains. At low drug concentrations, there are many free receptors and as the drug concentration increases, the drug can bind to the free receptors and response can increase proportionally. At higher concentrations, more and more of the receptors are occupied. As a result, increases in the drug concentration produce much less increase in effect. Eventually, all of the receptors are occupied (or saturated) and a maximum effect is observed. To accommodate a wide range of concentrations, the relationship between effect and concentration is usually plotted on a semilogarithmic scale, which transforms the plot to a sigmoidal shape (Figure 1.4b).

Many agonists are able to produce the system's maximum response without fully occupying all the receptors. In these systems, the maximum response of the drug must be the result of some other saturable, capacity-limited process that occurs after receptor binding. These tissues or systems are said to have *spare receptors*. Experimentally, the presence of spare receptors can be demonstrated by destroying some of the receptors. If an agonist is still able to produce a maximum response, the system must contain spare receptors.

The efficiency with which a drug's interaction with the receptor is converted into the initial stimulus or biosignal is a function of the number of receptors at the site of action and a drug's *intrinsic efficacy*. Intrinsic efficacy can be defined as the magnitude of the stimulus produced per unit receptor occupied. The value of the stimulus that results from a specific concentration of a drug is also a function of the drug's affinity for its receptors. *Affinity* can be defined as the extent or fraction to which a drug binds to receptors at any given drug concentration. Drugs that have high affinity require less drug to produce a certain degree of binding and to elicit a certain response compared to drugs with low affinity. Affinity is one of the factors that determines *potency* (see Chapter 19).

A drug that binds to a receptor but does not activate it is referred to as an *antagonist*. The presence of an antagonist at the receptor site blocks the action of the agonist (Figure 1.5). Higher concentrations of the agonist are needed to displace the antagonist and to produce the effect that is elicited when the antagonist was absent. The antagonist shifts the concentration–response curve of an agonist to the right (Figure 1.6). At sufficiently high concentrations of the antagonist, the agonist's action may be blocked completely and the effect of even high concentrations of the agonist is reduced to zero. Some drugs bind to

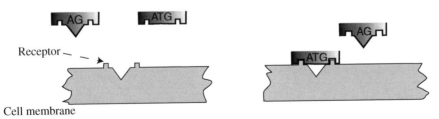

FIGURE 1.5 Diagrammatic representation of the action of an antagonist. The antagonist (ATG) binds to the receptor but does not produce a signal. Its presence on the receptor blocks the action of agonists (AG), including the natural ligand.

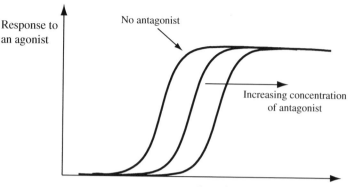

FIGURE 1.6 Plot of response versus logarithm concentration for an agonist in the absence and presence of increasing concentrations of an antagonist.

receptors, but the binding is less efficient and a full response cannot be achieved even when the drug's concentration is very high and all the receptors are occupied (Figure 1.7). These drugs are referred to as *partial agonists*. A partial agonist will block the effect of a full agonist. In the presence of high concentrations of a partial agonist, the action of a full agonist can be reduced to the maximum response elicited by the partial agonist. Clinically, partial agonists are used to act as buffers to avoid full stimulation of a system. Examples of partial agonists include several β-blockers, including pindolol, and the opioid buprenorphine. The latter is a partial agonist on the μ-opioid receptors and is considered a safer alternative to morphine because it does not produce as much respiratory depression (see Chapter 19).

In summary, drug action is mediated primarily by the interaction of a drug with membrane-bound receptors at its site of action. This produces conformational changes in the receptor, which lead to the generation of an initial signal. The signal is then relayed to the intracellular environment by means of a variety of transduction processes. The response increases with increases in drug concentration until enough receptors are occupied to generate the maximal response. The response to a specific concentration of drug is dependent on drug-specific properties (e.g., intrinsic efficacy and affinity) and tissue-specific properties (e.g., number or density of receptors and amplification or diminution of the initial signal during transduction). An important goal in a study of pharmacodynamics is to derive

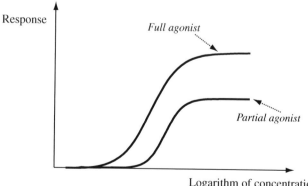

FIGURE 1.7 Plot of response versus logarithm concentration for a full and a partial agonist.

a mathematical expression for the magnitude of drug response as a function of drug concentration:

$$E = f_{PD}(C) \tag{1.1}$$

where E is the drug effect or response, C is the drug concentration, and f_{PD} is a pharmacodynamic function that links these two variables and contains the drug-specific parameters of intrinsic efficacy and affinity. In equation (1.1), E is the *dependent variable* because it is dependent on all the other components of the equation. The drug concentration at the site of action (C) is the *independent variable* because it is independent of all the other components of equation (1.1). This expression would allow the effect to be estimated at any drug concentration and allow the required concentrations for optimum response to be identified.

1.3   INTRODUCTION TO PHARMACOKINETICS

Pharmaco- comes from the Greek word for "drug," *pharmackon*, and *kinetics* comes from the Greek word for "moving," *kinetikos. Pharmacokinetics (PK) is the study of drug movement into, around, and out of the body. By extension, it involves the study of drug absorption, distribution, and elimination (metabolism and excretion) (ADME).*

Pharmacokinetics involves the study of how drugs enter the body, distribute throughout the body, and leave the body. It is concerned with the driving forces for these processes and the rate at which they occur. Pharmacokinetics is the study of the *time course of drug concentrations in body compartments.* From a therapeutic perspective, the drug concentration at the site of action is by far the most important: Concentrations should be sufficiently high to produce a response but not so high as to produce toxicity. Since it is not possible to routinely measure this concentration clinically, the *plasma concentration* of the drug is the main focus in pharmacokinetics. It is often assumed that the *plasma concentration reflects the drug concentration at the site of action.* This is generally true and the relationship is often linear. Increases or decreases in the plasma concentration will be reflected by proportional increases or decreases at the site of action, respectively. However, as discussed in subsequent chapters, this is not always the case and a more complex relationship between these two concentrations may exist. It is important to note that although changes in the plasma concentration will usually result in proportional changes in the drug concentration at the site of action, the reverse is not true. Because the amount of drug that is delivered to the site of action is usually such a very small fraction of the total amount of drug in the body (in other tissues and the systemic circulation), local changes in the amount of drug at the site of action are generally not reflected by noticeable changes in the plasma concentration.

1.3.1   Plasma Concentration of Drugs

As stated above, pharmacokinetics is concerned with the body's exposure to a drug and how drug concentrations change over time. For the most part, drug concentrations in the plasma are the focus in pharmacokinetics. The rationale for this is twofold. First, blood is one of the few body fluids that can be obtained and analyzed repeatedly for drug concentrations at specified times after the administration of a dose. The concentration of drug in whole blood is not commonly used in pharmacokinetics because blood is a complex physical system that consists of red blood cells, white blood cells, and platelets suspended in plasma water. Blood with the cellular elements removed, either by centrifugation (plasma) or clotting

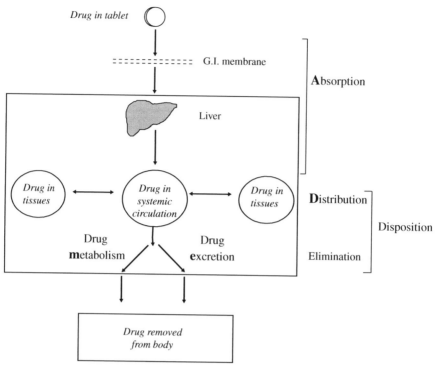

FIGURE 1.8   Processes of drug absorption, distribution, and elimination (metabolism and excretion) (ADME). Drug contained within the tablet must undergo absorption. It must penetrate the gastrointestinal membrane and pass through the liver before reaching the systemic circulation. Once in the blood, it has the opportunity to distribute to the tissues, including the site of action. As soon as drug is present in the systemic circulation, it is subject to elimination. This occurs primarily in the liver and kidneys, where drugs undergo metabolism and/or excretion, respectively. The fate of a drug in the systemic circulation (distribution and elimination) is referred to as drug disposition.

(serum), is preferred. The collection of plasma requires the use of an anticoagulant such as heparin. However, heparin can interfere with the assay of some drugs. In these cases (e.g., for measuring digoxin concentration), serum rather than plasma is used as the reference fluid. In this book, no distinction will be made between plasma and serum, and the term *plasma concentration* will be used almost universally.

The second rationale for focusing on plasma concentrations in pharmacokinetics is that the circulatory system is the central fluid for the receipt and distribution of drugs (Figure 1.8). All drug input processes conclude when drug reaches the plasma, and all *disposition* (distribution and elimination) *processes* begin once drug is present in the plasma. Thus, drugs at absorption sites such as the gastrointestinal tract or subcutaneous tissue are absorbed into the circulatory system. Once in the blood, drugs undergo distribution to various tissues in the body and undergo elimination primarily through the liver and/or kidneys.

Plasma or plasma water consists of small dissolved molecules (e.g., glucose, ions, nutrients, and drugs) and suspended substances such as proteins, which are too large to dissolve. Many drugs can *bind* or *associate* with the plasma proteins. The binding is reversible and may be expressed according to the *law of mass action*:

$$[D] + [P] \underset{k_2}{\overset{k_1}{\rightleftharpoons}} [DP] \tag{1.2}$$

where D is the free drug concentration, P is the concentration of the protein not involved in binding, DP is the concentration of the drug–protein complex, and k_1 and k_2 are the rate constants for the forward and backward reaction, respectively.

Thus, many drugs exist in the plasma in an equilibrium between two forms: one component dissolved in the plasma water (*free drug*) and one component associated with or bound to plasma proteins (*bound drug*). The term *plasma concentration (Cp)* in pharmacokinetics refers to the total drug concentration of the drug, that is, the bound plus the free drug. Total drug concentrations are reported routinely because they are much easier and less expensive to measure than free drug concentrations. However, as presented in subsequent chapters, the free concentration is the clinically important component: Only free unbound drug is able to pass biological membranes, interact with the receptor, and generate a pharmacological response.

1.3.2 Processes in Pharmacokinetics

Pharmacokinetics involves the study of the processes that affect the plasma concentration of a drug at any time after the administration of a dose. These processes are summarized in Figure 1.8. Most drugs are administered orally as tablets. A *tablet* is a compressed powder mass that consists of the active drug, which usually comprises only a small portion of the overall tablet, and other compounds required for either the manufacture of the tablet (i.e., diluents and lubricants) or to optimize the characteristics of the finished product (i.e., color, taste, and hardness). Once a tablet is swallowed, it enters the stomach, where the drug contained within the hard powder mass must be exposed and released. The tablet must first disintegrate into small particles to enable the drug to dissolve in the gastrointestinal fluid. These initial processes of disintegration and dissolution are part of *biopharmaceutics*, which may be defined as the study of how a drug's chemical and physical properties influence both the administration of the drug and the pharmacokinetic behavior of the dosage form *in vivo*. When the drug is dissolved in the gastrointestinal fluid, it has the opportunity to pass across the epithelial cell lining of the gastrointestinal membrane and get taken up into the blood on the other side. Once in the circulatory system, the drug has to pass through the liver, which is a major organ of drug elimination. The absorbed drug may undergo elimination by *metabolism during its first pass through the liver*. After passing through the liver, the drug is taken to the heart, which pumps the drug throughout the entire circulatory system. At this point, the drug has been *absorbed*. The rate and extent of absorption of a drug are very important determinants of the early plasma concentrations of a drug. Rapid rates of absorption will promote high early plasma concentrations. Once the heart pumps the drug around the body, the drug is given the opportunity to *distribute* to all the tissues, including the biophase or site of action. A drug's distribution pattern, particularly the rate and extent to which it distributes to the tissues, is also an important determinant of the early plasma concentrations. If a drug distributes extensively to the tissues, little drug will be left in the plasma and the plasma concentration will be low. The plasma concentration will also be influenced by drug *elimination*, which occurs as soon as the drug is in the plasma. The main pathways of elimination are *hepatic metabolism* and *renal excretion*. The process of drug elimination will continue to affect the plasma concentration until the drug has been removed from the body completely.

In summary, a drug's pharmacokinetics are determined by the simultaneous processes of ADME (Figure 1.8). The combined processes of drug elimination and drug distribution or the fate of a drug once it is present in the body is referred to as *drug disposition*

TABLE 1.2 Pharmacokinetic Processes That Control the Dose–Plasma Concentration Relationship after the Consumption of a Tablet

	Process	Type of Process
1	Release of drug: tablet disintegration	Biopharmaceutics
2	Dissolution of tablet	Biopharmaceutics
3	Absorption of drug through gastrointestinal membrane into the blood	Absorption
4	Passage through the liver	Absorption
5	Entry to systemic circulation	Absorption
6	Distribution to the biophase	Biophase distribution
7	Distribution throughout the body	Distribution
8	Elimination (metabolism and excretion)	Elimination

(Figure 1.8). The individual pharmacokinetic steps associated with the administration of a tablet are summarized in Table 1.2.

The goal of pharmacokinetics is to study each of the ADME processes with the aim of:

1. Identifying the drug and patient factors that determine the rate and extent of each process. Topics to be considered include:
   - How does a drug's lipophilicity influence absorption, distribution, and elimination?
   - What factors determine a drug's distribution pattern?
   - Is the whole of a dose absorbed into the body?
   - Does a drug get to every tissue in the body?
   - To what extent, do drugs undergo renal as opposed to hepatic elimination?
   - How are pharmacokinetic processes affected by patient characteristics, such as the age of the patient, renal or hepatic impairment, ethnicity, and genetics?
2. Identifying a way to quantify or summarize each process in ADME using a single parameter. Issues to be considered include:
   - How can the extent of absorption of a drug be quantified?
   - How can the extent to which a drug distributes the tissues be quantified?
3. Deriving a mathematical expression for the rate of each process in ADME and for the overall relationship between a drug's plasma concentration and time after any dose:

$$Cp = f_{PK} \text{ (dose, time)} \tag{1.3}$$

where Cp is the plasma concentration, and f_{PK} is a function that contains expressions and parameters for ADME. In equation (1.3), Cp is the dependent variable because it is dependent on all the other components of the equation, time is the independent variable, and dose is a constant in a given situation.

1.4 DOSE–RESPONSE RELATIONSHIPS

It will become apparent in subsequent chapters that for most drugs, *the drug concentration in the body at any time is proportional to the dose*. As a result, plots of response at a certain time as a function of dose (Figure 1.9) resemble the plots of response versus concentration

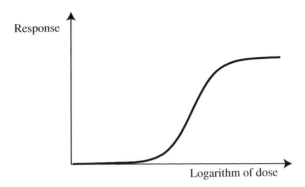

FIGURE 1.9   Graph of response versus logarithm of dose.

(Figure 1.4): A hyperbolic plot is often observed on the linear scale, and a sigmoidal plot is observed on the semilogarithmic scale. Thus, dose–response curves are analogous, but not identical, to pharmacodynamic concentration–effect curves.

In contrast to the plots of response versus concentration, which are purely dependent on a drug's pharmacodynamics, a dose–response curve is a function of both the drug's pharmacodynamic characteristics (intrinsic efficacy and affinity) and its pharmacokinetic characteristics (the fraction of the dose absorbed, the extent to which a drug distributes throughout the body, etc.). Note that low doses produce no effect, and as the maximum response is approached, increasing the dose produces little change in the response (limiting returns). Based on the characteristics shown in Figure 1.9, doses must be selected to avoid the subtherapeutic areas of the plot and to avoid doses that approach or lie on the plateau that provide little or no additional benefit over lower doses. Most drugs also produce toxicity at higher concentrations, and it is important that doses are selected that minimize this toxicity. The toxicity may be an extension of the drug's pharmacological action (e.g., the major adverse effects of warfarin, digoxin, and anticholinergic drugs), in which case it is important to avoid areas on the dose–response curve close to the maximum effect. Alternatively, the toxicity may arise because the drug may interact with multiple receptors of different types, particularly at higher concentrations, to produce undesired effects. Examples of this type of toxicity include muscle toxicity associated with the statins and drowsiness associated with first-generation antihistamines. The development of models and mathematical expressions of the pharmacokinetic and pharmacodynamic phases of drug response provides an opportunity for the rational selection of optimum dosing regimens.

The expression for a drug's pharmacokinetics [equation (1.3)] can be combined with the expression for a drug's pharmacodynamics [equation (1.1)] to produce a *complete expression for the dose–response relationship*:

$$E = f_{\text{PD}}\left(f_{\text{PK}}\left(\text{dose}, \text{time}\right)\right) \tag{1.4}$$

Note that in this equation, the plasma concentration of the drug (Cp) has been substituted for the drug concentration at the site of action (C) in the pharmacodynamic equation. This assumes that the concentration at the site is always proportional to the plasma concentration. The validity and limitations of this are discussed in subsequent chapters. Equation (1.4) enables the full time course of drug response to be estimated after any dose. It could also be used to estimate the dose and dosing interval to produce optimum response. If these relationships are identified early in the course of drug development, they can be used to determine optimum doses for clinical trials. This in turn will increase the efficiency of trials, reduce the time for drug development, and decrease the price of these highly costly studies. The expressions can also be used to simulate response data for situations not yet studied clinically. For example, if a drug's pharmacokinetics and pharmacodynamics are known after a single dose, it is possible to use a combined PK–PD equation to simulate the response that may be expected during multiple dosing therapy. Simulations can be performed using different dosing regimens to try to obtain an estimate of what may be the most effective dosing regimen.

1.5 THERAPEUTIC RANGE

In vivo pharmacodynamic studies aimed at developing mathematical expressions of drug response are relatively new. Historically, *in vivo* pharmacodynamic studies have been very difficult to perform. Some reasons for this are presented below:

1. It is difficult to obtain precise measurements of drug response. Meaningful models and mathematical expressions for drug response require that response data be collected on a continuous scale. The data must also possess a reasonable degree of precision. All-or-none responses and subjective data, based largely on a patient's or a physician's opinion, have limited value in this application. The response to only a handful of drugs (e.g., anticoagulants and hypoglycemic agents) meets these criteria. In the last 10–20 years, this problem has been overcome by the development and use of biomarkers (see Chapter 19) of drug response. *Biomarkers* are parallel changes in the levels or intensities of concrete measurable biological molecules or other effects that have been found to be predictably associated with a drug's biological response. Examples of biomarkers may include cells, proteins, antibodies, body temperature, or features of an electroencephalograph.

2. The mathematical expressions derived from pharmacodynamic models are mainly nonlinear and could not be applied to clinical data until computer software became available for nonlinear regression analysis.

3. Each drug or drug class has a unique mechanism of action and way of relaying or coupling the initial drug effect. Signal transduction may take less than a second for some drugs, several minutes for others, or up to several hours for others. As a result, summarizing the characteristics of the concentration–response relationship can be complex.

4. In many cases, a drug's response lags behind the plasma concentration. This can confound the concentration–response relationship and add an additional layer of complexity to modeling response as a function of plasma concentration.

By contrast, pharmacokinetic studies are relatively simple to perform. Blood is easily sampled, drug assays for most drugs are fairly easily developed, and the data analysis is relatively straightforward and could be performed even before the wide availability of computers and software for pharmacokinetic analysis, by linearizing the mathematical expressions and analyzing the data using simple linear regression analysis. Furthermore, the pharmacokinetics of most drugs can be modeled using one of about three basic well-established models. As a result, pharmacokinetic studies and modeling have been a central part of the drug development process for decades. In order to use pharmacokinetic models for the design of dosing regimens, it is necessary to have target-optimal plasma concentrations

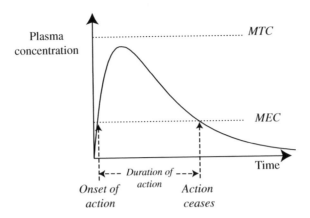

FIGURE 1.10   Therapeutic range. The therapeutic range of a drug is the range of plasma concentrations bounded by a lower minimum effective concentration (MEC) and an upper maximum tolerated concentration (MTC). The typical plasma concentration–time profile observed with the administration of a single oral dose is also shown. The therapeutic range allows the onset and duration of action of a drug to be estimated.

or some idea of the concentration–response relationship. In the absence of mathematical expressions for this relationship, a very simple approach for linking drug concentrations to response was developed and termed the *therapeutic range*. The therapeutic range is defined as the range of plasma concentrations that are associated with optimum response and minimal toxicity in most patients. Most commonly, the goal of therapy is to maintain drug concentrations within the therapeutic range at all times. There are a small number of drugs for which this is not desirable, such as certain antibiotics and drugs like nitroglycerin, where tolerance develops with continuous exposure to the drug.

The therapeutic range is illustrated in Figure 1.10, which shows:

- The *minimum effective concentration* (MEC) is the lower boundary for effective drug concentrations; plasma concentrations below the MEC have a high probability of being subtherapeutic.
- The *maximum tolerated concentration* (MTC) is the upper boundary for optimum drug concentrations; plasma concentrations above the MTC have a high probability of producing adverse effects or toxicity.
- The *onset of action* of a drug, which may be estimated as the time it takes for plasma concentrations to reach the MEC.
- The *duration of action* of a drug, which may be estimated as the time during which plasma concentrations remain within the therapeutic range.

1.5.1 Determination of the Therapeutic Range

To apply the therapeutic range appropriately, and to understand both its value and limitations, it is necessary to appreciate how it is typically derived. It is usually determined by studying the effects of a drug in a large population and noting the plasma concentrations at which patients:

- experience therapeutic effects;
- experience side effects or toxicity.

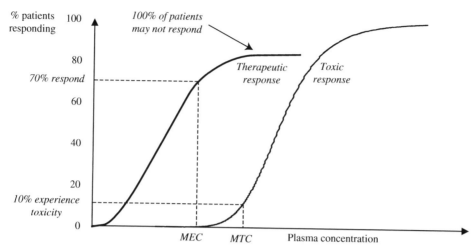

FIGURE 1.11 Identification of the therapeutic range. A drug's therapeutic range is based on studying the concentrations associated with response and toxicity in a large group of patients. The MEC is selected at a concentration at which a large fraction of the population respond (70% is used in the diagram). The MTC is selected at a concentration where a significant fraction of the population experience toxicity. In the diagram, the MTC was selected at the concentration where 10% of the population experience toxicity.

The cumulative plot of the percentage of all patients who experience a therapeutic response is then plotted as a function of plasma concentration (Figure 1.11). The cumulative plot of the percentage of patients experiencing adverse effects at the various concentrations is then added to the same graph (Figure 1.11). Similar sigmoidal shapes are obtained for both curves, but the plot for toxicity is always displaced to the right. Higher concentrations are needed for adverse compared to therapeutic effects (if this were not the case, the drug would not be of therapeutic value). A frequent characteristic of these plots is that although 100% of patients experience toxicity if concentrations are high enough, fewer than 100% of patients experience therapeutic effects even at high concentrations. Patients who do not respond therapeutically even to high concentrations are referred to as *nonresponders*.

This plot is then used to estimate a drug's therapeutic range. The MEC and MTC are usually chosen at concentrations where a high percentage of patients experience a therapeutic effect and a small percentage of patients experience toxicity, respectively. The specific concentrations selected for the MEC and the MTC will depend on the margin of safety and the risk–benefit ratio acceptable for a given indication. For example, the MTC for an over-the-counter analgesic or nonsteroidal anti-inflammatory drug will be chosen at a concentration associated with much less toxicity than that of a drug used to treat a life-threatening condition such as cancer. In Figure 1.11, the MEC was selected as the concentration at which 70% of the population experienced a therapeutic benefit, and the MTC was selected as the concentration at which 10% of the population experienced some adverse effects.

The therapeutic range has been enormously useful clinically, particularly in helping clinicians determine optimum doses of drugs that have both narrow therapeutic ranges and wide interpatient variability in dose requirements. Examples of these drugs are shown in Table 1.3. A dose that is optimum for one patient (i.e., a dose that gives plasma concentrations in the therapeutic range) may produce concentrations below the MEC in a second patient and produce concentrations above the MTC in a third patient. As a result, doses are

TABLE 1.3   Therapeutic Ranges of Example Drugs [1]

Drug	Therapeutic Range
Cyclosporine	100–400[a] µg/L, whole blood HPLC[b] analysis
Digoxin	0.5–2[c] µg/L
Lithium	0.6–1.5 mEq/L
Phenytoin	10–20 mg/L
Tacrolimus	5–20[a] µg/L, whole blood
Theophylline	5–15 mg/L

[a]Depending on the time after transplant, the type of transplant, and the preference of the center.
[b]High-performance liquid chromatography.
[c]Depending on the indication.

frequently individualized by measuring plasma concentrations achieved by a typical dose and then applying pharmacokinetic principles to calculate a dose that will provide concentrations in the therapeutic range.

It is, however, important to recognize that the therapeutic range has limitations, which include:

1. It represents the range of concentrations that are optimum for most people. Certain patients will, however, experience therapeutic effects at concentrations below the MEC, and others will experience toxicity below the MTC. Some patients never respond therapeutically to a drug even at concentrations well above the MTC.

2. It does not incorporate a graded concentration-related response (i.e., a response that increases with increases in concentration). It is an all-or-nothing response: Patients are predicted to respond when the plasma concentration is within the established therapeutic plasma concentration range and not to respond when the plasma concentration is below the MEC.

3. It only applies to plasma concentrations that are in equilibrium with the drug concentrations at the site of action. It can take a long time for some drugs to distribute to their site of action. For example, it takes about 6–8 h for digoxin to fully distribute to its site of action (the myocardium of the heart). During this distribution period, the therapeutic range will not apply. For example, serum concentrations above the MTC in this period will not necessarily be associated with toxicity.

Therapeutic Index (TI) or Therapeutic Ratio   Like the therapeutic range, the TI or therapeutic ratio is a way to express the safety margin offered by a drug. It is the ratio of the dose of the drug that produces toxicity in 50% of patients to the dose of the drug that produces therapeutic response in 50% of patients:

$$TI = \frac{TD_{50}}{ED_{50}} \tag{1.5}$$

where TD_{50} is the dose that produces toxicity in half the patients, and ED_{50} is the therapeutic or effective dose in half the patients. If, for example, a drug has a TI of 100, the toxic dose is about 100 times larger than the effective dose and the drug has a wide safety margin. Conversely, a TI of 3 would indicate a small margin of safety. A drug with a small therapeutic ratio will have a narrow therapeutic range.

1.6 SUMMARY

In summary:

- *Pharmacokinetics* may be defined as a study of the relationship between drug concentration and time after the administration of a given dose. It involves the study of all the processes that affect this relationship: that is, a drug's ADME. Pharmacokinetics represents the first stage in the process of drug response.

- In pharmacokinetics, the plasma concentrations of a drug are usually studied. A goal is to derive a mathematical expression for the relationship between the plasma concentration, dose, and time:

$$Cp = f_{PK} \,(\text{dose}, \text{time}) \tag{1.6}$$

where Cp is the plasma concentration of the drug, and f_{PK} is a function that describes the relationships among Cp, dose, and time. The function incorporates the drug's pharmacokinetic parameters.

- *Pharmacodynamics* may be defined as a study of the relationship between drug concentration at the site of action and the onset, duration, and intensity of response to the drug. The pharmacodynamic phase constitutes the second and final step in drug response.

- A goal is to derive a mathematical expression for the relationship between the response and the drug concentration:

$$E = f_{PD} \,(C) \tag{1.7}$$

where E is the drug effect or response, C is the concentration at the site of action, and f_{PD} is a function that describes the relationship between the two and incorporates a drug's pharmacodynamic parameters.

- Integrating pharmacokinetics and pharmacodynamics covers the entire dose–response relationship. Mathematical expressions for the pharmacokinetic and pharmacodynamic phases can be combined to provide a complete mathematical expression of the dose–response relationship:

$$E = f_{PD} \left(f_{PK} \,(\text{dose}, \text{time}) \right) \tag{1.8}$$

- Equation (1.8) provides a complete expression for the time course of drug response. It will allow the drug response to be calculated at any time after any dose. It will allow optimum dosing regimens to be determined and can be used to simulate drug response data in situations not studied clinically.

REFERENCE

1. Bauer, L. A. (2008) *Applied Clinical Pharmacokinetics*, 2nd ed., McGraw-Hill, New York.

2

PASSAGE OF DRUGS THROUGH MEMBRANES

Sara E. Rosenbaum

Objectives

The material in this chapter will enable the reader to:

1. Distinguish passive diffusion and transporter-mediated passage
2. Distinguish transcellular and paracellular transport
3. Identify membrane and drug factors that control passive diffusion
4. Distinguish uptake and efflux transporters
5. Become familiar with members of the SLC and ABC superfamilies
6. Understand how transporters affect pharmacokinetics and pharmacodynamics

Basic Pharmacokinetics and Pharmacodynamics: An Integrated Textbook and Computer Simulations,
Second Edition. Edited by Sara E. Rosenbaum.
© 2017 John Wiley & Sons, Inc. Published 2017 by John Wiley & Sons, Inc.

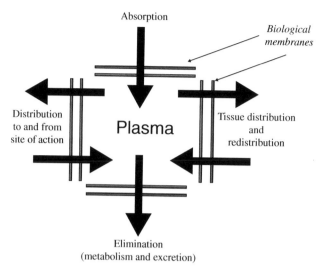

FIGURE 2.1   Points of membrane penetration in pharmacokinetics. Drugs must pass one or more membranes during absorption, distribution, metabolism, excretion, and delivery to the site of action.

2.1   INTRODUCTION

A knowledge of how drugs penetrate membranes is fundamental to understanding the processes of drug absorption, distribution, metabolism, and excretion (ADME). The systemic circulation is the central transport medium for drugs. The process of drug *absorption* results in drugs entering the systemic circulation from the place of drug administration (e.g., gastrointestinal tract and intramuscular site). Drug *distribution* is the transport of drugs from the circulatory system to other parts of the body. Drug elimination (*metabolism* and *excretion*) is a process by which drugs in the circulatory system are removed from the body (either by chemical modification, primarily in the liver, or by excretion of the parent drug, which occurs primarily in the kidney). *All of these processes require that drugs penetrate membranes* (Figure 2.1). Drugs taken orally must penetrate the gastrointestinal membrane. The first step in drug distribution involves the passage of drugs across the membranes of the capillaries that bathe the various tissues. Drug metabolism requires that drugs penetrate the hepatocyte membrane. Finally, the ability of drugs to pass across the glomerular membrane and the membranes in the renal tubule controls a drug's renal excretion. Most important, drugs must pass all the membranes that separate the site of action from the systemic circulation. Centrally acting drugs must penetrate the blood–brain barrier, drugs that act within a cell must penetrate cell membranes, and drugs used in the treatment of solid tumors must penetrate the tumor mass and remain within a cancer cell long enough to elicit a response.

2.2   STRUCTURE AND PROPERTIES OF MEMBRANES

To get into the body and get taken up by the tissues, drugs have to penetrate the *epithelial membranes* that line the major organs and body cavities. Epithelial membranes consist of a series of cells joined by water-filled junctions (Figure 2.2). The membranes of these cells consist of a bimolecular layer of phospholipids. The two layers of phospholipids are

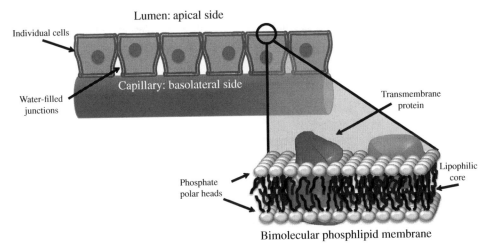

Lumen: apical side

Individual cells

Capillary: basolateral side

Water-filled
junctions

Transmembrane
protein

Lipophilic
core

Phosphate
polar heads

Bimolecular phosphlipid membrane

FIGURE 2.2   Cell membrane. Individual epithelial cells are joined together by water-filled junctions. The membranes of the cells consist of bimolecular layers of lipoproteins. The phosphate polar portion of the phospholipids points toward the outer side of the membrane, and the lipid component makes up the inner core of the membrane. The apical side of the membrane points toward the outside, or lumen, and the remaining sides are known as the basolateral sides.

oriented such that the polar phosphate ends of the molecule point out toward the aqueous medium or the outside of the membrane, and the lipid component makes up the inner core or the matrix of the membrane. Various protein molecules are embedded at different points in the membranes (Figure 2.2). The portion of the epithelial membrane that faces the outside of the organ or body (i.e., the side facing the gastrointestinal lumen) is called the *apical side*. The remaining sides, including the side that faces the circulatory system, are the *basolateral sides*. Individual membranes may consist of a single layer or multiple layers of cells. During each process in ADME, a drug may have to pass across several membranes. For example, orally administered drugs must pass through the gastrointestinal wall into the interstitial fluid and then through the capillary membrane to enter the blood. From there, they may have to pass several other membranes to access their site of action and to be removed from the body. Drugs penetrate these membranes by either passive diffusion or by a transport-mediated process.

2.3 PASSIVE DIFFUSION

Passive diffusion is the most common way for drugs to pass through biological membranes. The concentration gradient across a membrane is the driving force for the process, which tries to equalize the drug concentrations on either side of the membrane. As a result, there is a net movement of drug from the side with a high concentration to the side with a low concentration. Any drug that is bound to tissue macromolecules or plasma proteins is essentially taken out of circulation and does not participate in the concentration gradient. The process of diffusion is governed by Fick's law and may be expressed as:

$$\frac{dA_b}{dt} = P_m \cdot SA_m \cdot \left(C_{u1} - C_{u2}\right) \tag{2.1}$$

where dA_b/dt is the amount of drug diffusing per unit time (mg/h), P_m is the permeability of the drug through the membrane (cm/h), SA_m is the surface area of the membrane (cm^2), C_{u1} is the higher unbound drug concentration (mg/mL), and C_{u2} is the lower unbound concentration (mg/mL).

In most situations (e.g., during drug absorption and the initial phases of drug distribution), drug that diffuses across the membrane is diluted into a very large volume. Thus, C_{u2} can be considered to be considerably smaller than C_{u1}:

$$C_{u1} \gg C_{u2} \text{ and } C_{u1} - C_{u2} \approx C_{u1}$$

Thus, equation (2.1) may be written as:

$$\frac{dA_b}{dt} = P_m \cdot SA_m \cdot C_{u1} \tag{2.2}$$

From equation (2.2), it can be seen that under these circumstances, the rate of diffusion approximates a first-order process:

$$\frac{dA_b}{dt} = \text{Constant} \cdot C_{u1} \quad \text{where} \quad \text{Constant} = P_m \cdot SA_m \tag{2.3}$$

The rate of diffusion is proportional to the driving force for the process: that is, the concentration of drug. The constant of proportionality is the product of a drug's permeability (the relative ease with which the drug passes the membrane) and the surface area of the membrane.

Surface Area   According to equation (2.2), the rate of diffusion increases as a membrane's surface area increases. The importance of surface area is illustrated by considering the structure of the membrane of the small intestine, a tissue whose function is to absorb essential nutrients from digested foods. To assist in this function, the membrane of the small intestine is folded into villi, or fingers, which are estimated to increase the surface area of the small intestine about 10-fold. Each of the villi is folded further into microvilli (Figure 2.3), which are estimated to increase the surface area an additional 20-fold. This extremely large surface area greatly enhances the absorptive properties, a feature that can also be taken advantage of by drugs administered orally. The very favorable absorption of the small intestine results in its being the primary site for the absorption of drugs taken orally.

Permeability   Permeability reflects the ability or speed with which a drug can pass through a membrane. It is dependent on both the characteristics of the membrane and the physicochemical properties of the drug: specifically, lipophilicity, charge, and size. The impact of these variables on diffusion depends on whether a drug passes through the membrane by the transcellular route or by the paracellular route. In *transcellular transport*, drugs diffuse through the matrix or core of the membrane. In *paracellular transport*, drugs diffuse through the water-filled gaps between adjacent cells (Figure 2.4).

The nature of the core of the membrane is essentially constant from one type of membrane to another. As a result, the principles of transcellular diffusion are the same for all membranes, including the gastrointestinal membrane, the blood–brain barrier, and the renal tubular membrane. Paracellular diffusion is controlled by the nature of the junctions between adjacent cells of the membrane. These vary from tissue to tissue. As a result, and

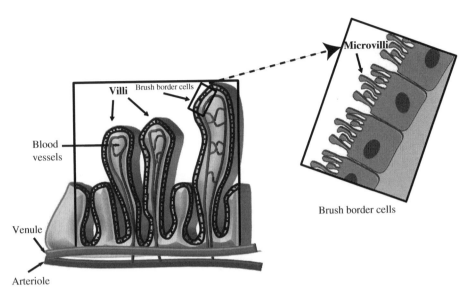

FIGURE 2.3   Villi and microvilli in the small intestine. The membrane of the small intestine is folded into villi, which are then folded further into microvilli. This provides the membrane with a very large surface area, ideally suited for the absorption of nutrients and drugs. Courtesy of Linnea E. Anderson.

in contrast to transcellular diffusion, the ability of a drug to pass through a membrane by the paracellular route will vary from one tissue to another.

2.3.1   Transcellular Passive Diffusion

The ease of transcellular diffusion is determined by a drug's permeability across the lipophilic matrix of the membrane. As such, it depends on the lipophilicity, polarity, and

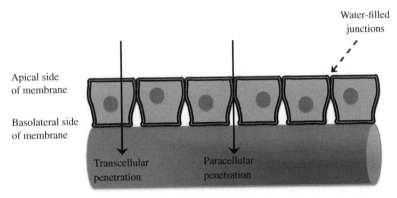

FIGURE 2.4   Transcellular and paracellular diffusion. Passive diffusion is the most common way that drugs penetrate membranes. They can pass through the matrix of the cell (transcellular passage) or through the water-filled junctions between adjacent cells (paracellular transport). Courtesy of Linnea E. Anderson.

TABLE 2.1   Calculated Values of Log P, Log $D_{7.4}$, and Log $D_{6.0}$ of Several Drugs

Drug	Log P	Log $D_{7.4}$	Log $D_{6.0}$
Atenolol	0.10	−1.66	−2.74
Famotidine	−0.40	−1.02	−2.06
Felodipine	4.83	4.83	4.82
Furosemide	3.00	−0.12	0.26
Ibuprofen	3.72	0.80	2.12
Ondansetron	2.49	2.14	1.02
Pindolol	1.97	0.18	−0.88
Theophylline	−0.17	−0.20	−0.18
Valproic acid	2.72	0.16	1.51

Source: Reference [1].

size of the drug molecule. A drug's lipophilicity is probably the most important determinant of permeability. A drug's *lipophilicity*, or fat-loving nature, is traditionally assessed by measuring its distribution between the immiscible phases of *n*-octanol and water. The ratio of the drug's concentration in *n*-octanol and water is the drug's *partition coefficient* (P):

$$P = \frac{C_{n-octanol}}{C_{water}} \tag{2.4}$$

Because of the very wide range of P values among therapeutic drugs, P values are expressed most conveniently on a log scale. Table 2.1 provides the log P values of some therapeutic drugs.

Drugs with large positive log P values (felodipine) preferentially partition into the lipid layer. They are lipophilic, would have high permeability across the lipophilic core of the membrane, and would be expected to diffuse easily. As the log P value decreases among a series of drugs, lipophilicity and permeability both decrease and transcellular membrane penetration would become increasingly difficult. Drugs with very low or negative log P values (e.g., atenolol and famotidine) partition primarily into the aqueous phase, are more polar in nature, and would be expected to have poor membrane permeability.

The disadvantage of the partition coefficient is that it measures the distribution of drugs between the two phases when the drug is completely in the nonionized state. Thus, it is a measure of a drug's inherent or intrinsic lipophilicity. But most drugs are either weak acids or bases and, as a result, exist in biological fluids in equilibrium between their ionized and nonionized forms. For example, a drug that is a weak acid would ionize as follows in an aqueous medium:

$$DH \rightleftarrows D^- + H^+ \tag{2.5}$$

The degree of ionization will influence a drug's permeability because only the nonionized form of the drug would be able to penetrate a lipophilic membrane. A more useful measure of membrane permeability is the partition coefficient measured at a specific, biologically relevant pH. The partition coefficient of a drug between a lipid phase and an aqueous phase at a specific pH is referred to as the *distribution coefficient* (D), or log D on the log scale. The log $D_{7.4}$ and log $D_{6.0}$ values of several drugs are shown in Table 2.1. It can be seen that a drug's log D value is generally less than its log P value, which reflects the fact that when the drug is partially ionized, the ionized form cannot partition into the lipid phase, which makes the drug effectively less lipophilic than the totally nonionized form of the drug. It can also be seen that the log D values of drugs that are weak acids (e.g., ibuprofen, furosemide, and valproic acid) are higher at the more acidic pH of 6.0 than at pH 7.4. This reflects the fact that drugs are less ionized at more acidic pHs. Conversely, the log D values of drugs that are weak bases (e.g., atenolol and ondansetron) are lower at a more acidic pH of 6.0, owing to the greater degree of ionization.

The size or mass of the drug molecules also affects the permeability, as large molecules experience difficulty in diffusing. Studies suggest, however, that mass does not appear to be important if it is below about 400 Da, which includes many of the drugs presently used therapeutically. Transcellular diffusion has been studied most extensively in the context of the absorption of orally administered drugs. Pharmaceutical companies want to maximize the possibility that newly developed drugs can be given orally, and much research has been conducted to try to identify critical physiochemical properties of drugs. Studies have emphasized the importance of a high log D value. These studies also indicate that mass and polarity are important and suggest that drugs with a molecular mass greater than 500 Da are likely to have poor membrane permeability, particularly if they also possess additional adverse physicochemical characteristics, such as polarity or poor lipophilicity [2].

In summary, transcellular permeability is highest for small lipophilic, nonpolar drugs.

2.3.2 Paracellular Passive Diffusion

Paracellular transport involves the passage of drugs through the junctions between the cells of the membrane (Figure 2.4). It is dependent on the size of the junction and on the size of the drug molecule. The junctions between adjacent cells of the epithelium membrane vary from one tissue to another. The junctions between the cells in the gastrointestinal membrane and skin are very tight and serve to hold transcellular proteins in place and also, presumably, to protect the body from the penetration of foreign substances across these outside membranes. As a result, paracellular diffusion of drugs across the intestinal membrane is a very minor route of absorption. Atenolol (molecular weight or molecular mass [MW] = 266 Da; log $D_{6.5} = -2$) and terbutaline (MW = 180 Da; log $D_{6.5} = -1.3$) were thought to be absorbed by this route. However, recent evidence has cast doubt on this [3] and suggests that they may be too large for paracellular diffusion across the intestinal membrane. The aminoglycoside antibiotics, which are both too polar (log $D_{7.4} \approx -10$) and too large (MW 450 to over 1000) for transcellular or paracellular diffusion, must be administered parenterally for the treatment of systemic infections. The gaps between adjacent cells in the nasal membrane are looser in nature, and the cutoff for paracellular absorption is around 1000 Da. However, even at this site, paracellular diffusion of polar drugs is much less efficient than transcellular absorption of lipophilic drugs. A very high percentage of a dose of a lipophilic drug such as pentazocine and fentanyl can be absorbed by the transcellular route through the nasal membrane, compared to only about 10% of a polar drug such as morphine. The use of absorption enhancers to improve the intranasal delivery of polar drugs has met with some success. Chitosan, a compound derived from crustacean shells, has produced substantial increases in morphine penetration through the nasal membrane [4]. It is believed that the effect of chitosan is due in part to a transient opening of the tight junctions and increased paracellular diffusion. Clinical trials of intranasal morphine preparations containing chitosan suggest that it will offer an alternative to intravenous morphine for the treatment of postoperative pain [5].

Capillary membranes in most tissues have fairly loose membrane junctions that allow free passage of even large molecular mass (high molecular weight) peptides and polypeptides into and out of the circulatory system. Large molecular mass drug molecules such as the aminoglycosides are able to pass through these membranes by the paracellular route. The hydrophilicity of the aminoglycosides will prevent them from diffusing passively through the membranes within the tissues, and as a result their distribution is limited primarily to extracellular fluid. The aminoglycosides are active against bacteria because bacterial cell membranes contain an oxygen-dependent transport process that carries the drugs to the inside of the bacterial cell. The membrane in the renal glomerulus is another example of a very loose membrane that allows the paracellular passage of even large drug molecules. Plasma water and solutes undergo paracellular filtration across this membrane into the renal tubule. The paracellular space in the glomerular membrane allows the passage of molecules with molecular weights up to about 5000 Da. For example, insulin is able to pass through the glomerular membrane. In contrast, in certain sensitive or delicate tissues, such as the central nervous system (CNS), the retina, the placenta, and the testes, the capillary epithelial membrane is very tightly knit and limits paracellular diffusion, presumably to protect these tissues from potentially toxic drugs and other xenobiotics.

2.4   CARRIER-MEDIATED PROCESSES: TRANSPORT PROTEINS

Transporters are proteins that reside in cell membranes and serve to facilitate the passage of chemicals into or out of a cell. It is likely that transporters have evolved to protect cells against potentially harmful xenobiotics and to assist in the absorption and distribution of essential nutrients. Over the last 15–20 years, it has become apparent that drug transporters exert a profound influence on the body's exposure to drugs and on the access of drugs to their site of action and/or toxicity. Transporters located in the intestinal membrane, the hepatocyte, and the renal tubular membrane influence drug absorption, metabolism, and excretion, respectively, and as a result, the body's overall exposure to drugs. In other locations, such as the CNS, the placenta, and the testis, transporters may have only subtle or negligible influence on the body's overall exposure to a drug, but by virtue of their control of the access of a small fraction of the dose to these areas are critical in controlling therapeutic and/or toxicological effects.

There are two broad classes of transporters: *uptake transporters*, which transport drugs into the cell, and *efflux transporters*, which extrude or transport drugs out of the cell. In gastrointestinal, hepatocytic, and renal tubular membranes, transporters may reside on either the basolateral (blood) side or on the apical (luminal) side of the membrane. The four possible arrangements of drug transporters in an epithelial membrane such as the gastrointestinal tract are shown in Figure 2.5. The location of a transporter in the membrane determines its impact on the body's exposure to a substrate. For example, an efflux transporter on the apical side of a membrane would restrict the body's exposure to its substrates. In contrast, an efflux transporter on the basolateral side would serve to enhance absorption a drug. If the drug were a substrate for both an efflux transporter on the basolateral side of the membrane and an uptake transporter on the luminal side, the two transporter systems could work in concert to absorb and/or retain the drug in the body.

A very large number of transporters have been identified in human tissue, but the role of many is not fully understood at this time. The discussion that follows is restricted to those transporters whose involvement in drug response and/or pharmacokinetics has been demonstrated in clinical studies. The role of specific transporters in drug absorption, drug

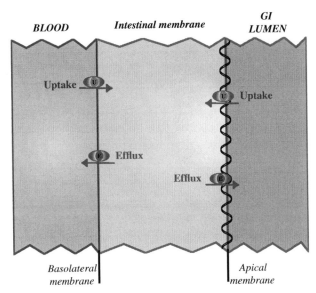

FIGURE 2.5   Theoretical placements of uptake and efflux transporters in an epithelial cell membrane such as the intestinal membrane. E represents an efflux transporter such as permeability glycoprotein (P-gp) or breast cancer-resistance protein (BCRP); U represents an uptake transporter such as organic anion transporting polypeptide (OATP) or organic cation transporter (OCT). Uptake transporters on the apical membrane and efflux transporters on the basolateral side promote the retention of drugs in the body. Uptake transporters on the basolateral side of the membrane and efflux transporters on the apical side promote the removal of drug from the body. Courtesy of Linnea E. Anderson. *(For a color version of this figure, see the color plate section.)*

excretion in the kidney, drug elimination in the liver, and drug uptake into the CNS is discussed in greater detail in later chapters.

2.4.1   Uptake Transporters: SLC Superfamily

The main uptake transporters belong to the *solute carrier* (SLC) *superfamily* and operate primarily by bidirectional facilitated diffusion, although in some cases the transport may be active and unidirectional. As a result, these proteins generally transport drug molecules along their concentration gradient but at a higher rate than that observed for passive diffusion. These transporters do not require adenosine triphosphate (ATP), and they transport substances into the cell. Of the very large number of SLC transporters that have been identified, four transporter families have been found to be important for the absorption and disposition (distribution and elimination) of drugs in humans: the *organic anion transporting polypeptide* (OATP, gene symbol SLCO), the *organic anion transporter* (OAT, gene symbol SLC22), the *organic cation transporter* (OCT, gene symbol SLC22), and the *peptide transporter* (PEPT; gene SLC15A). Some examples of specific transporters, their tissue distribution, and some example of substrates are shown in Table 2.2.

Organic anions are transported by the OATP and the OAT families. The OAT1 and OAT3 are important in the kidney, where they facilitate the uptake of drugs from the blood into the renal tubular cells. The OATP family is important in drug absorption in the intestine and the uptake of drugs into the hepatocyte, where they subsequently undergo metabolism. Small organic cations such as metformin, cisplatin, procainamide, and cimetidine are transported

TABLE 2.2   Primary Locations of Major Drug Uptake Transporters and Some Example of Substrates and Inhibitors[a]

Transporter	Gene Name	Location	Example of Substrates	Inhibitors
OATP1A2	SLCO1A2	Brain: AS Intestine: AS Renal: AS	Fexofenadine, digoxin, and saquinavir	Fruit (apple, grapefruit, and orange) juices
OATP1B1	SLCO1B1	Liver: BS	Statins, angiotensin II receptor antagonists, and ACE inhibitors	Cyclosporine, rifampin, and gemfibrozil
OATP1B3	SLCO1B3	Liver: BS	Similar to OATP1B1	Similar to OATP1B1
OAPT2B1	SLCO2B1	All tissues	Statins and benzylpenicillin	
OCT1	SLC22A1	Liver: BS	Metformin and cimetidine	Ritonavir and cimetidine
OCT2	SLC22A2	Kidney: BS	Metformin, cimetidine, and cisplatin	Cimetidine
OAT1	SLC22A6	Kidney: BS	Overlaps with OAT3: furosemide, adefovir, acylcovir, and cephalosporins	Probenecid and cephalosporins
OAT3	SLC22A8	Kidney: BS	Overlaps with OAT1: furosemide, adefovir, pravastatin, olmesartan, fexofenadine, H2-receptor blockers, and benzylpenicillin	Probenecid, cimetidine, NSAIDs, and cephalosporins
PEPT1	SLC15A1	Intestine: AS	Cephalosporins, penicillins, and valacyclovir	Cephalosporins

Source: Data from References [6–11].

[a]AS is the apical or luminal side of the membrane; BS is the basolateral side of the membrane; NSAIDs are nonsteroidal anti-inflammatory drugs.

by the OCT family (OCT1, OCT2, and OCT3), which have very similar specificity and have some though not complete overlap in the substrates they transport. They differ in their expression in the body. OCT1 is highly expressed in the liver, where it enhances hepatic uptake of drugs, and OCT2 is highly expressed in the kidney, where it enhances the uptake of its substrates into the renal tubular membrane from the blood. OCT3 is found in the liver, kidney, and intestinal epithelial cells.

The location of the main uptake transporters in the intestinal, hepatocytic, and proximal renal tubular cells is shown in Figure 2.6.

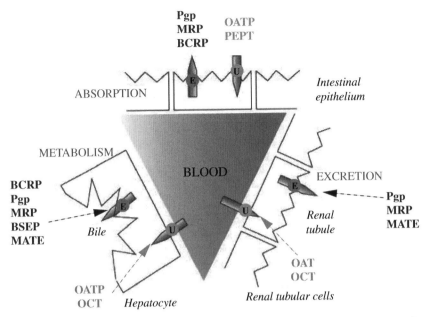

FIGURE 2.6 Location of some of the major uptake (U) and efflux (E) transporters involved in drug absorption, metabolism, and excretion. Efflux transporters include permeability glycoprotein (P-gp), multidrug resistance-associated protein family (MRP), breast cancer resistance protein (BCRP), bile salt export pump (BSEP), and multidrug and toxin extrusion protein (MATE). Uptake transporters include organic anion transporting polypeptide (OATP), organic anion transporter (OAT), organic cation transporter (OCT), and peptide transporter (PEPT). An interactive version of this diagram Model 2, Transporter Model may be found at http://web.uri.edu/pharmacy/research/rosenbaum/sims/Model2 and can be used to observe how transporters at the various locations influence the plasma concentration–time profile.

2.4.2 Efflux Transporters: ABC Superfamily

Efflux transporters were first identified in the 1970s when a glycoprotein was found to provide some cancer cells with resistance to certain anticancer drugs. The protein, known as *permeability glycoprotein* (P-gp) or *multidrug resistance protein 1* (MDR 1; gene ABCB1), was found to operate by reducing cellular exposure to a particular drug by actively extruding it from the cell. Since that time, P-gp and several other efflux transporters have been found not only in cancer cells, but also in many normal tissues, where they are thought to function to protect healthy cells from damage by drugs and other xenobiotics. The efflux transporters primarily belong to the *ATP-binding cassette* (ABC) *superfamily*. The exception is the transporters in the MATE (*multidrug and toxin extrusion protein*) family, which function as efflux transporters but are members of SLC superfamily.

The efflux transporters facilitate the removal of drugs from cells by an active transport process. Clinically important members of this superfamily include P-gp, multidrug resistance-associated protein (MRP; gene ABCC) family, breast cancer resistance protein (BCRP; gene ABCG2), bile salt export pump (BSEP; gene ABCB11; also known as sister P-glycoprotein), and MATE (gene SLC47A). The location of the efflux transporters and some examples of substrates and modifiers are shown in Tables 2.3 and 2.4.

P-gp is found in many areas of the body, including the intestinal membrane, the blood–brain barrier, the placenta, the kidney, and the liver. In these locations, it serves either to

TABLE 2.3   Primary Locations of Major Drug Efflux Transporters and Some Example of Substrates[a]

Transporter	Gene Name	Location	Example of Substrates	Inhibitors
P-gp	MDR1 and ABCB1	Brain: AS Liver: AS Kidney: AS Intestine: AS Placenta Testis	See Table 2.4	See Table 2.4
MRP2	ABCC2	Liver: AS Kidney: AS Intestine: AS	Pravastatin, olmesartan, indinavir, conjugates of gluathione, and glucuronide sulfasalazine	Cyclosporine
MRP3	ABCC3	Liver: BS Intestine: BS	Methorexate and glucoronides	
MRP4	ABCC4	Liver: BS Kidney: AS	Methotrexate and adefovir	
BCRP	ABCG2	Brain: AS Liver: AS Intestine: AS	Irinotecan, topotecan, daunorubicin, imatinib, mitoxantron, quinolones, pravastatin, rosuvastatin, and sulfasalazine	Proton pump inhibitors, protease inhibitors, and elacridar
BSEP	ABCB11	Liver: AS	Pravastatin, vinblastine, and tamoxifen	Cyclosporine, troglitazone, and glyburide
MATE1	SLC47A1	Liver: AS Kidney: AS	Cimetidine and metformin	
MATE2-K	SLC47A2	Kidney: AS	Cimetidine and metformin	

Source: Data from References [6, 7, 12, 13].
[a]AS is the apical or luminal side of the membrane; BS is the basolateral side of the membrane.

prevent drugs from being absorbed into the body or to facilitate their removal from the body or to protect individual cells from potentially toxic chemicals. It transports such a wide variety of different molecules that it has been termed the "promiscuous" transporter. This broad substrate specificity, combined with the large number of compounds known to modify its activity, makes P-gp an important target for *drug–drug interactions (DDIs)*. In view of its importance and the relatively large body of information on this transporter, a separate list of its substrates, inhibitors, and inducers is provided in Table 2.4. The very large overlap in the substrates, inducers, and inhibitors of P-gp with those of cytochrome P450 3A4 (CYP3A4), a hepatic and intestinal drug metabolizing enzyme, suggests that P-gp and CYP3A4 may have evolved to work in concert to reduce the body's exposure to harmful chemicals. MRP2 is found in the apical membrane in the kidney, liver, and intestine. In the liver, it promotes the biliary excretion of anionic drugs and conjugates of glucoronide, glutathione, and sulfate. Some of the MRP transporters, such as MRP4 in the hepatocyte and intestine, are located

TABLE 2.4   Examples of Substrates, Inhibitors, and Inducers of P-gp

Substrates

Anticancer drugs	Cardiovascular drugs	H2-receptor antagonists
Paclitaxel	Verapamil	Cimetidine
Doxorubicin	Diltiazem	Ranitidine
Vinblastine	Digoxin	Immunosuppressants
Etoposide	Talinolol	Cyclosporine
Irinotecan	Quinidine	Tacrolimus
Antiemetics	Amiodarone	Protease inhibitors
Ondansetron	Losartan	Indinavir
Antihistamines	Atorvastatin	Nelfinavir
Fexofenadine		Saquinavir
		Ritonavir
Inhibitors		
Cyclosporine	Second generation	Third generation
Verapamil	Valspodar	Elacridar
Quinidine		
Itraconazole		
Ketoconazole		
Ritonavir		
Inducers		
Rifampin	St. John's wort	

Source: Data from References [8, 12, 14].

on the basolateral side of the membrane, where they promote the absorption or retention of substrates in the systemic circulation. BCRP is found in many tissues, including the intestinal membrane, liver, brain, and placenta, and has been studied primarily in relation to cancer treatment because several anticancer drugs, including irinotecan and topotecan, are substrates. However, many other drugs, including cimetidine, pravastatin, and rosuvastatin, are substrates of BCRP. BSEP is located canalicular side of the hepatocyte membrane and is important for the biliary secretion of bile salts, drugs, and drug metabolites. The transporters in the MATE family have substrate and inhibitor specificities that overlap with those of the OCTs. For example, both cimetidine and metformin are substrates for both. The location of the main efflux transporters in the intestine, hepatocytic, and proximal renal tubular cells is shown in Figure 2.6.

2.4.3   Characteristics of Transporter Systems

Transporter-mediated membrane permeation differs in several ways from diffusion-mediated transport. First, transporters are substrate-specific and only carry drugs that have specific molecular features. Second, there is only a finite amount of a transporter at a given location, and if the substrate concentration is high, it may saturate the transporter. For example, consider a drug that is a substrate for an intestinal efflux transporter, which limits its absorption. If the concentration of the drug in the intestine becomes so high that it saturates the transporter, the efflux process will no longer work efficiently and the drug will be able to undergo a greater degree of absorption. Competition between two drugs for the same transporter can also result in reduced transport of a drug and may result in adverse DDIs. Finally, because transporters are biological in nature, their expression is under genetic control and their activity may vary substantially within a population. Their activity can be further modified by concomitant drugs, nutritional products, foods, and environmental factors that either inhibit or induce transport systems.

2.4.4 Simulation Exercise: http://web.uri.edu/pharmacy/research/rosenbaum/sims

An interactive model of the major uptake and efflux transporters involved in absorption and elimination (Model 2, Transporter Model) is provided at the following link:
 http://web.uri.edu/pharmacy/research/rosenbaum/sims/Model2
 Simulations can be performed to observe how the transporters in the membranes of the intestine, hepatocyte and renal tubule influence the plasma concentration–time profile.

1. *Go to the Single Oral Dose page and perform a simulation with all the transporter systems switched on. Run six more simulations in which each of the transporters is switched off in turn. Observe how the plasma concentration profile and half-life are affected in each case.*
2. *Repeat the exercise with multiple oral and intravenous doses.*
3. *Digoxin is a substrate for P-gp in the intestinal membrane and renal tubule. Use the single oral dose model to observe how digoxin's plasma concentration–time relationship and half-life may be affected when:*
   (a) intestinal P-gp is inhibited;
   (b) renal P-gp is inhibited.
   Comment on any differences in the two profiles.
4. *Repeat the above exercise with multiple intravenous model.*
5. *How would it be possible to distinguish between effects on intestinal P-gp and renal P-gp?*
6. *Give four examples of modifiers of P-gp.*

2.4.5 Clinical Examples of Transporter Involvement in Drug Response

In an effort to identify clinically important drug transporters and delineate their role in drug response, there has been an explosive growth in the number of research papers published in this area during the past 15 years. It is likely that our knowledge of these systems and the specific functions of individual transporters will grow at a rapid rate in the coming years. The transporters are frequently studied *in vitro*, using human cells and tissues, and in animals, in which the activity of a transporter is altered either by chemical inhibitors or by breeding animals deficient in the transporter (e.g., knockout mice). Clinical studies are then performed to try to confirm the findings of the *in vitro* and animal studies.

 The clinical role played by transporters is usually studied by observing the effects of altered activity, either in people who have genetically determined low activity or using chemical modifiers (inhibitors and inducers) of specific transport systems. These studies have revealed many interesting and important characteristics of transporters. Inhibitors of intestinal P-gp have been found to increase the absorption of many drugs, which in some cases (e.g., digoxin) can lead to toxicity. Conversely, inducers of P-gp, such as rifampin, can reduce the absorption of P-gp substrates and in some cases (e.g., cyclosporine) can lead to dangerously low, subtherapeutic blood concentrations of a drug. Metformin, a polar drug, relies on OCT1 for its delivery to its site of action in the liver and reduced activity of this transporter has been associated with a diminished impaired response to the drug [11]. The hepatic transporters OATP1B1 and OATP1B3 are very important for the uptake of the HMG-CoA reductase inhibitors (statins) to the hepatocyte where they subsequently undergo metabolism and biliary elimination. Reduced activity or inhibition of these transporters by other drugs has been associated with reduced elimination of the many of the statins. This in turn can lead to large increases in systemic concentrations of these drugs, and an increased risk of statin-induced muscle toxicity. Several of the hepatic efflux transporters facilitate the secretion of drugs, their metabolites, and other metabolic waste products into the bile. Inhibition of the activity of these transporters can lead to a buildup of these compounds in the liver and predispose patients to cholestasis and drug-induced liver disease. Uptake and efflux transporters on the basolateral and apical sides, respectively, of the renal tubular membrane can act in concert to enhance the renal excretion of drugs. The uptake transporters carry drugs from the circulatory system into the tubular membrane, and the efflux transporters continue the elimination process by secreting the drugs into the renal tubule. However, the high drug concentrations in renal tabular cells that result from this uptake have been implicated as a possible cause of the renal toxicity of cisplatin, cidofovir, and cephaloridine.

Transporters at the blood–brain barrier restrict the uptake of potentially toxic substances into this very sensitive organ. The opioid loperamide is devoid of central effects because P-gp prevents its accumulation in the brain, and as a result it is readily available over the counter for the treatment of traveler's diarrhea. However, when coadministered with quinidine, an inhibitor of P-gp, loperamide, produces respiratory depression, which demonstrates that significant amounts are able to access the CNS. P-gp may also play a role in excluding the nonsedating, second-generation antihistamines from the CNS [15], which raises the possibility that inhibitors of P-gp could produce sedation from these drugs. By limiting access to the CNS, the efflux transporters also create a significant barrier for the treatment of such conditions of the brain as cancer, neurological diseases, mood disorders, and infections.

REFERENCES

1. Linnankoski, J., Makela, J. M., Ranta, V. P., Urtti, A., and Yliperttula, M. (2006) Computational prediction of oral drug absorption based on absorption rate constants in humans, *J Med Chem*, *49*, 3674–3681.

2. Lipinski, C. A., Lombardo, F., Dominy, B. W., and Feeney, P. J. (2001) Experimental and computational approaches to estimate solubility and permeability in drug discovery and development settings, *Adv Drug Deliv Rev*, *46*, 3–26.

3. Lennernas, H. (2007) Intestinal permeability and its relevance for absorption and elimination, *Xenobiotica*, *37*, 1015–1051.

4. Illum, L., Watts, P., Fisher, A. N., Hinchcliffe, M., Norbury, H., Jabbal-Gill, I., Nankervis, R., and Davis, S. S. (2002) Intranasal delivery of morphine, *J Pharmacol Exp Ther*, *301*, 391–400.

5. Stoker, D. G., Reber, K. R., Waltzman, L. S., Ernst, C., Hamilton, D., Gawarecki, D., Mermelstein, F., McNicol, E., Wright, C., and Carr, D. B. (2008) Analgesic efficacy and safety of morphine–chitosan nasal solution in patients with moderate to severe pain following orthopedic surgery, *Pain Med*, *9*, 3–12.

6. Ho, R. H., and Kim, R. B. (2005) Transporters and drug therapy: implications for drug disposition and disease, *Clin Pharmacol Ther*, *78*, 260–277.

7. Kusuhara, H., and Sugiyama, Y. (2009) In vitro–in vivo extrapolation of transporter-mediated clearance in the liver and kidney, *Drug Metab Pharmacokinet*, *24*, 37–52.

8. Oostendorp, R. L., Beijnen, J. H., and Schellens, J. H. (2009) The biological and clinical role of drug transporters at the intestinal barrier, *Cancer Treat Rev, 35*, 137–147.

9. United States Food and Drug Administration. (2006) *Drug Development and Drug Interactions: Table of Substrates, Inhibitors and Inducers*, U.S. FDA, Washington, DC.

10. Yasui-Furukori, N., Uno, T., Sugawara, K., and Tateishi, T. (2005) Different effects of three transporting inhibitors, verapamil, cimetidine, and probenecid, on fexofenadine pharmacokinetics, *Clin Pharmacol Ther, 77*, 17–23.

11. Choi, M. K., and Song, I. S. (2008) Organic cation transporters and their pharmacokinetic and pharmacodynamic consequences, *Drug Metab Pharmacokinet, 23*, 243–253.

12. Marchetti, S., Mazzanti, R., Beijnen, J. H., and Schellens, J. H. (2007) Concise review: clinical relevance of drug drug and herb drug interactions mediated by the ABC transporter ABCB1 (MDR1, P-glycoprotein), *Oncologist, 12*, 927–941.

13. Murakami, T., and Takano, M. (2008) Intestinal efflux transporters and drug absorption, *Expert Opin Drug Metab Toxicol, 4*, 923–939.

14. Eyal, S., Hsiao, P., and Unadkat, J. D. (2009) Drug interactions at the blood–brain barrier: fact or fantasy?, *Pharmacol Ther, 123*, 80–104.

15. Polli, J. W., Baughman, T. M., Humphreys, J. E., Jordan, K. H., Mote, A. L., Salisbury, J. A., Tippin, T. K., and Serabjit-Singh, C. J. (2003) P-glycoprotein influences the brain concentrations of cetirizine (Zyrtec), a second-generation non-sedating antihistamine, *J Pharm Sci, 92*, 2082–2089.

3

DRUG ADMINISTRATION AND DRUG ABSORPTION

STEVEN C. SUTTON

Basic Pharmacokinetics and Pharmacodynamics: An Integrated Textbook and Computer Simulations, Second Edition. Edited by Sara E. Rosenbaum.
© 2017 John Wiley & Sons, Inc. Published 2017 by John Wiley & Sons, Inc.

Objectives

The material in this chapter will enable the reader to:

1. Define local and systemic drug administration
2. Describe common routes of drug administration and their characteristics
3. Characterize the steps involved in oral absorption
4. Define the bioavailability factor (F)
5. Categorize the components of F: F_a, F_g, and F_h
6. Identify the drug, formulation, and biological determinants of bioavailability
7. Understand the determinants of drug absorption
8. Define the biopharmaceutical classification system
9. Understand how the BCS and BDDCS can be applied

3.1 INTRODUCTION: LOCAL AND SYSTEMIC DRUG ADMINISTRATION

Drugs can be administered using a variety of routes. The route must be selected so that the drug is delivered to its site of action in a time frame appropriate for the clinical indication. For some indications, such as the treatment of life-threatening cardiac arrhythmias, it is critical that a drug reaches its site of action within a few minutes of administration. In other situations, the patient will not be adversely affected if it takes 0.5–1 h or more for the drug to elicit an effect. Drug administration may be broadly classified as local or systemic. Local administration refers to the direct application of a drug to its site of action, and it is much less common than systemic administration. Examples of *local administration* include the use of creams, ointments, or gels to apply drugs topically: for example, the use of lidocaine gel to provide anesthesia at the site of application. Other examples are the treatment of ulcerative colitis with oral sulfasalazine, a drug that is not absorbed through the intestinal membrane and is delivered to the colon; and the treatment of asthma with inhaled β-agonists and corticosteroids. In contrast, the vast majority of drugs rely on the circulatory system to deliver drugs to their site of action. This is referred to as *systemic administration*, and in many cases the uptake or absorption of the drug into the systemic circulation is a critical first step in response process. In pharmacokinetics, *drug absorption* refers specifically to the uptake of drug to the systemic circulation and not just its entry into the body. For example, in the case of orally administered drugs, drug absorption is not simply passage of the drug across the intestinal membrane—this is only an intermediary step in the overall absorption of the drug into the systemic circulation.

3.2 ROUTES OF DRUG ADMINISTRATION

3.2.1 Common Routes of Local Drug Administration

3.2.1.1 *Topical*
The above example of lidocaine gel to provide anesthesia requires that the site of application is accessible. Commonly accessible sites of application are the skin (including scalp), hair, and nails. The intended drug target is usually one or a few layers of cells from the application site. The same drug formulation is often used for one or more of these sites.

3.2.1.2 *Targeted, NonSystemic*
This section addresses specialized drug formulations that may be used to reach tissues not readily accessible, or that required special handling. With the exception of the orally administered drug products, all of these formulations need to be rendered sterile for use.

Colon   Ulcerative colitis and Crohn's disease can be treated with an orally administered drug product that is designed to release the drug in the colon. Sulfasalazine is a pro-drug composed of 5-aminosalicylic acid (5-ASA) linked to sulfapyridine through an azo bond (Figure 3.1). Following oral administration of sulfasalazine, the drug is not absorbed through the gastrointestinal tract and is delivered to the colon, where the enzyme azoreductase, excreted by bacteria, breaks the azo bond, releasing sulfapyridine and 5-ASA. 5-ASA is poorly absorbed from the colon and so remains in the colon, where its anti-inflammatory properties alleviate some of the symptoms of colitis.

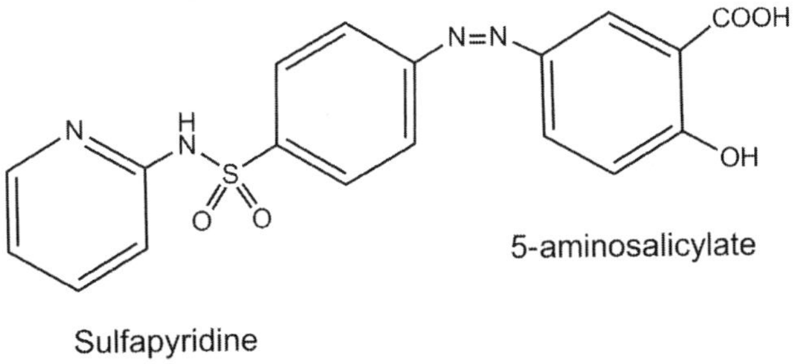

FIGURE 3.1   The chemical structure of sulfasalazine.

Ocular   Wet age-related macular degeneration is a debilitating disease where a type of vascular endothelia growth factor (VEGF) produces defective capillaries that leak blood components into retina, causing scarring and damage to rods and cones. Treatment is accomplished through the periodic intravitreal injection of the anti-VEGF drug aflibercept. Open-angle glaucoma is usually caused by an elevated vitreous pressure that damages the optic nerve. Ocular topical formulations ("eye drops") include prostaglandins (latanoprost), β-blockers (timolol maleate), α-adrenergic agonists (brimonidine tartrate).

Otic   For most common afflictions of the ear (e.g., otitis media), topical antibiotics (e.g., ofloxacin) instilled into the ear are the first-line treatment.

3.2.2   Common Routes of Systemic Drug Administration

3.2.2.1   *Intravascular Direct Systemic Administration*

Intravenous and Intraarterial   The administration of drugs directly into the systemic circulation using the intravenous route, or the less common intraarterial route, bypasses the absorption process completely. These routes of administration are invasive and require a skilled health professional and are generally not used unless there is a specific reason. *Intravenous administration* is often used when an immediate effect is desired and/or when it is important that the dose be administered with a high degree of accuracy. It may also be used for drugs that are poorly or incompletely absorbed from other routes. *Intraarterial administration* is not common but may be used if a therapy is to be directed to a specific organ. For example, it has been used to administer anticancer drugs to target liver tumors. Intravascular administration is the only route that guarantees that the entire dose administered will reach the systemic circulation. For all other routes of drug administration, poor membrane penetration and/or loss of drug at the absorption site may result in the incomplete absorption of a dose. An extreme example of this is provided by alendronate, used in the treatment of osteoporosis. Only about 0.7% of an oral dose of this drug reaches the systemic circulation. Doses of drugs given intravenously are often much lower than those used in other routes, where absorption may be incomplete. For example, the intravenous dose of morphine is about one-third of the oral dose.

3.2.2.2   *Extravascular Parenteral Routes*

Intramuscular and Subcutaneous Administration   Like intravenous and intraarterial, intramuscular and subcutaneous drug delivery are examples of parenteral routes. *Parenteral* is defined as "outside the gastrointestinal tract" and, strictly speaking, would include all nonoral routes. However, in the pharmaceutical field, the term is limited to injectable routes. The *intramuscular and subcutaneous routes* are frequently used to avoid the gastrointestinal tract, either because the drug would be destroyed in the gastrointestinal fluid or because a drug is too polar or too large to penetrate the gastrointestinal membrane. Drugs administered by the intramuscular and subcutaneous routes must still undergo absorption into the bloodstream, but generally, loose capillary membranes at their site of administration, allows paracellular penetration even of polar and/or large drug molecules. Drugs administered by the intramuscular and subcutaneous routes often reach the bloodstream faster than do orally administered drugs. However, the physicochemical properties of a drug (e.g., particle size and solubility) can be manipulated to provide a more gradual absorption from these routes.

3.2.2.3   *Other Extravascular Routes*

The convenience of oral administration makes it the most common route of drug administration. As such, the bulk of this chapter is devoted to discussing the principles of oral drug absorption. However, many drugs cannot be administered orally, either because they are destroyed in the gastrointestinal fluid, unable to penetrate the intestinal membrane, or eliminated in the liver during the absorption process. Most of the other extravascular routes of drug administration were developed initially to provide a nonparenteral alternative for the administration drugs that cannot be given orally.

Buccal and Sublingual   The *buccal* (between the gums and cheek) and *sublingual* (under the tongue) routes of administration take advantage of relatively porous, well-perfused mucous membranes in the mouth. The major advantage of these routes is that the capillaries in this area do not drain into the hepatic artery, and thus they offer an alternative oral route for drugs such as nitroglycerin that undergo extensive metabolism in the liver and are essentially removed from the body before they reach the systemic circulation (see Section 3.5.10). Drug absorption from these routes is sometimes—but not always—fairly rapid. As shown in Figure 3.2, the time for a maximum systemic concentration for drugs ranged from under 5 min for nitroglycerin to almost 2 h for lorazepam [1].

Fast-dissolving films and tablets   These dosage forms usually contain a small dose of a drug, which has a high aqueous solubility (e.g., Claritin® RediTabs® 10 mg loratidine). The formulation excipients include sweeteners to disguise the taste of the drug. These dosage forms do not require water to swallow—they disintegrate and dissolve in the mouth in seconds. The drug is swallowed, and it eventually enters the gastrointestinal tract. The drug usually is not absorbed from the oral cavity. Unlike the buccal and sublingual routes of administration, the fast-dissolving film and tablet formulations are not designed for avoiding the metabolism in the intestines and liver. These drug products are primarily

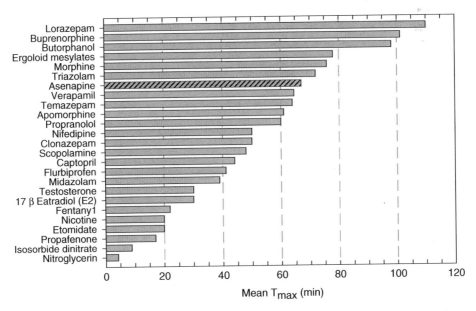

FIGURE 3.2   The mean T_{max} of active drugs administered to humans as an oral mucosa dosage form. *Source:* Bartlett 2012, pp. 1110–1115 [1]. Reproduced with permission of Springer.

employed as a convenience to the patient, and generally are expected to improve patient compliance.

Rectal   The rectal route of administration has the advantage of bypassing the liver. It is also a particularly useful route for patients who cannot take drugs orally, either because they are experiencing nausea and vomiting or are unconscious. Prochlorperazine, for example, is available in suppository form for the treatment of nausea and vomiting.

Transdermal   The transdermal route was initially developed as a way to bypass the liver and administer drugs that experienced extensive hepatic first pass extraction, but it has become popular because of the convenience it offers. A single patch can provide continuous and constant delivery of drug over an extended period, making it particularly attractive for drugs that are eliminated rapidly and usually require frequent administration. Examples of drugs that are available as transdermal patches include methylphenidate, estradiol/norethindrone, fentanyl, and nitroglycerin. This route is limited to small lipophilic drugs, which can penetrate the poorly perfused, tightly knit stratum corneum layer of the skin. For the practical reason of accommodating the drug in the patch, this route is also limited to drugs that are used in relatively small doses. Rotigotine, a new drug for the treatment of Parkinson's disease, was recently launched as a transdermal patch because it experienced extensive hepatic extraction from the oral route. Unfortunately, the product had to be withdrawn due to crystallization of the drug in the patch.

Intranasal   Drugs administered by the intranasal route take advantage of the large surface area and highly permeable nature of the nasal membrane. This area is also very well perfused with blood, which enables drugs to be absorbed rapidly. The intranasal route has been pursued aggressively as a means of administering protein and peptide drugs, which generally have to be administered parenterally. Intranasal formulations of calcitonin and desmopressin are currently on the market, and the intranasal delivery of insulin is being pursued. The rapid absorption of traditional small drug molecules from this route has resulted in its use when a rapid onset of action is required. For example, nasal formulations are available for analgesics (morphine), antimigraine drugs (sumatriptan and zolmitriptan), and the intranasal delivery of naloxone has been used as an alternative to the intravenous route in the treatment of heroin overdose. Because a portion of the dose administered by the intranasal route gains direct access to the central nervous system (CNS), this route is being investigated as a means of avoiding the blood–brain barrier in the delivery of drugs used in the treatment of such diseases as Alzheimer's disease and Parkinson's disease [2]. Intranasal delivery is limited by the local irritation caused by the drugs and excipients, and constraints on the amount of drug that can be formulated in the small volume of an intranasal unit dose.

Pulmonary   The pulmonary route is used primarily for the local administration of agents to treat asthma and other respiratory conditions. The large surface area, good permeability, and extremely high perfusion of the alveolar membrane make it ideally suited for drug absorption. As a result, it has been investigated as a route for the administration of therapeutic agents, particularly proteins and peptides, which generally must be administered parenterally. An inhalation form of insulin (Exubera) was approved by the US Food and Drug Administration (FDA) but subsequently withdrawn due to poor sales, as it failed to gain acceptance among health professionals and patients. Concern has also been expressed about the long-term health effects of using the delicate alveoli to transport proteins.

3.3   OVERVIEW OF ORAL ABSORPTION

Orally administered drugs are formulated into convenient, palatable dosage forms, such as tablets (compressed powder mass), capsules, solutions, suspensions, and emulsions. The remainder of the chapter is devoted to discussing the absorption of drugs from the oral route. The discussion focuses on absorption from standard dosage forms rather than the more specialized topic of controlled-release products. When an individual dose is consumed, the drug must go through a series of processes and steps before reaching the systemic circulation. These steps control both the amount of the dose that is eventually absorbed into the systemic circulation and the rate of drug absorption.

After a patient has swallowed a tablet, it enters the stomach and is wet by the gastric fluid. The tablet must break up or *disintegrate* in the fluid so that the drug contained within its matrix is exposed or released. Thus, disintegration of the tablet is the first step in drug absorption. Once the tablet breaks up into small particles, the drug must *dissolve* in the gastrointestinal fluid. Once in solution, the drug now has the opportunity to *pass through the gastrointestinal membrane*. Drug absorption through the membrane most commonly occurs by passive diffusion, driven by the concentration gradient across the membrane. *Uptake transporters* in the luminal side of the enterocyte (intestinal epithelial absorptive cell) membrane may facilitate absorption. Once in the enterocyte the drug may be subject to the action of *efflux transporters*, which will reduce absorption by secreting the drug back into the lumen. The enterocytes of the intestine also contain some *drug-metabolizing enzymes*, which may metabolize and inactivate a drug before it passes through the basolateral (blood-side) membrane. When the drugs pass through the basolateral membrane, they are taken up into the capillaries bathing the tissue. These capillaries ultimately drain into the hepatic artery, which takes drugs through the liver before they reach the systemic circulation. The liver is a major organ of drug elimination, and any drug that is metabolized extensively by the liver may be eliminated before reaching the systemic circulation.

The key steps involved in drug absorption are summarized in Figure 3.3 and listed below.

1. Disintegration of tablet.
2. Dissolution of drug.
3. Diffusion of drug across the gastrointestinal membrane.
4a. Active uptake of drug across the gastrointestinal membrane.
4b. Active efflux of drug from the enterocyte back into the lumen.
5. Metabolism of drug in the enterocyte.
6. Metabolism of drug during the first passage through the liver (first pass).

Drugs that are already either in the dispersed state (suspension formulations) or in solution (solution formulations, e.g., syrups) will be farther along the absorption chain than solid dosage forms such as tablets. As a result, drugs formulated as suspensions and solutions, in particular, often display more rapid and/or more complete absorption than do their solid dosage formulations. The absorption of itraconazole, for example, which has poor dissolution properties, is better from a solution formulation than from a tablet.

3.3.1   Anatomy and Physiology of the Oral-Gastric-Intestinal Tract and Transit Time

The pathway that an orally administered drug product takes from the mouth is through the esophagus, stomach, and intestines. For most patients, swallowing a solid oral dosage form

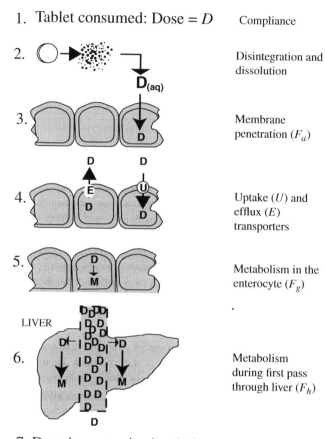

1. Tablet consumed: Dose = D — Compliance

2. — Disintegration and dissolution

   $D_{(aq)}$

3. — Membrane penetration (F_a)

4. — Uptake (U) and efflux (E) transporters

5. — Metabolism in the enterocyte (F_g)

6. LIVER — Metabolism during first pass through liver (F_h)

7. Drug in systemic circulation:

   Effective dose = $F_a \cdot F_g \cdot F_h \cdot D$

FIGURE 3.3   Steps involved in the oral absorption of a dose of a drug formulated as an oral tablet. After consumption, the tablet must disintegrate in the gastrointestinal fluid so that the drug can dissolve. Once in solution, the drug has the opportunity to pass the intestinal membrane. The fraction of the dose penetrating the membrane is F_a. In the membrane, the drug may be subject to uptake and efflux transporters. In the enterocyte cell, the drug may be subject to metabolism. The fraction of the drug in the enterocyte that escapes metabolism is F_g. When the drug passes into the capillary vessels, it is taken to the liver where it may undergo metabolism. F_h is the fraction of the drug entering the liver that escapes metabolism.

with a full glass of water results in the rapid delivery of the dosage form to the stomach in 5–15 s. But for the elderly, the coordination of the tongue, oropharynx, and esophagus begins to fail. For example, capsules can separate from the water, resulting in a "dry swallow" that can result in the capsule sticking to the throat. This can result in an ulceration from certain medications. This condition can be studied with gamma (γ) scintigraphy [3]. A series of images using γ scintigraphy is shown in Figure 3.4 [4] Starting in the left panel (a), all the dose is in the mouth (white color); swallowing takes place in the middle panel (b); most of the dose has made it into the stomach in the right panel (c). In the elderly, an additional drink of water is required for the dose to make it all the way into the stomach [3].

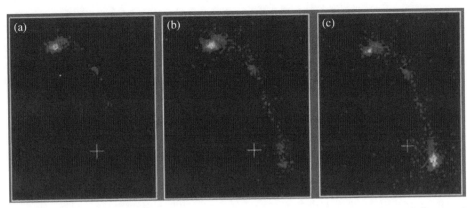

FIGURE 3.4   A series of γ scintigraphs showing the transit in the human esophagus following the administered of a liquid [4]. Courtesy of Clive Wilson, D.o.P.S., Strathclyde Institute for Biomedical Sciences. *(For a color version of this figure, see the color plate section.)*

From the esophagus, everything enters into the stomach, which is a low acid environment. The pH in healthy young adults ranges from 1.5 to 6. Figure 3.5 shows the range in stomach pH repeatedly measured in adults. While most subjects had a consistent pH less than 2, wide variability was reported [5].

The stomach is a storage and grinding organ that also secretes acid and enzymes to aid in the digestion of food. Periodic muscular contractions in the stomach result in a mixing and grinding of tablets and food into particles. The muscular pylorus sphincter regulates gastric emptying. When food is present in the stomach, the pyloris can tightly clamp shut, preventing even liquids from passing into the duodenum. The nutrients contained in a meal are metered out as semisolids or as particles reduced in size to about 2 mm in diameter.

The duodenum is a short segment of the small intestine consisting of (i) feedback receptors responsible for control of the pylorus sphincter, (ii) transporters responsible for the absorption of nutrients, and (iii) port responsible for entry into the intestine for bile acids and pancreatic enzymes. The pH of the duodenum ranges from 5.8 to 6.5. Transit through the duodenum is very rapid, as shown in a short video (http://simconserv.com/2.html) of a magnetically tagged capsule as it transits through the duodenum of a volunteer [6]. In this video, a magnetically tagged capsule is shown emptying from the stomach and traveling

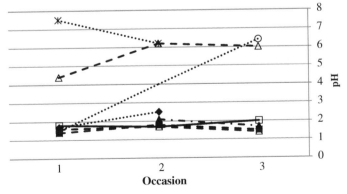

FIGURE 3.5   Day-to-day variations in the pH of gastric fluids from nine healthy human subjects in the fasted state. *Source:* Lindahl 1997, pp. 497–502 [5]. Reproduced with permission of Springer.

through the duodenum and into the jejunum. On this web page is shown a figure of the gastrointestinal tract with the approximate configuration of the stomach and duodenum in the volunteer. When the video starts, the capsule tumbles in the stomach before it makes an abrupt exit left into the duodenum, and then traverses the entire 10 cm length of the duodenum left to right in about 8 s. As the capsule then begins to loop, it has entered the jejunum. The entire "trip" took less than half a minute, as shown in the real-time counter visible in the video.

Although the small intestine begins at the duodenum, most of the small intestine is jejunum (pH ranges from 6 to 8) and ileum (pH range of 7–8). At the end of the ileum is the ileocecal sphincter, which controls the rate at which the ileal contents empty into the colon. As discussed in Chapter 2, the small intestine (duodenum, jejunum, and ileum) has an extremely large absorptive area, which results in it being the primary site for drug absorption. The colon—or large intestine—consists of the ascending, transverse, and descending portions. The colon has a pH range of 5.5–7. Water and some nutrients (e.g., fatty acids) are absorbed in the ascending colon. The transverse colon is usually empty (except for gas), and the descending colon stores the waste material until it is excreted.

Transit and Residence Time, Migrating Myoelectric Complex   The contents of the small intestine are mixed by a combination of circular and longitudinal muscle contractions. In the fasting state, a migrating myoelectric complex (MMC) propagates from the stomach all the way to the ileal-cecal junction. This so-called *housekeeper wave* moves the unabsorbed intestinal contents toward the colon and is repeated every 2 h or so. The time it takes for most fluids, particulates, or tablets to transit the entire small intestine (the *transit time*) is about 3 h.

3.4   EXTENT OF DRUG ABSORPTION

3.4.1   Bioavailability Factor

The extent of drug absorption is assessed by means of its bioavailability factor, which is usually referred to simply as "bioavailability," although strictly speaking, a drug's bioavailability refers to both the rate and extent of drug absorption. The *bioavailability factor F* is the fraction of the dose that reaches the systemic circulation intact. As a factor, it can achieve a value between zero (none of the dose reaches the systemic circulation) and 1 (the entire dose reaches the systemic circulation). Thus, if a drug's F value is 0.80, 80% of the dose administered reaches the circulation as intact drug. Since the body is exposed only to the dose that is absorbed, the *effective dose* of a drug may be defined as the product of the bioavailability and the dose administered:

$$\text{effective dose} = F \cdot \text{dose administered}$$

Thus, if 100 mg of a drug is administered and if $F = 0.8$,

$$\text{effective dose} = 0.8 \times 100 = 80 \, \text{mg}$$

As pharmacokinetic equations are introduced throughout the book, all formulas will include the bioavailability factor as a potential qualifier of the dose. The factor will even be included in a formula specifically derived for intravenous administration, where bioavailability is always 1. This is because an intravenous formula may be applied to other routes of administration that may not have complete bioavailability, and the presence of the factor in the formula serves as a reminder to account for bioavailability if necessary.

The determinants of the bioavailability factor can be classified into three broad areas:

1. Physicochemical characteristics of the drug.
2. Biological factors such as whether or not a drug is a substrate for the membrane transporters, and the drug-metabolizing enzymes.
3. The manufacturing process and formulation of a specific dosage form. As such, this component of bioavailability may vary from one brand of dosage form to another.

Under normal circumstances, the bioavailability factor for a given brand is constant and, very important, does not change with dose. A dose-dependent bioavailability factor is an example of nonlinear pharmacokinetics, discussed in Chapter 15.

3.4.2 Individual Bioavailability Factors

A portion of the drug dose may be lost at several points during the absorption process. Overall, the losses are usually classified into three categories, which results in three types of bioavailability (Figure 3.3):

1. *Fraction absorbed* (F_a): the fraction of the dose that is absorbed intact across the apical membrane into the cells (enterocytes) of the intestinal membrane.
2. *Intestinal bioavailability* (F_g): the fraction of the drug in the enterocytes that escapes metabolism.
3. *Hepatic bioavailability* (F_h): the fraction of the drug that enters the liver that escapes metabolism during the first pass.

Overall bioavailability (F) may thus be expressed as:

$$F = F_a \cdot F_g \cdot F_h \tag{3.1}$$

Example 3.1 Consider a drug that has the following characteristics: 20% dose of a drug is destroyed by acid in the stomach, the remaining drug is able to penetrate the apical membrane completely, 10% of the drug passing through the membrane is metabolized, and 40% of the drug entering the liver is metabolized. Find the effective dose when 100 mg is administered.

Solution

$$\begin{aligned} F &= F_a \cdot F_g \cdot F_h \\ &= 0.8 \times 0.9 \times 0.6 = 0.432 \end{aligned}$$

If 100 mg was administered, the effective dose would be $F \cdot D = 43.2$ mg.

This categorization is useful because it separates the physicochemical factors that control F_a from the biological factors that control F_g and F_h. It is useful to distinguish F_g from F_h because they are influenced by different factors. For example, F_h may be altered by changes in hepatic blood flow, which would have no effect on F_g.

3.5   DETERMINANTS OF THE FRACTION OF THE DOSE ABSORBED (*F*)

As introduced in Chapter 1, an immediate release tablet must first disintegrate before it can dissolve. The formulation excipients largely account for these actions. Disintegrants (e.g., starch) are highly water soluble, swell on contact with water, and result in the tablet breaking apart. Surfactants (e.g., tweens) help to wet the drug particles in the formulation. As the drug particles become wet, they begin to dissolve. Many of the same excipients can be found in a capsule. The tablet or capsule often also has a coating that has been sprayed on the surface of the unit. Most often the coating is hydrophilic, and serves to mask the bitter taste of the drug. Sometimes, the coating is *enteric* in that it does not dissolve until it comes into contact with the pH 5–7 fluids of the intestine; thereby, protecting the dosage form from disintegration and dissolution in the stomach. This type of coating serves to protect the drug from the stomach acid and can prevent the drug from irritating the stomach.

3.5.1   Disintegration

The disintegration of the tablet into small particles suitable for drug dissolution is an essential step in the absorption process. If disintegration does not occur, or if it is very slow, the absorption of the drug will be compromised. Most tablets contain special ingredients or excipients called *disintegrants* (e.g., starch), which swell when wet by the gastric fluid. As a result, tablet disintegration is usually a straightforward, unproblematic step in the absorption process. Additional excipients are discussed in Section 3.5.3.

3.5.2   Dissolution

The dissolution characteristics are determined primarily by a drug's aqueous solubility, which in turn is determined primarily by its hydrophilicity or lipophilicity, with more hydrophilic drugs dissolving in the aqueous gastrointestinal fluid more readily than do lipophilic drugs. Other factors that determine dissolution include the crystalline form of the drug and the particle size of the powdered drug. See Section 3.5.2.4 for additional discussion about particle size.

3.5.2.1   Importance of pKa for Drug Absorption

Any drug that has an ionizable group will have a pKa for that group. For example, the basic secondary amine on ephedrine has a pKa of about 9.5, and the carboxylic acid group in salicylic acid has a pKa of 3. The base in this case will become more ionized at pHs below 9.5, while the acid will become more ionized at a pH above its pKa. Recall the distribution coefficient *D* describes the partitioning of a compound as between a lipophilic solvent and a hydrophilic solvent at a specific pH (see Chapter 2, Section 2.3.1). As the pH for ephedrine is lowered from 7.4 to 5, its value for *D* decreases; whereas the value of *D* for salicylic acid increases as the pH is lowered. When we consider that the lipid core in the lipid bilayer of the absorptive cell's membrane is the rate-limiting barrier for the absorption of many drugs, then we would expect the absorption rate for these drugs to correlate with their values for their log D. This is shown in Figure 3.6 for ephedrine and salicylic acid in the rat intestine [7].

3.5.2.2   Impact of pH and Ionization on Passive Diffusion

The observation just described for ephedrine and salicylic acid is the basis of the *pH-partition hypothesis,* which states that the nonionized species will more readily partition

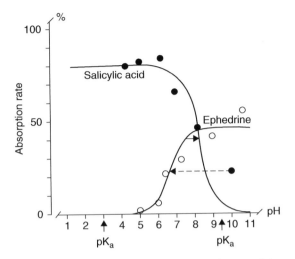

FIGURE 3.6   Drug absorption as a function of pH for a weak base and weak acid.

into a lipophilic solvent than the ionized species. For an acid drug with a pKa of 3, 50% of the drug will be ionized at a pH of 3. At a pH < 3 —as in the stomach—most of the drug will be nonionized, yet for many weakly acidic drugs, very little is absorbed from the stomach. Most of the weakly acidic drug is absorbed in the small intestine where at a pH > 5, where most (but not all) of the drug is ionized. The reason why most absorption occurs in the small intestine is that there are several orders of magnitude more surface area for absorption in the small intestine than in the stomach. Any nonionized species will be readily absorbed, upsetting the equilibrium between ionized and nonionized species, driving the equilibrium to form more nonionized drug. The sequence continues until most of the drug is absorbed.

Most drugs that are either weak acids or weak bases are often formulated as salts, to improve the *wetting* of the drug (see Section 3.5.3.1). This is accomplished by virtue that the drug is ionized when in the salt form and therefore hydrophilic. Table 3.1 shows some commonly used salts [8]. Improved wetting leads to faster dissolution and an increased rate and extent of absorption of the drug. The specific salt form can be selected to optimize these qualities. Examples of salts include propranolol hydrochloride, phenytoin sodium, naproxen sodium, and aminophylline, which is the ethylenediamine salt of theophylline.

3.5.2.3 *Attributes of the Crystalline Solid that Impact Dissolution*
For the dissolution of a drug crystal, three processes must occur: sublimation, cavitation, and hydration. Sublimation is the process whereby a solid becomes a gas without existing in the intermediate liquid phase. It involves the breaking of bonds to remove a molecule from its crystal lattice. Depending on the type and number of intermolecular bonds that make up the crystal, sublimation may require a significant amount of energy. For some crystals, pharmaceutical scientists have made amorphous forms of the drug. These amorphous forms do not have the long-range order consisting of strong intermolecular bonds found in crystals. The amount of sublimation energy is much less than for the crystalline material, and they usually readily dissolve. Some forms of crystals, called polymorphs, may have a solubility that is intermediate of the crystal and amorphous forms, due to an intermediate crystal lattice strength.

TABLE 3.1 Salt Forms of New Chemical Entities (NCEs) Approved by the FDA from 1995 to 2006

Salts of Basic Drugs	Total Number
Hydrochloride	54
Methanesulfonate (mesylate)	10
Hydrobromide/bromide	8
Acetate	5
Fumarate	5
Sulfate/bisulfate	3
Succinate	3
Citrate	2
Phosphate	2
Maleate	2
Nitrate	2
Tartrate	2
Benzoate	1
Carbonate	1
Pamoate	1
Total of all salts of basic drugs	101
Salts of acidic drugs	**Total number**
Sodium	12
Calcium	4
Potassium	2
Tromethamine	1
Total of all salts of acidic drugs	19

Source: Serajuddin 2007, pp. 603–616 [8]. Reproduced with permission of Elsevier.

During cavitation, a cavity is created in the solvent for the drug molecule. Molecules with a smaller molecular weight (which for some molecules can be correlated to molecular volume) will require a smaller cavity and less energy.

In hydration, the drug molecule moves into the space in the solvent. This step requires the formation of hydrogen bonds between the drug and water. It also requires close contact between the drug and the water—a process called *wetting* (see 3.5.3.1).

3.5.2.4 Impact of Particle Size and Nanoparticles on Dissolution

The rate of dissolution of a drug is described by the *Noyes–Whitney equation* [9]. Accordingly, the rate may be expressed as:

$$\frac{dC}{dt} = \frac{D \cdot S}{V \cdot h} \cdot (Cs - C) \tag{3.2}$$

where C is the concentration of the drug in the gastrointestinal fluid, t is the time, S is the surface area of the solid undergoing dissolution, h is the thickness of a diffusion layer surrounding the solid, D is the diffusion coefficient of the drug, V is the volume of the gastrointestinal fluid, and Cs is the solubility of the drug in the gastrointestinal fluid.

As shown in Figure 3.7, surface area S is a property of particle size: cutting the diameter of a particle in half results in a doubling of its surface area.

The dissolution properties of poorly soluble drugs can be improved by using a process known as *micronization* to greatly reduce the particle size. This method is used to

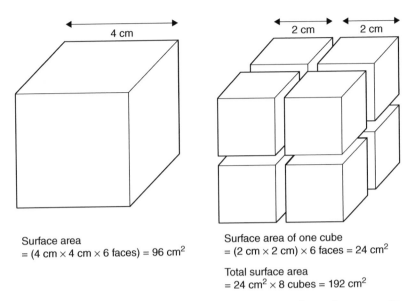

Surface area
= (4 cm × 4 cm × 6 faces) = 96 cm^2

Surface area of one cube
= (2 cm × 2 cm) × 6 faces = 24 cm^2

Total surface area
= 24 cm^2 × 8 cubes = 192 cm^2

FIGURE 3.7 Illustrative example where subdividing increases the surface area of a particle. *Source:* Public access.

increase the dissolution of cilostazol. By decreasing particle size, surface area is increased, and this in turn increases the number of contact points between solid and solvent, resulting in an increase in the dissolution rate. Figure 3.8 shows the impact of the reduced particle size on the percent dissolved over time (the dissolution rate) for powders of the poorly water soluble compound cilostazol [10]. The median particle diameters of the powders are 13 μm (squares), 2.4 μm (diamonds), and 0.22 μm (triangles). The initial slope of the 2.4 μm particles is much steeper than for the 13 μm particles (nanoparticles), reflecting a much faster dissolution rate. Interestingly, the 0.23 μm nanoparticles seem to dissolve almost instantly. When nanoparticles are made from powders, imperfections are introduced into the crystal

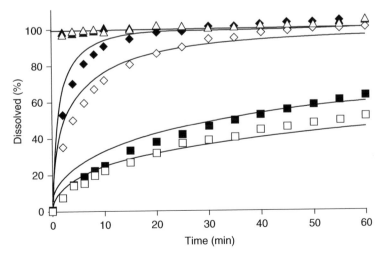

FIGURE 3.8 *In vitro* dissolution profiles of cilostazol. See text for the description of symbols. *Source:* Jinno *et al.* 2006, pp. 56–64 [10]. Reproduced with permission of Elsevier.

lattice—decreasing the energy required for sublimation—and resulting in almost instantaneous dissolution. If the short-range ordered structure is sufficiently disrupted, the material becomes *amorphous*. Amorphous materials are also known as liquid crystals or solid dispersions. These materials—such as cilostazol—behave as if they are liquids, and their aqueous solubility is greatly enhanced.

3.5.3 Formulation Excipients

Dosage forms contain many other ingredients in addition to active drug. These ingredients, or excipients, are pharmacologically inert and are added to assist in the manufacture of the dosage form or to impart certain properties to the finished product. For example, many powder-based dosage forms (tablets and capsules) contain *lubricants* (e.g. talc, magnesium stearate) to improve the flow properties of the powders so that they can be poured and transferred more easily during manufacture. Most solid dosage forms also contain diluents to increase the size of the unit dosage form, to make it a more manageable size. The importance of assessing the potential influence of inert excipients on bioavailability was demonstrated very poignantly in 1968 when over 50 Australian patients developed serious phenytoin toxicity after the manufacturer simply changed the diluent in the formulation from calcium sulfate to the more hydrophilic lactose.

3.5.3.1 *Impact of Wetting*
If a molecule is hydrophobic, it will not easily wet with water. One way to improve wetting is to add a *surfactant*. The surfactant has a portion of its structure that is lipophilic and a portion that is hydrophilic. The surfactant molecules self-assemble in water, forming a spherical micelle, with the lipophilic part of the molecule pointing toward the center. The center is a more favorable environment for the lipophilic drug molecule, while the surfactant hydrophilic portion bonds with water resulting in the structure dissolving.

3.5.4 Adverse Events within the Gastrointestinal Lumen

The gastrointestinal lumen is an extremely harsh environment. It contains enzymes, foods in various stages of digestion, and displays fairly wide changes in pH. This hostile environment can be beneficial in that it can destroy potentially harmful bacteria but can also be very detrimental for drugs.

3.5.4.1 *Acid Degradation*
The pH along the gastrointestinal tract varies from around 1.5 to 7. The gastric pH can approach about 1.5 in the presence of a small amount of food as a result of gastric acid secretion stimulated by gastrin and histamine. However, a large meal may result in a transient, high pH (near pH 6) depending on its buffering effect on the stomach acid. In the fasting state, the pH generally rests at around a pH of 2–6 (Figure 3.5). The high acidity of the stomach can be particularly problematic for drugs. The early or natural penicillins are very susceptible to acid hydrolysis, particularly penicillin G, which as a consequence is best administered parenterally. Oral preparations of penicillin V should be administered on an empty stomach (1–2 h before food) to minimize hydrolysis. The newer semisynthetic penicillins such as amoxicillin are much less susceptible to hydrolysis and provide better and more consistent oral bioavailability. Drugs susceptible to acid hydrolysis in the stomach can be formulated into enteric-coated tablets. The coating protects the drug from the acid in the stomach, since it will dissolve only in the higher

pH of the small intestine, which generally lies in the region of 6–7. In another approach to protecting acid-labile drugs, antacids can be included in their formulation. This is used for the acid-labile reverse transcriptase inhibitor didanosine. The increase in the gastric pH brought about by treatment with proton pump inhibitors, H2 antagonists, and antacids can affect the dissolution and bioavailability of some drugs. The absorption of drugs such as delavirdine and the poorly soluble antifungal agents, itroconazole and ketoconazole, which display much better dissolution in acidic pH, has been found to be reduced by low gastric acidity. The absorption of other drugs, such as alendronate, has been found to be increased [11]. The less acidic environment created by proton pump inhibitors may also reduce the absorption of calcium, which can make patients who take these drugs for extended periods more susceptible to bone fractures and osteoporosis [12].

3.5.4.2 *Enzymatic Attack*
Digestive enzymes such as pepsin, trypsin, and chymotrypsin in the gastrointestinal fluid are the main enzymes that affect drug absorption. These enzymes have severely limited the success of protein drugs such as insulin being given orally. The importance of the microflora (bacteria) of the gastrointestinal tract has recently been recognized for the management of health (such as probiotic supplements, yogurt). While the subject is beyond the scope of this book, the interested reader might read published reviews [13] and [14]. Drugs can also affect and be affected by the enzymes of the microflora, which are found primarily in the large intestine. Since most drugs are absorbed before they reach the large intestine, these enzymes generally do not affect the fraction of the dose absorbed initially. They can be important for drugs that are conjugated with a glucuronide during hepatic metabolism and subsequently excreted in the bile and then into the intestine. The gut flora can hydrolyze the conjugates and release the drug, which can then be reabsorbed back into the body. This process, known as *enterohepatic recirculation* often results in the appearance of a secondary peak in the plasma concentration–time profile of a drug (Figure 3.9). The process results

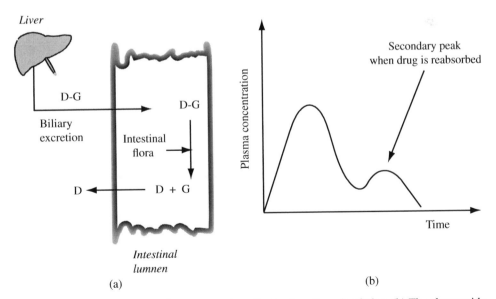

FIGURE 3.9 (a) Diagrammatic representation of enterohepatic recirculation. (b) The glucuronide conjugate of the drug is hydrolyzed by the gut flora. The reabsorption of the drug results in a second peak on the plasma concentration–time curve.

in the reabsorption of drug that has been eliminated from the body. Thus, in theory, entero-heaptic recirculation could result in a drug having a bioavailability factor greater than 1. The concurrent administration of broad-spectrum antibiotics such as the quinolones can reduce the population of the gut flora, which in turn can lead to reduced enterohepatic recirculation and a reduction in the body's exposure to a drug. The enterohepatic recirculation of ethinyl estradiol, a component in oral contraceptives, can be reduced by concurrent antibiotics, which could compromise the effectiveness of the drug. Generally, this is thought to be a problem only in patients who are already predisposed to low bioavailability of ethinyl estradiol, or when the antibiotic rifampin is used. In addition to reducing the gut flora, rifampin induces liver enzymes and can increase the metabolism of estradiol to further reduce the body's exposure to estradiol.

3.5.4.3 Interaction with Other Components of the Gastrointestinal Fluid
Drugs may interact adversely with other components of the gastric fluid, such as digested and undigested foods and other drugs. The classical example of this type of interaction is the *complexation reaction* between tetracycline and di- and trivalent ions (Ca^{2+}, Mg^{2+}, and Al^{3+}) found in dairy products and antacids. The tetracycline complex is insoluble and therefore the drug cannot be absorbed. Similar complexes are formed with the quinolone antibiotics. Antacids can reduce the absorption of so many other drugs, including pheny-toin, several β-blockers, isoniazid, and digoxin, that as a general rule, patients should be advised to stagger the dosing of antacids and other prescription drugs by a period of at least 2 h.

3.5.4.4 Food Effects
Food can affect drug absorption through effects on gastrointestinal physiology and through physical effects on drugs in the lumen. The magnitude and direction of a food effect depends on the specific characteristics of the meal, including the composition of the meal (proteins, carbohydrates, or fats), calorie content, and the total volume of food and fluid ingested. Physiological changes brought about by food include a delay in gastric emptying, changes in gastrointestinal pH, stimulation of bile flow, and increased liver blood flow, all of which can affect drug absorption. Absorption can also be affected by the physical presence of food in the gastrointestinal lumen. Food can impede drug diffusion to the membrane and reduce absorption; and constituents in food, such as ions, can chelate drugs and reduce absorption. Increased gastric residence time may increase dissolution in gastric fluid but can also increase the destruction of acid-labile drugs. As a general rule, the delay in gastric emptying brought about by food delays the absorption of most drugs because it slows their delivery to the small intestine, which is where most drugs are absorbed. The effect of food on the extent of absorption is more variable. A classification system in which drugs are categorized according to their permeability and dissolution characteristics has been used to help predict whether food will increase, decrease, or not affect the absorption of individual drugs (see Section 3.7).

3.5.4.5 Absorption Window
If, as we will see, the active drug is primarily absorbed by specialized transporters located in a specific region of the small intestine, then we say the absorption of the drug is subject to an *absorption window*. For drugs with an absorption window, the impact of the transit time and the MMC (Section 3.3.1) needs to be considered. For example, the drug must be in close proximity to the transporters for a minimum amount of time. If the MMC propagates

the drug along the small intestine past the transporters before it can be absorbed, the consequence could be a reduced bioavailability (see also Section 3.7).

3.5.5 Transcellular Passive Diffusion

Most drugs penetrate the gastrointestinal membrane by transcellular passive diffusion, driven by the concentration gradient across the membrane. As discussed in Chapter 2, the small intestine (duodenum, jejunum, and ileum) has an extremely large absorptive area, which results in it being the primary site for drug absorption. The small intestine is also highly perfused with blood. This allows absorbed drug to be rapidly carried away from the absorption site, and enables a high concentration gradient to be maintained across the intestinal membrane. Because of the more extensive absorption of the drug from the intestine, the rate of stomach emptying plays an important role in controlling the speed with which drugs are absorbed. Slow stomach emptying delays the delivery of drug to the primary site of absorption and slows down absorption, whereas rapid stomach emptying can speed up the onset of drug absorption.

A drug's transcellular permeability is determined primarily by its lipophilicity, which as discussed in Chapter 2, can be quantified using the drug's partition coefficient (P) or distribution coefficient (D). Drugs with negative log P or log D values, indicative of high hydrophilicity and poor lipophilicity, cannot easily penetrate the lipid core of a bilayer membrane. Conversely, drugs with high log P or log D values generally have good permeability. A study of almost 500 therapeutic drugs found that 50% had log $P > 2$ and 80% had log $P > 0$ [2]. However, compounds with high log P or log D values are also most likely to have poor dissolution in aqueous media. As a result, values of log $D_{7.4}$ in the range of about 1–3 are considered optimum for balancing permeability and dissolution. The size of a drug molecule is also important. Large molecules such as peptides and proteins are unable to penetrate the intestinal membrane. Drugs with a molecular mass greater than 500 Da are predicted to have poor membrane permeability, particularly if they also possess additional adverse physicochemical characteristics, such as polarity or low lipophilicity [15]. Studies indicate that for drugs with molecular masses below around 400 Da, size is not an important factor for membrane penetration [16]. Under these circumstances, a drug's log P or log D value at a physiological pH, combined with a measure of the drug's polarity (polar surface area or number of hydrogen bond donors), can be used to predict transcellular passive diffusion.

3.5.6 Particulate Uptake

In addition to the absorptive epithelia cells discussed in Section 2.2, the small intestine also has *mucous secreting cells* and *lymphoid follicles* (*M* cells). The *M cells* are responsible for antigen sampling of the intestinal contents and for a high transcytotic capacity (e.g., vaccines and nanoparticles). Besides M cells, nanoparticles that exhibit specific physicochemical properties (e.g., size, charge, and coating with PEG groups—pegylation) are found to be taken up by micropinocytosis, phagocytosis, and endocytosis in the absorptive epithelia cells.

3.5.7 Paracellular Passive Diffusion

Each epithelial cell is connected to neighboring cells by a ring of cytoskeletal filaments—much like a six-pack of cans is held together with a plastic ring. In the intestine, this ring is called the *terminal web*, and includes aqueously filled channels called *tight junctions*. The tight junctions are negatively charged and function like a 4–8 angstrom pore, which makes it extremely difficult for all but very small drugs to penetrate. Furthermore, the gaps between adjacent cells in the small intestine constitute only a very small fraction (0.01%) of the total absorptive area, which makes it a very unappealing and inefficient route of drug penetration [17]. Small polar drugs such as atenolol (MW 266 Da; log $D_{7.4} \approx -1.5$) were believed to be absorbed by this route. However, recent work has cast doubt on this and suggests that the enormous absorptive area available for transcellular absorption may enable small hydrophilic drugs such as atenolol to undergo some transcellular absorption [17]. The aminoglycoside antibiotics, which are both very polar (log $D_{7.4} \approx -10$) and very large (MW 450 to >1000 Da), are unable to penetrate the intestinal membrane by either route. These drugs must be given parenterally and are usually administered as short, intermittent intravenous infusions for the treatment of systemic infections.

The use of excipients to increase the size of the tight junctions in the intestinal lumen is being investigated as a means of opening up the paracellular route to large and/or polar drugs, which normally cannot penetrate the membrane. However, these excipients often display a cationic charge, which has been shown to be toxic to absorptive cells [18, 19].

3.5.8 Uptake and Efflux Transporters

Drug transporters within the enterocyte membrane can also play an important role in the absorption process. Over 400 individual transporters have been identified on the apical and basolateral sides of the cell membrane. The clinical role of many of these has yet to be established, and this discussion will generally be limited to uptake and efflux transporters, whose role in drug absorption has been demonstrated in clinical studies. Many of these were introduced in Chapter 2 (Section 2.4). The main transporters involved in drug and nutrient absorption from the gastrointestinal tract are solute carrier (SLC) OATPs, PEPT1, and PEPT 2; ABC superfamily MDR1 (P-gp), MRP2, and breast BCRP (Figure 3.10), and they are all located on the apical side of the membrane [20]. Thus, the uptake transporters (OATPs and PEPT) enhance drug absorption, and the efflux transporters (P-gp, BCRP, and MRP2) impede absorption. The uptake transporter SLC superfamily OCT1, located on the basolateral side of the membrane, enhance intestinal cell uptake of substrates from blood, and could potentially contribute to the secretion of the substrates into the intestine. The efflux ABC superfamily MRP3, located on the basolateral side of the membrane, would in theory serve to enhance the absorption of its substrates.

3.5.8.1 Uptake Transporters

OATP1A2 and OATP2B1 are present on the apical and basal sides of the intestinal membrane, and there appears to be some overlap in their substrate specificity. Fexofenadine and saquinavir are transported by OATP1A2, and the concomitant administration of fruit (apple, grapefruit, or orange) juices, which inhibit OATP1A2, decreases the absorption of fexofenadine by between 30% and 50% [21, 22]. Atorvastatin and other HMG-CoA reductase inhibitors (statins) are substrates for OATP2B1, but its role, if any, in the absorption of these drugs is not known at this time. The PEPT1 transporter plays an important role in the absorption of digested proteins (dipeptides and tripeptides). However, it can also transport drugs that possess di- and tripeptide-like structures such as cephalosporins, penicillins, and angiotensin-converting enzyme inhibitors like captopril [23]. Valacylovir, the L-valine ester prodrug of acyclovir, was developed specifically to take advantage of the

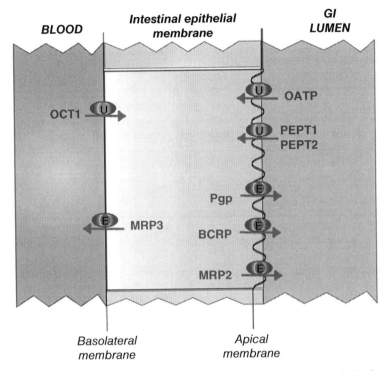

FIGURE 3.10 Transporters in the intestinal epithelia. *(For a color version of this figure, see the color plate section.)*

PEPT1 carrier. The absorption of the valacyclovir is about double that of acyclovir [24]. Some of the substrates of PEPT1 (e.g., the cephalosporins) also act as inhibitors of the transporter. Generally, information on the role of uptake transporters in drug absorption in humans is still rather limited. The transporter apical sodium-dependent bile acid transporter (ASBT) is responsible for the bile acid uptake in the ileum. A mutation of the ASBT gene results in steatorrhea and congenital diarrhea due to a malabsorption of bile acids in these patients [25].

3.5.8.2 Efflux Transporters
The efflux transporters on the apical side of the intestinal membrane serve to reduce the absorption of drugs by pumping substances that have penetrated the cell membrane back into the lumen (Figure 3.10). The greatest amount of clinical evidence is available on the role of MDR1 (ABCB1 and P-gp), which is able to transport a wide variety of drugs with diverse chemical structures. Clinical studies have demonstrated that P-gp plays an important role in limiting the oral absorption of many drugs, including lipophilic, cationic compounds, and the list of its substrates/inhibitors includes anticancer agents (e.g., paclitaxel and irinotecan), antivirals, calcium channel blockers, immunosuppressive agents (e.g., cyclosporine and tacrolimus), talinolol, and digoxin [23, 26–28]. Many of these drugs have a narrow therapeutic range, and Table 3.2 lists some examples for clinically significant drug–drug interactions (DDIs).

The levels of P-gp vary throughout the intestine and are present in greater amounts in the distal portion (ileum) than in the proximal portion (duodenum and jejunum) of the small intestine. A drug's exposure to the higher P-gp concentration in the distal portion of the

TABLE 3.2   Examples of Clinically Important Changes in Bioavailability Resulting from Altered P-gp Activity

Drug	Concomitant Drug	Outcome	Mechanism Proposed
Digoxin	Quinidine	Increased F	Inhibition of P-gp
	St. John's wort	Decreased F	Induction of P-gp
Cyclosporine	Rifampin	Decreased F	Induction of P-gp
Tacrolimus	Rifampin	Decreased F	Induction of P-gp
Paclitaxel	Cyclosporine	Increased F	Inhibition of P-gp
	Elacridar	Increased F	Inhibition of P-gp
Docetaxel	Cyclosporine	Increased F	Inhibition of P-gp
Topotecan	Elacridar	Increased F	Inhibition of P-gp, inhibition of BCRP

Source: Data from References [23, 27].

small intestine will depend on how rapidly it is absorbed. Highly soluble, lipophilic P-gp substrates such as diltiazem and verapamil are absorbed rapidly in the upper small intestine and their bioavailability is less affected by P-gp efflux. Additionally, highly soluble, lipophilic P-gp substrates may be absorbed so rapidly that they saturate P-gp during absorption and limit its negative effects on bioavailability. The higher concentration of P-gp in the distal small intestine has been postulated to explain why the extent of absorption of talinolol is lower from slow-release than from immediate-release preparations: The greater exposure of the drug to the distal small intestine in the slow-release preparation leads to greater P-gp efflux and less absorption [26]. The greater bioavailability of cyclosporine from the Neoral® formulation compared to Sandimmune® is also believed to result, in part, from less P-gp efflux. Cyclosporine is absorbed faster from Neoral®, which results in less drug reaching the distal intestine, where the concentration of P-gp is greatest [26].

It is difficult to quantify definitively the effect of P-gp on drug absorption because there is extensive overlap of its substrates, inhibitors, and inducers with those of the cytochrome P450 (CYP3A4) drug metabolizing enzyme, which can also reduce drug absorption. Thus, metabolism by intestinal CYP3A4 will also play a role in limiting the absorption of many of the drugs listed in Table 3.2. Indeed, the wide overlap in the substrate specificity of these two systems suggests that they may have evolved to work together to provide a concerted effort to limit the absorption of foreign chemicals (xenobiotics) into the body. Talinolol, digoxin, and fexofenadine have been used in clinical studies as probes for P-gp because these drugs do not undergo substantial metabolism by CYP3A4. Intestinal P-gp reduces the bioavailability of digoxin, but digoxin is also a substrate for renal P-gp, which, like intestinal P-gp, reduces the body's exposure to digoxin, in this case by promoting elimination. Reduced P-gp activity at either site would increase the body's exposure to digoxin (increased absorption and/or decreased elimination), and increased P-gp activity would have the opposite effect. Rifampin, an inducer of P-gp activity, was indeed found to decrease the systemic concentrations of digoxin [29]. Three observations indicated that the effects on intestinal, as opposed to renal, P-gp appeared to dominate. First, digoxin's renal clearance and half-life were not altered by rifampin. Second, rifampin had much less effect on the pharmacokinetics of intravenous digoxin. Third, the increase in intestinal P-gp content mediated by rifampin correlated with the increase in digoxin concentration after oral administration. In other studies, the relative contribution of altered renal and/or intestinal P-gp on digoxin's pharmacokinetics is not clear. From a clinical standpoint, modifiers of P-gp should be used cautiously with digoxin. Irrespective of the mechanism, inhibitors and inducers may increase and decrease, respectively, the body's exposure to digoxin. Similarly, modifiers of P-gp and CYP3A4 should be used cautiously with the compounds listed in Table 3.2. Irrespective of the mechanism (P-gp or CYP3A4), inhibitors will tend to increase absorption and inducers will tend to reduce absorption.

Some of the changes in bioavailability brought about by modifiers of P-gp activity are small. For example, pretreatment with St. John's wort or rifampin, both of which induce P-gp, reduced the bioavailability of talinolol by 25% and 35%, respectively [30, 31]. In other cases, modifiers can bring about large changes in bioavailability. For example, cyclosporine, an inhibitor of P-gp, increased the bioavailability of the anticancer drugs paclitaxel and docetaxel from a negligible value (0.04 and 0.08, respectively) to a substantial value (0.47 and 0.88, respectively) [23]. Clinically, the coadministration of P-gp inhibitors with anticancer drugs not only offers the advantage of improving oral bioavailability, but could also improve their effectiveness by preventing the efflux of drugs from cancer cells and/or the CNS. The use of cyclosporine as an inhibitor P-gp is limited by its immunosuppressant activity, and newer P-gp inhibitors have been developed that are devoid of this activity. Second-generation inhibitors such as valspodar cause unacceptable side effects because they inhibit the elimination of some drugs. Third-generation P-gp inhibitors such as zosuquidar and elacridar are potent P-gp inhibitors but do not inhibit hepatic enzymes. They are being tested clinically as a means of increasing the effectiveness and bioavailability of anticancer drugs [32] Elacridar, an inhibitor of both P-gp and BCRP, increased the bioavailability of topotecan from 0.4 to 0.97 [23].

Other efflux transporters that have been shown to have clinically important effects on absorption include the organic solute transporter (OSTα and OSTβ), which is responsible for the transport of bile acids across the intestinal epithelium [33]; the equilibrative nucleoside transporter (ENT1 and ENT2), which regulates ethanol intoxication [34] and can predict pancreatic cancer survival in patients treated with gemcitabine [35]. Additionally, inhibition of this transporter is thought to be responsible for cannabidiol-mediated immunosuppression [36].

BCRP is one of the most abundant efflux transporters in the human intestinal lumen, particularly the jejunum. Animal studies have demonstrated that BCRP reduces the absorption of a number of anticancer drugs, including topotecan and irinotecan. Clinical studies in people with a genetically determined low activity level of BCRP were found to have markedly higher plasma concentrations of atorvastatin and rosuvastatin [37]. These patients had higher peak plasma concentrations but not altered elimination half-lives, which suggests that BCRP affects the absorption but not the elimination of these drugs. Sulfasalazine, a drug used in the treatment of ulcerative colitis and Crohn's disease, is a substrate for both BCRP and MRP2. Despite good inherent membrane permeability characteristics (log $P =$ 3.88), only a small fraction of the dose is absorbed after oral administration. It is thought that BCRP and/or MRP2 [38–40] reduces its absorption and enables a large portion of the dose to reach its site of action in the colon, where bacteria cleave to its active metabolites, sulfapyridine and 5-ASA. Indomethacin, an inhibitor of MRP2, was found to increase the absorption of sulfasalazine [39]. Thus, the concomitant consumption of indomethacin with sulfasalazine may reduce the effectiveness of sulfasalazine.

3.5.8.3 Characteristics of Transporter-Mediated Transport

There are four facts that distinguish transporters from passive diffusion. Firstly, all compounds that are absorbed via a transporter are also absorbed by passive diffusion. But not all compounds that are absorbed by passive diffusion are also absorbed via a transporter.

Transporters recognize specific substrates. Some transporters may have a broader selection criterion than others. While passive diffusion has no specific selectivity, remember that good oral absorption is more likely when the compound adheres to the Lipinski's "rule of five": molecular weight < 500 Da, $\log P < 5$, less than five hydrogen bond donors (e.g., –OH and –NH), and less than 10 hydrogen bond acceptors. Secondly, there are also a limited number of transporters on any membrane. Therefore, it is extremely likely that the transporter-mediated uptake will become saturated at higher substrate concentrations. Thirdly, similar substrates will compete for the same transporter. This could result in either an inhibition of the substrate transport, or induce the synthesis of additional amino acids, and their assembly into transporter protein. Finally, genetic variance in a population may result in an over- or underexpression of a particular transporter.

Summary of the Impact of Efflux Transporters on the Oral Absorption of Drugs   The substrates of efflux transporters normally are absorbed at a certain basal rate. This basal rate represents the net rate that reflects any absorptive flux minus any efflux (contra-absorption) flux. Consider what would happen to the net rate if the efflux transporter(s) are inhibited or induced.

If an inhibitor of the efflux is present, less substrate will be effluxed. The result is a more efficient substrate absorption—an increase over the basal rate—manifested as an increase in its absorption.

If an induction of the efflux occurs, more efflux transporters will be present. If during the basal efflux some saturation of the efflux transporters normally occurs, then the addition of more efflux transporters will alleviate this saturation. This means that more substrate will be effluxed—a decrease in the basal rate. The result is a less efficient substrate absorption, manifested as a decrease in its absorption. These principles are demonstrated in the transporter simulation model found at http://web.uri.edu/pharmacy/research/rosenbaum/sims/Model2.

3.5.9   Presystemic Intestinal Metabolism or Extraction

The enterocytes of the small intestine contain several enzymes that can metabolize drugs that get inside the cell. These include cytochrome P450 (CYP) isozymes, glucuronosyltransferases, and alcohol dehydrogenase. For many drugs, intestinal extraction is the least important component of overall bioavailability. However, for some drugs, the fraction of a dose lost at this point in absorption is substantial and results in a large loss of dose. Extensive intestinal extraction makes the subject drugs susceptible to clinically important DDIs. CYP3A4 and CYP2C9 are the most abundant phase I enzymes in the enterocytes, comprising 80% and 15% of total intestinal CYP, respectively. The high concentration of CYP3A4 and the large number of drugs metabolized by this isozyme combine to make CYP3A4 metabolism the most important intestinal extraction process. In contrast to P-gp, the levels of CYP3A4 are higher in the upper part of the small intestine (duodenum) and decrease progressively to the distal ileum. There appears to be wide interindividual variability in its expression, which will result in wide interindividual variability in the bioavailability of drugs that undergo significant intestinal metabolism [41]. Despite its low concentration relative to the liver (about 1%) [42], intestinal CYP3A4 can metabolize a very substantial part of an oral dose of its substrates. Table 3.3 shows the values of F_g for several drugs [43]. The values were estimated using grapefruit juice to inhibit intestinal CYP3A4. It can be seen that buspirone, lovastatin, and simvastatin undergo substantial intestinal extraction. Others, such as atorvastatin and midazolam, undergo significantly less intestinal extraction though

TABLE 3.3   Values of Intestinal (F_g) for Several CYP3A4 Substrates. Estimated Using Grapefruit as an Inhibitor [43]

Drug	F_g
Atorvastatin	0.56^a
Buspirone	0.11
Cyclosporine	0.65
Lovastatin	0.07
Midazolam	0.56
Nifedipine	0.62
Simvastatin	0.14
Tacrolimus	0.14^b
Verapamil	0.71

[a]Was reported to be as low as 0.24.
[b]Estimated from iv and oral data [43].

still lose about half of their dose as they pass through the intestinal membrane. Note statins, such as pravastatin and rosuvastatin that are not substrates of CYP3A4, do not undergo intestinal extraction.

Drugs that undergo significant intestinal extraction will be particularly susceptible to clinically important DDIs. For example, in theory, if the intestinal extraction of tacrolimus was completely inhibited, its bioavailability would increase from around 0.14 to almost 1, which translates into a sevenfold (1/0.14) increase in the effective dose.

Table 3.4 illustrates that drugs with high intestinal extraction, for example, simvastatin, are much more sensitive to changes in intestinal extraction than drugs with lower intestinal extraction, for example, atovastatin. The effect of a 10% decrease in intestinal extraction on bioavailability is shown. It can be seen that there is little change in the effective dose of the low extraction drug. In contrast, the 10% reduction in the extraction of a highly extracted drug essentially doubles the effective dose. Large increases (in some cases over 10-fold) in the bioavailability of buspirone, tacrolimus, sirolimus, lovastatin, and simvastatin have been observed in the presence of inhibitors. Reduced P-gp activity as well as reduced hepatic CYP3A4 activity could also contribute to these effects.

TABLE 3.4   Effect of a 10% Reduction in Intestinal Extraction on the Effective Oral Dose of High- and Low-Extraction Drugs

	Control		10% Reduction in Extraction	
	Drug 1	Drug 2	Drug 1	Drug 2
Fraction of dose extracted in membrane	0.1	0.9	0.09	0.81
F_g	0.9	0.1	0.91	0.19
Effective dose from a 100 mg dose	90 mg	10 mg	91 mg	19 mg
Change in effective dose	—	—	1.1%	90%

It is assumed that the entire dose is absorbed into the membrane.

Many of the drugs that are substrates for intestinal CYP3A4 are also substrates for P-gp, and as mentioned previously, the two processes may have evolved to work synergistically within the enterocyte to prevent the absorption of drugs and other xenobiotics. The efflux of a drug by P-gp followed by its reabsoprtion creates a recycling effect that can prolong the overall time that a drug spends in the enterocyte and provide CYP3A4 with more opportunity to metabolize it. This may explain, in part, why despite its relatively low concentration compared to the liver, intestinal CYP3A4 is able to metabolize such a large fraction of the dose of some drugs. There are drugs, however, such as midazolam, felodipine, and nifedipine, which are CYP3A4 substrates but do not appear to be substrates for intestinal P-gp, whereas others, including talinolol, digoxin, and fexofenadine, are substrates for P-gp but not CYP3A4 [32].

Clinical studies have demonstrated that inhibitors of CYP3A4, such as HIV antivirals (e.g., indinavir, nelfinavir, and ritonavir), macrolide antibiotics (e.g., clarithromycin, erythromycin, and NOT azithromycin), and "azole" antifungals (e.g., ketoconazole and itroconazole), increase the bioavailability of many CYP3A4 substrates. There is wide interindividual variability in the magnitude of the effect of inhibitors, presumably because of interpatient variability in the expression of intestinal CYP3A4 as a result of genetic and environmental factors.

Grapefruit juice is an irreversible inhibitor of CYP3A4, and evidence suggests that it affects primarily intestinal rather than hepatic CYP3A4, although consumption of large quantities may also inhibit hepatic CYP3A4. Thus, concomitant administration of drugs with grapefruit juice may provide a good indication of the role of intestinal CYP3A4 in drug absorption. While there is no strong evidence that it inhibits P-gp [22], grapefruit juice along with other fruit juices or green tea inhibits OATP. Unlike its effects on CYP3A4, its effects on OATP seem to last no more than 4 h. Grapefruit juice increases the oral bioavailability of many drugs, including simvastatin, lovastatin, atorvastatin, felodipine, cyclosporine, and buspirone. The effect appears to be concentration dependent, as double-strength juice has a greater effect than regular-strength juice. Large increases of more than 10-fold have been observed in the plasma concentrations of simvastatin, lovastatin, and buspirone [44–46]. However, since OATP aids in the absorption of its substrates, inhibiting OATP may decrease the absorption of atenolol (40%), ciprofloxacin (20%), fexofenadine (40%), and nadolol (85% by green tea).

3.5.10 Presystemic Hepatic Metabolism or Extraction

After drugs pass through the basolateral side of the intestinal membrane, they are taken up into the mesenteric vessels surrounding the small intestine. These vessels drain into the hepatic portal system, which then takes them directly to the liver. The liver is a major organ for drug elimination and contains the full complement of the drug-metabolizing enzymes (see Chapter 5), which are present in a higher concentration than anywhere else in the body. As a result, a portion of an oral dose can be lost before it reaches systemic circulation during this first pass through the liver. The extent of presystemic hepatic extraction (the *first-pass effect*) depends on the ability of the liver enzymes to metabolize a specific drug. This is expressed using the drug's *hepatic extraction ratio* (E), which is defined as the fraction of the incoming drug that is metabolized during a single pass through the liver. As a fraction, E can achieve values between 0 and 1, and under normal circumstances it is a constant for a particular drug. If the liver enzymes have a large capacity to metabolize a particular drug, its extraction ratio will be large, and a large fraction of the incoming drug will be lost during its first pass through the liver. Recall that a drug's hepatic bioavailability (F_h) is defined as the fraction of the dose entering the liver that escapes extraction. Thus, F_h is equal to $1 - E$ and a high level of extraction will be associated with a small degree of hepatic bioavailability. For example, when

$$E = 0.8, \quad 80\% \text{ of the drug entering the liver is eliminated by metabolism during its first pass}$$

F_h is the fraction of the drug entering the liver that escapes metabolism:

$$F_h = 1 - E = 1 - 0.8 = 0.2 \quad 20\% \text{ of the drug entering the liver escapes metabolism and reaches the systemic circulation}$$

Poor oral bioavailability due to extensive first-pass extraction may preclude the oral route of administration for some drugs. Examples of drugs that experience extensive first-pass extraction and cannot be given orally include lidocaine, nitroglycerin, and naloxone. Alternative routes for these three drugs include the parenteral, buccal, intranasal, and transdermal routes. Interestingly, an oral preparation containing the opiate antagonist naloxone is available. It is present in combination with the opioid, pentazocine in Talwin tablets. The tablets were developed specifically to prevent the misuse of pentazocine to produce a heroin substitute. When Talwin tablets were taken orally, naloxone is inactive because of extensive first-pass extraction in the liver. However, if attempts are made to administer the preparation intravenously or subcutaeously, naloxone will be completely bioavailable and will block the action of pentazocine. Despite extensive first-pass metabolism, many other drugs, including propranolol, meperidine, and verapamil, are still administered orally. Oral doses of these drugs greatly exceed the value of intravenous doses.

The factors that influence hepatic metabolism and first-pass extraction are discussed in more detail in Chapter 5.

3.6   FACTORS CONTROLLING THE RATE OF DRUG ABSORPTION

Drug absorption involves several steps, including tablet disintegration, drug dissolution, and membrane penetration. The overall rate of drug absorption is controlled by the slowest step in the process, usually either dissolution or membrane penetration. As discussed previously, owing to its large surface area and extremely large blood supply, the small intestine is the primary site for drug absorption. When dissolution is rapid and absorption is controlled by membrane penetration, stomach emptying can exert an important influence on the rate of drug absorption. Stomach-emptying time varies widely. Food is a particularly important factor (see section 3.8). The consumption of food, particularly high-fat meals, slows stomach emptying to allow digestion to occur and generally delays drug absorption. Opiates and anticholinergic drugs such as propanthiline also delay stomach emptying. In contrast, in the fasting state, when there is less need to hold drug in the stomach, emptying time is much shorter. Metoclopramide increases gastrointestinal motility and speeds up stomach emptying. The relationship between stomach emptying and the rate of drug absorption is particularly strong for drugs that have a rapid dissolution rate and permeability-controlled absorption.

The absorption of these drugs, such as acetaminophen, can be used to assess stomach-emptying time. Figure 3.11 shows how the absorption of acetaminophen was influenced by the coadministration of either metoclopramide or propantheline. Propantheline, which slows stomach emptying, slowed the absorption of acetaminophen. The size and time of the

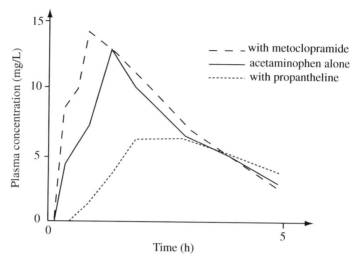

FIGURE 3.11 Use of acetaminophen to assess the rate of drug absorption. Acetaminophen (1500 mg) was administered alone and concurrently with propantheline or metoclopramide in a 22-year-old man. *Source:* Nimmo 1973 [48]. Adapted with permission from BMJ Publishing Group Limited.

peak plasma concentration were smaller and longer, respectively. In contrast, when coadministered with metoclopramide, acetaminophen's absorption was faster: The peak plasma concentration was larger and occurred earlier than in the absence of metoclopramide. Even pregnancy can have an impact on gastric emptying and subsequently on the onset of action from such drugs. Figure 3.12 shows the urinary excretion rate of acetaminophen in a healthy woman on the last day of pregnancy and 38 days after parturition. The authors

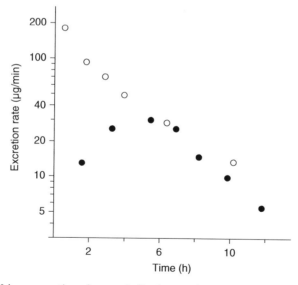

FIGURE 3.12 Urinary excretion of unmetabolized acetaminophen as a function of time after ingestion of 1 g as three tablets on the last day of pregnancy (filled circles) and 38 days after partition (empty circles). From [47], with permission.

stated that because of a delay in gastric emptying in pregnancy, acetaminophen absorption was delayed, and subsequently, acetaminophen excretion was also delayed [47].

The determinants of dissolution and permeability controlled absorption will now be presented.

3.6.1 Dissolution-Controlled Absorption

The rate of dissolution of a drug is described by the *Noyes–Whitney equation*. Accordingly, the rate may be expressed as:

$$\frac{dC}{dt} = \frac{D \cdot S}{V \cdot h} \cdot (Cs - C) \tag{3.2}$$

where C is the concentration of the drug in the gastrointestinal fluid, t is the time, S is the surface area of the solid undergoing dissolution, h is the thickness of a diffusion layer surrounding the solid, D is the diffusion coefficient of the drug, V is the volume of the gastrointestinal fluid, and Cs is the solubility of the drug in the gastrointestinal fluid.

When absorption is dissolution controlled, any dissolved drug is rapidly absorbed and removed from the intestinal fluid. As a result, C will be much, much less than Cs. Thus, the equation reduces to

$$\frac{dC}{dt} = \frac{D \cdot S}{V \cdot h} \cdot Cs \tag{3.3}$$

As dissolution proceeds, the surface area of the solid will decrease and the dissolution will decrease proportionally. Under these circumstances, dissolution approximates a first-order process.

3.6.2 Membrane Penetration-Controlled Absorption

Since passive diffusion is the most common method of membrane penetration, the rate of penetration-controlled absorption can be approximated by Fick's law of diffusion [equation (2.2)]. Diffusion is driven by the concentration gradient across the intestinal membrane. However, as discussed in Chapter 2, because the drug absorbed is rapidly diluted into a very large volume, diffusion approximates a first-order process driven by the concentration of drug in the intestinal fluid [equation (2.3)].

3.6.3 Overall Rate of Drug Absorption

As discussed above, both dissolution and membrane penetration approximate first-order processes. As a result, the *absorption of orally administered drugs is often assumed to follow first-order kinetics*. The rate of drug absorption is proportional to the amount of drug in the gastrointestinal tract:

$$\frac{dAb}{dt} = A_{GI}.k_a \tag{3.4}$$

where Ab is the amount of drug in the body, A_{GI} is the amount of drug in the gastrointestinal tract, k_a is the first-order rate constant for absorption, and t is the time.

This simplistic approach to a complex process that involves several steps, each of which can be influenced by a variety of factors, may not hold on all occasions. The rate of absorption of some drugs may require more complex approaches, which could include absorption lag times, zero-order absorption, and multiple concurrent first- and/or zero-order processes.

3.7   BIOPHARMACEUTICS CLASSIFICATION SYSTEM

In view of the importance of dissolution and gastrointestinal permeability in controlling the rate and extent of drug absorption, several attempts at simplifying or categorizing the processes have been suggested. Among these are the *reserve length*, biopharmaceutics classification system (BCS) and biopharmaceutics drug disposition classification system (BDDCS).

3.7.1   Intestinal Reserve Length

The first use of the intestinal reserve length in drug absorption is attributed to Normon Ho [49]. In this model, the point in the small intestine at which 95% of the drug is absorbed is noted, and the remaining length of the small intestine—not needed for its absorption—was a "reserve." The model applies only if certain simplifying assumptions were made about the small intestine and the way the drug was absorbed: Small intestine contents moved along small intestine at a constant rate, and there are no differences in the absorptive capacity of a part of the small intestine to the drug. But the physiological differences in small intestine transit of different meal components (e.g., carbohydrates and fats) are variable, and if semisolid then the components may alter the reserve length for a drug. Furthermore, any drug that is carrier mediated would not have the same absorptive capacity along the entire small intestine. Perhaps in part because of the physiologic complexity of the gastrointestinal tract, the more useful models focused on the *solubility* and *permeability* of drugs.

3.7.2   Biopharmaceutics Classification System (BCS)

In view of the importance of dissolution and gastrointestinal permeability in controlling the rate and extent of drug absorption, the *Biopharmaceutics Classification System* (BCS) has been developed, in which drugs are placed into one of four groups, depending on whether they possess high or low solubility and permeability [50] (Table 3.5). Drugs are defined as highly soluble if the highest dose strength is soluble in 250 mL or less of an aqueous medium over the pH range 1–7.5 at 37°C. Drugs are defined as highly permeable if the extent of absorption (parent drug plus metabolites) is greater than or equal to 90%.

TABLE 3.5   Biopharmaceutics Classification System

Class	Solubility	Permeability	Examples
I	High	High	Acetaminophen, desipramine, and fluoxetine
II	Low	High	Digoxin, ibuprofen, naproxen, and warfarin
III	High	Low	Atenolol, cimetidine, nadolol, and penicillins
IV	Low	Low	Amphotericin B, chorothiazine, and neomycin

Source: Data from Reference [51].

Drugs in class I (high solubility and high permeability) are absorbed rapidly and extensively unless they are subject to presystemic extraction, and the rate of absorption is controlled by dissolution, or stomach emptying if dissolution is very fast. In the case of class II drugs (low solubility and high permeability), dissolution is the rate-controlling step in absorption. In contrast, the absorption rate of class III drugs (high solubility and low permeability) is controlled by membrane permeability. The poor solubility and low membrane permeability of class IV drugs make oral administration problematic. The classification system has been used by the US FDA to simplify the assessment of the bioavailability of immediate-release oral preparations. In the case of class I drugs (highly permeable and highly soluble), if the product can exhibit rapid dissolution, it is assumed that the absorption process should be straightforward, and the requirements for human trials to demonstrate the equivalence of their bioavailability (bioequivalence) with other products may be waived. For example, the innovator company may wish to change an excipient in the formulation the manufacturing location for a drug product. If the active drug and its drug product can be classified as BCS class I with rapid dissolution, and it is shown that the new formulation and/or drug product has an equivalent *in vitro* performance, then the FDA may waive the requirement of a clinical study for proving bioequivalence of the marketed and new drug product. It turns out that this is a significant saving in time and cost for the company, with no sacrifice in safety to the public. Interestingly, the so-called "biowaiver" can also be used by a company to show bioequivalency of their generic drug product.

3.7.3 Biopharmaceutics Drug Disposition Classification System (BDDCS)

Benet and his colleagues noted that most of the drugs in classes I and II (highly permeable) are eliminated primarily by metabolism, and that drugs in classes III and IV (low permeability) are almost all eliminated by the renal or biliary excretion of unchanged drug. They proposed a modification of the BCS in which the route of elimination is substituted for permeability [51]. In this system, which is known as the *Biopharmaceutics Drug Disposition Classification System* (BDDCS), if a drug is $\geq 90\%$ eliminated in the form of metabolites in the urine or feces, it is classified as being highly permeable, because in order to be metabolized, it must have been absorbed through the intestinal membrane. The BDDCS system has the advantage of making it easier to classify drugs because assessment of the extent of metabolism is much more straightforward than the assessment of permeability, and it is evaluated routinely during drug development. The BDDCS system has also been used to make predictions about a drug's distribution, elimination, and food effect.

3.8 FOOD EFFECTS

As shown in Table 3.6, the biopharmaceutical classifications have also been used to predict the potential effect of food (high-fat meals) on the extent of drug absorption [51] (Table 3.6). Accordingly, the extent of absorption of class I drugs is predicted to be least affected by food because they dissolve rapidly and their high permeability allows them to be absorbed quickly. However, since the presence of food delays stomach emptying, the absorption of these drugs may be delayed by food. The extent of absorption of class II drugs (low solubility and high permeability) is predicted to increase in the presence of high-fat meals as a result of increased solubility due to increased bile flow. Drugs in class III dissolve easily but have poor membrane permeability, and the presence of food

TABLE 3.6   Use of the BCS and BDDCS Classification Systems to Predict the Effect of Food on Drug Absorption

Class	Solubility	Permeability	Effect of Permeability on Extent of Absorption
I	High	High	↔
II	Low	High	↑
III	High	Low	↓
IV	Low	Low	?

is only predicted to impede membrane permeability further and reduce absorption of these drugs. The effect of food on the absorption of class IV drugs is more difficult to predict. As mentioned previously, the delay in gastric emptying brought about by food generally delays the absorption of most drugs.

Beyond these relatively straight forward predictions, there are always a few exceptions— primarily explained by the complexation and/or competition of food stuffs with the carrier-mediated uptake and/or efflux of the drug. For example, the complexation of tetracycline with dairy products will decrease the extent of absorption for the active drug. Orange juice–often administered with the FDA standard high-fat breakfast—can inhibit OATP-2B1-mediated absorption [52] and P-gp efflux [53]. This will potentially decrease and increase, respectively, the absorption of their respective substrates. For example, this could result in increased absorption of the P-gp substrate estrone-3-sulfate, a conjugated estrogen found in Premarin.

Finally, the BCS and BDDCS models have strict definitions of solubility, and solubility enabling formulations (e.g., nanocrystalline suspensions and solid dispersions) do not easily fit into these definitions. The effects of food are therefore much more difficult to predict for these drug products.

PROBLEMS

3.1 A drug has a log $D_{6.0}$ value of 3.7 and is poorly soluble in aqueous media. When administered orally, approximately 30% of a dose is lost due to incomplete dissolution.

It encounters no further problems during absorption, but it is a CYP3A4 substrate, and about 25% of the drug passing through the membrane undergoes intestinal metabolism. During its initial pass through the liver, about 70% of the drug is lost due to metabolism.

(a) Calculate F_a, F_g, F_h, and F for this drug.

(b) Determine the effective dose when 50 mg is given orally.

(c) Determine the value of an intravenous dose that is equivalent to a 100-mg oral dose.

3.2 Three fictitious drugs are used as examples throughout this book: lipoamide, nosolatol, and disolvprazole. Details of these drugs are provided in Appendix E. Lipoamide is a novel antipyretic drug, nosolatol is a cardioselective β_1-adrenergic antagonist, and disolvprazole is a proton pump inhibitor. Table P3.2 lists the physicochemical characteristics of the three drugs.

TABLE P3.2 Properties of Lipoamide, Nosolatol, and Disolvprazole

	Lipoamide	Nosolatol	Disolvprazole
Acid or Base	Base	Acid	Base
Molecular mass	396 Da	365 Da	221 Da
Highest dose strength	150 mg	250 mg	50 mg
$\log P$	3.2	2.1	0.2
$\log D_{6.0}$	3.0	1.8	−2.8
Solubility pH 1–7.5	High: 1.0 g/1000 mL	Low: 0.5 g/1000 mL	High: 5 g/1000 mL
Fraction of oral dose recovered as metabolites in humans	99.0%	99.2%	3–5%
Main enzyme involved in its metabolism	CYP2C9	CYP3A4	None
Substrate for intestinal uptake transporter	None known	None known	OATP1A2
Substrate for intestinal efflux transporter	None known	P-gp	None known
Bioavailability factor (F)	0.21	0.7	0.5

(a) Use this information to discuss their potential for oral administration. Address in detail how the information provides insight into how they may penetrate the intestinal membrane, their expected extent of absorption, and how they would be classified according to the BCS or BDDCS system.

(b) Discuss how you would predict food to affect their absorption.

(c) Suggest possible explanations for the value of bioavailability reported for each drug.

REFERENCES

1. Bartlett, J., and Voort Maarschalk, K. (2012) Understanding the oral mucosal absorption and resulting clinical pharmacokinetics of asenapine, *AAPS Pharm Sci Tech*, *13*, 1110–1115.

2. Costantino, H. R., Illum, L., Brandt, G., Johnson, P. H., and Quay, S. C. (2007) Intranasal delivery: physicochemical and therapeutic aspects, *Int J Pharm*, *337*, 1–24.

3. Perkins, A. C., Wilson, C. G., Blackshaw, P. E., Vincent, R. M., Dansereau, R. J., Juhlin, K. D., Bekker, P. J., and Spiller, R. C. (1994) Impaired oesophageal transit of capsule versus tablet formulations in the elderly, *Gut*, *35*, 1363–1367.

4. Clive Wilson, D. O. P. S. Strathclyde Institute for Biomedical Sciences.

5. Lindahl, A., Ungell, A.-L., Knutson, L., and Lennernas, H. (1997) Characterization of fluids from the stomach and proximal jejunum in men and women, *Pharm Res*, *14*, 497–502.

6. Werner Weitschies, D. O. B. University of Greifswald, Greifswald, Germany.

7. Winne, D. (1977) The influence of unstirred layers on intestinal absorption, in *Intestinal Permeation, Workshop Conference Hoechst*, (Kramer, M., and Lauterbach, F., Eds.), pp. 58–64.

8. Serajuddin, A. T. M. (2007) Salt formation to improve drug solubility, *Adv Drug Deliv Rev*, *59*, 603–616.

9. Noyes, A., and Whitney, W. (1897) The rate of solution of solid substances in their own solutions, *J Amer Chem Soc*, *19*, 930–934.

10. Jinno, J.-I., Kamada, N., Miyake, M., Yamada, K., Mukai, T., Odomi, M., Toguchi, H., Liversidge, G. G., Higaki, K., and Kimura, T. (2006) Effect of particle size reduction on dissolution and oral absorption of a poorly water-soluble drug, cilostazol, in beagle dogs, *J Control Release*, *111*, 56–64.

11. Lahner, E., Annibale, B., and Delle Fave, G. (2009) Systematic review: impaired drug absorption related to the co-administration of antisecretory therapy, *Aliment Pharmacol Ther*, *29*, 1219–1229.

12. Yang, Y. X. (2008) Proton pump inhibitor therapy and osteoporosis, *Curr Drug Saf*, *3*, 204–209.

13. Sutton, S. C., and Smith, P. L. (2011) Animal model systems suitable for controlled release modeling, in *Controlled Release in Oral Drug Delivery*, (Wilson, C. G., and Crowley, P. J., Eds.), pp. 71–90, Springer, Glasgow.

14. Rowland, I. R., Mallett, A. K., and Wise, A. (1985) The effect of diet on the mammalian gut flora and its metabolic activities, *Crit Review Toxicol*, *16*, 31–103.

15. Lipinski, C. A., Lombardo, F., Dominy, B. W., and Feeney, P. J. (2001) Experimental and computational approaches to estimate solubility and permeability in drug discovery and development settings, *Adv Drug Deliv Rev*, *46*, 3–26.

16. Linnankoski, J., Makela, J. M., Ranta, V. P., Urtti, A., and Yliperttula, M. (2006) Computational prediction of oral drug absorption based on absorption rate constants in humans, *J Med Chem*, *49*, 3674–3681.

17. Lennernas, H. (2007) Intestinal permeability and its relevance for absorption and elimination, *Xenobiotica*, *37*, 1015–1051.

18. Pawar, V. K., Meher, J. G., Singh, Y., Chaurasia, M., Reddy, B. S., and Chourasia, M. K. (2014) Targeting of gastrointestinal tract for amended delivery of protein/peptide therapeutics: strategies and industrial perspectives, *J Control Release*, *196*, 168–183.

19. Eleonore, F. (2012) The role of surface charge in cellular uptake and cytotoxicity of medical nanoparticles, *Int J Nanomedicine*, *7*, 5571–5591.

20. Hillgren, K. M., Keppler, D., Zur, A. A., Giacomini, K. M., Stieger, B., Cass, C. E., and Zhang, L. (2013) Emerging transporters of clinical importance: an update from the international transporter consortium, *Clin Pharmacol Ther*, *94*, 52–63.

21. Glaeser, H., Bailey, D. G., Dresser, G. K., Gregor, J. C., Schwarz, U. I., McGrath, J. S., Jolicoeur, E., Lee, W., Leake, B. F., Tirona, R. G., and Kim, R. B. (2007) Intestinal drug transporter expression and the impact of grapefruit juice in humans, *Clin Pharmacol Ther*, *81*, 362–370.

22. Farkas, D., and Greenblatt, D. J. (2008) Influence of fruit juices on drug disposition: discrepancies between in vitro and clinical studies, *Expert Opin Drug Metab Toxicol*, *4*, 381–393.

23. Oostendorp, R. L., Beijnen, J. H., and Schellens, J. H. (2009) The biological and clinical role of drug transporters at the intestinal barrier, *Cancer Treat Rev*, *35*, 137–147.

24. Rautio, J., Kumpulainen, H., Heimbach, T., Oliyai, R., Oh, D., Jarvinen, T., and Savolainen, J. (2008) Prodrugs: design and clinical applications, *Nat Rev Drug Discov*, *7*, 255–270.

25. Hruz, P., Zimmermann, C., Gutmann, H., Degen, L., Beuers, U., Terracciano, L., Drewe, J., and Beglinger, C. (2006) Adaptive regulation of the ileal apical sodium dependent bile acid transporter (ASBT) in patients with obstructive cholestasis, *Gut*, *55*, 395–402.

26. Murakami, T., and Takano, M. (2008) Intestinal efflux transporters and drug absorption, *Expert Opin Drug Metab Toxicol*, *4*, 923–939.

27. Marchetti, S., Mazzanti, R., Beijnen, J. H., and Schellens, J. H. (2007) Concise review: clinical relevance of drug drug and herb drug interactions mediated by the ABC transporter ABCB1 (MDR1, P-glycoprotein), *Oncologist*, *12*, 927–941.

28. Terada, T., and Hira, D. (2015) Intestinal and hepatic drug transporters: pharmacokinetic, pathophysiological, and pharmacogenetic roles, *J Gastroenterology*, *50*, 508–519.

29. Greiner, B., Eichelbaum, M., Fritz, P., Kreichgauer, H. P., Von Richter, O., Zundler, J., and Kroemer, H. K. (1999) The role of intestinal P-glycoprotein in the interaction of digoxin and rifampin, *J Clin Invest*, *104*, 147–153.

30. Schwarz, U. I., Hanso, H., Oertel, R., Miehlke, S., Kuhlisch, E., Glaeser, H., Hitzl, M., Dresser, G. K., Kim, R. B., and Kirch, W. (2007) Induction of intestinal P-glycoprotein by St John's wort reduces the oral bioavailability of talinolol, *Clin Pharmacol Ther*, *81*, 669–678.

31. Westphal, K., Weinbrenner, A., Zschiesche, M., Franke, G., Knoke, M., Oertel, R., Fritz, P., Von Richter, O., Warzok, R., Hachenberg, T., Kauffmann, H. M., Schrenk, D., Terhaag, B., Kroemer, H. K., and Siegmund, W. (2000) Induction of P-glycoprotein by rifampin increases intestinal secretion of talinolol in human beings: a new type of drug/drug interaction, *Clin Pharmacol Ther*, *68*, 345–355.

32. Fischer, V., Einolf, H. J., and Cohen, D. (2005) Efflux transporters and their clinical relevance, *Mini Rev Med Chem*, *5*, 183–195.

33. Rao, A., Haywood, J., Craddock, A. L., Belinsky, M. G., Kruh, G. D., and Dawson, P. A. (2008) The organic solute transporter α-β, Ostα-Ostβ, is essential for intestinal bile acid transport and homeostasis, *Proc Nat Acad Sci*, *105*, 3891–3896.

34. Choi, D.-S., Cascini, M.-G., Mailliard, W., Young, H., Paredes, P., McMahon, T., Diamond, I., Bonci, A., and Messing, R. O. (2004) The type 1 equilibrative nucleoside transporter regulates ethanol intoxication and preference, *Nat Neurosci*, *7*, 855–861.

35. Giovannetti, E., Del Tacca, M., Mey, V., Funel, N., Nannizzi, S., Ricci, S., Orlandini, C., Boggi, U., Campani, D., and Del Chiaro, M. (2006) Transcription analysis of human equilibrative nucleoside transporter-1 predicts survival in pancreas cancer patients treated with gemcitabine, *Cancer Res*, *66*, 3928–3935.

36. Carrier, E. J., Auchampach, J. A., and Hillard, C. J. (2006) Inhibition of an equilibrative nucleoside transporter by cannabidiol: a mechanism of cannabinoid immunosuppression, *Proc Nat Acad Sci*, *103*, 7895–7900.

37. Keskitalo, J. E., Zolk, O., Fromm, M. F., Kurkinen, K. J., Neuvonen, P. J., and Niemi, M. (2009) ABCG2 polymorphism markedly affects the pharmacokinetics of atorvastatin and rosuvastatin, *Clin Pharmacol Ther*, *86*, 197–203.

38. Urquhart, B. L., and Kim, R. B. (2009) Blood-brain barrier transporters and response to CNS-active drugs, *Eur J Clin Pharmacol*, *65*, 1063–1070.

39. Dahan, A., and Amidon, G. L. (2009) Small intestinal efflux mediated by MRP2 and BCRP shifts sulfasalazine intestinal permeability from high to low, enabling its colonic targeting, *Am J Physiol Gastrointest Liver Physiol*, *297*, G371–G377.

40. Dahan, A., and Amidon, G. L. (2010) MRP2 mediated drug-drug interaction: indomethacin increases sulfasalazine absorption in the small intestine, potentially decreasing its colonic targeting, *Int J Pharm*, *386*, 216–220.

41. Thelen, K., and Dressman, J. B. (2009) Cytochrome P450-mediated metabolism in the human gut wall, *J Pharm Pharmacol*, *61*, 541–558.

42. Paine, M. F., Khalighi, M., Fisher, J. M., Shen, D. D., Kunze, K. L., Marsh, C. L., Perkins, J. D., and Thummel, K. E. (1997) Characterization of interintestinal and intraintestinal variations in human CYP3A-dependent metabolism, *J Pharmacol Exp Ther*, *283*, 1552–1562.

43. Galetin, A., Gertz, M., and Houston, J. B. (2010) Contribution of intestinal cytochrome p450-mediated metabolism to drug-drug inhibition and induction interactions, *Drug Metab Pharmacokinet 25*, 28–47.

44. Bressler, R. (2006) Grapefruit juice and drug interactions. Exploring mechanisms of this interaction and potential toxicity for certain drugs, *Geriatrics*, *61*, 12–18.

45. Neuvonen, P. J., Backman, J. T., and Niemi, M. (2008) Pharmacokinetic comparison of the potential over-the-counter statins simvastatin, lovastatin, fluvastatin and pravastatin, *Clin Pharmacokinet*, *47*, 463–474.

46. Ando, H., Tsuruoka, S., Yanagihara, H., Sugimoto, K., Miyata, M., Yamazoe, Y., Takamura, T., Kaneko, S., and Fujimura, A. (2005) Effects of grapefruit juice on the pharmacokinetics of pitavastatin and atorvastatin, *Br J Clin Pharmacol*, *60*, 494–497.

47. Galinsky, R., and Levy, G. (1984) Absorption and metabolism of acetaminophen shortly before parturition, *The Annals Pharmacother*, *18*, 977–979.

48. Nimmo, J., Heading, R. C., Tothill, P., and Prescott, L. F. (1973) Pharmacological modification of gastric emptying: effects of propantheline and metoclopromide on paracetamol absorption, *Br Med J*, *1*, 587–589.

49. Ho, N. F. H., Merkle, H. P., and Higuchi, W. I. (1983) Quantitative, mechanistic and physiologically realistic approach to the biopharmaceutical design of oral drug delivery systems, *Drug Dev Ind Pharm*, *9*, 1111–1184.

50. Amidon, G. L., Lennernas, H., Shah, V. P., and Crison, J. R. (1995) A theoretical basis for a biopharmaceutic drug classification: the correlation of in vitro drug product dissolution and in vivo bioavailability, *Pharm Res*, *12*, 413–420.

51. Wu, C. Y., and Benet, L. Z. (2005) Predicting drug disposition via application of BCS: transport/absorption/ elimination interplay and development of a biopharmaceutics drug disposition classification system, *Pharm Res*, *22*, 11–23.

52. Shirasaka, Y., Shichiri, M., Murata, Y., Mori, T., Nakanishi, T., and Tamai, I. (2013) Long-lasting inhibitory effect of apple and orange juices, but not grapefruit juice, on OATP2B1-mediated drug absorption, *Drug Metab Dispos*, *41*, 615–621.

53. Di Marco, M. P., Edwards, D. J., Wainer, I. W., and Ducharme, M. P. (2002) The effect of grapefruit juice and seville orange juice on the pharmacokinetics of dextromethorphan: the role of gut CYP3A and P-glycoprotein, *Life Sci*, *71*, 1149–1160.

4

DRUG DISTRIBUTION

Sara E. Rosenbaum

Objectives

The material in this chapter will enable the reader to:

1. Understand the factors that control a drug's distribution from the plasma to the tissues
2. Know the main physiological volumes that a drug may access
3. Understand the influence of plasma protein and tissue binding on the distribution profile

Basic Pharmacokinetics and Pharmacodynamics: An Integrated Textbook and Computer Simulations,
Second Edition. Edited by Sara E. Rosenbaum.
© 2017 John Wiley & Sons, Inc. Published 2017 by John Wiley & Sons, Inc.

4. Understand how the apparent volume of distribution expresses the distribution of a drug between plasma and the rest of the body

5. Understand the factors that control plasma protein binding

6. Appreciate the clinical significance of altered protein binding

7. Understand the factors that control the rate of drug distribution

8. Appreciate some unique aspects of drug distribution to the central nervous system

4.1 INTRODUCTION

As a result of either direct systemic administration or absorption from an extravascular route, drug reaches the systemic circulation, where it very rapidly distributes throughout the entire volume of plasma water and is delivered to tissues around the body. Two aspects of drug distribution need to be considered: *how rapidly*, and *to what extent*, the drug in the plasma gets taken up by the tissues. Clinically, it is rarely possible to measure tissue concentrations of a drug, and consequently, distribution patterns have to be inferred from measurements of the plasma concentrations of the drug. A lot of information on the rate of drug distribution can be obtained by observing the pattern of the changes in the plasma concentrations in the early period following drug administration. Information about the extent of drug distribution can be obtained by considering the value of the plasma concentration once distribution is complete. Thus, the plasma concentration constitutes a "window" for obtaining information on the distribution of the bulk of the drug in the body and how it changes over time.

4.2 EXTENT OF DRUG DISTRIBUTION

Two aspects of a drug's distribution pattern are of greatest interest:

- the access of the drug to its site of action;
- the relative distribution of a drug between plasma and the rest of the body.

A drug must reach its site of action to produce an effect. Generally, this involves only a very small amount of the overall drug in the body, and access to the site of action is generally a problem only if the site is located in a specialized area or space. For example, drug access to certain poorly perfused areas such as inner ear fluid or solid tumor masses may be problematic. Additionally, the specialized membrane (the blood–brain barrier [BBB]) that separates the brain from the systemic circulation limits the access of many drugs to the central nervous system (CNS).

The second important aspect of the extent of drug distribution is the relative distribution of a drug between plasma and the rest of the body. This affects the plasma concentration of the drug and is important because:

1. As discussed above, the plasma concentration is the "window" through which we are able to "see" the drug in the body. It is important to know how a measured plasma concentration is related to the total amount of drug in the body.

2. Drug is delivered to the organs of elimination via the blood. If a drug distributes extensively from the plasma to the tissues, the drug in the plasma will constitute only a small fraction of the drug in the body. Little drug will be delivered to the organs of

elimination, and this will hamper elimination. Conversely, if a drug is very limited in its ability to distribute beyond the plasma, a greater fraction of the drug in the body will be physically located in the plasma. The organs of elimination will be well supplied with drug, which will enhance elimination.

It is important to appreciate that as long as the drug reaches its site of action, within reason there is no "good" or "bad" distribution pattern. It is simply important to understand the distribution pattern for a given drug.

Drug distribution to the tissues is driven primarily by the passive diffusion of free, unbound drug along its concentration gradient. Consider the administration of a single intravenous dose of a drug. In the early period after administration, the concentration of drug in the plasma is much higher than that in the tissues, and there is a net movement of drug from the plasma to the tissues (Figure 4.1); this period is known as the distribution phase. Eventually, a type of equilibrium is established between the tissues and plasma, at which point the ratio of the tissue to plasma concentration remains constant and the tissue and plasma concentrations rise and fall in parallel. At this time, the distribution phase is complete and we are now in the *postdistribution phase* (Figure 4.1), where plasma and tissue concentrations fall in parallel as drug is eliminated from the body. It should be noted that after a single dose, true equilibrium between the tissues and the plasma is not achieved in the postdistribution phase because the plasma concentration falls continuously as drug is eliminated from the body. This continuously breaks the equilibrium between the two spaces and results in the redistribution of drug from the tissues to the plasma.

Uptake and efflux transporters in certain tissues may also be involved in the distribution process and may enhance or limit a drug's distribution to specific tissues. Our discussion of

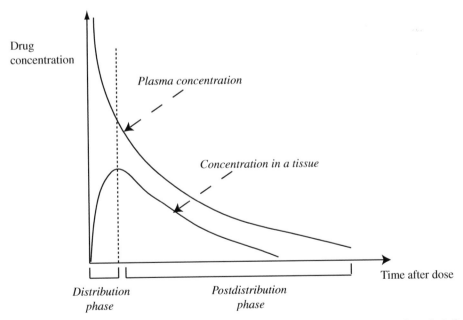

FIGURE 4.1   Drug concentrations in the plasma and a theoretical tissue during the early period after an intravenous dose of a drug. The plasma concentration falls steeply and the tissue concentration rises during the distribution phase. During the postdistribution phase, distribution is complete and the plasma and tissue concentrations fall in parallel.

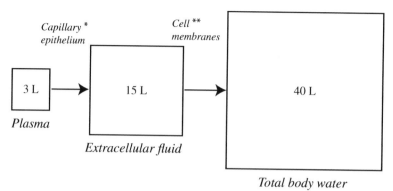

FIGURE 4.2   Physiological volumes drugs may access. *Most capillary membranes are loose and permit the paracellular passage of even large polar drugs. Notable exceptions include the brain, testes, and placenta. **Possible only for lipophilic drugs unless a specialized transport system is present for a drug. Efflux transporters may extrude drugs that penetrate the membrane. Note that the three volumes are drawn to scale.

the factors controlling drug distribution is presented through a consideration of the major physiological volumes that drugs can potentially access.

4.2.1   Distribution Volumes

Three important physiological volumes—plasma water, extracellular fluid, and total body water—are shown in Figure 4.2. In the figure, these volumes are drawn to scale.

Plasma   In the systemic circulation, drugs distribute throughout the volume of plasma water (about 3 L) (Figure 4.2). Where a drug goes beyond this, including distribution to the cellular elements of the blood, depends on the physicochemical properties of the drug and the permeability characteristics of individual membranes.

Distribution to the Extracellular Fluid   The membranes of the capillary epithelial cells are generally very loose in nature and permit the paracellular passage of even polar and/or large drug molecules, including the aminoglycosides (log $D_{7.4} \approx -10$; MW 450–1000 Da) and protein molecules. Thus, essentially all drugs are able to distribute throughout the volume of extracellular fluid, a volume of about 15 L (Figure 4.2). However, the capillary membranes of certain tissues, notably delicate tissues such as the CNS, the placenta, and the testes, have much more tightly knit membranes, which may limit the access of certain drugs, particularly large and/or polar drugs.

Distribution to Intracellular Fluid   Once in the extracellular fluid, drugs are exposed to the individual cells of tissues. The ability of drugs to penetrate the membrane of these cells is dependent on a drug's physicochemical properties (Figure 4.2). Polar drugs and large molecular mass drugs will be unable to pass cell membranes by passive diffusion. For example, the extremely polar aminoglycosides cannot penetrate cell membranes and, as a result, distribute into a volume that is approximately equal to that of extracellular fluid. Polar drugs may enter cells if they are substrates for specialized uptake transporters. The antidiabetic drug metformin is a small polar molecule (MW 129 Da; log $D_{7.4} \approx -3.4$) that would be expected to have difficulty diffusing through cell membranes. However, it is able to access its site of action in the hepatocyte because it is a substrate for the hepatic OCT1 uptake transporter, which transports it across the hepatocyte membrane. On the other hand, efflux transporters will restrict the distribution of their substrates. For example, P-gp at the BBB limits the access of a large number of drugs, including ritonavir, loperamide, and many anticancer drugs. Small lipophilic drugs that can easily penetrate cell membranes can potentially distribute throughout the total body water, which is around 40 L.

In summary, drugs are able to pass through most of the capillary membranes in the body and distribute into a volume approximately equal to that of the extracellular fluid (about 15 L). The ability of a drug to distribute beyond this depends primarily on its physicochemical characteristics. Small, lipophilic drug molecules should penetrate biological membranes with ease and distribute throughout the total body water (about 40 L). A drug's distribution to specific tissues may be enhanced by uptake transporters. Conversely, efflux transporters will restrict the tissue distribution of their substrates. Total body water, about 40 L, represents the maximum volume into which a drug can distribute.

4.2.2 Tissue Binding, Plasma Protein Binding, and Partitioning: Concentrating Effects

Given that drug distribution is driven primarily by passive diffusion, it would be reasonable to assume that once distribution has occurred, the concentration of drug would be the same throughout its distribution volume. This is rarely the case because of *tissue and plasma protein binding*. Drugs frequently bind in a reversible manner to sites on proteins and other macromolecules in the plasma and tissues (binding is discussed in more detail in Section 4.2.4). As mentioned earlier, distribution is driven by the concentration gradient of the unbound drug. Bound drug cannot participate in the concentration gradient that drives the distribution process and can be considered to be secreted away or hidden in tissue or plasma. Binding has a very important influence on a drug's distribution pattern. Consider a drug that binds extensively (90%) to the plasma proteins but does not bind to tissue macromolecules. In the plasma, 90% of the drug is bound and only 10% is free and able to diffuse to the tissues. At equilibrium, the unbound concentrations in the plasma and tissues will be the same, but the total concentration of drug in the plasma will be much higher than that in the tissues. Plasma protein binding has the effect of limiting distribution and concentrating drug in the plasma (Figure 4.3). Conversely, consider a drug that binds extensively to macromolecules in the tissues but does not bind to the plasma proteins. Assume that overall 90% of the drug in the tissues is bound and only 10% is free. As the distribution process occurs, a large fraction of the drug in the tissues will bind and be removed from participation in the diffusion gradient. As a result, more and more drug will distribute to the tissues. When distribution is complete, the unbound concentrations in the plasma and tissues will be the same, but the total (bound plus free) tissue concentration will be much larger than the plasma concentration (Figure 4.3). Tissue binding essentially draws drug from the plasma and concentrates it in the tissues. High tissue concentrations may also result if a lipophilic drug partitions into the lipid components of tissues. This phenomenon can be particularly significant in adipose tissue. Drugs that concentrate in tissues as a result of binding and/or partitioning may also bind to the plasma proteins. In this case, the final distribution pattern will be determined by the relative magnitude of the three effects.

In summary, the binding of drugs to plasma proteins and tissue macromolecules exerts an important influence on the pattern of drug distribution. Plasma protein binding tends to concentrate drug in the plasma and limit its distribution to the tissues. Tissue binding tends to

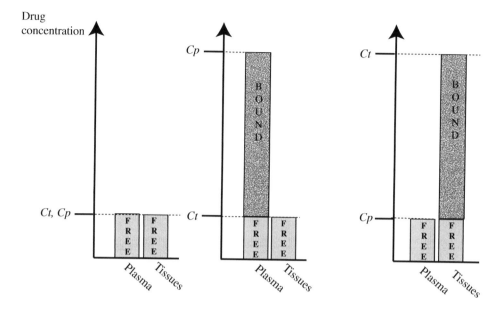

FIGURE 4.3 Influence of plasma protein binding and tissue binding on a drug's distribution between the plasma and tissues. The histograms show the total plasma (Cp) and tissue (Ct) concentrations of a drug partitioned into free and bound drug. At equilibrium, the free drug concentration is the same in the plasma and tissues. If a drug does not bind either to plasma proteins or tissue macromolecules, the total concentrations in the tissues and plasma will be the same (a). Plasma protein binding concentrates drug in the plasma (b) and tissue binding concentrates drug in the tissues (c).

concentrate a large amount of drug in a tissue. Similar concentrating effects are observed if a drug partitions into lipid components of tissues. Drug concentration will vary from tissue to tissue and be greatest in those tissues where binding and/or partitioning is most extensive.

Overall, drug distribution is driven primarily by the passive diffusion of a drug along the concentration gradient created by the unbound drug in the plasma and tissues. The overall pattern of drug distribution is determined by the physiological volumes that a drug is able to access and by the concentrating effects of drug binding and partitioning within these spaces. Once distribution is complete, the unbound drug concentration should be the same throughout the physiological volumes where the drug is found.

Uptake and efflux transporters may also be involved in drug distribution and may, respectively, either promote or limit a drug's distribution beyond that predicted by passive diffusion alone.

4.2.3 Assessment of the Extent of Drug Distribution: Apparent Volume of Distribution

Once distribution has gone to completion, the ratio of the tissue concentration (Ct) to the total plasma concentration (Cp) remains constant. This ratio (Ct/Cp) *is* known as the tissue to plasma partition coefficient (Kp). This ratio (Kp) will vary from one tissue to another depending on the extent of tissue binding and partitioning that occurs within the tissue.

It is important to find a way to express a drug's distribution characteristics using a number or distribution parameter that can easily be estimated clinically. The tissue to plasma partition coefficient discussed above expresses distribution, but it is not convenient as it cannot be easily measured and varies from tissue to tissue. The ideal requirements for the distribution parameter are:

- Overall distribution is expressed by a single parameter.
- It assesses or reflects the relative distribution of the drug between the plasma and the rest of the body once distribution is complete.
- It must be based on the plasma concentration of the drug, as this is usually the only drug concentration that can be measured routinely.

The *apparent volume of distribution (Vd)* is the primary distribution parameter for a drug. It is a constant for a drug and it is the ratio of the amount of drug in the body (*Ab*) at any time to the plasma concentration (*Cp*) at the same time:

$$Vd = \frac{\text{amount of drug in the body at any time}}{\text{plasma concentration at the same time}} : \frac{Ab \text{ mg}}{Cp \text{ mg/L}} \text{ L units} \qquad (4.1)$$

Note, although *Vd* has units of volume, it is important to recognize that it is a **ratio** and **not a physiological volume**. This point is underscored by the fact that the value of the volume of distribution of many drugs greatly exceeds the maximum physiological volume (total body water ~40 L).

Understanding Vd *and the Significance of its Size*   An understanding of the significance of the value of a drug's *Vd* is conveniently addressed by imagining that the body is a well-stirred entity, and that drug distribution throughout the body occurs so quickly that it can be viewed as instantaneous. Assume that an 80 mg intravenous dose is administered. The drug then distributes instantaneously into the spaces or volumes it can access. The only window into the drug's distribution, that is, the only thing that can be measured on a routine basis, is the drug's plasma concentration, *Cp*.

Imagine further that total body water (assumed to be 40 L) is segmented into the plasma (3 L, which we can "see") and the remaining body water (~37 L, which we cannot see). Further, assume that these two volumes are like two immiscible liquids in a separating flask (Figure 4.4).

Case 1. Suppose the drug can access the whole of total body water and that it distributes evenly throughout this space (Figure 4.4a). At time zero, the drug concentration throughout will be 80 mg/40 L = 2 mg/L. The concentration measured in the plasma at time zero will be 2 mg/L. Based on these values, at time zero:

$$Vd = Ab/Cp = 80 \text{ mg}/2 \text{ mg/L} = 40 \text{ L}$$

In this case, the *Vd* is equal to the actual volume of total body water, 40 L.

Case 2. Suppose the plasma concentration at time zero was found to be 5 mg/L.

$$Vd = Ab/Cp = 80 \text{ mg}/5 \text{ mg/L} = 16 \text{ L}$$

Sampling volume (plasma)

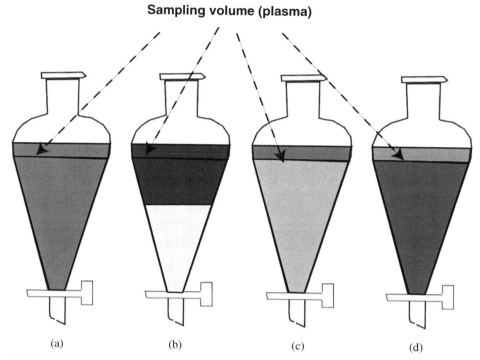

(a)   (b)   (c)   (d)

FIGURE 4.4 Two immiscible liquids in a separating flask. The upper layer is sampled and represents the plasma (3 L). The lower layer represents the remaining body water (37 L) into which a drug could distribute.

In this case, Vd is much smaller than total body water. What are the possible explanations for this?

Explanation 1. The drug distributes evenly, but only throughout a volume of 16 L (Figure 4.4b)

Example. The Vd of aminoglycosides, such as gentamicin (~20 L), is less than total body water. This is because these large polar molecules cannot access the intracellular space, so their distribution is primarily limited to extracellular fluid.

Explanation 2. The drug distributes throughout total body water but concentrates in the plasma (the concentration in the plasma is greater than that outside) (Figure 4.4c). This phenomenon would occur if the drug binds extensively to plasma proteins and not within the tissues.

Example. Warfarin's Vd (~8 L) is less than total body. This is because warfarin binds extensively to proteins and other components in the plasma, which concentrates the drug in the plasma volume.

Case 3. Suppose the plasma concentration at time zero was found to be 0.2 mg/L.

$$Vd = Ab/Cp = 80\,\text{mg}/0.2\,\text{mg/L} = 400\,\text{L}$$

In this case, Vd is much greater than total body water. What are the possible explanations for this?

Explanation. The concentration outside the plasma (i.e., in the tissues) is greater than that in the plasma (Figure 4.4d). This phenomenon would occur if a drug binds extensively and/or partitions within the tissues.

Example. Digoxin's Vd (~500 L) is much greater than total body water because it binds extensively in tissues, primarily to the enzyme Na^+, K^+ ATPase. This causes it to concentrate in the tissues.

In summary, the volume of distribution is simply *a ratio that has units of volume*. It is not a physiological volume and, despite its name, it is *not* the volume into which a drug distributes. If, for example, a drug had a Vd value of 20 L, it does not mean that the drug distributes into a volume of 20 L, which is greater than extracellular fluid and less than the total body water. In theory, this could be the case if the drug did not bind to plasma proteins or tissue macromolecules and could not access most of the intracellular fluid. On the other hand, a Vd of 20 L would also result if a drug distributes throughout the total body water (40 L) and binds to plasma proteins. If a drug has a Vd of 100 L, it would be physically impossible for it to distribute into this volume as total body water, which represents the maximum volume into which a drug can distribute, and is only around 40 L. A drug can achieve a Vd of 100 L if it preferentially distributes to the tissues, as a result of tissue binding and/or partitioning into tissue components.

The Vd is a ratio that reflects the relative distribution of a drug between the plasma and the rest of the body. It is a constant for a drug. If a drug preferentially binds to tissue macromolecules, the tissue concentrations will be higher than those in the plasma and its volume of distribution may greatly exceed the volume of total body water, the maximum volume into which a drug can distribute. Conversely, if a drug preferentially binds to plasma proteins, the plasma concentration will be greater than the tissue concentrations, which will result in an apparent volume that is less than the volume of total body water and less than the actual volume throughout which the drug distributes. Under the unusual circumstances that a drug does not bind to plasma proteins or tissue macromolecules, its volume of distribution will be equal to the volume into which it distributes. This is the case for ethanol, which distributes throughout the total body water, does not bind to plasma proteins or tissue macromolecules, and has a volume of distribution of around 40 L.

Because of its dependence on physiological volumes, the volume of distribution is dependent on body size and is usually expressed on a per kilogram of body weight basis. This value is then multiplied by body weight to obtain a person's volume of distribution. A 35-kg child will thus have a volume of distribution of a drug half that of a typical 70-kg standard adult male. The volume of distribution expressed in this way is assumed to be a constant for a drug under normal conditions and health. Its value may be affected by conditions that affect either body volumes (e.g., dehydration, overhydration, and the presence of ascites), plasma protein binding, or tissue binding.

Table 4.1 shows the values of the volume of distribution of some drugs. Some commonly encountered volumes are presented to provide some perspective. A consideration of some of the values in the table clearly illustrates that the volume of distribution cannot possibly be equal to the volume into which a drug distributes. Chloroquine has a volume of distribution approximately equal to the volume of an average dumpster or aboveground swimming pool. A drug's volume of distribution exceeds physiological volumes because of tissue binding, which draws a large fraction of the drug from the plasma and results in an average tissue concentration that exceeds the plasma concentration. The volume of distribution could be considered to be the hypothetical volume into which the drug distributes if the concentration of drug throughout the volume was the same and equal to the plasma concentration.

TABLE 4.1   Volume of Distribution of Selected Drugs

Drug/Physiological Volume	Vd (L/70 kg) or Volume	Example of Volume
Plasma	*3*	
Heparin	4.2	Gallon of milk
Warfarin	8	
Extracellular fluid	*15*	Water cooler vessel
Aminoglycosides	20	
Total body water	*40*	
Phenytoin	45	Approximately a "half-barrel" keg
Atenolol	65	
Diazepam	77	
Digoxin	500	Large refrigerator
Felodipine	700	
Nortriptyline	1260	
Amiodarone	4600	
Chloroquine	14,000	Dumpster/aboveground pool

4.2.3.1 Fraction of Drug in the Plasma and Tissues

The value of a drug's volume of distribution can be used to estimate the fraction of the drug in the body that is physically present in either the plasma or the tissues. The drug in the body (Ab) may be partitioned into drug in the plasma (Ap) and drug outside the plasma or in the tissues (At):

$$Ab = Ap + At \tag{4.2}$$

The fraction of the drug in the plasma,

$$\text{fraction in plasma} = \frac{Ap}{Ab} \tag{4.3}$$

The amount of drug in the plasma is the product of the plasma concentration and the volume of the plasma.

The amount of drug in the body is the product of the volume of distribution and the plasma concentration [see equation (4.1)]:

$$\text{fraction in plasma} = \frac{Vp \cdot Cp}{Vd \cdot Cp} = \frac{Vp}{Vd} \tag{4.4}$$

In a standard 70-kg adult male, $Vp = 3$ L:

$$\text{fraction in plasma} = \frac{3}{Vd} \tag{4.5}$$

The fraction of the drug in the body located in the tissues:

$$\text{fraction in tissue} = 1 - \text{fraction in plasma}$$
$$= 1 - \frac{Vp}{Vd} = 1 - \frac{3}{Vd} \tag{4.6}$$

TABLE 4.2 Relative Distribution of Drugs Between the Plasma and Tissues for Different Values of *Vd*

Vd (L/70 kg)	Drug in Plasma (%)[a]	Drug in Tissues (%)
12	25	75
21	14	86
42	7	93
300	1	99
12,000	0.025	99.98

[a]Assumes that $Vp = 3$ L for a standard 70-kg person.

Table 4.2 shows the relative distribution of drugs between the tissues and plasma for different values of volume of distribution.

4.2.3.2 Influence of Tissue and Plasma Protein Binding

As expressed in equation (4.2), drug in the body is located in either the plasma or the tissues. The amount of drug in either of these spaces is the product of the concentration of drug and the volume of the space. Equation (4.2) can be rewritten as:

$$Cp \cdot Vd = Cp \cdot Vp + Ct \cdot Vt \qquad (4.7)$$

where Vt is the volume outside the plasma into which the drug distributes. Drug diffusion is driven by the concentration gradient created by the unbound drug in the plasma and tissues. The unbound drug concentrations are expressed as:

$$\begin{aligned} Cp_u &= Cp \cdot fu \\ Ct_u &= Ct \cdot fu_t \end{aligned} \qquad (4.8)$$

where Cp_u and Ct_u are the unbound drug concentrations in the plasma and tissue, respectively, and fu and fu_t are the fractions unbound in the plasma and tissues, respectively.

When distribution is complete, the unbound drug concentrations in the tissue and plasma are equal:

$$Cp_u = Ct_u \qquad (4.9)$$

Substituting for the expressions of Cp_u and Ct_u given in equation (4.8) into equation (4.9) yields

$$Cp \cdot fu = Ct \cdot fu_t \qquad (4.10)$$

Rearranging gives

$$Ct = \frac{Cp \cdot fu}{fu_t} \qquad (4.11)$$

Substituting the expression of Ct given in equation (4.11) into equation (4.7), we have

$$Cp \cdot Vd = Cp \cdot Vp + Vt\frac{Cp \cdot fu}{fu_t}$$

$$Vd = Vp + Vt\frac{fu}{fu_t} \qquad (4.12)$$

TABLE 4.3   Compounds That Do Not Bind to Plasma Proteins or Tissue Macromolecules

Compound	Vd (L) in 70-kg Male	Distribution Volume
Evans blue	3	Plasma
Br⁻	15	Extracellular fluid
Antipyrene	40	Total body water
Ethanol	40	Total body water

Equation (4.12) shows that a drug's volume of distribution is dependent on both the volume into which a drug distributes and on tissue and plasma protein binding. It also shows that increased tissue binding ($fu_t \downarrow$) or decreased plasma protein binding ($fu \uparrow$) will result in an increase in the volume of distribution.

Equation (4.12) can also be used to show that if a drug binds to neither the plasma proteins ($fu = 1$) nor the tissues ($fu_t = 1$), its volume of distribution will be equal to that of the volume into which the drug distributes. Table 4.3 lists some compounds that have volumes of distribution that approximate the volumes into which they distribute. The volume of distribution of these substances can be used to estimate the respective physiological volumes.

Summary of Volume of Distribution

1. Vd is a ratio that reflects a drug's relative distribution between the plasma and the rest of the body.
2. It is dependent on the volume into which a drug distributes and a drug's binding characteristics.
3. It is a constant for a drug under normal conditions.
4. Conditions that alter body volume may affect its value.
5. Altered tissue and/or protein binding may alter its value.
6. It provides information about a drug's distribution pattern. Large values indicate extensive distribution of a drug to the tissues.
7. It can be used to calculate the amount of drug in the body if a drug's plasma concentration is known.

4.2.4   Plasma Protein Binding

A very large number of therapeutic drugs bind to certain sites on the proteins in plasma to form drug–protein complexes. The binding process occurs very rapidly, it is completely reversible [see equation (4.14)], and equilibrium is quickly established between the bound and unbound forms of a drug. If the unbound or free drug concentration falls due to distribution or drug elimination, bound drug dissociates rapidly to restore equilibrium. Clinically, although the total drug concentration is measured routinely, pharmacological and toxicological activity is thought to reside with the free unbound drug (Cp_u). It is only this component of the drug that is thought to be able to diffuse across membranes to the drug's site of action and to interact with the receptor. Binding is usually expressed using the parameter fraction unbound (fu), and the unbound pharmacologically active component can be calculated:

$$Cp_u = Cp \cdot fu \tag{4.13}$$

TABLE 4.4   Common Proteins Involved in Drug Binding in Plasma

Protein	Average MW (Da)	Typical Average Concentration		Types of Drugs That Bind	Examples of Drugs That Bind
		g/L	μM		
Albumin	66,000	~40	600	Acid, neutral, and some basic	Diflunisal, phenytoin, salicylic acid, valproic acid, and warfarin
α_1-Acid glycoprotein	43,000	~1	23	Basic, some acid, and neutral	Alfentanil, meperidine, saquinavir, and verapamil
Lipoproteins	200,000– 3,000,000	–	Wide variation	Neutral and basic	Amiodarone and cyclosporine
High-density lipoprotein		~1.50			
Low-density lipoprotein		~3.00			

Albumin, α_1-acid glycoprotein (AAG), and the lipoproteins are the plasma proteins principally involved in the binding of drugs. Some characteristics of these plasma proteins are provided in Table 4.4. Albumin is the most abundant and has a concentration of about 40 g/L. Many drugs bind to albumin, particularly weak acids and neutral drugs.

AAG is present in lower concentration than albumin and binds primarily neutral and basic drugs. It is referred to as an *acute-phase reactant protein* because its concentration increases in response to a variety of unrelated stressful conditions, such as cancer, inflammation, and acute myocardial infarction. The lipoproteins consist of a heterogeneous group of very large molecular mass proteins, including the high-density lipoproteins and low-density lipoproteins. Their concentrations vary widely within the population, depending on diet and genetic factors, and they tend to bind neutral and basic lipophilic drugs, including cyclosporine and propranolol. Other specialized proteins may be involved in the binding of a small number of other drugs. For example, corticosteroid-binding globulin or transcortin is important in the plasma protein binding of corticosteroids such as prednisolone.

Given that the unbound concentration is the clinically important fraction and that it is the total concentration that is routinely measured, it is important to know how and when the unbound fraction may change for a drug. If *fu* were to vary widely, it would have to be considered every time that a plasma concentration was interpreted. On the other hand, if it remained constant, it would not have to be considered because the unbound concentration would always be proportional to the total concentration.

4.2.4.1 *Factors Controlling Binding*
The binding of drugs to plasma proteins is an example of a capacity-limited process that is governed by the law of mass action. This is a very important type of process that will be

encountered many times in pharmacokinetics and pharmacodynamics. The interaction of the drug with the protein is given by the *law of mass action:*

$$[D] + [P] \underset{k_2}{\overset{k_1}{\rightleftharpoons}} [DP] \tag{4.14}$$

where [D] is the concentration of free drug, [P] is the concentration of free protein binding sites, [DP] is the concentration of the drug–protein complex, and k_1 and k_2 are the rate constants for the forward and backward processes, respectively.

The process is referred to as *capacity limited* because there are only a finite number of binding sites on a protein: Binding is limited by the total capacity of the proteins. Substituting the more familiar symbols in equation (4.14) gives us

$$Cp_u + (P_T - Cp_b) \underset{k_2}{\overset{k_1}{\rightleftharpoons}} Cp_b \tag{4.15}$$

where Cp_u is the unbound drug concentration, P_T is the total concentration of protein-binding sites, and Cp_b is the concentration of the drug–protein complex or the concentration of bound drug.

Equating the rates of the forward and backward reactions, which are equal at equilibrium, and rearranging the expression yield

$$Cp_b = \frac{P_T \cdot Cp_u}{K_d + Cp_u} \tag{4.16}$$

where K_d is the dissociation constant equal to k_2/k_1, which is a reciprocal measure of the drug's affinity for the protein. As K_d increases, affinity decreases, and vice versa. Note from equation (4.16) that when $Cp_b = P_T/2$, $Cp_u = K_d$.

Figure 4.5 shows the typical relationship between the product of a capacity-limited process (in this case, the bound drug: Cp_b) and the concentration driving the process (free drug concentration: Cp_u). At low concentrations, binding increases in direct proportion to an increase in the free drug (*fu* remains constant as Cp_u increases). As the free drug concentration increases further, some saturation of the proteins occurs, and proportionally less drug can bind (*fu* will increase as Cp_u increases). Eventually, at high drug concentrations, all the binding sites on the protein are taken and binding cannot increase further.

Affinity   The affinity of the drug for the protein is the main determinant of *fu*. In equation (4.16), affinity is expressed by K_d, which is a reciprocal form of affinity. As affinity increases, K_d gets smaller. Drugs with small K_d values bind extensively, whereas those with large K_d values will not bind extensively.

Influence of Drug Concentration on fu   As shown in Figure 4.5, the therapeutic plasma concentrations of most drugs are much less than their K_d values. As a result, over therapeutic concentrations, binding is able to increase in proportion to increases in the total concentration: *fu* remains *constant* over therapeutic plasma concentrations. There are, however, a few drugs that have therapeutic plasma concentrations that are around the range of their K_d values. These drugs, which tend to be drugs that have very high therapeutic plasma concentrations, include valproic acid (therapeutic concentrations range from 40 to 100 mg/L) and salicylates (100–400 mg/L), both of which bind to albumin, and disopyramide

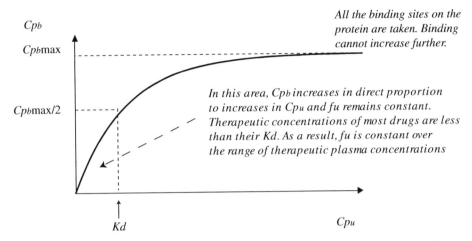

Cpb

Cpbmax

All the binding sites on the
protein are taken. Binding
cannot increase further.

In this area, Cpb increases in direct proportion
to increases in Cpu and fu remains constant.
Therapeutic concentrations of most drugs are less
than their Kd. As a result, fu is constant over
the range of therapeutic plasma concentrations

Cpbmax/2

Kd

Cpu

FIGURE 4.5   Binding of drugs to plasma proteins: a capacity-limited process. The graph shows the relationship between the bound drug concentration (Cp_b) and the free drug concentration (Cp_u). At low free drug concentrations, there are many free binding sites, and binding can increase in direct proportion to increases in the free drug concentration (fu is constant). But as some saturation of the binding sites occurs, proportionally less drug can bind (fu increases). Eventually, at very high drug concentrations, all the binding sites are taken, and the concentration bound remains constant at its maximum value (Cp_b, max).

(2–8 mg/L), which binds to AAG. The binding of these drugs uses a substantial amount of protein, and as a result they display concentration-dependent binding. As the drug concentration increases, some degree of saturation is observed, and the fraction unbound gets larger. At concentrations of 40 and 130 mg/L, valproic acid is about 10% and 20% free, respectively. Disopyramide is about 20% free at 2 mg/L and about 50% free at 8 mg/L. Variations in the degree of binding over therapeutic plasma concentrations affect the dose–response relationship of these drugs and complicate their clinical use.

Influence of Protein Concentration on fu   As predicted by the law of mass action and equation (4.16), changes in the protein concentration will produce changes in the degree of binding. Factors that increase the protein concentration will increase binding (decrease *fu*). Conversely, factors that decrease the protein concentration will decrease binding. A variety of conditions can reduce albumin concentration, including liver disease, age, pregnancy, burns, and other trauma. In the case of AAG, increases in the concentration are more common. Physiological stress caused by myocardial infarction, cancer, and surgery can lead to four- to fivefold increases in the AAG concentration and a corresponding decrease in *fu*. Lipoprotein concentrations vary widely in the population. They can decrease as a result of diet and therapy with HMG-CoA reductase inhibitors (statins), and increase due to alcoholism and diabetes mellitus.

Displacement   The binding of one drug may displace a second drug from its binding site. This displacement occurs because two drugs compete for a limited number of binding sites on the protein. Not surprisingly, displacers tend to be those drugs that achieve high concentrations in the plasma, use up a lot of protein, and display concentration-dependent binding. Examples of displacing drugs include valproic acid, phenylbutazone, and salicylic acid.

TABLE 4.5 Binding Characteristics of Some Example Drugs

Drug	Percent Bound	fu
Amiodarone	>99	<0.01
Amoxicllin	18	0.82
Carbamazepine	74	0.26
Diazepam	98.7	0.013
Digoxin	25	0.75
Felodipine	>99	<0.01
Gentamicin	<10	>0.90
Ibuprofen	>99	<0.01
Imipramine	90	10
Lovastatin	>95	<0.05
Methotrexate	46	0.54
Propranolol	87	0.13
Ritonavir	98	0.02
Tamoxifen	>98	<0.02

Renal and Hepatic Disease   The binding of drugs to albumin is often decreased in patients with severe renal disease. This appears to be the result of both decreased albumin levels and the accumulation of compounds that are normally eliminated, which may alter the affinity of drugs for albumin and/or compete for binding sites. The binding of several acidic drugs, including phenytoin and valproic acid, is reduced in severe renal disease. Plasma protein binding may also be reduced in hepatic disease. It is likely that the reduced albumin and AAG concentrations, particularly those observed in chronic liver disease, explain a large part of this observation.

In summary, the degree to which drugs bind to the plasma protein is generally constant throughout the range of therapeutic concentrations of most drugs. Binding will change if the protein concentration changes and will change if a drug is displaced by either a concomitant medication or by compounds that may accumulate in renal disease. Examples of the binding characteristics of some drugs are shown in Table 4.5.

4.2.4.2 Clinical Consequences of Changes in Plasma Protein Binding

Changes in *fu* as a result of altered protein concentration or displacement will result in a change in the fraction of the total drug that is unbound. Two issues need to be addressed when considering the clinical consequences of this: the potential changes in the unbound drug concentration at the site of action, and the interpretation and evaluation of the routinely measured total plasma concentrations.

Changes in Unbound Concentration   When binding decreases, the pharmacologically active unbound component increases, and in theory, the response or toxicity could increase. However, the clinical consequences of altered plasma protein binding are minimized by two factors: (1) increased elimination and (2) little change in drug concentrations outside the plasma.

INCREASED ELIMINATION   In many cases, only the unbound drug is accessible to the organs of elimination. This is known as *restrictive elimination* because elimination is restricted by protein binding and is limited to the unbound drug. For drugs that display restrictive clearance, the increase in the unbound concentration that occurs when binding decreases results in an increase in elimination of the drug. The increase in elimination is usually proportional to the increase in unbound concentration. As a result, the unbound drug concentration in the plasma eventually falls to exactly the same value as that before the change in binding. In other words, the increase in the unbound concentration is canceled out by increased elimination.

Example 4.1   A drug is 90% bound to the plasma proteins and has a resting total concentration of 10 mg/L:

$$Cp = 10 \text{ mg/L} \quad fu = 0.1 \quad Cp_u = 1 \text{ mg/L}$$

Note that the unbound pharmacologically active concentration is 1 mg/L.
A second drug is coadministered and displaces the first drug. Only 80% is now bound:

$$Cp = 10 \text{ mg/L} \quad fu = 0.2 \quad Cp_u = 2 \text{ mg/L}$$

The displacement has caused a doubling of the unbound pharmacologically active concentration, but elimination of the drug now increases proportionally to this increase. The doubling of elimination results in a halving of the resting Cp, which decreases from 10 to 5 mg/L:

$$Cp = 5 \text{ mg/L} \quad fu = 0.2 \quad Cp_u = 1 \text{ mg/L}$$

Note that the unbound pharmacologically active concentration is equal to its original value before the displacement.

The time it takes for the unbound concentration to return to its normal level is determined by the rate of elimination of the drug (the *elimination half-life*) (this is explained in Section 11.3.5). If the drug is eliminated rapidly (short half-life), the unbound concentration returns to its original level quickly. If the drug is eliminated slowly, it takes a long time for the unbound concentration to return to its original level. The time it takes to return can be important for drugs that have a narrow therapeutic index.

CHANGES IN DRUG CONCENTRATION OUTSIDE THE PLASMA   The plasma comprises a relatively small physiological volume (3 L). This is shown clearly in Figure 4.2, in which the main physiological volumes are drawn to scale. Even when plasma protein binding is extensive, the fraction of the drug in the body that is located in the plasma is much less than that in the tissues. As a result, when the fraction unbound (in plasma) increases, the extra drug that distributes to the tissues is often very small in comparison to the amount of drug already present. This is particularly the case for drugs that have large volumes of distribution, where the majority of the drug in the body is in the tissues and only a very small fraction resides in the plasma.

Example 4.2   Consider a drug with $Vd = 60$ L and $fu = 0.10$. For this drug, $3/60 \times 100 = 5\%$ of the drug in the body is in the plasma, and 95% of the drug is in the tissues. If the drug were displaced and fu increased to 0.2, equation (4.12) can be used to predict that Vd would increase to 117 L and the fraction of drug in the plasma would decrease to about 2.5%. At the same time, the fraction in the tissues would increase by only about 2.5% to achieve a value of 97.5%.

Thus, displacement of drugs from their plasma protein binding sites often has little effect on the concentration of drug outside the plasma.

WARFARIN   The anticoagulant warfarin has a very narrow therapeutic range and there are very serious clinical consequences of being outside the range. Subtherapeutic concentrations put patients at risk for blood clots and stroke. High concentrations predispose patients to dangerous bleeding episodes. It is very important that therapeutic plasma concentrations be achieved at all times. Warfarin binds extensively to the plasma proteins (~99%) and is displaced by several drugs, including diflunisal and phenylbutazone. The clinical significance of changes in the protein binding of warfarin is controversial, and there is evidence that the interaction with phenylbutazone has its roots in a reduction in the metabolism of warfarin rather than a displacement [1]. In theory, any displacement will lead to only a transient increase in the fraction unbound. However, warfarin has two characteristics that could make displacement more clinically significant than normal. First, warfarin's volume of distribution (8 L) is among the smallest of all therapeutic drugs. As a result, about 37.5% of the drug in the body is in the plasma, and changes in the unbound plasma concentration may produce clinically important changes in the unbound concentration outside the plasma. Second, the active S-isomer of warfarin is metabolized by cytochrome P450 2C9 (CYP2C9), which displays genetic polymorphism, and within the population there are individuals who have a mutant type of CYP2C9 that is associated with an impaired ability to metabolize warfarin. After a displacement in these patients, it will take a very long time for the unbound concentration to return to the resting level. During this prolonged period, the patient may be exposed to potentially dangerously high concentrations of unbound warfarin. As a result, a displacement in these patients may have clinical consequences.

Interpreting Cp   In clinical practice, drug therapy may be monitored by ensuring that plasma concentrations lie within the therapeutic range. The therapeutic range of a drug is expressed most conveniently in terms of concentration routinely measured, the total plasma concentration (Cp). But since the unbound concentration is the pharmacologically active component, the therapeutic range should more correctly be expressed in terms of this unbound concentration.

For example, the therapeutic range of phenytoin is usually expressed as 10–20 mg/L total plasma concentration. This is based on an optimum unbound (pharmacologically active) concentration range of 1–2 mg/L and the assumption of normal binding ($fu = 0.1$). If binding is altered in a patient due to altered protein concentration or renal disease, the therapeutic range based on the unbound concentration will not be affected, but the range based on total concentration will be different. Table 4.6 shows the therapeutic range of phenytoin based on

TABLE 4.6   Phenytoin's Therapeutic Range in Patients with Normal and Reduced Binding

	Normal Binding	Reduced Binding
Therapeutic range based on Cp_u (mg/L)	1–2	1–2
fu	0.1	0.2
Therapeutic range based on Cp (mg/L): $Cp = Cp_u/fu$	10–20	5–10

total plasma concentration for a normal patient ($fu = 0.1$) and a patient with reduced binding ($fu = 0.2$). When evaluating a plasma concentration (total drug concentration) and assessing whether it is within the therapeutic range, it is important to be aware of any potential changes in protein binding.

Example 4.3   G.Y. is a 45-year-old male who has been taking 400 mg of phenytoin twice daily for several years. He has recently developed serious hepatic disease, and his albumin concentration is abnormally low. The reduced albumin concentration is predicted to reduce the binding of phenytoin to the plasma proteins. Based on G.Y.'s albumin concentration, fu is estimated to be 0.2. During a routine clinic visit, G.Y.'s phenytoin concentration (total concentration) is found to be 8 mg/L. Is this within the therapeutic range, or should the dose be increased to get plasma concentrations in the range of 10–20 mg/L?

Solution   The therapeutic range of phenytoin is 1–2 mg/L based on the unbound concentration. In patients with normal binding ($fu = 0.1$), this is equivalent to 10–20 mg/L total phenytoin. Since G.Y. has altered binding, the range of 10–20 mg is not applicable. G.Y.'s fu value is 0.2 and the therapeutic range based on total phenytoin may be calculated as:

$$Cp = \frac{Cp_u}{fu} \quad \text{if} Cp_u = 1, \quad Cp = \frac{1}{0.2} = 5 \quad \text{if } Cp_u = 2, \quad Cp = \frac{2}{0.2} = 10$$

The therapeutic range based on total phenytoin is 5–10 mg/L. This patient's phenytoin level (8 mg/L) is within the therapeutic range.

Formulas have been developed for some drugs that will convert a total plasma drug concentration measured in the presence of altered protein concentration to the equivalent value when the protein concentration is normal. For example, if a phenytoin plasma concentration is measured in a patient with low albumin, it can be converted to the value that would be expected with normal albumin using the formula [2]

$$Cp_{\text{normal}} = \frac{Cp_{\text{observed}}}{0.2\text{Alb} + 0.1} \tag{4.17}$$

where Cp_{normal} is the plasma concentration in the presence of a normal albumin concentration, and Cp_{observed} is the measured plasma concentration in a patient with an albumin concentration of Alb g/dL. When the plasma concentration is converted in this way, the usual therapeutic range of 10–20 mg/L may be used.

In summary, decreased protein binding usually results in only a very small increase in the tissue distribution of a drug. Furthermore, any changes in the unbound concentration should only be temporary, due to the resulting increase in elimination, which in theory should return the unbound concentration to its normal level. It is important to consider altered binding when interpreting plasma concentrations. A drug's therapeutic range based on total plasma concentrations will change if the fraction unbound changes.

4.3   RATE OF DRUG DISTRIBUTION

The factors that determine the extent of drug distribution have now been addressed. The second part of the discussion of drug distribution considers the time it takes for a drug to distribute in the tissues. Figure 4.1 shows the plasma concentration and the typical tissue concentration profile after the administration of a drug by intravenous injection. It can be

TABLE 4.7   Approximate Blood Flow and Perfusion Rates for Several Tissues in a Standard 70-kg Male

Tissue	Blood Flow (mL/min)	Perfusion Rate (mL/min/100 g tissue)
Lung	5400	400
Kidney	1230	350
Liver	1550	85
Heart	250	84
Brain	750	55
Skeletal muscle	600	2
Skin	400	5
Fat	250	3

seen that during the distribution phase, the tissue concentration increases as the drug distributes to the tissue. Eventually, a type of equilibrium is reached, and following this, in the postdistribution phase, the tissue concentration falls in parallel with the plasma concentration. *How long does the distribution phase last?*

Drug distribution is a two-stage process that consists of:

1. delivery of the drug to the tissue by the blood;
2. diffusion or uptake of drug from the blood to the tissue.

The overall rate of distribution is controlled by the slowest of these steps. The delivery of drug to the tissue is controlled by the blood flow to a given tissue. This is expressed as tissue *perfusion*, the volume of blood delivered per unit time (mL/min) per unit of tissue (g). Table 4.7 shows the perfusion of some tissues. Once at the tissue site, uptake or distribution from the blood is driven by the passive diffusion of the unbound drug across the epithelial membrane of the capillaries and the membrane of the cell. Most capillary membranes are very loose, so drugs can usually diffuse from the plasma very easily. Additionally, most drugs are small lipophilic molecules that can easily penetrate cell membranes. Consequently, in most cases, *drug distribution is perfusion controlled.* The rate of drug distribution will vary from one tissue to another, and drugs will distribute fastest to the tissues that have the higher perfusion rates.

4.3.1   Perfusion-Controlled Drug Distribution

Drug is presented to the tissues in the arterial blood, and any uptake of drug by the tissue will result in a lower concentration of drug leaving the tissue in the venous blood (Figure 4.6). The amount of drug delivered to the tissue per unit time or rate of presentation of a drug to a tissue is given by

$$\text{Rate In} = Q \cdot Ca \tag{4.18}$$

where Ca is the drug concentration in the arterial blood, and Q is the blood flow to the tissue.

The rate a drug leaves a tissue is given by:

$$\text{Rate Out} = Q \cdot Cv_t \tag{4.19}$$

where Cv_t is the drug concentration in the venous blood leaving the tissue.

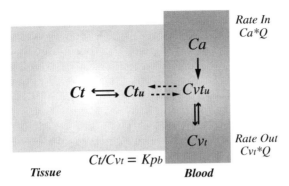

FIGURE 4.6 Diagrammatic representation of the delivery of drug in the blood to a tissue. Drug is delivered to the tissue in the arterial blood with a concentration of Ca. The concentration in the emergent blood is Cv_t. The drug concentration in the tissue is Ct. The blood flow to the tissue is Q and the volume of the tissue is Vt. Thus, the tissue perfusion is Q/Vt. The tissue is assumed to be in equilibrium with the venous blood, and $Kp_b = Ct/Cv_t$.

The rate of uptake is given by the difference between the rate into and out of the tissue:

$$\text{Rate of Uptake} = Q \cdot (Ca - Cv_t) \qquad (4.20)$$

Note, initially, there is little in the tissue and there is extensive uptake from the arterial blood. Thus, $Ca \gg Cv_t$, $(Ca - Cv_t) \approx (Ca)$ and the rate of uptake expressed in equation (4.20) approximates a first-order process.

It is assumed that drug in the tissue rapidly equilibrates with that in the blood. As a result, the drug concentration in the emerging venous blood is in equilibrium with that in the tissue. The unbound concentrations will be equal (Figure 4.6). The ratio of the tissue and blood concentrations is expressed using the tissue to blood partition coefficient $(Kp_b)^*$:

$$Kp_b = \frac{Ct}{Cv_t} \qquad (4.21)$$

where Ct is the tissue concentration. The value of Kp_b will depend on binding and the relative affinity of a drug for the blood and tissues. Tissue binding will promote a large value of Kp_b, whereas extensive binding within the blood will promote a small Kp_b.

The amount of drug in the tissue (At) at any time is

$$At = Ct \cdot Vt \qquad (4.22)$$

But $Ct = Kp_b \cdot Cv_t$ [see equation (4.21)]:

$$At = Kp_b \cdot Cv_t \cdot Vt \qquad (4.23)$$

As discussed earlier, during the initial stages of drug distribution, the rate approximates that of a first-order process. The first-order rate constant for distribution is k_d. It would be valuable to know the physiological and drug-specific determinants of k_d. This is best

---

* Note, Kp_b is similar to the tissue to *plasma* partition coefficient (Kp) introduced earlier in this chapter. Their relative values depend on how a drug distributes plasma and the cellular elements in blood. If the plasma and blood concentration are equal, $Kp = Kp_b$.

approached by considering Cv_t and the redistribution process, which is governed by the same physiological factors, and has the same rate constant (k_d) as the distribution process. Redistribution will be isolated by assuming that the drug concentration in arterial blood suddenly becomes zero:

$$\text{Rate of Redistribution} = k_d \cdot At \tag{4.24}$$

Substituting for At from equation (4.23) into equation (4.24) yields

$$\text{Rate of Redistribution} = k_d \cdot Kp_b \cdot Cv_t \cdot Vt \tag{4.25}$$

But the rate of redistribution is equal to the rate at which the drug leaves the tissue:

$$\text{Rate of Redistribution} = Q \cdot Cv_t \tag{4.26}$$

Thus,

$$Q \cdot Cv_t = k_d \cdot Cv_t \cdot Vt \cdot Kp_b$$
$$k_d = \frac{Q/Vt}{Kp_b} \tag{4.27}$$

The first-order rate constant for distribution is equal to tissue perfusion divided by the tissue to blood partition coefficient. The corresponding distribution half-life is

$$t_{1/2,d} = \frac{0.693}{k_d} \quad \text{or} \quad t_{1/2,d} = \frac{0.693\,Kp_b}{Q/Vt} \tag{4.28}$$

As with any first-order process (see Appendix B), it will take about four distribution half-lives for distribution to go to completion in a tissue. Thus, the actual time for this to occur will depend on the tissue:blood partition coefficient and the tissue perfusion (Q/Vt). These expressions illustrate some important points for perfusion-controlled distribution:

1. The time it takes for distribution to occur is dependent on tissue perfusion. Generally, drugs distribute to well-perfused tissues such as the lungs and major organs faster than they do to poorly perfused tissues such as resting muscle and skin.

2. The duration of the distribution phase is also dependent on Kp_b. If a drug has a high Kp_b value, tissue concentrations are high and it may take a long time to achieve equilibrium even if the tissue perfusion is relatively high. If on the other hand, a drug has a high Kp_b value in a tissue with low perfusion, it will require an extended period of drug exposure to reach equilibrium. An example of this is the distribution of lipophilic drugs to fat tissue.

3. The amount of drug in tissue at equilibrium depends on Kp_b (the affinity of the drug for the tissue) and on the size of the tissue [equation (4.23)]. A drug may concentrate in a tissue (high Kp_b), but if the tissue is only small, the total amount of drug present in the tissue will be low. The distribution of a drug to such a tissue may not have a noticeable impact on the plasma concentration of the drug.

4. Redistribution of a drug from the tissues back to the blood is controlled by exactly the same principles. Thus, redistribution takes less time when the Kp_b value is low and

the perfusion is high, and will take a long time when the Kp_b is high and the perfusion is low. For example, highly lipophilic drugs can partition into fat, where they achieve very high concentrations (the Kp_b value is very high). Fat is poorly perfused, and as a result it takes a long time to achieve equilibrium (assuming continued exposure to the compound; otherwise, equilibrium may never be achieved). Once the drug is withdrawn, redistribution will be slow and the compound may persist in the fat for an extended period. At later times, fat may be the only tissue in the body that holds any significant amounts of drug. As a result, its redistribution may control the drug's plasma concentration and the rate of elimination.

These concepts are illustrated in the physiologically based pharmacokinetic simulation model found in Chapter 18.

4.3.2 Diffusion or Permeability-Controlled Drug Distribution

The epithelial junctions in some tissues, such as the brain, placenta, and testes, are very tightly knit, and the diffusion of more polar and/or large drugs may proceed slowly. As a result, drug distribution in these tissues may be diffusion or permeability controlled. In this case, drug distribution will proceed more slowly for polar drugs than for more lipophilic drugs. It must be pointed out that not all drug distribution to these sites is diffusion controlled. For example, small lipophilic drugs such as the intravenous anesthetics can easily pass membranes by the transcellular route and display perfusion-controlled distribution to the brain.

Diffusion-controlled distribution may be expressed by Fick's law [equation (2.1)]:

$$\text{rate of uptake} = P_m \cdot SA_m \cdot (Cp_u - Ct_u) \tag{4.29}$$

Or

$$\text{rate of uptake} = PS_m \cdot (Cp_u - Ct_u)$$

where P_m is the permeability of the drug through the membrane (cm/h), SA_m is the surface area of the membrane (cm^2), Cp_u is the unbound drug concentration in the plasma (mg/mL), Ct_u is the unbound concentration in the tissue (mg/mL), and PS_m is the permeability surface area product (mL/h).

Initially, the drug concentration in the tissue is very low, $Cp_u \ggg Ct_u$, so the equation may be written as:

$$\text{rate of uptake} = PS_m \cdot Cp_u \tag{4.30}$$

From equation (4.30), it can be seen that under these circumstances, the rate of diffusion approximates a first-order process. A more detailed and complete model for permeability-controlled distribution is presented in Chapter 18, Section 18.7.

4.4 DISTRIBUTION OF DRUGS TO THE CENTRAL NERVOUS SYSTEM

Drug distribution to the CNS is limited by the BBB and the *blood–cerebrospinal fluid* (CSF) *barrier*. These two gatekeepers that guard drug access to the brain severely hamper the development of drugs for the treatment of such diseases of the CNS as cancer, neurological conditions, mood disorders, and infections. As a result, far fewer drugs are available

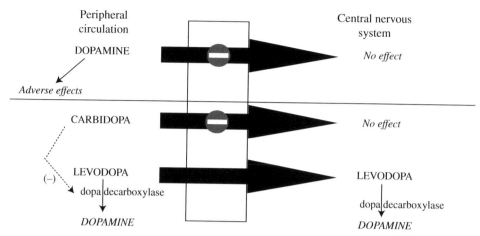

FIGURE 4.7   Use of the combination of levodopa and carbidopa in the treatment of Parkinson's disease. Dopamine, which cannot penetrate the blood–brain barrier (BBB), is administered as its precursor levodopa, which can penetrate the BBB. Levodopa is converted to dopamine by dopa decarboxylase. In the peripheral system, dopamine produces unwanted adverse effects. Carbidopa inhibits dopa decarboxylase but is not able to penetrate the BBB. Thus, it inhibits the formation of dopamine in the periphery but not in the central nervous system (CNS). Combining carbidopa with levodopa reduces peripheral side effects to dopamine and increases the amount of dopamine available to the CNS.

for the treatment of conditions of the CNS than for non-CNS conditions. It is estimated that about 98% of newly developed centrally acting drugs fail during development, due to their inability to penetrate the BBB and the blood–CSF barrier [3]. Consequently, much research is directed to trying to increase drug access to the CNS. The use of a combination of levodopa and carbidopa for the treatment of Parkinson's disease provides an old but creative example of how the BBB cannot only be circumvented, but also used for therapeutic advantage (Figure 4.7).

Parkinson's disease is characterized by reduced dopamine levels in the substantia nigra. A logical treatment would be the administration of dopamine, but dopamine does not penetrate the BBB. Instead, Parkinson's disease is treated using a dopamine precursor, levodopa, which is able to penetrate the BBB. Once inside the CNS, it undergoes decarboxylation by dopa decarboxylase to dopamine (Figure 4.7). Dopa decarboxylase is present throughout the body, and the formation of dopamine outside the CNS is associated with two problems. First, peripheral dopamine causes unpleasant adverse effects, such as nausea and vomiting. Second, the peripheral conversion reduces the amount of levodopa available to the CNS. These problems have been overcome by the coadministration of carbidopa, an inhibitor of dopa decarboxylase that cannot penetrate the BBB (Figure 4.7). By including it in the formulation with levodopa, side effects are reduced as a result of reduced peripheral exposure to dopamine, and the amount of levodopa that is available to the brain is increased.

The BBB is made up of a structural component and a biological component or transporter system [4]. The *structural component* consists of the capillary endothelial cells, joined together by extremely tight junctions which prevent paracellular passage for all but extremely small molecules (Figure 4.8). This essentially restricts membrane diffusion of drugs to the transcellular route, which in turn limits diffusion to small lipophilic drug molecules and prevents polar molecules from diffusing into the brain. The *biological component* consists primarily of uptake and efflux transporter systems (Figure 4.8).

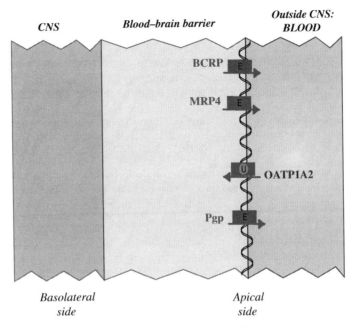

FIGURE 4.8 Drug transporters at the blood–brain barrier. Efflux transporters such as BCRP, P-gp, and MRP4 are expressed on the apical side and reduce the CNS exposure of their substrates. The OATP1A2 uptake transporter is also expressed on the apical side and increases the CNS exposure of its substrates. *(For a color version of this figure, see the color plate section.)*

Drug-metabolizing enzymes have also been found to be part of the BBB, but their role in controlling drug access to the brain is not completely understood. Uptake transporters allow essential nutrients to gain entry to the CNS and are probably critical for the transport of polar drugs. OAPT1A2 has been found on the apical side of the capillary endothelial cells of the BBB (Figure 4.8) and appears to function by transporting drugs from the blood into the brain. Levofloxacin and methotrexate are OATP1A2 substrates, and it has been suggested that the transporter at the BBB may be an important factor in their CNS toxicity [5].

The efflux transporters P-gp, MRP4, and BCRP expressed on the apical side of the capillary endothelial cells (Figure 4.8) serve as gatekeepers to limit the access of xeno-biotics to the CNS. They are highly effective, but unfortunately cannot distinguish between harmful chemicals and therapeutically useful drugs. Thus, many potentially useful drugs pass through the capillary membrane only to be returned back to the systemic circula-tion by this system of efflux transporters. The role of P-gp in limiting access of drugs to the CNS has been demonstrated primarily in studies in mice deficient in P-gp (knockout mice) and other breeds of animals that are naturally deficient in P-gp (e.g., collie dogs). These studies have demonstrated greater CNS penetration of many P-gp substrates (see Table 2.3) in the absence of P-gp. Studies in humans are difficult to perform, but evi-dence supports a similar role of P-gp in the human brain. For example, the opioid lop-eramide normally has no central effects and it is available over the counter for the treat-ment of diarrhea. It is a substrate for P-gp, which is believed to limit its access to the CNS. In support of this theory, coadministration of quinidine, an inhibitor of P-gp, results in the emergence of central effects from loperamide [6]. Additionally, CSF concentrations of ritonavir, which is also a substrate for P-gp, have been shown to increase when it was coadministered with a P-gp inhibitor (ketoconazole). Additional evidence of the involvement of P-gp *in vivo* has been obtained from positron-emission tomography (PET) studies. For example, PET studies demonstrated a greater CNS penetration of ^{11}C-labeled verapamil when P-gp was inhibited by cyclosporine [4]. There appears to be overlap in the substrate specificity of P-gp and BCRP. For example, the CNS uptake of topotecan appears to be limited by both P-gp and BCRP [5]. P-gp and other transporters have been found in the epithelium of the choroid plexus, which makes up the blood–CSF barrier, but at this time there is limited information on the clinical impact of these transporters.

The development of a new drug intended to treat a condition of the CNS may be halted if it is found to be a substrate for P-gp. Inhibition of the efflux transporters at the BBB presents a way to bypass the BBB and potentially increase the number of drugs available to treat conditions of the CNS. Studies in animals have found that the brain uptake of paclitaxel, docetaxel, and imatinib was increased when they were administered with inhibitors of P-gp and BCRP such as cyclosporine and elacridar [4, 7] The effectiveness and safety of this strategy are being evaluated in humans.

The rate of drug uptake to the CNS is important for intravenous anesthetic induction agents such as thiopental, propofol, and ketamine. These drugs are all small lipophilic molecules that easily penetrate the BBB and exert their effects within 0.5–2 min following administration. The magnitude and duration of effect of these drugs is determined by drug distribution rather than drug elimination [8]. In the seconds after an intravenous injection of thiopental, for example, the drug travels to the heart, through the pulmonary circulation, and is then pumped through the systemic circulation. This first-pass concentration is very high, and at the BBB the small highly lipophilic drug distributes rapidly to the CNS, where the high perfusion and small volume of the organ result in a very high initial concentration and a rapid onset of action. As the drug distributes to other, less well-perfused tissues, the plasma concentration quickly falls and thiopental redistributes from the brain along its concentration gradient back into the plasma. As the concentration in the CNS falls, the effect of the drug is terminated. Response to intravenous anesthetics is highly dependent on blood volume, cardiac output, and cerebral blood flow. Reduced blood volume and/or reduced cardiac output increases response to these agents by increasing the fraction of the dose that is taken up by the brain. Thus, smaller doses are required in patients in septic shock and in the elderly. Increased cerebral blood flow was found to increase the depth but not the duration of anesthesia [9]. The use of standard doses of thiopental on severely hypovolemic victims of the Pearl Harbor attack resulted in so many fatalities that it was referred to as "an ideal form of euthanasia" [8, 10].

PROBLEMS

4.1 The values of the volume of distribution of three drugs (A, B, and C) are given below. For each drug, discuss the information provided by the value of this parameter. Address specifically the potential volume into which the drugs distribute, the relative distribution of the drugs between plasma and tissues, and the binding to the tissues and the plasma proteins.

Drug A: 0.5 L/kg or 35 L in a 70-kg person

Drug B: 0.143 L/kg or 10 L in a 70-kg person

Drug C: 14.3 L/kg or 1000 L in a 70-kg person

4.2 Theophylline has a volume of distribution of 0.50 L/kg.

    (a) A 40-kg child has a theophylline plasma concentration of 10 mg/L. How much drug is in the child's body?

    (b) A therapeutic plasma concentration of 12 mg/L theophylline is desired in a 110-kg male patient. How much drug will be in his body at this plasma concentration?

4.3 A drug binds extensively to the albumin. When it is administered with valproic acid, it is displaced from its protein binding site and the fraction unbound in the plasma (fu) increases. How will this affect the volume of distribution?

4.4 Amiodarone has a volume of distribution of 4600 L. If the plasma concentration is 1 mg/L:

    (a) How much drug is in the body?

    (b) How much drug is in the plasma? (Assume that the volume of plasma is 3 L.)

    (c) How much drug is in the tissues?

    (d) What percentage of the drug in the body is in the tissues?

4.5 Warfarin has a volume of distribution of 8 L. If the plasma concentration is 1 mg/L:

    (a) How much drug is in the body?

    (b) How much drug is in the plasma? (Assume that the volume of plasma is 3 L.)

    (c) How much drug is in the tissues?

    (d) What percentage of the drug in the body is in the tissues?

4.6 R.S. is a pregnant woman who has been stabilized on phenytoin for 15 years. She is in her third trimester and her phenytoin plasma concentration is found to be 7.0 mg/L. The therapeutic range of phenytoin is 10–20 mg/L when the plasma protein binding is normal ($fu = 0.1$). R.S.'s albumin level is measured and found to be low, and her fu value for phenytoin is estimated to be 0.15. Is the measured phenytoin concentration therapeutic, toxic, or subtherapeutic?

4.7 The volume of distribution and protein binding of the three drugs introduced in Chapter 3 are listed in Table P4.7. Use this information to summarize their distribution characteristics.

TABLE P4.7 Volume of Distribution and Protein Binding of Lipoamide, Nosolatol, and Disolvprazole

Drug	Vd (L/kg)	fu
Lipoamide	4	0.05
Nosolatol	2	0.6
Disolvprazole	1	>0.95

4.8 Nosolatol binds extensively in skeletal muscle, and the equilibrium tissue/blood ratio is 3. Assume perfusion-controlled distribution. Given that the blood perfusion to muscle is 0.02 mL/min/g:

    (a) What is the distribution half-life for nosolatol in muscle?

    (b) How long will it take for the drug to distribute to the muscle?

4.9 The tissue to equilibrium tissue/blood ratio of disolvprazole in heart, kidney, and lungs is 1. Assume perfusion-controlled distribution. Given that the perfusion of these tissues is 0.84, 3.5, and 4 mL/min/g, respectively, calculate the time it takes for distribution to go to completion in these tissues.

REFERENCES

1. Sands, C. D., Chan, E. S., and Welty, T. E. (2002) Revisiting the significance of warfarin protein-binding displacement interactions, *Ann Pharmacother*, *36*, 1642–1644.

2. Winter, M. E., and Tozer, T. N. (2006) Phenytoin, in *Applied Pharmacokinetics and Pharmacodyamics*, 4th ed. (Burton, M. E., Shaw, L. M., Schentag, J. J., and Evans, W. E., Eds.), Lippincott Williams and Wilkins, Baltimore.

3. Nicolazzo, J. A., and Katneni, K. (2009) Drug transport across the blood–brain barrier and the impact of breast cancer resistance protein (ABCG2), *Curr Top Med Chem*, *9*, 130–147.

4. Eyal, S., Hsiao, P., and Unadkat, J. D. (2009) Drug interactions at the blood–brain barrier: fact or fantasy?, *Pharmacol Ther*, *123*, 80–104.

5. Urquhart, B. L., and Kim, R. B. (2009) Blood–brain barrier transporters and response to CNS-active drugs, *Eur J Clin Pharmacol*, *65*, 1063–1070.

6. Ho, R. H., and Kim, R. B. (2005) Transporters and drug therapy: implications for drug disposition and disease, *Clin Pharmacol Ther*, *78*, 260–277.

7. Breedveld, P., Beijnen, J. H., and Schellens, J. H. (2006) Use of P-glycoprotein and BCRP inhibitors to improve oral bioavailability and CNS penetration of anticancer drugs, *Trends Pharmacol Sci*, *27*, 17–24.

8. Henthorn, T. K., Krejcie, T. C., and Avram, M. J. (2008) Early drug distribution: a generally neglected aspect of pharmacokinetics of particular relevance to intravenously administered anesthetic agents, *Clin Pharmacol Ther*, *84*, 18–22.

9. Ludbrook, G. L., and Upton, R. N. (1997) A physiological model of induction of anaesthesia with propofol in sheep: 2. Model analysis and implications for dose requirements, *Br J Anaesth*, *79*, 505–513.

10. Halford, F. J. (1943) A critique of intravenous anesthesia in war surgery, *Anesthesiology*, *21*, 40–45.

5

DRUG ELIMINATION AND CLEARANCE

SARA E. ROSENBAUM

Basic Pharmacokinetics and Pharmacodynamics: An Integrated Textbook and Computer Simulations, Second Edition. Edited by Sara E. Rosenbaum.
© 2017 John Wiley & Sons, Inc. Published 2017 by John Wiley & Sons, Inc.

Objectives

The material in this chapter will enable the reader to:

1. Identify the major routes of drug elimination
2. Apply first-order kinetics to drug elimination
3. Understand how clearance is used to express drug elimination
4. Understand the relationships among clearance, volume of distribution, and the rate of elimination
5. Understand the factors that control renal clearance: glomerular filtration, tubular secretion, and tubular reabsorption
6. Identify the major enzymes involved in drug metabolism
7. Identify the characteristics of metabolism-based drug–drug interactions
8. Know the role of the major drug transporters in hepatic clearance
9. Understand the factors that control hepatic clearance
10. Understand restrictive and nonrestrictive hepatic clearance
11. Distinguish the effects of modifiers of drug metabolism on the pharmacokinetics of nonrestrictively and restrictively cleared drugs
12. Determine total body and renal clearance from clinical data

Note: This chapter assumes that the reader possesses a knowledge and understanding of the characteristics of first-order processes. Readers who are not familiar with this topic should review this material, which is presented in Appendix B.

5.1   INTRODUCTION

Drug elimination is a general term that incorporates all the processes that may be involved in removing a parent drug from the body. *Renal excretion and metabolism* (which occurs primarily in the liver) are the major processes of drug elimination. Collectively, they are responsible for the elimination of over 90% of drugs [1] (Figure 5.1). The excretion of the parent drug into the bile, the third-most-prevalent process, is involved in the elimination of less than 10% of parent drugs. Other forms of elimination, such as the excretion of parent drug in the sweat, or exhalation of the drug by the lungs, may exist, but they generally constitute very minor pathways.

Renal elimination involves the transfer or excretion of the parent drug from the blood to the renal tubule, from where it is subsequently eliminated in the urine. Metabolism, which takes place primarily in the liver, involves the conversion of the parent drug to another molecular species (metabolite) through the action of an enzyme. Metabolites may undergo further metabolism, renal excretion, and/or biliary excretion. It is important to note that

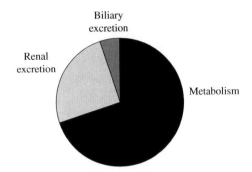

FIGURE 5.1   Routes of elimination of the top 200 drugs.

when the parent drug is altered chemically and converted to a metabolite, the drug is considered to be eliminated, and that the subsequent fate of the metabolite is not part of the pharmacokinetic profile of the parent drug. If the metabolite possesses some therapeutic and/or toxic activity, a separate study of its pharmacokinetics would be of clinical importance.

5.1.1   First-Order Elimination

Renal excretion and metabolism are first-order processes for over 90% of all drugs. Elimination that is not first order results in nonlinear pharmacokinetics, which is discussed in Chapter 15. As first-order processes, the rates of excretion and metabolism may be expressed as:

$$\text{rate of excretion} = k_r \cdot Ab \tag{5.1}$$

$$\text{rate of metabolism} = k_m \cdot Ab \tag{5.2}$$

where k_r and k_m are the first-order rate constants (units, time^{-1}) for renal excretion and metabolism, respectively, and Ab is the amount of drug in the body.

The rate of overall elimination, which is the sum of all component processes, may be expressed as:

$$\text{rate of elimination} = \text{rate of (excretion + metabolism + other processes)}$$

$$= (k_r \cdot Ab) + (k_m \cdot Ab) + (k_{\text{other}} \cdot Ab) = (k_r + k_m + k_{\text{other}}) \cdot Ab \tag{5.3}$$

$$-\frac{dAb}{dt} = k \cdot Ab$$

where k_{other} is the sum of the first-order rate constants for any processes other than renal excretion or metabolism, and k, *the sum of all the rate constants, is known as the overall elimination rate constant.* Because most drugs are eliminated by renal excretion or metabolism, $k \approx k_r + k_m$.

Elimination of a drug can also be expressed in terms of its *elimination half-life* $(t_{1/2})$ (see Appendix B):

$$t_{1/2} = \frac{0.693}{k} \tag{5.4}$$

The half-life and the elimination rate constant are both measures of the speed with which a drug is eliminated. One is the reciprocal form of the other. Under normal circumstances, they are constants for a drug and their values can be obtained from the literature. A drug that has a large elimination rate constant will have a short half-life and will be eliminated rapidly. Conversely, a drug that has a small elimination rate constant will have a long half-life and will be eliminated slowly. Clinically, the half-life is used more frequently because it has more meaning. For example, if a drug has a half-life of 7 h, it is clear that the plasma concentration and the amount of drug in the body will fall by half every 7 h. An elimination rate constant of 0.1 h^{-1} provides the same information but has much less direct practical meaning.

5.1.2   Determinants of the Elimination Rate Constant and the Half-Life

The half-life and the elimination rate constant are simply parameters of a first-order process. It is important to understand how they are related to physiological processes in the body and the disposition characteristics of a drug. The half-life and the elimination rate constant are known as *secondary* or *derived parameters*, because they are derived from, or determined by, two primary drug parameters: the primary parameter for elimination (clearance) and the primary parameter for distribution (volume of distribution).

Clearance is a measure of the efficiency with which the liver and/or kidney can extract a drug from the plasma and eliminate it from the body. High values of clearance will promote large elimination rate constants. However, in order for the liver and kidney to have the opportunity to eliminate a drug, the drug must be present in the plasma. As a result, a drug's volume of distribution, which reflects the relative distribution of a drug between the plasma and the rest of the body, is also an important determinant of the elimination rate constant and half-life. If a drug has a large volume of distribution, a large fraction of the drug in the body will be located in the tissues and will not be accessible to the organs of elimination. This will impede the body's efforts to remove the drug and will promote a long half-life.

- A large clearance and a small volume of distribution will promote rapid elimination and a short half-life.
- A small clearance and a large volume of distribution will promote slow elimination and a long half-life.

5.2   CLEARANCE

Clearance is the most important of all the pharmacokinetic parameters. As we show in Chapter 11, it controls the average plasma concentration achieved from a particular rate of drug administration. If a patient is suspected to have altered clearance for a drug, the dose may have to be adjusted appropriately or the drug may have to be avoided altogether.

5.2.1   Definition and Determinants of Clearance

Clearance is the primary or fundamental pharmacokinetic parameter for elimination. It expresses the collective ability of the organs of elimination to remove drug from plasma. Because drugs are eliminated primarily by renal excretion and/or hepatic metabolism, total clearance is made up primarily of renal clearance and hepatic clearance, which express the ability of the kidney and liver, respectively, to eliminate drug presented to them in the

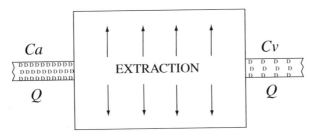

FIGURE 5.2 Extraction unit. Drug (D) in solution is extracted as it flows through the unit. The concentration of drug entering the extraction unit is Ca (mg/L) and the concentration of drug leaving the unit is Cv (mg/L). The solution flows through at a rate of Q (L/h).

blood. A drug's clearance is a constant under normal circumstances but can be altered by diseases of the liver and/or kidney, concomitant medications, and other factors that affect renal and/or hepatic function.

Clearance, by definition, is the constant of proportionality between the rate of elimination and the plasma concentration:

$$\text{rate of elimination} = Cl \cdot Cp \tag{5.5}$$

Although the processes of renal and hepatic clearance are very different, both elimination processes involve the extraction of drug from the blood as it flows through the organ.

The overall clearance of an organ of elimination is a function of both the blood flow to the organ and the efficiency with which the processes within the liver or kidney can eliminate a drug. Its characteristics and determinants are most conveniently presented using a hypothetical elimination organ (Figure 5.2). Drug enters the organ in arterial blood (blood flow = QvL/h) with a concentration of Ca mg/L and leaves the organ in venous blood with a concentration of Cv mg/L. It is assumed that extraction is the only process that accounts for the change in drug concentration as the blood moves through the unit. As a result of extraction, $Ca > Cv$.

The rate of presentation of the drug to the extraction organ is expressed as:

$$\text{rate of presentation} = Ca \text{ (mg/L)} \cdot Q(\text{L/h}) = Ca \cdot Q(\text{mg/h}) \tag{5.6}$$

The rate of which the drug leaves the elimination organ is

$$\text{rate of exit} = Cv \text{ (mg/L)} \cdot Q(\text{L/h}) = Cv \cdot Q(\text{mg/h}) \tag{5.7}$$

The rate of extraction or elimination is calculated as:

$$\text{rate of elimination} = \text{rate of presentation} - \text{rate of exit}$$
$$= (Ca - Cv) \cdot Q(\text{mg/h}) \tag{5.8}$$

The fraction of drug entering that is extracted is the *extraction ratio*, E:

$$E = \frac{(Ca - Cv) \cdot Q}{Ca \cdot Q} = \frac{Ca - Cv}{Ca} \tag{5.9}$$

The fraction of incoming drug extracted or eliminated is a measure of the efficiency of the processes within the organ to extract a given drug. It is independent of Ca and is a constant (elimination is first order) that reflects the ability of the unit to extract drug that is presented to it. For example, if E is high (>0.7), a large fraction (more than 70%) of incoming drug is extracted as it flows though the unit.

As defined above, clearance is the constant of proportionality between the rate of elimination and concentration:

$$\text{rate of elimination} = Cl^*Ca \tag{5.10}$$

$$Cl = \frac{\text{rate of elimination}}{Ca} \tag{5.11}$$

Substituting for the rate of elimination given in (5.8) gives

$$Cl = \frac{Ca - Cv}{Ca} {}^*Q \text{L/h} \tag{5.12}$$

or

$$Cl = E^*Q \text{L/h} \tag{5.13}$$

Equation (5.13) shows that clearance has units of blood flow (e.g., L/h) (recall E is a fraction and has no units). Note, if E is equal to its maximum value, 1: all of the incoming drug is removed, and clearance achieves its maximum value, Q, the blood flow to the organ.

Equation (5.13) also shows that clearance can be viewed as the fraction of incoming blood completely cleared of drug per unit time as it flows through the organ. This can be demonstrated by example. For a hypothetical extraction unit, assume $Q = 10$ L/h and $Ca = 100$ mg/L. Table 5.1 uses different values of the extraction ratio to calculate: Cl ($E * Q$); the amount of drug eliminated in a 1-h period; and the volume of the blood entering (concentration 100 mg/L) that would be completely cleared to achieve this extent of elimination.

5.2.2   Total Clearance, Renal Clearance, and Hepatic Clearance

Total clearance (Cl), which is referred to as *total body clearance* or *systemic clearance*, is sum of all the component clearances:

$$Cl = Cl_r + Cl_h + Cl_{\text{other}} \tag{5.14}$$

TABLE 5.1   Demonstration that Clearance is Equivalent to the Volume of Blood Completely Cleared of Drug Per Unit Time. The Calculations are Based on a Hypothetical Extraction Unit with a Blood Flow of 10 L/h and an Entering Concentration of 100 mg/L

E	Cl (L/h)	Amount Eliminated in 1 h (mg)	Volume (L) of Blood, Concentration 100 mg/L Containing the Amount Eliminated
	$E * Q$	$Cl * Ca$	*Amount Eliminated/Ca*
1	10	1000	10
0.7	7	700	7
0.5	5	500	5
0.25	2.5	250	2.5

where Cl is the total body clearance, Cl_r is the renal clearance, Cl_h is the hepatic clearance, and Cl_{other} represents any other form of clearance. As we demonstrate later in the chapter, total body clearance and renal clearance are easily measured, and values for specific drugs are usually widely available. In contrast, other forms of clearance, including hepatic clearance, are much more difficult to quantify. As a result, clearance is often expressed as:

$$Cl = Cl_r + Cl_{nr} \tag{5.15}$$

where Cl_{nr}, which is the sum of all nonrenal forms of clearance, is the difference between measured total body clearance and renal clearance.

As discussed previously, hepatic clearance is the major form of nonrenal clearance, and as a result,

$$Cl_{nr} \approx Cl_h \tag{5.16}$$

and the expression for total clearance is often presented as:

$$Cl = Cl_r + Cl_h \tag{5.17}$$

In summary:

1. Clearance is the primary parameter for elimination and expresses the ability of the kidneys and liver to remove drug from the systemic circulation.
2. Clearance is expressed in terms of the equivalent volume of blood or plasma completely cleared of drug per unit time at it passes through the organ.
3. Clearance is dependent on the blood flow to the organ (Q) and on the ability of the organ to extract the drug from the bloodstream and eliminate it (E).
4. Clearance is the constant of proportionality between the rate of drug elimination and the plasma concentration.
5. Clearances are additive, and total body clearance is often expressed as the sum of its two main component clearances: renal and hepatic clearances.

5.2.3 Relationships among Clearance, Volume of Distribution, Elimination Rate Constant, and Half-Life

Renal excretion and hepatic metabolism are first-order processes, and the rate of elimination can be expressed using first-order kinetics:

$$-\frac{dAb}{dt} = k \cdot Ab \quad (\mathrm{mg/h}) \tag{5.18}$$

But elimination can also be expressed using clearance (Cl):

$$-\frac{dAb}{dt} = Cl \cdot Cp \quad (\mathrm{mg/h}) \tag{5.19}$$

Combining equations (5.18) and (5.19) gives us

$$k \cdot Ab = Cl \cdot Cp \tag{5.20}$$

But $Ab = Cp \cdot Vd$:

$$k \cdot Cp \cdot Vd = Cl \cdot Cp$$

$$\boxed{k = \frac{Cl}{Vd}} \tag{5.21}$$

Since $t_{1/2} = 0.693/k$

$$\boxed{t_{1/2} = 0.693\,\frac{Vd}{Cl}} \tag{5.22}$$

Equations (5.21) and (5.22) show the relationship between the two parameters for the rate of drug elimination (k and $t_{1/2}$) and the parameters for elimination (clearance) and distribution (volume of distribution). The boxes around equations (5.21) and (5.22) indicate they are important and should be memorized.

5.2.4 Primary and Secondary Parameters

It is very important to distinguish between the dependent (secondary parameters) and independent (primary parameters) in equations (5.21) and (5.22). Clearance and volume of distribution are the primary pharmacokinetics parameters for elimination and distribution, respectively. Primary parameters are independent parameters. Thus, clearance will not change if distribution changes. Likewise, volume of distribution will not change if clearance changes. In contrast, the elimination rate constant and the half-life are secondary or derived parameters. They are dependent on the primary parameters of clearance and volume of distribution, and their value will change with changes in elimination (*Cl*) and/or distribution (*Vd*). As derived parameters, the elimination rate constant and half-life *cannot* change independent of clearance and volume of distribution, and cannot change either of these primary parameters.

It is also important to appreciate that clearance is *not* a measure of the rate of drug elimination. It is one of the two factors (*Vd* is the other) that determines how quickly or slowly a drug is eliminated from the body. Many drugs that have high values of clearance are eliminated rapidly (short half-lives). For example, buspirone, didanosine, metoprolol, and morphine all have high clearances and short half-lives in the region of 1–2 h. Similarly, many drugs that have low clearances are eliminated slowly; for example, phenobarbital has a very low clearance and a half-life of around 4 days. But a drug's volume of distribution is also a factor. For example, diltiazem and felodipine have similar values for clearance (around 800 mL/min), but felodipine's elimination half-life is about four times larger than diltiazem's because its volume of distribution is about four times larger than that of dilitazem. Also, chloroquine and amiodarone both have moderate clearances but have exceptionally long half-lives ($\sim$1 month) because they both have very large volumes of distribution ($\sim$14,000 and 4500 L, respectively). In both cases, the majority of the drug in the body is located in the tissues and is inaccessible to the organs of elimination.

5.2.5 Measurement of Total Body Clearance

Total body clearance can easily be determined from plasma concentration–time data. Figure 5.3 shows a typical plasma concentration–time profile obtained after administration of

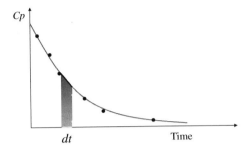

FIGURE 5.3   Plot of plasma concentration against time. The amount of drug eliminated during the very small period *dt* is equal to the area under the curve over that period (the shaded area).

an intravenous dose of a drug. The solid circles indicate the measured data points. Consider a very small time frame, *dt* (Figure 5.3). Note that *dt* has been magnified in the figure for clarity.

The rate of elimination during the period *dt* is

$$- \frac{dAb}{dt} = Cl \cdot Cp \tag{5.23}$$

The amount of drug eliminated during the period *dt* is

$$- dAb = Cl \cdot Cp \cdot dt \tag{5.24}$$

But $Cp \cdot dt$ is the area under the plasma concentration–time curve (AUC) for the period *dt*:

$$- dAb = Cl \cdot \text{AUC}_{dt} \tag{5.25}$$

By extension, the amount of drug eliminated from time zero to infinity is the sum of all the small areas from time zero to infinity:

$$\text{Amount eliminated by infinity} = Cl \cdot \sum_{0}^{\infty} \text{AUC}_{dt} = Cl \cdot \text{AUC}_{0}^{\infty} \tag{5.26}$$

But the effective dose is eliminated by infinity:

$$D_{\text{IV}} = Cl \cdot \text{AUC}_{0}^{\infty} \tag{5.27}$$

Rearranging yields

$$Cl = \frac{D_{\text{IV}}}{\text{AUC}} \tag{5.28}$$

When extravascular route of administration, such as oral, is used and/or a salt of a drug is administered, a more general expression is

$$Cl = \frac{S \cdot F \cdot D}{\text{AUC}_0^\infty}$$ (5.29)

where S is the salt factor (see Section 6.2), and F is the bioavailability. The box around equation (5.29) signifies that it is a very important and useful equation in pharmacokinetics. Familiarity with the equation is strongly recommended.

Pure clearance can only be determined when a drug is given intravenously. When a drug is administered orally, it is not possible to separate the contributions of clearance and bioavailability to the AUC. As a result, only Cl/F, which is known as oral clearance, can be determined.

$$\frac{Cl}{F} = \frac{S \cdot D_{p0}}{\text{AUC}_0^\infty}$$ (5.30)

Thus, clearance is calculated by measuring the AUC. A drug is administered to a subject and plasma samples are taken at various times and analyzed for the parent drug. A graph of plasma concentration versus time is constructed. The AUC is most commonly calculated using the trapezoidal rule, which uses the measured plasma concentration–time data points to divide the curve into a series of trapezoids. The area of each trapezoid is calculated and the total area is determined from the sum of the area of each trapezoid. The measurement of the AUC using the trapezoidal rule is described in Appendix C, which also provides the instructions to set up an Excel worksheet to determine the AUC and clearance.

The AUC is a measurement of a patient's exposure to the drug, the larger the value of the AUC the greater the exposure. It follows, based on equation (5.29) that a patient's exposure to the drug is dependent on the dose, clearance, and bioavailability. *A patient's exposure to a dose will increase if clearance decreases or bioavailability increases.*

5.3 RENAL CLEARANCE

In the kidney, the parent drug may be eliminated by excretion into the urine. Approximately 32% of the top 100 drugs in 2010 are cleared renally, which is defined as when $\geq 25\%$ of the dose is excreted unchanged in the urine (see [2]). A drug's renal clearance is a measure of the efficacy with which the kidney can accomplish this process. The value of renal clearance is determined by blood flow to the part of the kidney involved in drug excretion and on the ability of the kidney to excrete the drug. The ability of the kidney to excrete the drug is a function of renal physiology and the physicochemical properties of the drug.

The nephron is the functioning unit of the kidney, and each kidney possesses about 1–1.5 million of these. A simplified diagram of the nephron is shown in Figure 5.4. In the glomerulus, plasma water is filtered (*glomerular filtration*) into the renal tubule, the contents of which eventually drain into the bladder. However, as the filtrate passes through the tubule, components such as water and dissolved substances, including drugs, may move back and forth across the renal tubule membrane between the blood and the lumen of the tubule. The movement of compounds from the capillaries surrounding the tubules (peritubular capillaries) into the tubule is referred to as *tubular secretion*. The movement in the

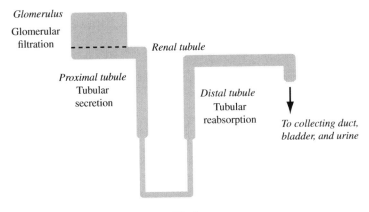

Loop of Henle

FIGURE 5.4   Simplified diagrammatic representation of the nephron. Three processes in the kidney participate in drug excretion: glomerular filtration in the glomerulus; tubular secretion, which takes place primarily in the proximal renal tubule; and tubular reabsorption, which occurs primarily in the distal renal tubule.

opposite direction, from the tubules back into the blood, is referred to as *tubular reabsorption*. During transit through the tubule, much of the plasma water is reabsorbed back into the bloodstream.

5.3.1   Glomerular Filtration

About 20% of the renal blood supply (about 1.2 L/min) is directed to the glomerulus. In the glomerulus, the blood is subjected to hydrostatic pressure, which forces plasma water and small solutes, including most drugs, through the capillary membrane and into the renal tubule. The glomerular capillaries are extremely permeable and permit the free passage of neutral molecules below 4 nm in diameter. The filtration of compounds with diameters between 4 and 8 nm is inversely proportional to their size. Compounds greater than 8 nm are excluded completely. The glomerular capillary wall appears to possess a negative charge, which repels negatively charged molecules. As a result, the permeability of anions is less than that of neutral molecules. Plasma proteins, including albumin, which has a negative charge and a diameter of about 7 nm, do not undergo any appreciable filtration [3]. Small proteins such as insulin (MW $\sim$ 5000 Da) are able to undergo filtration.

The normal glomerular filtration rate (GFR) in the standard 70-kg young adult male is about 120–130 mL/min per 1.73 m^2 (about 7.5 L/h or 180 L/day), and it declines with age. If a drug does not bind to plasma proteins and it is small enough to be filtered in the glomerulus, its clearance by glomerular filtration is equal to the GFR (at this point, the filtrate, and any drug it contains, is eliminated and removed from the circulation). It represents the volume of plasma completely cleared of drug:

$$Cl_{GF} = GFR$$

where Cl_{GF} is clearance by glomerular filtration.

However, many drugs bind to the plasma proteins, and bound drug will not be filtered. For example, if a drug is bound completely (100%), its clearance by glomerular filtration will be zero. If, on the other hand, a drug is 70% bound to the plasma proteins ($fu = 0.3$), only 30% of the drug in the plasma will be filtered and

$$Cl_{GF} = fu \cdot \text{GFR}$$
$$= 0.3 \times 120 = 36 \, \text{mL/min}$$

In summary:

$$Cl_{GF} = fu \cdot \text{GFR} \tag{5.31}$$

5.3.2 Tubular Secretion

Drug elimination can be further augmented by tubular secretion brought about by various transporters, primarily located in the proximal tubular cell membranes. Renal secretion is an important part of renal clearance as it is estimated that at least 92% of drugs cleared renally undergo some secretion [2]. Several reviews of the role of transporters in renal excretion can be found in the literature [2, 4–8].

Uptake transporters (OAT1, OAT3, and OCT2) are primarily located on the basolateral side of the membrane and the efflux transporters (P-gp, MRP2, MRP4, and MATE) on the apical side. In these locations, both transporter systems serve to promote the urinary excretion of their substrates (Figure 5.5). For some drug substrates, the two transporter systems act together and coordinate, first the uptake into the tubular cells and then the subsequent efflux into the tubule. Examples of compounds whose tubular secretion appears to involve

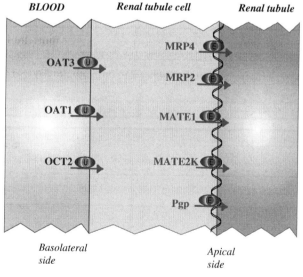

FIGURE 5.5 Drug transporters in the human renal tubule. The uptake transporters (U) organic cation transporter (OCT2) and organic anion transporters (OAT1 and OAT3) are found on the basolateral side of the renal tubular membrane. These transporters promote excretion by transporting drugs from the blood into the tubular cells. The efflux transporters (E), permeability glycoprotein (P-gp), multidrug resistance-associated protein family (MRP2 and MRP4), and multidrug and toxin extrusion protein (MATE) can conclude the process by transporting drugs from the tubular cells into the tubule. (*For a color version of this figure, see the color plate section.*)

TABLE 5.2   Some Examples of Substrates and Inhibitors of Renal OAT and OCT2/MATE1 Transporter Systems (See [7,8])

Transporter	Substrate	Inhibitors
OAT	β-Lactam antibiotics diuretics (furosemide) NSAIDs (aspirin and indomethacin) antiviral drugs (acyclovir, cidofovir, and zidovudine) methotrexate	Probenecid penicillins
OCT2/MATE1	Metformin creatinine procainamide cisplatin	Cimetidine trimethoprin ciprofloxacin antiviral drugs cobicistat

the coordinated efforts of uptake and efflux transporters include fexofenadine, which is a substrate for renal OAT3 and P-gp [9, 10], and adefovir and tenofovir, which are substrates for OAT1 and MRP4. Interestingly, creatinine, which is used to estimate renal function and the GFR, is subject to this type of coordinated secretion primarily by OCT2 uptake and MATE1 efflux [8]. This secretion accounts for 10–40% of creatinine clearance, and the percentage can increase in patients with severe impairment.

In addition to the role they play in drug excretion, by virtue of their control on intracellular drug levels, transporter systems may be important determinants of the cellular toxicity of drugs and environmental chemicals. For example, the OAT uptake and the resultant high intracellular levels of adefovir, cidofovir, and cephaloridine are believed to be factors responsible for the renal toxicity of these drugs. In order to reduce the toxicity of cidofovir, patients taking this drug are now recommended to also take probenecid, an inhibitor of OAT, to reduce the accumulation of cidofovir in the renal tubular cells.

OATs   The major renal OAT drug transporters are OAT1 and OAT3, which serve to primarily secrete weak acids. Examples of substrates are shown in Table 5.2 and a more exhaustive list can be found in the literature [2]. There is some overlap in the substrate specificity of the OATs, but OAT1 appears to be more important for small molecular mass drugs such as adefovir, and OAT3 appears to be more important for larger drugs such as the penicillin G and for sulfate and glucoronide conjugates such as estradiol glucoronide. OAT3 can also carry positively charged molecules, such as the H2-receptor antagonists (famotidine), and molecules with both positive and negative charges, such as fexofenadine. In the coordinated uptake and efflux of OAT substrates, efflux is usually mediated by MRP.

OCTs   OCT2 is the predominant renal OCT transporter. Cationic substrates include the H2 antagonists (cimetidine and famotidine), cisplatin, creatinine, and metformin, which is almost completely eliminated by renal excretion. Again the high concentration of drugs in the renal tubular cells that results from OCT2-mediated uptake has been associated with toxicity. In support of this, cimetidine, an OCT2 inhibitor, was found to reduce the renal toxicity of cisplatin, an OCT2 substrate. The significant overlap in the substrate specificity of OCT2 and MATE1 suggests that these two transporters serve to coordinate the complete transport of their substrates from the blood to the renal lumen. Examples of OCT2 and MATE1 transporters are shown in Table 5.2.

Interestingly, the peptide transporter, present in the gastrointestinal lumen, is also present on the apical side of the renal tubular membrane, where it is believed to function to scavenge di- and tripeptides in the urine and facilitate their return to the blood. A role in drug elimination has not been identified.

Efflux Transporters   The efflux transporters P-gp, MRPs, and BCRP have been discussed elsewhere in this book. They are all located on the apical side of the membrane where they transport their substrates from the tubular cells into the lumen. As discussed above, MRP (MRP2 and MRP4) and MATE (MATE1 and MATE2-K) appear to work with OAT and OCT, respectively, to coordinate the transport of drugs from the blood into the renal tubule.

Drug–Drug Interactions at the Transporter Level   Given the large number (~92%) of renally excreted drugs that undergo some secretion, modification of activity of the renal transporters by concomitant medications is an important source of drug–drug interactions (DDIs). Some examples of inhibitors of the uptake transporters are shown in Table 5.2 and a more exhaustive list can be found in the literature [2]. Inhibitors generally reduce the excretion of those drugs that are substrates for the transporters. This results in reduced renal clearance, increased plasma concentrations of the drug, and increased risk of adverse effects. Probenecid inhibits several uptake transporters and was first marketed for the treatment of gout because of its inhibition of the Urate transporter on the apical side of the renal tubular membrane, which reduced the reuptake of uric acid back into the blood. Probenecid inhibits OAT and reduces the clearance of many drugs. For example, it reduces the renal clearance of acylovir and fexofenadine by 32% and 68%, respectively, (see [7]). Probenecid's inhibition of OAT was used to advantage to prolong the half-life of penicillins during periods when the drug was in short supply. In the case of methotrexate, inhibition of OAT by either probenecid or penicillin is associated with an increased risk of methotrexate-induced bone marrow suppression.

As discussed above, OCT2 and MATE1 appear to work in a coordinated manner to promote the excretion of their substrates. Examples of drugs that inhibit one or both of these transporters are shown in Table 5.2. Cimetidine has been found to reduce the renal clearance of metformin and procainamide by 14% and 44%, respectively, (see [7]). Inhibition of OCT2/MATE1-mediated secretion of creatinine can create a special problem when serum creatinine levels are used to assess renal function. The inhibitors cimetidine and trimethoprin were found to increase serum creatinine and to decrease the value of the calculated creatinine clearance by 15% and 16%, respectively. Ignoring this effect will lead to an underestimation of renal function. This effect can complicate the assessment of renal function in patients taking nephrotoxic drugs in combination with drugs that inhibit the renal transport of creatinine. For example, tenofovir, disoproxil, fumarate, or atazanavir, which can all cause renal toxicity are often combined with cobicisat, a CYP3A inhibitor that also inhibits the OCT2/MATE1 transporter system [8].

Less is known about DDIs originating at the level of renal efflux transporters. Many of the known inhibitors are fairly weak and may not achieve sufficiently high concentrations to exert a large effect in the kidney [7]. Digoxin is often used as a model P-gp substrate because it does not undergo any metabolism by CYP3A4. As discussed in Chapter 3, digoxin is also a substrate for intestinal P-gp. In theory, inhibition of P-gp could increase the absorption of digoxin in the intestine and/or decrease its elimination in the kidney. Both would increase the serum concentrations of digoxin. Rifampin, which induces P-gp, was found to have a greater effect on the intestinal efflux of digoxin than on the renal efflux. In other studies, the relative contribution of altered renal and/or intestinal P-gp on digoxin's pharmacokinetics is not clear. From a clinical standpoint, modifiers of P-gp should be used cautiously with digoxin. Irrespective of the mechanism, inhibitors and inducers may increase and decrease, respectively, the body's exposure to digoxin.

5.3.3 Tubular Reabsorption

As the filtrate moves through the proximal tubule and the loop of Henle, water is reabsorbed back into the systemic circulation. When the filtrate reaches the distal tubule, about 80% of the filtered water has been reabsorbed. As a result, the concentration of drugs in the filtrate becomes higher than that in the blood in the surrounding capillaries, and drugs diffuse along their concentration gradient back into the systemic circulation. The extent of this tubular reabsorption is controlled by:

1. *The drug's lipophilicity.* Lipophilic drugs will readily pass through the tubular membrane and be reabsorbed back into the circulation. This highlights the importance of hepatic metabolism in producing more polar, less lipophilic molecules that are much less susceptible to tubular reabsorption.
2. *pH.* Most drugs are weak acids or bases and exist in solution in an equilibrium between their ionized and nonionized forms. The pH of the filtrate and the drug's pK_a control the equilibrium. Since only the nonionized form is able to diffuse through the tubular membrane, urinary pH could, in theory, influence tubular reabsorption. An alkaline pH will favor the ionized form of weak acids and inhibit their reabsorption:

$$\text{HA} \;\rightleftharpoons\; \text{A}^- \;+\; \text{H}^+$$
$$\vdots \cdots\cdots\cdots >$$
$$\text{OH}^- \tag{5.32}$$

(The dotted lines represent the direction in which the equilibrium changes.)

An acidic pH will favor the ionized form of weak bases and inhibit their reabsorption:

$$\text{B} \;+\; \text{H}^+ \;\rightleftharpoons\; \text{BH}^+$$
$$\vdots \text{--------}>$$
$$\text{H}^+ \tag{5.33}$$

(The dashed line shows the direction of change of the equilibrium.)

Urinary pH can be modified by several compounds. Potassium citrate and sodium bicarbonate increase urinary pH, and ammonium chloride and the thiazide diuretics decrease pH. In practice, however, variation in urinary pH affects the renal clearance of only a limited number of drugs because of the constraint placed on possible pH changes. For example, ammonium chloride treatment produces pH values in the range 5–6, and sodium bicarbonate treatment leads to pH values in the range 7–8. This limited pH range will only influence the ionization of weak acids and bases with midrange pK_a values. Amphetamine and phenobarbital are examples of drugs with midrange pK_a values. The tubular reabsorption of amphetamine (weak base) can be decreased (and its clearance increased) by acidifying the filtrate using ammonium chloride. Conversely, the tubular reabsorption of phenobarbital (weak acid) can be decreased (and its clearance increased) by making the filtrate more alkaline using potassium citrate or sodium bicarbonate. Methadone is another example of a drug that displays pH sensitive reabsorption. Normally, little of this basic drug undergoes renal excretion, but the acidification of the urine decreases it reabsorption resulting in the excretion of around 30% of a dose. This effect is associated with an increase in methadone's half-life.

3. *Filtrate/urine flow.* The faster the filtrate flows through the tubules, the more limited the opportunity for reabsorption. Thus, tubular reabsorption can be decreased, and renal clearance increased, by the consumption of large amounts of water and coadministration of diuretics, including ethanol and caffeine.

5.3.4 Putting Meaning into the Value of Renal Clearance

A drug's overall renal clearance is a function of glomerular filtration, tubular secretion, and tubular reabsorption. It may be expressed as:

$$Cl_r = Cl_{GF} + Cl_{TS} - TR \quad \text{or} \quad Cl_r = GFR \cdot fu + Cl_{TS} - TR \quad (5.34)$$

where Cl_{TS} is clearance by tubular secretion, and TR represents tubular reabsorption.

Example 5.1 Consider a hypothetical drug that does not bind to the plasma proteins ($fu = 1$) and has a renal clearance of 50 mL/min (Figure E5.1). Use this information to gain insight into the processes involved in its renal clearance.

Solution Assuming that GFR = 120 mL/min, the clearance by glomerular filtration is

$$Cl_{GF} = GFR \cdot fu$$
$$= 120 \times 1 = 120 \, mL/min$$

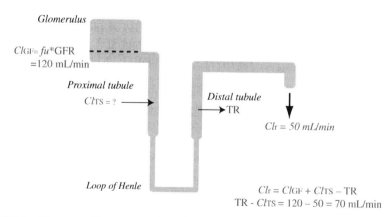

FIGURE E5.1 Diagrammatic representation of renal clearance of a hypothetical drug. The drug's clearance by glomerular filtration is 120 mL/min, but its ultimate renal clearance is 50 mL/min. Thus, tubular reabsoprtion must exceed any clearance by tubular secretion by 70 mL/min.

TABLE 5.3   Interpretation of the Renal Clearance of Some Drugs

Drug	Cl_r (mL/min)	fu	Cl_{GF} (mL/min)	Comments
Atenolol	170	0.95	114	Some tubular secretion
Ciprofloxacin	500	0.6	72	Significant tubular secretion
Methotrexate	120	0.5	60	Some tubular secretion; OAT family involved

Substituting into equation (5.34) yields

$$50 = 120 + Cl_{TS} - TR$$
$$TR - Cl_{TS} = 70 \, ml/min$$

Although it is not possible to know exactly how much tubular secretion and/or reabsorption occurs, it is clear from equation (5.34) and Figure E5.1 that tubular reabsorption must exceed any tubular secretion by 70 mL/min.

Example 5.2   A second drug, which is 20% bound to proteins, has a renal clearance of 300 mL/min. What are the relative values of active secretion and tubular reabsorption?

Solution   Substituting into equation (5.34) gives us

$$300 = 120 \times 0.8 + Cl_{TS} - TR$$
$$Cl_{TS} - TR = 204 \, ml/min$$

For this drug, tubular secretion must exceed any tubular reabsorption by 204 mL/min.

Table 5.3 provides the interpretation of the renal clearance of some example drugs.

5.3.5   Measurement of Renal Clearance

Several methods are available to determine a drug's renal clearance. They are all based on the relationship between the excretion rate and the plasma concentration:

$$\frac{dAu}{dt} = Cl_r \cdot Cp \tag{5.35}$$

where Au is the amount of drug in the urine. One of the most straightforward methods for the determination of renal clearance is to collect urine samples over successive periods of time and measure the average rate of excretion of a drug during each period. As shown in equation (5.35), renal clearance is the constant of proportionality between the rate of excretion and the plasma concentration. Thus, a plot of the rate of excretion against the corresponding plasma concentration yields a straight line with a slope equal to renal clearance (Figure 5.6).
  Experimentally:

- Urine is collected over successive time periods after a dose.
- The urine is analyzed for unchanged drug and the average rate of excretion over each time period is calculated.

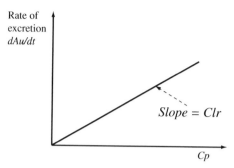

FIGURE 5.6   Determination of renal clearance. Renal clearance is the slope of a plot of the rate of excretion against plasma concentration (*Cp*).

- During a collection period, the plasma concentration changes continuously as drug is excreted. Since excretion is a first-order process, the rate of excretion will also change continuously during the collection period. The excretion rate calculated above represents the average excretion rate over a collection period and will correspond most closely to the plasma concentration at the midpoint of the collection period. This plasma concentration is determined.
- The rate of excretion for each time period is then plotted against the plasma concentration at the midpoint of the collection period. The slope of the line is the renal clearance (Figure 5.6).

Example 5.3   The fictitious drug disolvprazole is almost completely eliminated by renal excretion. A 10-mg dose was administered intravenously to a healthy subject. Urine samples were collected over various periods and the plasma concentration was measured at the midpoint of each collection period. The data are given in Table E5.3A. Determine the renal clearance of disolvprazole in this patient.

Solution   The average rate of excretion over a collection period is calculated as follows:

$$\text{average rate of excretion} = \frac{\text{volume of urine} \cdot \text{urinary concentration}}{\text{duration of collection period}}$$

For the first collection period in Table E5.3A:

$$\text{average rate of excretion} = \frac{200\,\text{mL} \times 15\,\mu\text{g/mL}}{1\,\text{h}} = 3000\,\mu\text{g/h} \quad \text{or} \quad 3\,\text{mg/h}$$

TABLE E5.3A   Urinary and Plasma Concentrations of Disolvprazole After a 10-mg Dose

Urine Data			Plasma Data	
Collection Period	Volume of Urine (mL)	Urinary Concentration (μg/mL)	Time (h) (Midpoint of Urine Collection Period)	*Cp* (μg/L)
0−1	200	15	0.5	240
1−3	180	19.4	2	142
3−5	140	12.8	4	71
5−10	400	3.5	7.5	21

TABLE E5.3B   Rate of Excretion and Corresponding Plasma Concentrations for Disolvprazole

Urine Data		Plasma Data	
Collection Period (h)	Rate of Excretion (µg/h)	Time (h)	Cp (µg/L)
0–1	3000	0.5	240
1–3	1746	2	142
3–5	896	4	71
5–10	280	7.5	21

The plasma concentration that most closely corresponds to the time when the excretion rate is 3 mg/h is the plasma concentration at the midpoint of the period (Cp at 0.5 h).

The remaining average excretion rates are calculated and the data tabulated prior to plotting are listed in Table E5.3B.

The average rate of excretion is plotted against the plasma concentration (Figure E5.2) and yields a slope of 12.4 L/h. Thus, the renal clearance of disolvprazole is 12.4 L/h.

Single-Point Determination of Renal Clearance   Under steady-state conditions, when the plasma concentration of a drug is constant, the rate of excretion will be constant and renal clearance can be estimated using a simpler single-point determination:

- The steady-state plasma concentration of the drug is determined.
- One large urine sample rather than individual urine samples is collected over an extended period (3–5 elimination half-lives of the drug).
- The average rate of excretion over the entire collection period is calculated.
- Renal clearance is calculated by dividing the excretion rate determined above by the steady-state plasma concentration of the drug.

This method should be used only under steady-state conditions, when the plasma concentration is constant. If the plasma concentration undergoes wide changes during the study period, the rate of excretion will change constantly, and by averaging the rate over an extended period, a bias value of renal clearance will be obtained. This is the method used to calculate the clearance of creatinine, an endogenous compound produced from

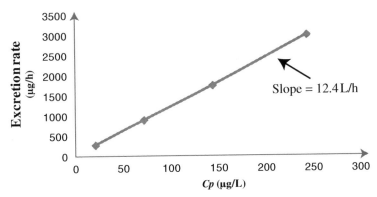

FIGURE E5.2   Plot of rate of average excretion of disolvprazole against plasma concentration.

muscle metabolism. Under normal circumstances, the concentration of creatinine in the blood is constant. It does not bind to proteins, and normally undergoes minimal tubular secretion and tubular reabsorption. As a result, its renal clearance approximates the GFR [see equation (5.34)], and it is used to assess renal function. Because creatinine is eliminated exclusively by the renal route, its total body clearance is equal to its renal clearance.

Example 5.4   Creatinine clearance is to be determined in a 55-year-old 65-kg female patient. Her urine was collected over a 24-h period, and the urinary concentration of creatinine was determined. The patient's serum concentration of creatinine was measured at the beginning of the study. The data are as follows:

Collection period: 0–24 h
Volume of urine collected: 1050 mL
Urinary creatinine concentration: 1.14 mg/mL
Serum creatinine concentration: 1.0 mg/dL

Determine creatinine's clearance rate.

Solution

Amount of creatinine excreted in urine: 1197 mg
Average rate of drug excretion: 1197/24 mg/h = 49.9 mg/h
Renal clearance:

$$\text{excretion rate}/Sr_{cr} = 49.9\,\text{mg/h}/(10\,\text{mg/L})$$
$$= 4.99\,\text{L/h}$$
$$= 83.1\,\text{mL/min}$$

Note: Because it is assumed that serum creatinine is constant, the time of its determination is not important.

5.3.6 Fraction of the Dose Excreted Unchanged

Recall that the rate of excretion of a drug is

$$\frac{dAu}{dt} = Cl_r \cdot Cp \tag{5.36}$$

where Au is the amount of drug in the urine. Rearranging to obtain an expression for the amount of drug excreted in period dt gives

$$dAu = Cl_r \cdot Cp \cdot dt \tag{5.37}$$

But $Cp \cdot dt$ is the area under the plasma concentration–time curve (AUC) for the period dt:

$$dAu = Cl_r \cdot \text{AUC}_{dt} \tag{5.38}$$

By extension, the amount of drug excreted from time zero to infinity is the sum of all the areas from time zero to infinity:

$$\text{Amount excreted by infinity} = Cl_r \cdot \sum_0^\infty \text{AUC}_{dt} = Cl_r \cdot \text{AUC}_0^\infty \qquad (5.39)$$

The amount of drug excreted in the urine by infinity is Au^∞:

$$Au^\infty = Cl_r \cdot \text{AUC}_0^\infty \qquad (5.40)$$

Rearranging equation (5.29) gives

$$S \cdot F \cdot D = Cl \cdot \text{AUC}_0^\infty \qquad (5.41)$$

Dividing equation (5.40) by equation (5.41) yields

$$fe = \frac{Au^\infty}{S \cdot F \cdot D} = \frac{Cl_r}{Cl} \qquad (5.42)$$

where fe is the fraction of the dose excreted unchanged.

Equation (5.42) shows that the fraction of the dose excreted unchanged is also the fraction of total body clearance made up of renal clearance. Thus, if 10% of a dose is excreted unchanged, renal clearance is 10% of total body clearance. Also, since total body clearance is usually the sum of renal and hepatic clearance, $1 - fe$ will be the fraction of total body clearance that comprises hepatic clearance. Continuing the example above, $fe = 0.1$, so $1 - fe = 0.9$. Hepatic clearance is 90% of total clearance.

Note that equation (5.40) can be rearranged to provide an alternative approach to the assessment of renal clearance. Rearranging the equation gives

$$Cl_r = \frac{Au^\infty}{AUC_0^\infty} \qquad (5.43)$$

Thus, renal clearance can be determined from the amount of drug ultimately excreted unchanged in the urine divided by the area under the plasma concentration–time curve.

5.4   HEPATIC ELIMINATION AND CLEARANCE

Lipophilic drugs cannot be eliminated by renal excretion because they undergo tubular reabsorption in the distal tubule. They may undergo glomerular filtration, and this excretion can be augmented by drug transporters in the proximal tubule, but when they reach the distal tubule, the concentration gradient between the tubule and the blood, combined with their good membrane permeability properties, will result in extensive, if not complete, reabsorption of these molecules. The primary purpose of hepatic metabolism is to create more hydrophilic molecules that will not undergo tubular reabsorption and thus can be eliminated from the body in the urine. Most drugs are lipophilic in nature and are eliminated by metabolism or biotransformation. Around 73% of the 200 drugs most prescribed in the United States are eliminated by metabolism [11] (Figure 5.1). In the majority of cases, metabolites have greater water solubility than that of the parent drug, but occasionally, metabolites are less soluble. For example, some of the metabolites of the sulfonamides possess poor water solubility and can crystallize out in the renal tubule, which can lead to serious kidney damage and blood in the urine. Patients taking sulfonamides are advised to drink a lot of water and to avoid taking any compounds that acidify the urine, such as methenamine. Although drug metabolism may be referred to as "drug detoxification," this is misleading because drug metabolites can be pharmacologically active and/or toxic. There are many examples of prodrugs, whose pharmacological activity resides with their metabolite, including codeine, prednisone, and tamoxifen. Acetaminophen is a classic example of a drug that produces toxic metabolites. Normally, acetaminophen's toxic metabolite is inactivated by glutathione in the liver. In the event of acetaminophen overdose, the amount of the highly reactive toxic metabolite exceeds the capacity of hepatic glutathione, and it reacts with hepatic macromolecules to produce necrosis.

5.4.1   Phase I and Phase II Metabolism

Although many tissues contain some drug-metabolizing enzymes and have the ability to metabolize drugs, the liver has the greatest abundance and greatest variety of these enzymes. As a result, the liver is the major organ of drug metabolism. It should be noted that enzymes in other locations can affect a drug's pharmacokinetic characteristics. Notably, as discussed in Chapter 3, the enzymes in the intestinal enterocytes can cause significant presystemic extraction and drastically reduce the oral bioavailability of some drugs. The various enzymatic reactions that are involved in hepatic metabolism are categorized as either phase I or phase II processes. Phase I reactions generally result in small chemical modifications of the drug molecule. They often involve oxidation, such as the addition of a hydroxyl group or the removal of a methyl group, although some reductions can occur. Although several families of enzymes, such as flavin monooxygenase, alcohol dehydrogenase, aldehyde dehydrogenase, and xanthine oxidase, participate in phase I reactions, the cytochrome P450 (CYP) enzyme system is by far the most important. It is estimated that this enzyme system is responsible for the elimination of around 75% of the drugs eliminated by metabolism [11] (Figure 5.7). In phase II metabolism, the parent drug or the product of phase I metabolism is conjugated with a polar function, such as a glucuronide, sulfate, or glutathione molecule. The UDP-glucuronosyltransferases (UGTs) are the most important of the phase II enzymes and are estimated to be responsible for the elimination of around 10% of the drugs eliminated by metabolism [1] (Figure 5.7). The parent drug, a phase I metabolite or more often a phase II metabolite, may be excreted into the bile.

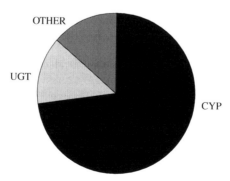

FIGURE 5.7   Relative contribution of different enzymes involved in the metabolism of the top 200 drugs. Here, CYP is the cytochrome P450 enzyme system and UGT represents UDP-glucuronosyltransferases.

TABLE 5.4   Characteristics of the Major Hepatic CYP Enzymes[a]

CYP Enzyme	Relative Abundance (%)	Clinically Significant Polymorphism
3A4	>35	Yes[b]
2D6	<5	Yes
2C9	>15	Yes
2E1	~15	No
1A2	>10	No
2A6	~10	Yes
2C19	<5	Yes
2C8	~5	Yes
2B6	<5	Yes

Source: Data from Reference [13].
[a]The table shows the relative abundance of the various CYP enzymes and identifies those that display significant genetic polymorphism.
[b]Recent studies have demonstrated genetic polymorphism.

5.4.2   The Cytochrome P450 Enzyme System

The CYP enzyme system is responsible for the elimination of around 55% of drugs used clinically [11] and as such plays a very important role in drug elimination. This function is carried out primarily by nine specific enzymes or isoforms within the CYP superfamily. The classification system for the families and subfamilies is based on the similarity of their amino acid sequencing. These enzymes and their relative abundance in the human liver are shown in Table 5.4. CYP 3A4 is the most abundant and is involved in the metabolism of the greatest number of drugs. The CYP3A family is responsible for around 46% of CYP-mediated metabolism [11]. Many drugs are metabolized by several enzymes, which makes it difficult to rank the enzymes in terms of their involvement in drug elimination. However, about 80% of the oxidative phase I reactions are thought to be mediated by four CYP enzymes: CYP3A4, CYP2D6, CYP2C9, and CYP2C19.

Note that the relative importance of an individual enzyme in metabolizing drugs does not necessarily parallel its relative abundance. CYP2D6 constitutes less than 5% of total hepatic CYP, yet is responsible for the metabolism of around 20% of the drugs metabolized by the CYP system. In contrast, CYP2E1 is relatively abundant but plays little role in the metabolism of drugs. This enzyme is induced by ethanol and acetone, which may be produced by diabetic patients, and is thought to be important in producing toxic metabolites, including that of acetaminophen. The activity of some of the individual enzymes is under genetic control (Table 5.4). Some people within the population may have extremely low activity of some of these enzymes, whereas others may have exceptionally high activity (see Chapter 16). Genetic polymorphism in CYP2D6 and CYP2C9 is particularly problematic because they metabolize a large number of drugs. Genetic polymorphism of CYP2C9, for example, is one of the important factors responsible for the wide variation in dose requirements of warfarin. Patients with low CYP2C9 activity often require lower doses. Tamoxifen is converted to its active antiestrogen metabolite, endoxifen, by CYP2D6, and women with a genetically determined low activity of CYP2D6 have been found to have a greater risk of breast cancer relapse than do women with normal CYP2D6 levels. In addition to CYP3A4, other forms of the CYP3A subfamily exist. CYP3A5 is a minor CYP3A enzyme that is only expressed in about 20% of human livers. There are ethnic differences in its expression, and it is more common in Africans. When present, it can make up 17–50% of CYP3A. Generally, it appears to have similar properties to CYP3A4 but some differences have been observed. For example, individuals with CYP3A5 may have increased susceptibility to certain cancers and have a higher clearance of tacrolimus [12]. CYP3A7 is the primary CYP3A enzyme expressed during the prenatal period and declines rapidly after birth and is barely measurable in adults.

5.4.3   Glucuronidation

It can be seen from Figure 5.7 that around 10% of drugs are metabolized by the UGTs to glucuronide metabolites. In addition, a large number of the products of phase I metabolism are also metabolized along this pathway. As drug companies strive to develop drugs that are eliminated by pathways other than CYP metabolism, it is likely that this route will become even more important in the future [14].

Examples of drugs that are metabolized by the UGTs include morphine, zidovudine, olanzapine, valproic acid, and codeine [1]. There are several isoforms of UGT, including UGT1A1, 1A4, 1A6, 1A9, 2B7, and 2B15, with UGT2B7 having the largest number of drug substrates. There appears to be wide interindividual variability in the activity of the different isoforms. This could predispose certain individuals to either toxic or subtherapeutic concentrations of the substrates of the UGTs. Genetic factors and induction by alcohol and smoking have been identified as factors contributing to their variability [14].

5.4.4   Metabolism-Based Drug–Drug Interactions

Changes in the hepatic metabolism of one drug (*victim drug*) as a result of the concomitant administration of a second medication (*perpetrator drug*) is the most common cause of DDIs. Perpetrator drugs usually either inhibit or induce one or more of the drug-metabolizing enzymes. Some perpetrators do both. Inhibitors reduce an enzyme's ability to metabolize other drugs, which can lead to increased concentrations of these drugs and toxicity. Inducers increase the amount of an enzyme. This can result in the more rapid metabolism and decreased, possibly subtherapeutic plasma concentrations of its substrates. DDIs present a serious health problem and are estimated to be responsible for up to 4% of hospitalizations annually.

Changes in the activity of any of the enzymes involved in drug metabolism can lead to DDIs but, as the primary enzyme system for the metabolism of drugs, the CYP enzymes are most commonly involved. The clinical outcome of changes in the activity of the phase II enzymes has received much less attention to date. This may be because altered activity of the UGTs appears to produce more modest changes in drug exposure. Rifampin (induction) and probenecid (inhibition) are both known modifiers of the UGTs. Interestingly, both these compounds also affect other enzymes and transporters, which complicates the interpretation of clinical data. Important substrates of the UGTs that may be victims of altered UGT activity include acetaminophen, zidovudine, lamotrigene, and lorazepam [15]. By contrast, there is a large body of research on substrates, inhibitors, and inducers of the various CYP enzymes and some common examples are shown in Table 5.5.

Perpetrators have been classified as strong, moderate, or weak, based on the change in exposure experienced by victim drugs. Strong inhibitors, such as fluvoxamine (CYP1A2), fluconazole (CYP2C9), fluoxetine (CYP2D6), and ritonavir (CYP3A4), can cause more than a fivefold increase in the AUC, or more than 80% decrease in oral clearance of victim drugs. Moderate inhibitors, such as amiodarone (CYP2C9), sertraline (CYP2D6), and erythromycin (CYP3A4), can cause greater than a twofold, but less than a fivefold increase in the AUC, or a 50–80% change in oral clearance. Weak inhibitors such as cimetidine

TABLE 5.5   Substrates, Inhibitors, and Inducers of the Major CYP Enzymes Involved in the Metabolism of Drugs

Enzyme	Substrates	Inhibitors	Inducers
CYP3A4	Benzodiazepines, immunosuppressants, statins (except pravastatin and rosuvastatin), and Ca^{2+} channel blockers	Macrolides (not azithromycin), azole antifungals, protease inhibitors, and cimetidine (weak)	Rifampin, efavirenz phenobarbital, phenytoin, and St. John's wort
CYP2D6	Debrisoquine, metoprolol, desipramine, codeine, tamoxifen, flecainide, and paroxetine	Quinidine, paroxetine, fluoxetine, ritonavir, and bupropion	Not inducible
CYP2C9	S-Warfarin, phenytoin, losartan, and fluvastatin	Fluconazole and amiodarone	Rifampin, phenytoin, and carbamazepine
CYP1A2	Theophylline, clozapine, and tizanidine	Fluvoxamine and quinolones	Smoking, omeprazole, and lansoprazole
CYP2C19	Proton pump inhibitors, S-mephenytoin, and diazepam	Omeprazole, fluvoxamine, and fluconazole	Rifampin and efavirenz
CYP2B6	Bupropion, efavirenz, and methadone	Ticlopidine and clopidogrel	Rifampin and phenobarbital
CYP2C8	Cerivastatin and paclitaxel	Gemfibrozil	Rifampin

Source: Data from References [13, 16].

(CYP1A2, CYP2D6, and CYP3A4) cause between a 2 and 1.25 change in the AUC, or a 20–50% change in oral clearance. The increase in exposure to the victim drugs can arise from reduced hepatic clearance, decreased intestinal extraction, and/or decreased hepatic extraction. Changes in bioavailability for drugs that undergo extensive extraction can produce profound changes in the AUC. For example, the AUC of saquinavir, which undergoes extensive presystemic extraction, can increase up to around 50-fold when coadministered with the potent inhibitor ritonavir. The clinical significance of a DDI will also depend on a drug's therapeutic range. Drugs with wide therapeutic ranges may tolerate large changes in exposure without clinical consequence. Conversely, drugs with narrow therapeutic ranges, such as digoxin and warfarin, may require dosage adjustment and/or monitoring when relatively modest changes in exposure occur. For example, although ritonavir increases digoxin's AUC by only about 36%, the drug combination necessitates careful monitoring of digoxin's levels and dose adjustment if necessary. Likewise, amoldipine increases exposure to simavastatin only about 1.3- to 1.6-fold. Yet, this is sufficient to increase the risk of muscle myopathy and has led several regulatory bodies, including the Food and Drug Administration, to cap simvastatin's daily dose at 20 mg when taken concurrently with amlodipine. In addition to increasing exposure to victim drugs, inhibitors may also reduce the efficacy of prodrugs that require metabolism to form the active species. For example, patients taking tamoxifen frequently suffer anxiety, depression, and hot flashes and are often prescribed SSRIs. Paroxetine and fluoxetine are both strong inhibitors of CYP 2D6 and should not be used in combination with tamoxifen because they can reduce the conversion of tamoxifen to the active metabolite, endoxifen, which would compromise the effectiveness of tamoxifen and lead to increased mortality rates. Genetic polymorphism can also influence the clinical outcome of DDIs. Poor and extensive metabolizers may display different sensitivities to inhibitors. Inhibition of CYP2D6 may have important clinical effects in extensive metabolizers but may have no effect in poor metabolizers, who are deficient in the enzyme. In poor metabolizers, alternative enzymatic pathways achieve greater significance, and inhibition of these pathways will be more clinically important in poor compared to extensive metabolizers.

Inhibitors may be either reversible or time dependent. These are discussed in more detail in Chapter 17. Reversible inhibitors act through a competitive mechanism and reduce the available active sites on an enzyme. This type of inhibition depends on the physical presence of the competitive inhibitor, which has a higher affinity for the enzyme than that of the victim drug. Thus, inhibition is usually apparent as soon as the inhibitor is introduced, although in some cases, the effect may require the inhibitor concentration to build up to reach steady-state levels, which takes about four elimination half-lives. Similarly, the inhibitory effect will persist as long as there is sufficient inhibitor present at the enzyme site. As a result, the effect may last for up to four elimination half-lives (time to eliminate the drug) after the inhibitor has been withdrawn. Inhibition from inhibitors with long half-lives, such as amiodarone ($t_{1/2} \approx 1$ month), can persist for prolonged periods after therapy with the inhibitor has been withdrawn. Examples of reversible inhibitors include cimetidine, fluconazole, and itraconazole. Time-dependent inhibitors (TDIs) or mechanism-based inhibitors are metabolized by the enzyme to reactive metabolic intermediates (MIs) that bind irreversibly to the enzyme and inactivate it. This results in a decrease in the amount of viable enzyme, a decrease in the efficiency of the system, and a decrease in the clearance of other drugs metabolized by the affected enzyme. The degree of inactivation and resulting inhibition of the system increases over time, as more MI is formed, hence the name, TDIs. Further, the inhibition will persist until new enzyme is synthesized, which is dependent on the rate constant or the half-life for enzyme degradation (see Chapter 17 and Appendix E). The range of the CYP3A4 degradation half-life has been reported to be 24–36 h (see Chapter 17), which would suggest that inhibition would persist for several days after the inhibitor has been eliminated. Examples of TDI include the macrolide antibiotics such as clarithromycin and erythromycin, diltiazem, ritonavir, and tamoxifen. TDI is responsible for some of the most serious DDIs. For example, erythromycin, a moderate inhibitor is associated with torsades de pointes when coadminstered with terfenadine and rhabdomylolyis when coadminstered with simvastatin. In addition to their destructive effect on enzymes, MI can be toxic. For example, the MI of tamoxifen has been thought to promote endometrial cancer.

Inducers of the enzymes act by stimulating the synthesis of additional enzyme and/or by inhibiting enzyme degradation. As a result, the full effect of these agents is usually not apparent immediately, and it may take between a few days to a few weeks for the maximum effect to be observed. The onset of the effect is dependent on the turnover time of the enzymes and on the time it takes the inducers to reach steady state. Inducers with short half-lives, such as rifampin, reach steady state more quickly and have faster onsets of action than do inducers with long half-lives, such as phenobarbital. It will also take an extended period for the enzyme activity to return to normal once an inducer is withdrawn from therapy.

Several software packages are available that allow health care professionals to screen for DDIs in patients taking more than one medication. Comprehensive lists of substrates, inhibitors, and inducers of the major CYP isoforms can be found in the literature [13, 17, 18] and on Web sites (e.g., [16]). Further details of DDIs can be found in Chapter 17, which presents a description of the models used to apply data obtained from *in-vitro* studies to predict the likelihood of clinically important DDIs *in vivo*.

5.4.5 Hepatic Drug Transporters and Drug–Drug Interactions

The uptake transporters OATP1B1, OATP1B3, OATP2B1, OAT2, and OCT1, and efflux transporters P-gp, MRPs, BCRP, and MATE1 are all found in the liver, where they participate in the hepatic clearance of drugs (Figure 5.8). The uptake transporters are expressed primarily on the sinusoidal (blood or basolateral) side of the hepatocyte membrane, where they assist in the hepatic clearance of drugs by transporting their substrates into the hepatocyte where they can then undergo metabolism and/or biliary excretion. The efflux transporters, reside primarily on the canalicular membrane and, participate in hepatic clearance by secreting unchanged drugs, drug metabolites, and conjugates of glucoronide, sulfate, and glutathione into the bile. The action of the uptake and efflux transporters has been referred to as phase 0 and phase III metabolism, respectively.

Although many drugs are able to diffuse passively across the hepatocyte membrane, the membrane can be a barrier for the uptake of hydrophilic and charged molecules (BDDCS and BCS class 3 and 4 drugs). For such drugs, the uptake transporters are an important first step for their subsequent metabolism. It is interesting to note that there is a movement in the pharmaceutical industry toward the development of drugs that are resistant to metabolism by the CYP enzymes. As a result, it is likely that an increasing number of BDDCS or BDS type 3 and 4 drugs will appear on the market in the future and that uptake transporters will play an increasing role in controlling the pharmacokinetics of drugs. OATP1B1 and the closely related OATP1B3 are found exclusively in the liver [19] and play a vital role in the hepatic elimination of several important drugs including the

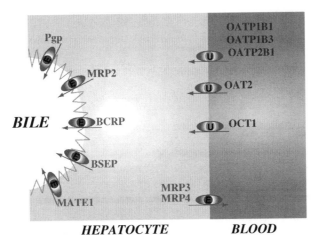

FIGURE 5.8 Drug transporters in the liver. The diagram shows a hepatocyte. The uptake transporters (U), organic anion transporting polypeptide (OATP), organic cation transporter (OCT), and organic anion transporter (OAT) are found on the basolateral side of the hepatocyte. The efflux transporters (E), permeability glycoprotein (P-gp), multidrug resistance-associated protein family (MRP), breast cancer-resistance protein (BCRP), bile salt export pump (BSEP), and multidrug and toxin extrusion protein (MATE) are found mainly on the canalicular membrane. Two efflux transporters (MRP3 and MRP4) are found on the basolateral membrane. (*For a color version of this figure, see the color plate section.*)

HMG-CoA reductase inhibitors (statins), angiotensin II receptor antagonists (sartans, e.g., olmesartan and valsartan), and the antidiabetic glinides (e.g., repaglinide). For some of these drugs, their transporter-mediated hepatic uptake is the rate determining step in their metabolism and/or biliary excretion, and low transporter activity as a result of genetics or the concomitant administration inhibitors can reduce their clearance and increase systemic concentrations. Gemfibrozil, cyclosporine, and rifampin are all potent inhibitors of the OATP family of transporters and when coadministered with the statins, sartans, and glinides can produce large (2- to 20-fold) increases in the AUC. The more polar statins pravastatin ($\log D_{7.4} = -0.7$) [20], rosuvastatin ($\log D_{7.4} = -0.25$), and pitavastatin ($\log D_{7.4} = 1.5$) undergo minimal metabolism and are mainly cleared by transporters followed by biliary excretion. As a result, inhibitors of OATP1B1 such as cyclosporine produce large increases (5- to 20-fold) in the AUC of these drugs. Even the more lipophilic statins, simvastatin acid and lovastatin acid are dependent on OATP uptake and experience clinically significant interactions with modifiers of the transporters. But the highly lipophilic lactone prodrugs of simvastatin ($\log D_{7.4} = 4.4$) and lovastatin ($\log D_{7.4} = 3.9$) are less dependent on OATP activity and more dependent on CYP3A4 activity. Increased plasma concentration of the statins is a serious clinical event because it increases patients' risk of muscle myopathy and rhabdomyolysis. Patients with genetically determined low activity of OATP1B1 have been found to have increased plasma concentrations of simvastatin acid and to be at increased risk of developing myopathy [21, 22]. The effect of polymorphism of OATP1B1 on the pharmacokinetics and safety profile of simvastatin acid is discussed further in Chapter 16. Altered hepatic uptake of statins may also impact their pharmacodynamics because their site of action is within the hepatocyte.

The OCT1 carrier is important for the uptake of various cations, including cimetidine, desipramine, and the hydrophilic antidiabetic drug metformin [5, 23]. The uptake facilitates metformin's access to its site of action in the hepatocyte but does not play a role in metformin's elimination, as it is primarily eliminated renally. Several protease inhibitors, including ritonavir, are inhibitors of both OCT1 and OCT2 (important in the kidney) and can impair the uptake of substrates of these transporters and cause drug interactions [24]. Substrates for the OAT transporter include endogenous and exogenous anions, such as *para*-aminohippurate, nonsteroidal anti-inflammatory drugs, and methotrexate [23].

The efflux transporters, located primarily on the canalicular (luminal) membrane of the hepatocyte, include BCRP, P-gp, MATE1 and MRP2 (Figure 5.8), where they play an essential role in facilitating the biliary excretion of drugs and their metabolites The low surface area of the canalicular membrane (<15% that of the hepatocyte) and the high polarity of many metabolites make passive diffusion across this membrane extremely challenging. Substrates for the efflux transporters include statins (e.g., rosuvastatin, pravastatin, and atorvastatin), irinotecan, its active metabolite SN38, and the glucoronide of SN38. Some efflux transporters, including MRP3 and MRP4, are located on the sinusoidal membrane, where they transport drugs and metabolites back into the bloodstream. As was the case in the kidney, hepatic MATE (MATE1) appears to work in conjunction with OCT (OCT1) for the transcellular transport of relatively hydrophilic small molecules into the bile [25]. Bile salt export pump (BSEP), which is also present in the canalicular membrane appears to have little role in the elimination of drugs in the liver. Its major role is the production and secretion of bile acids to help solubilize digested lipids [19]. Its inhibition by some drugs, however, is an important safety concern as the accumulation of bile acids in the liver is associated with cytotoxic events including cholestasis and drug-induced liver disease (DILD), which has been a major cause of drug withdrawals from the market over the last decade. Inhibitors of BSEP that are associated with DILD include cyclosporine, glyburide, troglitazone, sulindac, and nefazodone [23].

5.4.6 Kinetics of Drug Metabolism

Drug metabolism is an enzymatic process, which is initiated when the drug binds to the enzyme in a reversible manner. The enzyme converts the bound drug to a metabolite, and the metabolite and the enzyme are then released. The process is summarized as follows:

$$[D] + [E] \underset{k_2}{\overset{k_1}{\rightleftharpoons}} [DE] \xrightarrow{k_{cat}} [M] + [E]$$

where [D] is the unbound drug concentration, [E] is the free enzyme concentration, [DE] is the concentration of the drug–enzyme complex, [M] is the metabolite concentration, k_1 and k_2 are the forward and backward rate constants for the drug–enzyme interaction, and k_{cat} is the rate constant for the formation of the metabolite.

Metabolism is an example of a capacity-limited process and the rate or velocity (V) of metabolism is given by the Michaelis–Menten equation, which is derived and discussed in detail in Appendix E, It is expressed as follows:

$$V = \frac{V_{max} \cdot Ch_u}{K_m + Ch_u} \tag{5.44}$$

where V_{max} is the maximum rate of metabolism, which occurs when the enzyme is saturated, Ch_u is the unbound drug concentration in the hepatocyte, and K_m is the Michaelis–Menten constant, which is a dissociation constant and is equal to $(k_2 + k_{cat})/k_1$. Note that when $V = V_{max}/2$:

$$\frac{V_{max}}{2} = \frac{V_{max} \cdot Ch_u}{K_m + Ch_u}$$
$$K_m + Ch_u = 2 {}^* Ch_u \tag{5.45}$$
$$K_m = Ch_u$$

According to the Michaelis–Menten equation (5.44), the relationship between the drug concentration and the rate of the process is defined by a hyperbolic curve (Figure 5.9). This curve is explained by the fact that there is only a finite amount of enzyme. At low drug concentrations, the free enzyme concentration is high and the rate of metabolism can increase in proportion to increases in the drug concentration (first order) (Figure 5.7). As the drug concentration increases further, some degree of saturation occurs, and the rate of metabolism can no longer increase in proportion to increases in the drug concentrations. Eventually, all the enzyme is occupied by the drug and the rate of metabolism is constant (zero order) and at its maximum level (Figure 5.9).

Thus, at the extremes of low and high drug concentrations, the rate of metabolism is first order and zero order, respectively. This can be expressed mathematically as follows:

- *At low drug concentrations:* $Ch_u \ll K_m$, $K_m + Ch_u \approx K_m$, and the denominator in equation (5.44) simplifies to

$$V = \frac{V_{max} \cdot Ch_u}{K_m} = k \cdot Ch_u \tag{5.46}$$

where k is a constant equal to V_{max}/K_m. Thus, when $Ch_u \ll K_m$, the rate of metabolism is first order (Figure 5.9).

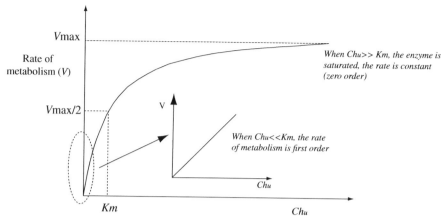

FIGURE 5.9   Plot of the rate of metabolism against the unbound drug concentration in the liver. The Michaelis–Menten constant (K_m) corresponds to the concentration where the rate is half the maximum rate (V_{max}). At low concentrations ($Ch_u \ll K_m$), the rate is first order. At high concentrations ($Ch_u \gg K_m$), the enzymes are saturated and the process is constant (zero order) and equal to V_{max}. Between these extremes, the rate is of mixed order and nonlinear.

- *At high drug concentrations:* $Ch_u \gg K_m$, $K_m + Ch_u \approx Ch_u$, and the denominator in equation (5.44) simplifies to

$$V = \frac{V_{max} \cdot Ch_u}{Ch_u} = V_{max} \qquad (5.47)$$

At high concentrations, the enzymes are saturated and the rate of metabolism occurs at its maximum possible rate (V_{max}), and it is zero order (Figure 5.9). Between these two extremes, the rate is a nonlinear, mixed-order process.

The unbound therapeutic concentrations of most drugs are well below their K_m values. As a result, the rate of metabolism for most therapeutic drugs is first order (Figure 5.9). A small number of drugs, however, have therapeutic concentrations that approach or can exceed their K_m value. These include ethanol and phenytoin (see Chapter 15). As a result of this, the pharmacokinetics of these drugs is more complicated and nonlinear.

5.4.7   Hepatic Clearance and Related Parameters

5.4.7.1   Hepatic Clearance
The model for hepatic clearance (Figure 5.10) is very similar to the extraction unit model shown in Figure 5.2 and discussed earlier in the chapter. As discussed previously, clearance is a function of blood flow to an organ and the ability of the organ to extract and eliminate the drug that is presented to it. Thus, hepatic clearance may be expressed as:

$$Clb_h = Q \cdot E \qquad (5.48)$$

where Clb_h is the hepatic blood clearance, Q is the hepatic blood flow, and E is the hepatic extraction ratio.

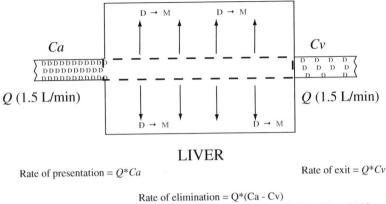

Rate of presentation = $Q*Ca$ Rate of exit = $Q*Cv$

Rate of elimination = Q*(Ca - Cv)
Fraction of incoming drug extracted $(E) = (Ca - Cv)/Ca$
Heaptic clearance = $Q*E$

FIGURE 5.10 Diagrammatic representation of hepatic clearance. Hepatic blood flow (Q) is 1.5 L/min. The concentration of drug in the arterial blood is Ca and the concentration leaving the liver is Cv. Drug (D) passing through the liver may be converted to metabolites (M) by hepatic enzymes.

Recall, clearance is defined as the volume of fluid completely cleared of drug per unit time. Thus, hepatic blood flow (about 1.5 L/min) represents the maximum value of hepatic clearance. A drug's hepatic clearance would achieve this value if all the drug entering the liver was metabolized ($E = 1$).

The extraction ratio (the fraction of the drug entering the liver that is eliminated) is a function of the ability of the drug in the blood to access the enzymes in the hepatocyte and the ability of the enzymes to metabolize the drug. The latter is known as *the drug's intrinsic clearance* (Cl_{int}), and it is a pure measure of the ability of the liver enzymes to metabolize a drug. It is not dependent on other factors, such as protein binding and hepatic blood flow that affect overall hepatic clearance. Intrinsic clearance is dependent only on the affinity of a drug for the enzyme(s) and the amount of enzyme present. Recall that the rate of metabolism can be expressed as the product of hepatic clearance and the blood concentration of the drug. When expressed in terms of intrinsic clearance, the rate of metabolism is equal to the product of intrinsic clearance and the drug concentration driving metabolism, the unbound drug concentration in the liver (Ch_u). The most common model used to develop an equation for the extraction ratio is the well-stirred venous equilibrium model [26]. This model is presented below for interested students.

Well-Stirred Venous Equilibrium Model
The well-stirred venous equilibrium model (Figure 5.11) assumes the following:

1. Steady state conditions apply. Distributional equilibrium has been achieved. Thus, the drug concentration in the tissues does not change.
2. The spaces within the liver are "well stirred": the drug concentration in the hepatocyte is uniform as is that in the blood in the liver.
3. Because of steady state conditions, the drug concentration in the liver does not change and any difference in the arterial and venous blood concentrations as the blood flows through the liver is the result of metabolism.

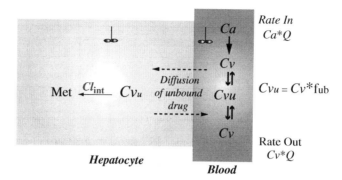

FIGURE 5.11   The well-stirred venous equilibrium model. The system is at steady state. The only loss of drug from the blood as it passes through the liver is the result of metabolism. Both the hepatocyte and blood are well-stirred spaces. The unbound drug concentration in the hepatocyte is equal to that in the venous blood. The unbound drug concentration in venous blood is equal to $Cv * fu_b$.

Thus,

Rate of metabolism = Rate of drug presentation to liver − Rate of drug exit from the liver

$$Cl_{int} * Chu = QCa − QCv \tag{5.49}$$

Distribution and redistribution are driven by the diffusion of the unbound drug and occur very quickly. As a result, the drug in the liver is in equilibrium with that in the venous blood leaving the liver (venous equilibrium), and the unbound concentrations in these two spaces are equal.

Thus,

$$Ch_u = Cv * fub \tag{5.50}$$

Where fub is the unbound fraction in blood. Substituting for Ch_u into equation (5.49)

$$Cl_{int} * Cv * fub = QCa − QCv \tag{5.51}$$

Rearranging

$$\frac{Cv}{Ca} = \frac{Q}{Q + Cl_{int} * fub} \tag{5.52}$$

The ratio Cv/Ca is the fraction of the drug entering the liver that leaves in the venous blood (fraction escaping metabolism). Thus, $1-(Cv/Ca)$ is the fraction of the drug extracted during the pass through the liver: the extraction ratio (E):

$$E = 1 - \frac{Cv}{Ca} = 1 - \frac{Q}{Q + Cl_{int} * fub} = \frac{Q + Cl_{int} * fub - Q}{Q + Cl_{int} * fub} = \frac{Cl_{int} * fub}{Q + Cl_{int} * fub}$$

In summary,

$$E = \frac{Cl_{\text{int}} * fub}{Q + Cl_{\text{int}} * fub} \qquad (5.53)$$

where Cl_{int} is an intrinsic clearance, fu_b is the fraction of the drug in the blood that is free, and Q is the hepatic blood flow.

Thus, according to the venous equilibrium model as shown in equation (5.53), the extraction ratio is dependent on intrinsic clearance (Cl_{int}), the fraction of the drug in the blood that is free (fu_b), and the hepatic blood flow (Q). Substituting this expression for E into equation (5.48) yields:

$$Clb_h = \frac{Q \cdot fu_b \cdot Cl_{\text{int}}}{Q + fu_b \cdot Cl_{\text{int}}} \qquad (5.54)$$

Hepatic clearance is also a function of intrinsic clearance, the fraction of the drug in the blood that is free, and the hepatic blood flow.

5.4.7.2 Hepatic Bioavailability

Metabolism in the liver also determines the extent of first pass hepatic extraction and the hepatic bioavailability of orally administered drugs. Hepatic bioavailability (Fh) is defined as the fraction of the dose that enters the liver and escapes extraction during its first pass through the liver. The extraction ratio (E) has been defined as the fraction of drug removed by metabolism during a single pass through the liver, so it follows that:

$$Fh = 1 - E$$

It was previously shown [equation (5.52)] above that the fraction of the drug entering the liver that escapes metabolism (Fh) is:

$$Fh = \frac{Q}{Q + fu_b \cdot Cl_{\text{int}}} \qquad (5.55)$$

Thus, hepatic bioavailability is also determined by intrinsic clearance, binding, and hepatic blood flow.

5.4.7.3 Hepatic Oral Clearance

The AUC is an expression of drug exposure. After an oral dose, the AUC is dependent both on Cl_h and Fh. The equation for the AUC after an oral dose has been presented earlier [equation (5.30)] and is shown below (assuming $S = 1$).

$$\frac{Cl}{F} = \frac{Dose_{po}}{AUC} \qquad (5.30)$$

Consideration of equation (5.30) demonstrates that after an oral dose, exposure is dependent both on hepatic clearance and hepatic bioavailability. Collectively, Cl_h/Fh is known as hepatic oral clearance and an expression for it can be obtained by dividing equation (5.54) by equation (5.55):

$$\frac{Clb_h}{Fh} = fu_b \cdot Cl_{int} \tag{5.56}$$

Equation (5.56) demonstrates that hepatic oral clearance and drug exposure from an oral dose are dependent only on intrinsic clearance and binding. If, for example, intrinsic clearance decreases, oral clearance will decrease proportionally and the AUC will increase in inverse proportion to the decrease in intrinsic clearance.

5.4.7.4 Sensitivity to Changes in Blood Flow Intrinsic Clearance and Binding: Nonrestrictive and Restrictive Clearance

Hepatic clearance and hepatic bioavailability are both dependent on hepatic blood flow, intrinsic clearance, and protein binding. Any one of these determinants may change under certain circumstances. For example, diseases such as hepatic cirrhosis and acute viral hepatitis are associated with decreases and increases, respectively, in hepatic blood flow. Inhibitors and inducers of the drug-metabolizing enzymes can alter intrinsic clearance, and concomitant medications can alter binding. It is important to be able to predict how these changes will affect hepatic clearance, bioavailability, and by extension a drug's pharmacokinetics and exposure. The factors controlling hepatic clearance, hepatic bioavailability, and oral hepatic clearance are expressed in equations (5.54), (5.55), and (5.56), respectively.

Equation (5.56) clearly demonstrates that a change in intrinsic clearance or the unbound fraction will result in proportional changes in Clb_h/Fh (oral hepatic clearance). It is not clear, however, from equations (5.54) and (5.55), how hepatic clearance and bioavailability will be individually affected. This is most conveniently addressed by considering drugs with extreme values of the extraction ratio. Drugs that have extraction ratios greater than 0.7 are considered high extraction drugs, and those with values less than 0.3 are considered low extraction drugs. Table 5.6 shows some examples of high and low extraction drugs as well as others that have intermediate values.

High Extraction: Nonrestrictive Clearance (Flow Dependent)   If a drug has a very high intrinsic clearance, the liver possesses an exceptional ability to metabolize the drug and can metabolize almost all that is presented to it in the blood. The hepatic clearance of high extraction drugs is not limited or restricted by processes in the liver. It is limited only by the delivery of drug to the liver (hepatic blood flow). If hepatic blood flow increases or decreases, the hepatic clearance will increase and decrease, respectively. Because the liver has excess capability to metabolize the drug it receives, small changes in the activity of the drug-metabolizing enzymes or intrinsic clearance (Cl_{int}) will essentially have no impact on overall clearance. Since clearance will not change, the half-life of high extraction drugs

TABLE 5.6   Examples of High, Low, and Intermediate Extraction Drugs [27]

Nonrestrictive Clearance High Extraction ($E > 0.7$)	Intermediate Extraction ($0.7 > E > 0.3$)	Restrictive Clearance Low Extraction ($E < 0.3$)
Metoprolol	Desipramine	Naproxen
Naloxone	Midazolam	Diazepam
Nifedipine	Codeine	Warfarin
Propranolol	Quinidine	Theophylline

TABLE 5.7   Values of Intrinsic Clearance and Fraction Unbound. The Table Shows Values for a High Extraction Drug (Propranolol), a Medium Extraction Drug (Desipramine) and a Low Extraction (Diazepam) Drug [27]

	Propranolol	Desipramine	Diazepam
Cl_{int} (mL/min)	31,780	11,690	1260
fu	0.16	0.16	0.04
E^a	0.77	0.6	0.03
Cl_{int} * fub (mL/min)	5085	2221	36

[a]The extraction ratio is calculated using Cl_{int} * $fub/(Q + Cl_{int}$ * $fub)$, and a hepatic blood flow of 1500 mL/min.

will not change in the presence of a modifier of Cl_{int}. Also, protein binding has little impact on clearance because any protein-bound drug is rapidly stripped from its binding site and metabolized.

Addressing this mathematically. Hepatic blood flow is much less than the product of intrinsic clearance and the fraction unbound. Thus, $Q \ll fu_b \cdot Cl_{int}$, and as a result the denominator in equation (5.54) simplifies: $Q + fu_b \cdot Cl_{int} \approx fu_b \cdot Cl_{int}$, giving:

$$Clb_h = \frac{Q \cdot fu_b \cdot Cl_{int}}{fu_b \cdot Cl_{int}} \approx Q \qquad (5.57)$$

This concept is illustrated using propranolol [27] as an example. Table 5.7 shows that it is a high extraction drug ($E = 0.77$) with a large intrinsic clearance. The value of fu_b * Cl_{int} for propranolol is 5085 mL/min, which is much greater than hepatic blood flow (1500 mL/min).

High extraction drugs have very poor bioavailability ($E > 0.7$ so $Fh < 0.3$), and oral doses will need to be much greater than intravenous doses. Because E is large and Fh is low, small changes in extraction will be magnified at the level of hepatic bioavailability. For example, let $E = 0.9$ and $Fh = 0.1$. Assume a small reduction of about 10% in extraction to 0.8. This would result in an increase in Fh from 0.1 to 0.2, which effectively doubles the dose. Thus, the hepatic bioavailability of high extraction drugs, in contrast to their hepatic clearance, is sensitive to changes in intrinsic clearance and protein binding as well as hepatic blood flow. As shown in equation (5.55), hepatic bioavailability will increase if intrinsic clearance or the unbound fraction decreases.

Changes in intrinsic clearance for high extraction drugs given intravenously will have a negligible effect on exposure and the AUC because hepatic clearance is unchanged. However, as discussed previously, based on equation (5.56), after oral administration, Clb_h/Fh will change in direct proportion to changes in intrinsic clearance. It can now be concluded that for high extraction drugs, this effect is primarily the result of increased bioavailability.

Low Extraction: Restrictive Clearance (System Dependent)   If a drug has a very low intrinsic clearance ($E < 0.3$), the liver enzymes possess only a poor or almost negligible ability to metabolize it. The system can only metabolize a small fraction of the drug delivered. Hepatic clearance is limited or restricted by the activity of the drug-metabolizing enzymes and by the extent to which the drugs bind to the plasma proteins. As a result, if, for example, intrinsic clearance decreased because of enzyme inhibition, hepatic clearance would decrease proportionally. The decrease in clearance would translate into an increase in the drug's half-life. The liver is presented with much more drug than it can metabolize. As a result, changes in the liver blood flow (delivery) will not affect the clearance of these drugs, provided that hepatic blood flow is not reduced to such an extent that it affects the oxygenation and function of the hepatocytes.

Low extraction drugs experience minimal first pass extraction and have excellent almost complete hepatic bioavailability. Any changes in hepatic bioavailability as a result of changes in intrinsic clearance, hepatic blood flow, and binding will be so modest that they can be ignored.

Addressing restrictive clearance mathematically. The hepatic blood flow is much greater than the product of intrinsic clearance and the fraction unbound, that is, $Q \gg fu_b \cdot Cl_{int}$, as a result, the denominator in equation (5.54) simplifies: $Q + fu_b \cdot Cl_{int} \approx Q$, giving:

$$Clb_h \approx \frac{Q \cdot fu_b \cdot Cl_{int}}{Q} \approx fu_b \cdot Cl_{int} \tag{5.58}$$

This concept is illustrated using diazepam [27] as an example. Table 5.7 shows that it is a low extraction drug ($E = 0.03$) with a small intrinsic clearance. The value of $fu_b{}^*Cl_{int}$ for diazepam is only 36 mL/min, which is much less than hepatic blood flow (1500 mL/min).

For low extraction drugs, changes in intrinsic clearance will bring about proportional changes in hepatic clearance but have no effect on hepatic bioavailability. Thus, the effect of altered intrinsic clearance will be the same for both intravenously and orally administered drugs. If intrinsic clearance decreases, exposure from both intravenously and orally administered drugs will increase. As discussed previously, based on equation (5.56), after oral administration, Clb_h/Fh will change in direct proportion to changes in intrinsic clearance. It can now be concluded that for low extraction drugs is primarily the result of an approximate proportional change in hepatic clearance with no change bioavailability.

The effects of a reduction in intrinsic clearance on the pharmacokinetics of high and low clearance drugs are summarized in Table 5.8. Note that these effects will also be observed by an increase in binding (a reduction in fu_b). Note that inducers of metabolism and decreased binding (increased fu_b) alter the same parameters as those shown in Table 5.8, but the direction of the change is the opposite. For example, an inducer of metabolism would increase hepatic clearance and decrease both the elimination half-life and the AUC of a restrictively cleared drug.

In summary, the hepatic clearance and hepatic bioavailability of high and low extraction drugs are controlled by hepatic blood flow, intrinsic clearance, and binding within the blood. The hepatic clearance of high extraction drugs is primarily influenced by hepatic blood flow.

TABLE 5.8 Theoretical Effect of a Reduction in Intrinsic Clearance on the Pharmacokinetics of High and Low Extraction Drugs

	High Extraction > 0.7	Low Extraction < 0.3
Cl_h	No change	Reduces proportionally
Fh	Increases in inverse proportion	No change
Cl_h/Fh	Reduces proportionally	Reduces proportionally
$t_{1/2}$	No change	Increases proportionally
Exposure to IV dose-AUC	No change	Increases proportionally
Exposure to PO dose-AUC	Increases proportionally	Increases proportionally

Note, these changes assume that the whole dose of the drug is eliminated by the affected enzymatic pathway. The same changes would be predicted if binding increased (decrease in the fraction bound). Recall $AUC_{IV} = Dose/Cl$ and $AUC_{PO} = Dose/(Cl/F)$.

In contrast, the hepatic clearance of low extraction drugs is primarily determined by intrinsic clearance and binding. The hepatic bioavailability of low extraction drugs is high and relatively insensitive to any changes in the system. In contrast, the hepatic bioavailability of high extraction drugs is very low and highly sensitive to changes in intrinsic clearance, binding, and hepatic blood flow. Changes in intrinsic clearance produce proportional changes in the Clb_h/Fh of all drugs given orally. For high extraction drugs, this is the result of an effect on hepatic bioavailability while for low extraction drugs, it is the result of altered hepatic clearance.

Drugs with Mid-Range Extraction Ratios   Although many therapeutic drugs have extraction ratios at the extreme ends of the spectrum, there are some drugs that have intermediate values of the extraction ratio (Table 5.6). For example, Table 5.7 shows that the extraction ratio of desipramine is around 0.6 and $Cl_{int} * fu_b$ is about 2221 mL/min, which is approaching the value of hepatic blood flow. As the extraction ratio increases beyond 0.3, the properties of the drugs gradually change from those typical of low, to those of high extraction drugs. Thus, in the presence of an enzyme inhibitor, for example, there will be a gradual shift from an effect on hepatic clearance to an effect on hepatic bioavailability. In parallel, the drug's half-life will become less and less affected by the changes in intrinsic clearance.

The concepts presented in this section are also addressed in the simulation model below.

5.4.7.5 *Simulation Model For Hepatic Clearance:*
http://web.uri.edu/pharmacy/research/rosenbaum/sims
(Open simulation model 3, Hepatic Clearance, which can be found at (http://web.uri.edu/pharmacy/research/rosenbaum/sims/Model3). The model has been created to demonstrate how intrinsic clearance, protein binding, and hepatic blood flow control the pharmacokinetics of high, low, and intermediate extraction ratio drugs. The model assumes a hepatic blood flow of 88.2 L/h and the following drug parameters: fe = 0; ka = 1.8 h^{-1}; Fa = 1; Fg = 1; fu = 0.1; BP = 1; Dose = 400 mg. In order to avoid wide variations in the half-lives among different simulations, a Vd of 200 and 20 L was used for values of Cl$_{int}$ greater than and less than 500 mL/min, respectively.

The model will simulate plasma concentrations after oral and intravenous administration and display the values of the following: Cl (note fe = 0, therefore Cl = Clh), Fh; Clh/Fh; AUC$_{po}$; AUC$_{iv}$; and t1/2.

1. ***Effect of Changes in Enzyme Activity (Altered Intrinsic Clearance).***

   1.A. Low Extraction Drugs. Select a Cl$_{int}$ of 10 L/h. Perform a run.

       i.   *Note, the extraction ratio is 0.01, which defines this as a low extraction drug.*

       ii.   *Record E, Cl, Fh, Cl/Fh; AUC$_{po}$, AUC$_{iv}$; and the half-life.*

       iii.   *Switch on "Reduce Cl$_{int}$ by 50%." Perform a simulation and note the change in the plasma concentration profiles after oral and intravenous administration, the changes in the half-life, E, Cl, Fh, Cl/Fh; AUC$_{po}$ and AUC$_{iv}$.*

       iv.   *Reset the model to its default parameters*

   1.B. High Extraction Drugs. Set the values of intrinsic clearance to 7000 L/h. Perform a run and note the extraction ratio is 0.89, which defines this as high extraction. Repeat steps ii. through iv. above.

1.C. Intermediate Extraction Drugs. Repeat the exercise for an intermediate extraction by setting Cl_{int} to 800 L/h, which gives an extraction ratio of 0.48.

Note for all three types of drugs, the AUC after oral administration doubled in response to the 50% reduction in intrinsic clearance. This was associated with a 50% reduction in oral clearance (Cl/Fh). For the low extraction drug, this was associated with an approximate proportional fall in clearance and an almost doubling of the half-life and the AUC. Hepatic bioavailability was not affected. Also note the AUC after IV administration almost doubled too. In contrast, for the high extraction drug, there was minimal change in clearance, the half-life, and the AUC after IV administration. After oral administration, however, the bioavailability and the AUC approximately doubled. The findings for the intermediate extraction drug fall between those of the low and high extraction drugs. As with all the drugs, the AUC after oral administration doubled, but Cl decreased by about 36%, and the half-life increased by 50%.

2. Effect of Changes in Protein Binding

Repeat the above exercise but instead of altering Cl_{int} alter binding using the "Reduce fu by 50%" button. Compare the pharmacokinetics parameters of the low, high, and intermediate extraction ratio drugs in the presence of altered binding.

Note the same results are obtained when the fraction unbound falls by 50% as when intrinsic clearance fell by 50%.

3. Effect of Changes in Hepatic Blood Flow

Repeat the first exercise again, but this time observe the pharmacokinetics changes when hepatic blood flow is reduced using the "Reduce Q by 50%" button. Compare the sensitivities of the low, high, and intermediate extraction ratio drugs to changes in hepatic blood flow.

Note that there is little change in the AUC and the pharmacokinetic parameters of low extraction drugs. For high extraction drugs, the clearance falls approximately in proportional to the fall in hepatic blood flow, and the half-life and the AUC_{IV} doubled. Note, although the Cp-time profile is different, the AUC_{po} does not change in response to the reduction in blood flow. This is because although the clearance falls by about 50%, the bioavailability also falls by about the same amount. As a result, there is no change in the AUC, but note the changes in the plasma concentration–time profile after oral administration. The observed fall in Cmax reflects the fall in bioavailability. Again the properties of drugs with intermediate extraction ratios fall between those of the high and low extraction drugs.

5.4.7.6 Relationship between Clearance and Michaelis–Menten Parameters

As presented in Section 5.4.6, the kinetics of drug metabolism are most commonly expressed using the Michaelis–Menten model. The therapeutic concentrations of most drugs are well below their K_m, and metabolism approximates a first-order process:

$$\text{Rate of Metabolism} = \frac{V \max}{K_m} * Ch_u \tag{5.59}$$

where Ch_u is the unbound drug concentration at the enzyme site.

Approaching metabolism from a clearance concepts perspective:

$$\text{Rate of Metabolism} = Cl_{int} * Ch_u \tag{5.60}$$

where Cl_{int} is the unbound intrinsic clearance of a drug. Equating equations (5.59) and (5.60), it follows therefore:

$$Cl_{int} = \frac{V\max}{K_m} \qquad (5.61)$$

Thus, intrinsic clearance is a function of a drug's maximum rate of metabolism, which is controlled by the amount of enzyme present, and the drug's K_m, which is an inverse measure of the drug's affinity for the enzyme.

5.4.7.7 Relationship between Blood and Plasma Hepatic Clearance

The model for the extraction ratio is based on blood and not on plasma concentrations of the drug. This is because a drug is presented to the liver in the blood, which gives the liver the opportunity to clear the entire amount of drug in the blood, not just that in the plasma. As a result, the model provides an expression for the blood clearance (Clb_h) of drugs. Clinically, because plasma concentrations, and not blood concentrations, are measured routinely, hepatic plasma clearance (Cl_h) and not blood clearance is used almost universally. Plasma clearance is the clearance that is most commonly measured in clinical studies, the clearance reported in the literature, and the clearance that is used to calculate dosing regimens. It is the clearance inferred when the term *hepatic clearance* without qualification is used. What is the relationship between blood and plasma clearance? Blood clearance and plasma clearance are the constants of proportionality between the rate of metabolism, and the blood and plasma concentrations, respectively:

$$\text{rate of metabolism} = Clb_h \cdot Cb \qquad (5.62)$$
$$\text{rate of metabolism} = Cl_h \cdot Cp \qquad (5.63)$$

Equating equations (5.62) and (5.63) and rearranging give:

$$Cl_h = \frac{Clb_h * C_b}{Cp} \qquad (5.64)$$

or

$$Cl_h = Clb_h * BP \qquad (5.65)$$

where BP is the drug's blood to plasma concentration ratio (C_b/Cp).

The model for hepatic clearance also expresses binding in terms of the fraction unbound in the blood (fu_b) rather than the more commonly determined and reported fraction unbound in the plasma (fu) value. On the basis that the unbound drug concentrations in the plasma and blood are the same:

$$fu = C_b * fu_b$$
$$fu_b = {fu}/{BP} \qquad (5.66)$$

The relationship between plasma and blood clearance (and fu and fu_b) depends on how a drug distributes between plasma and the cellular elements of the blood. If a drug distributes evenly throughout the blood, the plasma and blood concentrations will be about the same ($BP = 1$) and plasma and blood clearances will also be about the same. If a drug is unable to penetrate the cells of the blood and is concentrated in the plasma ($BP < 1$), according to equation (5.65), blood clearance will be greater than plasma clearance. Conversely, if a drug

TABLE 5.9   Determination of the Extraction Ratio from Blood Clearance[a]

	Drug 1	Drug 2
Cl_h	900	900
BP	2	0.7
Clb_h	450	1286
$E: (Clb_h/Q)$	0.3	0.86
Type of clearance	Restrictive	Nonrestrictive

[a]Cl_h and Clb_h are hepatic clearances based on plasma and blood, respectively. The calculation of E assumes a hepatic blood flow of 1.5 L/min.

concentrates in red blood cells, the blood concentration of the drug will be higher than that of the plasma ($BP > 1$) and plasma clearance will be greater than blood clearance. For most drugs, BP is between about 0.3 and 2. For example, the BPs for midazolam, alprazolam, and cylcosporine are 0.653, 0.85, and 1.36, respectively.

Oral hepatic clearance [see equation (5.56)] can also be expressed using hepatic plasma clearance by substituting Cl_h for Clb_h using equation (5.56) and fu for fu_b using equation (5.66). Accordingly:

$$\frac{Cl_h}{Fh} = Cl_{int} * fu \tag{5.67}$$

Clinically, blood clearance is rarely used. It is, however, important to use blood clearance in calculations to estimate an extraction ratio, and to back calculate a drug's intrinsic from a drug's hepatic clearance. For example, consider two hypothetical drugs (drugs 1 and 2) shown in Table 5.9, each has a hepatic clearance (plasma clearance) of 900 mL/min. Given that hepatic blood flow is about 1.5 L/min, it might be tempting to assume that they both have high extraction ratios and that both undergo nonrestrictive clearance. However, as can be seen in Table 5.9, when their respective blood clearances are determined, drug 1, which concentrates in the cellular elements of blood, in fact has a small blood clearance and extraction ratio, and its hepatic clearance would be classified as restrictive.

The value of a drug's intrinsic clearance can also be estimated by back calculation from its hepatic clearance. Blood clearance and not plasma clearance must be used for the calculation. Equation (5.54) demonstrated:

$$Cl_{h,b} = \frac{Q * Cl_{int} * fu_b}{Q + Cl_{int} * fu_b} \tag{5.54}$$

The relationship between plasma and blood clearance was given in equation (5.65):

$$Cl_h = Clb_h * BP \tag{5.65}$$

and the relationship between the unbound fractions in the blood and plasma was given in equation (5.66)

$$fu_b = {fu}/{BP} \tag{5.66}$$

Substituting these expressions for Cl_b and fu_b into equation (5.54) gives

$$Cl_h = \frac{Q * Cl_{int} * fu/BP}{Q + Cl_{int} * fu/BP} * BP = \frac{Q * Cl_{int} * fu}{Q + Cl_{int} * fu/BP}$$

Rearranging for Cl_{int} gives

$$Cl_{int} = \frac{Q * Cl_h}{fu(Q - Cl_h/BP)} \tag{5.68}$$

Example. Mitsui *et al.* 2014 [28] reported that midazolam has the following parameters: hepatic clearance (plasma) = 332 mL/min, BP = 0.653, and fu = 0.016. Calculate midazolam's intrinsic clearance.

Substituting values into equation (5.68) and using 1500 mL/min as hepatic blood flow give.

$$Cl_{int} = \frac{1500 * 332}{0.016 * (1500 - 332/0.653)} = 31,390 \, \text{mL/min}$$

The value of a drug's hepatic bioavailability can also be calculated from intrinsic clearance using equation (5.55) which is reproduced below.

$$F_h = \frac{Q}{Q + Cl_{int} \cdot fu_b}$$

Example. Using the data presented above, calculate midazolam's hepatic bioavailability

$$F_h = \frac{1500}{1500 + 31,390 * 0.016/0.653} = 0.66$$

PROBLEMS

5.1 Clearance is defined as a constant for a drug, but as a biological parameter it is expected to vary somewhat from patient to patient. Beyond this, what factors might cause a patient to have a clearance value that is either much greater than or much less than the population average value for a drug?

5.2 Gentamicin is eliminated almost completely in the kidneys ($fe > 0.9$), and its elimination half-life is about 2–3 h. Its elimination half-life is determined in a patient and found to be more than double the average value in the population. Suggest some potential explanations.

5.3 A drug that binds to the plasma proteins ($fu = 0.7$) has a total body clearance of 500 mL/min, and 75% of a dose is excreted unchanged.

(a) Calculate the drug's renal clearance.

(b) Calculate the drug's nonrenal clearance.

(c) Discuss possible processes in the kidney involved in its excretion.

(d) How may its excretion be modified?

5.4 A 36-year-old man who is 5 feet 11 inches tall is receiving a constant infusion of a drug. The steady-state plasma concentration is constant at 6 mcg/L. Over a 24-h period, 1200 mL of urine is collected. The drug concentration in the urine is

1.44 µg/mL. Calculate the drug's renal clearance in this patient. The drug does not bind to plasma proteins. Discuss the processes involved in the renal excretion of this drug.

5.5 Urine was collected over a 24-h period for a 32-year-old male patient. Serum creatinine was measured at the end of the collection period. Using the data given, calculate the creatinine clearance in this man. (*Note.* Under normal circumstances, serum creatinine is a constant value.) Assume that creatinine undergoes only renal clearance.

Serum creatinine: 1.1 mg/dL

Volume of urine collected: 1500 mL

Urine creatinine concentration: 140 mg/dL

5.6 A new drug under development has just undergone phase I trials to determine its human pharmacokinetics. These studies have obtained the following information:

$$Cl = 1200 \, \text{mL}/\min \qquad Vd = 25 \, \text{L/kg} \qquad fu = 0.85$$
$$fe = 0.05 \quad BP = 1 \quad \log D_{7.4} = 2$$

The drug is also a potent competitive inhibitor of CYP2D6. Discuss the drug's pharmacokinetics with particular reference to:

(a) Type of clearance: renal/hepatic and restrictive/nonrestrictive.

(b) Expected bioavailability.

(c) Distribution characteristics.

(d) Elimination half-life.

(e) Susceptibility to drug interactions from modifiers of drug metabolism.

(f) How long would it take after discontinuation of therapy for its inhibition of CYP2D6 to cease?

5.7 The volume of distribution of acetaminophen is about 1.0 L/kg in adults, and it is about 20% bound to plasma proteins. Almost all administered dose is metabolized by liver, primarily by glucuronidation and sulfation. The extraction ratio (E) of acetaminophen is 0.20 and its intrinsic clearance has been found to be about 6 mL/min/kg (see [29]). Estimate acetaminophen's half-life in a 70-kg adult after the administration of a 350-mg dose given as a suspension. Assume that the BP for acetaminophen is 1.

5.8 A drug has a hepatic clearance (plasma) of 900 mL/min. It concentrates in red blood cells, and its BP is 3.33. Assume that the hepatic blood flow is 1.5 L/min.

(a) What is the drug's extraction ratio?

(b) Does this drug undergo restrictive or nonrestrictive clearance?

5.9 Felodipine has the following characteristics: hepatic clearance = 770 mL/min, BP = 0.680, and $fu = 0.0.004$. Use 1500 mL/min for hepatic blood flow.

(a) Calculate its hepatic extraction ratio.

(b) Calculate its intrinsic clearance.

(c) Calculate its hepatic bioavailability.

5.10 Alprazolam has the following characteristics: total body clearance (plasma) = 73.5 mL/min, renal clearance 18.2 mL/min, BP = 0.818, and $fu = 0.268$. Calculate its hepatic intrinsic clearance. Use 1500 mL/min for hepatic blood flow.

5.11 Separate clinical studies were conducted on lipoamide, nosolatol, and disolvprazole. Each drug was administered as an intravenous dose to different groups of
healthy volunteers. Blood samples were obtained at various times after the dose.
Plasma samples were prepared and frozen until they could be analyzed for unchanged
drug. The data from a single patient for each drug are provided in Table P5.11.
Use the directions provided in Appendix C to create an Excel worksheet to determine the AUC and clearance of lipoamide, nosolatol, and disolvprazole in these
subjects.

**TABLE P5.11   Plasma Concentrations of Lipoamide, Nosolatol, and Disolvprazole After
Intravenous Doses**

Lipoamide		Nosolatol		Disolvprazole	
T (h)	Cp (µg/L)	T (h)	Cp (µg/L)	T (h)	Cp (µg/L)
0	23.8	0	476	0	286
0.5	22.1	0.5	462	0.2	266
1	20.5	1	448	0.4	249
1.5	19	1.5	435	0.8	216
2	17.6	2	422	1	202
3	15.2	2.5	409	1.2	188
5	11.3	5	352	1.6	163
7.5	7.82	8	294	2	142
10	5.39	12	231	3	100
15	2.57	15	193	5	50
20	1.22	20	143	8	18
24	0.68	24	112	12	4

The doses of lipoamide, nosolatol, and disolvprazole were 10, 100, and 10 mg,
respectively.

5.12 A 10-mg intravenous dose of disolvprazole was administered to a 70-kg male patient
with slight renal impairment. Urine was collected at various times over a 12-h period,
and the plasma concentration was measured at the midpoint of each collection period.
The data are given in Table P5.12. Use the data to calculate disolvprazole's renal
clearance in this patient.

**TABLE P5.12   Urinary and Plasma Concentrations of Disolvprazole
After a 10-mg Dose in a Patient with Renal Impairment**

Urine Data		Plasma Data	
Collection Period (h)	Amount Excreted (mg)	Time (h) (Midpoint of Urine Collection Period)	Cp (µg/L)
0–1	2.5	0.5	275
1–3	3.25	2	177
3–9	3.48	6	58
9–12	0.39	10.5	15

5.13   Lipoamide ($fe < 0.01$) and nosolatol ($fe < 0.01$) are potentially both subject to drug interactions when they are administered with ketoconazole. Use the clearance values calculated in Problem 5.11 to determine the type of hepatic clearance that these drugs display. Predict how ketoconazole may affect their pharmacokinetics after intravenous and oral administration. Complete details are given in Table P5.13.

TABLE P5.13   Predicted Effect of Ketoconazole on the Pharmacokinetics of Lipoamide and Nosolatol

	Lipoamide		Nosolatol	
Type of hepatic clearance				
	IV	PO	IV	PO
AUC				
F				
Cl				
$t_{1/2}$				

Note: Answers may be checked in Chapter 10, where data are provided for analysis of drug interaction studies on these two drugs.

5.14   Discuss how the pharmacokinetics of lipoamide, nosolatol, and disolvprazole may be affected by:

(a) Renal disease

(b) Hepatic disease

5.15   About 80% of a dose of theophylline is metabolized by CYP2D6. It has a total body clearance (plasma) of 2.73 L/h, the fraction unbound is 0.44.

(a) Calculate theophylline's clearance (plasma) for the CYP2D6 pathway.

(b) Using theophylline's *BP* of 0.85, calculate the blood clearance for the CYP2D6 pathway.

(c) Calculate the intrinsic clearance of the CYP2D6 pathway. Use 88.2 L/h for hepatic blood flow.

5.16   The hepatic clearance, *BP*, and fu for S-warfarin were reported as 4.20 mL/min, 0.55 and 0.01, respectively [27]. Calculate the intrinsic clearance of S-warfarin. Use 88.2 L/h for hepatic blood flow.

5.17   Desipramine is primarily (0.85%) metabolized along a CYP2D6 pathway. If the intrinsic clearance for this pathway is 1564 L/h:

(a) Calculate the blood hepatic clearance for the CYP2D6 pathway. Use 88.2 L/h for hepatic blood flow and 0.96 for desipramine's *BP* and 0.18 for the fraction unbound in the plasma, respectively.

(b) Calculate the plasma clearance for this pathway.

REFERENCES

1. Williams, J. A., Hyland, R., Jones, B. C., Smith, D. A., Hurst, S., Goosen, T. C., Peterkin, V., Koup, J. R., and Ball, S. E. (2004) Drug-drug interactions for UDP-glucuronosyltransferase

substrates: a pharmacokinetic explanation for typically observed low exposure (AUCi/AUC) ratios, *Drug Metab Dispos*, 32, 1201–1208.

2. Morrissey, K. M., Stocker, S. L., Wittwer, M. B., Xu, L., and Giacomini, K. M. (2013) Renal transporters in drug development, *Annu Rev Pharmacol Toxicol*, 53, 503–529.

3. Ganong, W. F. (1985) *Review of Medical Physiology*, pp. 581–606, Appleton and Lange, Norwalk.

4. Ho, R. H., and Kim, R. B. (2005) Transporters and drug therapy: implications for drug disposition and disease, *Clin Pharmacol Ther*, 78, 260–277.

5. Kusuhara, H., and Sugiyama, Y. (2009) In vitro-in vivo extrapolation of transporter-mediated clearance in the liver and kidney, *Drug Metab Pharmacokinet*, 24, 37–52.

6. Choi, M. K., and Song, I. S. (2008) Organic cation transporters and their pharmacokinetic and pharmacodynamic consequences, *Drug Metab Pharmacokinet*, 23, 243–253.

7. Lepist, E. I., and Ray, A. S. (2012) Renal drug-drug interactions: what we have learned and where we are going, *Expert Opin Drug Metab Toxicol*, 8, 433–448.

8. Gutierrez, F., Fulladosa, X., Barril, G., and Domingo, P. (2014) Renal tubular transporter-mediated interactions of HIV drugs: implications for patient management, *AIDS Rev*, 16, 199–212.

9. Yasui-Furukori, N., Uno, T., Sugawara, K., and Tateishi, T. (2005) Different effects of three transporting inhibitors, verapamil, cimetidine, and probenecid, on fexofenadine pharmacokinetics, *Clin Pharmacol Ther*, 77, 17–23.

10. Liu, S., Beringer, P. M., Hidayat, L., Rao, A. P., Louie, S., Burckart, G. J., and Shapiro, B. (2008) Probenecid, but not cystic fibrosis, alters the total and renal clearance of fexofenadine, *J Clin Pharmacol*, 48, 957–965.

11. Wienkers, L. C., and Heath, T. G. (2005) Predicting in vivo drug interactions from in vitro drug discovery data, *Nat Rev Drug Discov*, 4, 825–833.

12. Daly, A. K. (2006) Significance of the minor cytochrome P450 3A isoforms, *Clin Pharmacokinet*, 45, 13–31.

13. Pelkonen, O., Turpeinen, M., Hakkola, J., Honkakoski, P., Hukkanen, J., and Raunio, H. (2008) Inhibition and induction of human cytochrome P450 enzymes: current status, *Arch Toxicol*, 82, 667–715.

14. Court, M. H. (2010) Interindividual variability in hepatic drug glucuronidation: studies into the role of age, sex, enzyme inducers, and genetic polymorphism using the human liver bank as a model system, *Drug Metab Rev*, 42, 202–217.

15. Kiang, T. K., Ensom, M. H., and Chang, T. K. (2005) UDP-glucuronosyltransferases and clinical drug-drug interactions. *Pharmacol Ther*, 106, 97–132.

16. Division of Clinical Pharmacology Indiana University. (2016) P450 Drug Interaction Table, http://medicine.iupui.edu/clinpharm/ddis/main-table/.

17. Rendic, S. (2002) Summary of information on human CYP enzymes: human P450 metabolism data, *Drug Metab Rev*, 34, 83–448.

18. Rendic, S., and Guengerich, F. P. (2010) Update information on drug metabolism systems–2009, part II: summary of information on the effects of diseases and environmental factors on human cytochrome P450 (CYP) enzymes and transporters, *Curr Drug Metab*, 11, 4–84.

19. Terada, T., and Hira, D. (2015) Intestinal and hepatic drug transporters: pharmacokinetic, pathophysiological, and pharmacogenetic roles, *J Gastroenterol*, 50, 508–519.

20. Generaux, G. T., Bonomo, F. M., Johnson, M., and Doan, K. M. (2011) Impact of SLCO1B1 (OATP1B1) and ABCG2 (BCRP) genetic polymorphisms and inhibition on LDL-C lowering and myopathy of statins, *Xenobiotica*, 41, 639–651.

21. Link, E., Parish, S., Armitage, J., Bowman, L., Heath, S., Matsuda, F., Gut, I., Lathrop, M., and Collins, R. (2008) SLCO1B1 variants and statin-induced myopathy–a genomewide study, *N Engl J Med*, 359, 789–799.

22. Pasanen, M. K., Neuvonen, M., Neuvonen, P. J., and Niemi, M. (2006) SLCO1B1 polymorphism markedly affects the pharmacokinetics of simvastatin acid, *Pharmacogenet Genomics*, *16*, 873–879.

23. Funk, C. (2008) The role of hepatic transporters in drug elimination, *Expert Opin Drug Metab Toxicol*, *4*, 363–379.

24. Jung, N., Lehmann, C., Rubbert, A., Knispel, M., Hartmann, P., van Lunzen, J., Stellbrink, H. J., Faetkenheuer, G., and Taubert, D. (2008) Relevance of the organic cation transporters 1 and 2 for antiretroviral drug therapy in human immunodeficiency virus infection, *Drug Metab Dispos*, *36*, 1616–1623.

25. Yoshida, K., Maeda, K., and Sugiyama, Y. (2013) Hepatic and intestinal drug transporters: prediction of pharmacokinetic effects caused by drug-drug interactions and genetic polymorphisms, *Annu Rev Pharmacol Toxicol*, *53*, 581–612.

26. Wilkinson, G. R., and Shand, D. G. (1975) Commentary: a physiological approach to hepatic drug clearance, *Clin Pharmacol Ther*, *18*, 377–390.

27. Brown, H. S., Griffin, M., and Houston, J. B. (2007) Evaluation of cryopreserved human hepatocytes as an alternative in vitro system to microsomes for the prediction of metabolic clearance, *Drug Metab Dispos*, *35*, 293–301.

28. Mitsui, T., Nemoto, T., Miyake, T., Nagao, S., Ogawa, K., Kato, M., Ishigai, M., and Yamada, H. (2014) A useful model capable of predicting the clearance of cytochrome 3A4 (CYP3A4) substrates in humans: validity of CYP3A4 transgenic mice lacking their own Cyp3a enzymes, *Drug Metab Dispos*, *42*, 1540–1547.

29. Naritomi, Y., Terashita, S., Kagayama, A., and Sugiyama, Y. (2003) Utility of hepatocytes in predicting drug metabolism: comparison of hepatic intrinsic clearance in rats and humans in vivo and in vitro, *Drug Metab Dispos*, *31*, 580–588.

6

COMPARTMENTAL MODELS IN PHARMACOKINETICS

Sara E. Rosenbaum

Objectives

The material in this chapter will enable the reader to:

1. Understand how compartment models can be used to simplify drug disposition

Basic Pharmacokinetics and Pharmacodynamics: An Integrated Textbook and Computer Simulations,
Second Edition. Edited by Sara E. Rosenbaum.
© 2017 John Wiley & Sons, Inc. Published 2017 by John Wiley & Sons, Inc.

2. Apply the compartmental concept to develop pharmacokinetic models
3. Write equations to express how the amount of drug in a compartment will change with time

6.1 INTRODUCTION

Pharmacokinetics is the study of the time course of drug concentrations in the body. Usually, the plasma concentrations are the main focus of attention, and, as discussed in Chapter 1, a major goal is to express the time course of the plasma concentrations mathematically.

The plasma concentration of a drug can be viewed as the response over time to the dose of a drug that has been administered. The concentration at any time is controlled by the size of the dose and the processes of drug absorption, distribution, metabolism, and excretion (ADME), which may all be under way at the same time. Thus, the mathematical equation for the time course of the plasma concentrations must incorporate the dose and expressions for the rates of each of these processes. Drug ADME were discussed in detail in the initial chapters of the book, where expressions for each of their rates were presented. Compartmental models allow the dose and the individual processes of ADME to be combined in a logical, straightforward manner to create simple models of a complex physiological system. Mathematical expressions for the effective dose and rate of each of the processes in ADME are first reviewed in this chapter.

6.2 EXPRESSIONS FOR COMPONENT PARTS OF THE DOSE–PLASMA CONCENTRATION RELATIONSHIP

6.2.1 Effective Dose

In pharmacokinetic equations, the dose is referred to as a constant because its value is constant for a given administration. The *effective dose* is defined as the amount of parent drug that reaches the systemic circulation. This may differ from the dose administered for two reasons:

1. *Salt factor.* Many drugs are administered as salts. As such, the dose will consist of pure drug and its conjugate acid or base. For example, phenytoin sodium consists of 92% phenytoin and 8% sodium. Quinidine sulfate consists of 82% quinidine and 18% sulfate. To account for the fact that only a portion (usually a large portion) of a dose administered is pure drug, the dose is adjusted using the *salt factor* (S), defined as the fraction of the salt that is made up of pure drug. Thus, phenytoin sodium and quinidine sulfate have salt factors of 0.92 and 0.82, respectively.

2. *Bioavailability factor.* When drugs are administered by any route other than direct systemic administration (e.g., intravenous route), a portion of the dose may be lost prior to reaching the systemic circulation. In the case of orally administered drugs, some of the dose can be lost at several points during absorption, including destruction in the gastrointestinal fluid, poor membrane penetration, efflux and/or metabolism in the enterocyte, and hepatic first-pass extraction. The fraction of the parent drug that reaches the systemic circulation is the drug's *bioavailability* factor (F).

Overall, the dose reaching the systemic circulation or the effective dose is given by the expression

$$\text{effective dose} = S \cdot F \cdot D \tag{6.1}$$

where S is the salt factor, and F is the bioavailability factor or fraction of the dose administered (D) that reaches the systemic circulation.

Example 6.1 Theophylline is to be administered as its salt aminophylline ($S = 0.8$) in a sustained-release preparation ($F = 0.9$). What is the effective dose from a 400-mg tablet?

Solution

$$\begin{aligned} \text{Effective dose} &= S \cdot F \cdot D \\ &= 0.8 \times 0.9 \times 400 \text{ mg} \\ &= 288 \text{ mg} \end{aligned}$$

Example 6.2 A drug is administered orally as its hydrochloride salt ($S = 0.95$). It is susceptible to acid hydrolysis in the stomach and metabolism by CYP3A4 in the enterocytes and the liver. On average, only about 25% of a dose reaches the systemic circulation. What is the effective dose from a 5-mg tablet?

Solution

$$\begin{aligned} \text{Effective dose} &= S \cdot F \cdot D \\ &= 0.95 \times 0.25 \times 5 = 1.19 \text{ mg} \end{aligned}$$

6.2.2 Rate of Drug Absorption

The process of drug absorption occurs for all routes of administration except for the direct systemic routes, such as intravenous administration. As discussed in Chapter 3, absorption is usually a first-order process. For orally administered drugs, the rate of absorption is a function of the amount of drug in the gastrointestinal tract (A_{GI}), and the first-order rate constant for absorption (k_a) and can be expressed as:

$$\text{rate of absorption} = k_a \cdot A_{GI} \tag{6.2}$$

Absorption may begin as soon as the drug reaches and dissolves in the gastrointestinal fluid. The rate of drug absorption is greatest initially, when there is a lot of drug in the gastrointestinal tract. As drug is absorbed, the amount in the gastrointestinal tract decreases and the rate of absorption decreases proportionally. Eventually, the entire dose is absorbed and the absorption process ceases. At this point, drug absorption no longer has any influence on the plasma concentration–time profile. The time for absorption can be estimated as 3–5 absorption half-lives (where absorption $t_{1/2} = 0.693/k_a$).

The key pharmacokinetic parameters for absorption are the first-order rate constant for absorption (k_a), and the fraction of the dose that reaches the systemic circulation (F). Because the absorption of a drug can be influenced by the manufacturing process and the excipients contained in the dosage form, both k_a and F are dependent on the specific brand of the dosage form. Thus, in contrast to other pharmacokinetic parameters, they are not necessarily constant for a drug. For example, the rate and extent of absorption of cyclosporine differ in the Neoral preparation from those in the Sandimmune preparation. These parameters (F and k_a) can also be affected by anything that influences drug absorption, such as gastrointestinal motility and concomitant medications.

Other models that can be used for the rate of absorption include zero-order absorption, two parallel first-order processes, and a combination of zero- and first-order processes. If necessary, an absorption lag time can be incorporated into the absorption model.

6.2.3 Rate of Drug Elimination

As soon as drug is present in the plasma, the organs of elimination try to eliminate the drug. Elimination is a first-order process and is dependent on the plasma concentration of the drug and the amount of drug in the body. The rate is higher with higher plasma concentrations and lower with smaller plasma concentrations.

Elimination can be expressed as:

$$\text{rate of elimination} = k \cdot Ab \tag{6.3}$$

where k is the overall elimination rate constant, and Ab is the amount of drug in the body. Elimination can also be expressed using clearance:

$$\text{rate of elimination} = Cl \cdot Cp \tag{6.4}$$

where Cl is the total body clearance.

In the above equations, clearance is the primary pharmacokinetic parameter for elimination, and the overall elimination rate constant is the secondary or dependent pharmacokinetic parameter representing the rate of elimination. The elimination rate constant is dependent on the primary parameters of clearance and volume of distribution.

6.2.4 Rate of Drug Distribution

Once in the bloodstream, a drug is able to distribute to the tissues in the body. Some tissues will take up more drug than others, and there may be certain tissues that the drug cannot access at all. As distribution proceeds, the tissue/plasma concentration ratio increases in each tissue. Eventually, a form of equilibrium is achieved, the distribution phase is complete, and the tissue/plasma concentration ratio remains constant. Thereafter, the tissue concentrations and plasma concentration parallel each other. In Chapter 4, it was shown that the initial distribution of drugs is generally a first-order process and that tissue perfusion is an important determinant of the first-order rate constant for distribution. Thus, tissues take up drugs at different rates, depending on their perfusion rates. The physiological approach to pharmacokinetic modeling (see Chapter 18) considers different tissues separately and uses individual tissue perfusion rates to develop models that can then be used to estimate individual tissue concentrations. A simpler approach is adopted, however, in compartmental modeling, where tissues are grouped together based on the rate at which they take up the drug. The groups of tissues constitute a compartment. Thus, a *compartment is an imaginary unit that consists of a group of tissues that display similar rates of drug uptake.*

There are always some tissues, usually the well-perfused tissues, where drug uptake is extremely rapid. These tissues are grouped together. There may be another group of tissues, which take up the drug with similar uptake rates but where the rate is slower than that of the well-perfused tissues. There may be a third group where uptake is exceedingly slow, perhaps because the drug partitions slowly into the tissue(s). In practice, it has been found that the pharmacokinetics of almost all drugs can be described adequately using no more than three compartments; many can be described using two compartments; and when pharmacokinetics are applied to specific clinical situations (e.g., to individualize a dose for a patient), the one-compartment model can usually provide a sufficient degree of accuracy to predict the dose/plasma concentration relationship.

6.3 PUTTING EVERYTHING TOGETHER: COMPARTMENTS AND MODELS

A compartment is an imaginary unit that is used to represent a group of tissues with similar rates of drug distribution. The specific tissues that make up a compartment are unknown, and the number of compartments selected for a particular drug is based on the behavior of the plasma concentrations observed over time. A compartment is a homogeneous unit: *The drug concentration is uniform throughout at all times.*

As mentioned earlier, between one and three compartments are needed to produce the typical types of plasma concentration–time profiles observed clinically. One of the compartments in any model (the only one in a one-compartment model) is the *central compartment*, which always consists of the *plasma and tissues that take up the drug rapidly*. The concentration of drug in the central compartment is always equal to concentration routinely measured *in vivo*, the plasma concentration. One or two additional compartments may have to be added if, based on the behavior of the plasma concentrations, it appears that a significant amount of drug is distributing to some tissues at a slower rate. The organs of drug elimination are well-perfused tissues. Thus, elimination is usually, although not always, assumed to occur from the central compartment. The fundamental characteristics of each of the three compartment models are presented below.

6.3.1 One-Compartment Model

The body is viewed as a single compartment (Figure 6.1a). All the tissues where a drug goes have very rapid rates of drug uptake. The distribution of the drug to the tissues is so rapid that there is no evidence of it when plasma concentrations are observed over time. When

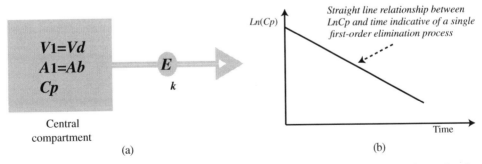

FIGURE 6.1   The one-compartment model. (a) The one-compartment model consists only of a central compartment. Distribution to those tissues that the drug can access occurs rapidly and appears to be an instantaneous process. The compartment is characterized by a volume (V_1), the amount of drug it contains (A_1), and the drug concentration, which is equal to the plasma concentration (Cp). In the one-compartment model, A_1 is equal to the amount of drug in the body (Ab) and V_1 is equal to the drug's volume of distribution (Vd). The first-order rate constant for elimination (E) is k. (b) Semilog plot Cp against time after intravenous administration.

a drug is administered intravenously, even during the initial period after the injection, the plasma concentrations appear only to be influenced by drug elimination and fall monoexponentially (Figure 6.1b). There is no evidence of a distribution phase. Thus, for all intents and purposes, drug distribution can be considered to be instantaneous. The compartment is characterized by a volume, the amount of drug it contains, and the concentration of the drug. In the one-compartment model, these quantities are given the symbols V_1, A_1, and C_1, respectively. However, since the single compartment of the one-compartment model is equivalent to the central compartment, the drug concentration is equal to the plasma concentration ($C_1 = Cp$). In the special case of a one-compartment model, A_1 is equal to the amount of drug in the body (Ab). Also V_1, which is $A_1/Cp =$ Ab/Cp in the one-compartment model, is the drug's volume of distribution (Vd).

6.3.2 Two-Compartment Model

The body is viewed as two compartments: the central and peripheral compartments (Figure 6.2). The *central compartment* consists of the plasma and tissues that take up the drug so rapidly that distribution can be considered to be instantaneous. Other tissues in the body take up the drug at a similar but slower rate than that for the tissues of the central compartment. These tissues constitute the *peripheral compartment*. The volume, amount, and concentration symbols for the peripheral compartment are qualified by the number 2 (e.g., A_2 is the amount of drug in the peripheral compartment) (Figure 6.2). Distribution to the peripheral compartment is modeled as a first-order process driven by the amount of drug in the central compartment, and redistribution of the drug from the peripheral compartment back to the central compartment is also modeled as a first-order process, in this case driven by the amount of drug in the peripheral compartment. The rate constants for distribution and redistribution are appropriately labeled k_{12} and k_{21}, respectively (Figure 6.2). After an intravenous dose, a steep initial fall in the plasma concentration is seen as drug distributes to the peripheral compartment (Figure 6.3a). Many drugs display two-compartmental pharmacokinetics.

6.3.3 Three-Compartment Model

The three-compartment model is an extension of the two-compartment model, where a sizable amount of the drug distributes to certain very poorly perfused tissues, such as fat

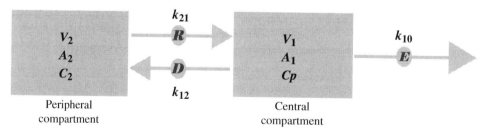

FIGURE 6.2 The two-compartment model. Drug distribution occurs very rapidly in the tissues that make up the central compartment, but the distribution of a significant amount of the drug to other tissues occurs at a noticeably slower rate. The latter tissues make up the peripheral compartment. The volumes (V), amounts (A), and concentrations (C) in each compartment are qualified by 1 and 2 for the central and peripheral compartment, respectively. Drug concentration in the central compartment is equal to the plasma concentration. The rate constants for distribution (D) and redistribution (R) are k_{12} and k_{21}, respectively. The first-order rate constant for elimination (E) is k_{10}.

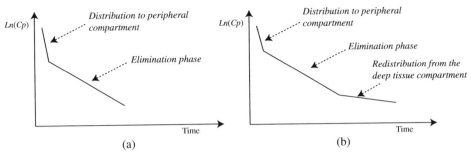

FIGURE 6.3 Plasma concentration–time profiles of the two- (a) and three-compartment (b) models. The main determinants of the different sections of the profiles are shown. After an intravenous injection, distribution to the tissues of the central compartment is essentially instantaneous and is not visible on the profile. Distribution to the peripheral compartment is associated with the steep initial fall in the plasma concentration. This is followed by the elimination phase, where a drug's elimination characteristics control the slope of the fall. In the three-compartment model, a third phase is observed at later times, when the drug in the deep tissue compartment comprises a large fraction of the total drug in the body. At this time, the redistribution of drug from the deep tissue compartment into the plasma controls the fall in the plasma concentration.

and bone, at an extremely slow rate. These tissues make up a third compartment, the *deep tissue compartment*. The volume, amount, and concentration symbols associated with the deep tissue compartment are qualified by the number 3 (Figure 6.4), and the first-order distribution and redistribution rate constants are labeled k_{13} and k_{31}, respectively (Figure 6.4). The three-compartment model has three groups of tissues. The groups of tissues that comprise the central compartment take up the drug very rapidly. There is no evidence of this distribution on the plasma concentration–time profile. Tissues in the peripheral compartment take up the drug more slowly and their distribution is associated with the steep

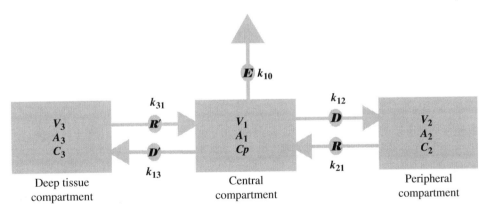

FIGURE 6.4 The three-compartment model. Compared to the two-compartment model, the three-compartment model has an additional compartment that is generally made up of very poorly perfused tissues, such as fat or bone, where distribution proceeds at an extremely slow rate. These tissues comprise the deep tissue compartment. The volumes (V), amounts (A), and concentrations (C) in each compartment are qualified by 1, 2, and 3 for the central, peripheral, and deep tissue compartment, respectively. Drug concentration in the central compartment is equal to the plasma concentration. The rate constants for distribution (D) and redistribution (R) to the peripheral compartment are k_{12} and k_{21}, respectively. The rate constants for distribution (D') and redistribution (R') to the deep tissue compartment are k_{13} and k_{31}, respectively. The first-order rate constant for elimination (E) is k_{10}.

initial fall in the plasma concentration, the distribution phase (Figure 6.4). Following the distribution phase, the fall in the plasma concentrations is controlled by elimination (the elimination phase, Figure 6.3b). The existence of a third group of tissues, the deep tissue compartment, only becomes apparent after a large fraction of the dose has been eliminated and plasma concentrations are very low. The initial distribution of drug to tissues in the third compartment is so slow that it has no discernible influence on the plasma concentrations. The redistribution of drug from this compartment is also slow. But at later times, the drug in this compartment constitutes a very large fraction of the drug in the body, and its redistribution into the plasma controls the fall in plasma concentrations (Figure 6.3b). Digoxin and the aminoglycosides are examples of drugs that display three-compartmental pharmacokinetics. From the model mapped in Figure 6.4, differential equations can readily be written for the rate of change of the amounts in each compartment. The solution of the differential equations and the clinical application of three-compartmental pharmacokinetics can get quite complex.

Selection of the most appropriate model for a given drug is driven by the characteristics of the plasma concentration–time profile. This, in turn, is dependent on the distribution characteristics of the drug and the timing of the plasma samples.

6.4 EXAMPLES OF COMPLETE COMPARTMENT MODELS

The three basic models discussed above can be used to develop models appropriate for any type of drug input or route of administration. Once the type of drug input has been added to a model, equations for the rate of change of the amount of drug in any of the compartments can readily be written. Applying calculus to develop explicit solutions to these expressions, however, can be quite complex. Some examples of complete models and the equations derived from them are provided below.

6.4.1 Intravenous Bolus Injection in a One-Compartment Model with First-Order Elimination

The model for an intravenous injection in a one-compartment model is shown in Figure 6.5. At time zero, the entire dose is placed into the body:

$$Ab_0 = S \cdot F \cdot D \tag{6.5}$$

where Ab_0 is the amount of drug in the body at time zero. Note that $F = 1$ for IV administration. The uptake of drug to those tissues where the drug distributes is so rapid that it can be considered to be instantaneous. Thus, at time zero, the drug is distributed uniformly throughout the homogeneous compartment and

$$Cp_0 = \frac{Ab_0}{Vd} = \frac{S \cdot F \cdot D}{Vd} \tag{6.6}$$

The only process that will influence the plasma concentration is elimination, a first-order process that can be expressed as:

$$\text{rate of elimination} - \frac{dAb}{dt} = k \cdot Ab \tag{6.7}$$

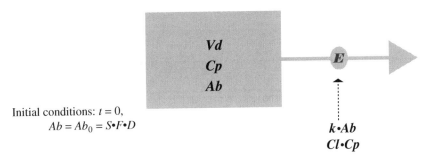

Initial conditions: $t = 0$,
$$Ab = Ab_0 = S \cdot F \cdot D$$

FIGURE 6.5   Model for an intravenous injection in a one-compartment model. The amount of drug in the compartment is equal to the amount of drug in the body (Ab), the concentration of drug in the compartment is equal to the plasma concentration (Cp), and the volume of the compartment (V_1) is equal to the drug's volume of distribution (Vd). Elimination (E) is a first-order process and can be expressed using the first-order elimination rate constant (k) or clearance (Cl). The effective dose is the product of the dose (D), the salt factor (S), and the bioavailability (F). Note that $F = 1$ for IV administration.

or

$$\text{rate of elimination} - \frac{dAb}{dt} = Cl \cdot Cp \qquad (6.8)$$

6.4.2 Intravenous Bolus Injection in a Two-Compartment Model with First-Order Elimination

The model for an intravenous injection in a two-compartment model is shown in Figure 6.6. At time zero, the entire dose is placed into the body. Distribution throughout the tissues that

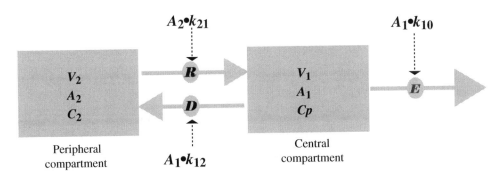

Initial conditions: $t = 0$,
$$A_1 = S \cdot F \cdot D, A_2 = 0$$

FIGURE 6.6   Model for an intravenous injection in a two-compartment model. Elimination (E) is a first-order process (rate constant, k_{10}) that occurs from the central compartment. Distribution (D) and redistribution (R) are also first-order processes with rate constants of k_{12} and k_{21}, respectively. Note that $F = 1$ for IV administration.

comprise the central compartment is so rapid that it can be considered instantaneous, but distribution to the tissues of the peripheral compartment is slower. At time zero,

$$A_{1_0} = S \cdot F \cdot D \text{ and } A_{2_0} = 0 \tag{6.9}$$

where A_{1_0} and A_{2_0} are the initial amounts in the central and peripheral compartments, respectively. Note that $F = 1$ for IV administration.

By definition, the concentration of drug throughout a compartment is uniform, and by definition, the concentration of drug in the central compartment is Cp. Thus, at time zero,

$$Cp = Cp_0 = \frac{A_{1_0}}{V_1} = \frac{S \cdot F \cdot D}{V_1} \tag{6.10}$$

Drug elimination is usually modeled from the central compartment (Figure 6.6). However, if appropriate in a specific situation, elimination could be modeled to arise from the peripheral compartment. Elimination in the two-compartment model is driven by the amount of drug in the central compartment (A_1), and the elimination rate constant is k_{10} (Figure 6.6).

The amount of drug in the central compartment (A_1) is the initial focus of a mathematical expression based on the model. Once an expression has been obtained, it can be converted to plasma concentration using the volume of the central compartment (V_1). The rate of change of A_1 with time is:

$$\begin{aligned}
\frac{dA_1}{dt} &= \text{rate of inputs} - \text{rate of outputs} \\
&= \text{rate of redistribution} - (\text{rate of elimination} + \text{rate of distribution}) \\
&= (k_{21} \cdot A_2) - (k_{10} \cdot A_1 + k_{12} \cdot A_1)
\end{aligned} \tag{6.11}$$

The rate of change of A_2 with time is

$$\begin{aligned}
\frac{dA_2}{dt} &= \text{rate of inputs} - \text{rate of outputs} \\
&= \text{rate of distribution} - \text{rate of distribution} \\
&= (k_{12} \cdot A_1) - (k_{21} \cdot A_2)
\end{aligned} \tag{6.12}$$

6.4.3 First-Order Absorption in a Two-Compartment Model with First-Order Elimination

The model for first-order absorption in a two-compartment model is similar to the model described above except that it incorporates drug absorption, which is represented by first-order drug input into the central compartment (Figure 6.7). The initial conditions of the system are also different:

$$A_{1_0} = 0 \quad \text{and} \quad A_{\text{GI}_0} = SFD$$

where A_{GI0} is the amount of drug in the gastrointestinal tract at time zero. Note that the initial amount in the gastrointestinal tract is considered to be the effective dose. The amount of drug $[S \cdot D \cdot (1 - F)]$ that never reaches the systemic circulation is not included in the initial amount in the gastrointestinal tract.

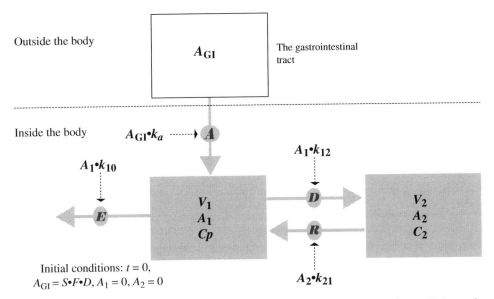

FIGURE 6.7   Model for first-order absorption in a two-compartment model. The symbols are the same as those defined in Figure 6.5. The gastrointestinal tract, which is outside the body, is symbolized as a compartment, and A_{GI} is the amount of drug it contains. The rate of absorption (A) is a first-order process controlled by A_{GI} and the first-order rate constant for absorption (k_a). The bioavailability factor (F) is the fraction of the dose that reaches the systemic circulation. S, F, and D are as defined in Figure 6.6.

An equation for the rate of change of the amount of drug in the central compartment can easily be obtained:

$$\frac{dA_1}{dt} = \text{rate of inputs} - \text{rate of outputs}$$
$$= (\text{rate of absorption} + \text{rate of redistribution}) \tag{6.13}$$
$$- (\text{rate of elimination} + \text{rate of distribution})$$
$$= [(k_a \cdot A_{GI}) + (k_{21} \cdot A_2)] - [(k_{10} \cdot A_1) + (k_{12} \cdot A_1)]$$

Similar expressions can be derived for the way in which the amounts in the gastrointestinal tract and peripheral compartment change over time.

6.5   USE OF COMPARTMENTAL MODELS TO STUDY METABOLITE PHARMACOKINETICS

In addition to simplifying drug distribution, compartment models can also be used to study the pharmacokinetics of a drug's metabolite. The distribution of the metabolite can be modeled using either a single- or a multiple-compartment model. The metabolite compartment(s) can then be attached to the compartmental model for the parent drug (Figure 6.8). Metabolites are formed primarily by a first-order process in the liver. Since the liver is usually part of the central compartment, the central compartment of the metabolite is usually attached to the central compartment of the parent drug. Figure 6.8 shows an integrated drug–metabolite model in which the distributions of both the parent drug and metabolite are

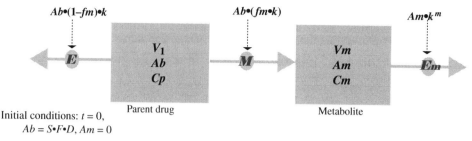

Initial conditions: $t = 0$,
$Ab = S{\cdot}F{\cdot}D, Am = 0$

FIGURE 6.8 Compartment model for a drug and its metabolite after the intravenous administration of the parent drug. The parent drug is assumed to follow one-compartmental pharmacokinetics. Elimination (E) is a first-order process with a rate constant of k. A fraction of the parent drug (f_m) is converted to the metabolite with a rate constant equal to $k \cdot f_m$. The rate constant for the other elimination processes for the parent drug is $k \cdot (1 - f_m)$. The metabolite is also assumed to follow one-compartmental pharmacokinetics. The plasma concentration of the metabolite is Cm, its volume of distribution is Vm, and the amount of metabolite in the compartment at any time is Am. The metabolite is eliminated (E_m) by a first-order process with a rate constant of k^m. S, F, and D for the parent drug are as defined in Figure 6.6.

represented as one-compartment models. The model applies to intravenous administration of the parent drug.

Equations can be developed for the rate of change of the amount of drug and metabolite:

$$\frac{dAb}{dt} = -k \cdot Ab$$

$$\frac{dAm}{dt} = [(k \cdot fm) \cdot Ab] - (k^m \cdot Am) \tag{6.14}$$

where Ab and Am are the amounts of parent drug and metabolite, respectively, k and k^m are the overall elimination rate constants of the parent drug and metabolite, respectively, and fm is the fraction of the parent drug converted to the metabolite. Note that the rate constant for the formation of the metabolite is $k \cdot fm$.

6.6 SELECTING AND APPLYING MODELS

Models are selected for a given drug by comparing the behavior of the model to the behavior of the data observed. Specifically, model-predicted plasma concentrations are compared to actual plasma concentrations measured at various times after a dose. This process is performed using robust mathematical and statistical procedures that provide numerical values of how well the data fit a model. Various models are tested and the simplest model that predicts the observed data adequately is selected. Once a satisfactory model has been found, it can be used to summarize a drug's properties and to estimate the model parameters (i.e., clearance and volume of distribution). The model can also be used to perform simulations to observe drug behavior and plasma concentrations in situations that have not yet been studied. For example, plasma concentrations can be simulated using various types of drug administration; parameters derived from single doses can be used to simulate steady-state conditions after multiple doses of a drug; and different doses and dosing intervals can be used to try to determine optimum regimens to target desired plasma concentrations.

PROBLEMS

6.1 Draw a two-compartment model for a drug that is to be administered orally and is thought to undergo constant zero-order absorption (rate $= k_0$). Assume that absorption and elimination are into and out of the central compartment, respectively. Write an expression for how the amount of drug in the central and peripheral compartments changes with time. What are the initial conditions of the system?

6.2 A drug follows one-compartment pharmacokinetics with first-order elimination with an overall elimination rate constant k. About 80% of the drug is excreted unchanged in the urine and 20% is metabolized to a metabolite. The metabolite also follows one-compartmental pharmacokinetics and has an overall elimination rate constant of k^m. About 70% of the metabolite is excreted unchanged into the urine and 30% is converted back to the parent drug. Draw an integrated parent drug–metabolite compartmental model for intravenous administration of the drug. Write expressions for the rate of change of the parent drug (Ab) and metabolite (Am). What are the initial conditions of the system?

SUGGESTED READINGS

1. Bourne, D. (1995) *Mathematical Modeling of Pharmacokinetic Data*, Technomic, Lancaster, PA.
2. Gibaldi, M., and Perrier, D. (1982) *Pharmacokinetics*, 2nd ed., Marcel Dekker, New York.
3. Wagner, J. G. (1993) *Pharmacokinetics for the Pharmaceutical Scientist*, Technomic, Lancaster, PA.

7

PHARMACOKINETICS OF AN INTRAVENOUS BOLUS INJECTION IN A ONE-COMPARTMENT MODEL

SARA E. ROSENBAUM

Objectives

The material in this chapter will enable the reader to:

1. Understand the derivation of a general equation that describes how a drug's plasma concentration at any time is related to the dose and the drug's pharmacokinetic parameters

Basic Pharmacokinetics and Pharmacodynamics: An Integrated Textbook and Computer Simulations,
Second Edition. Edited by Sara E. Rosenbaum.
© 2017 John Wiley & Sons, Inc. Published 2017 by John Wiley & Sons, Inc.

2. Apply an equation to determine plasma concentrations at any time after a dose and to determine doses necessary to achieve specific plasma concentrations
3. Understand how a drug's pharmacokinetic parameters influence the plasma concentration–time profile
4. Analyze plasma concentration–time data to obtain a drug's pharmacokinetic parameters
5. Apply the model to clinical situations

7.1 INTRODUCTION

The intravenous injection of a drug into a peripheral vein is the most common form of direct systemic drug administration. This route can provide immediate therapeutic plasma concentrations, and because it has 100% bioavailability, the intravenous route produces much more predictable concentrations than those for other routes. Consequently, intravenous administration is used when an immediate effect is desired and/or it is important that the dose be administered with a high degree of precision. Poor bioavailability from other routes is another reason that drugs may be given intravenously. Many drugs are administered intravenously, including antiarrhythmic drugs, narcotic analgesics, certain antibiotics, and anticancer drugs.

There are two main types of intravenous administration: the intravenous bolus injection and the intravenous infusion. The *intravenous bolus injection* involves administration of the entire dose at one time. Because a rapid injection can produce undesirable high plasma concentrations immediately after the injection, the injection is often given over a period of 1 min or more. For an *intravenous infusion*, the administration period is extended over a much more prolonged period, during which the drug is administered at a constant rate. Relatively short administration periods of around 0.5 to about 1–2 h can be used to give intermittent doses of a drug at regular intervals (e.g., every 8 or 12 h). This is referred to as an *intermittent infusion*. Alternatively, in hospitalized patients, an infusion may be continued over an extended period of up to several days. During this period, the patient receives the drug at a constant rate. This is referred to as a *continuous infusion*. The pharmacokinetics of intravenous infusions is discussed in subsequent chapters.

The intravenous injection of a single dose of a drug provides the simplest pharmacokinetic profile because there is no absorption or ongoing drug input. For simplicity, it will be assumed that the entire dose is injected instantaneously, even though, clinically, as discussed above, the dose is usually administered over a period of 1 min or more.

7.2 ONE-COMPARTMENT MODEL

The one-compartment model, the simplest of the pharmacokinetic models, applies when a drug distributes very rapidly throughout its total distribution volume. As a result, all the tissues that take up the drug achieve equilibrium with the plasma extremely quickly. Indeed, distribution is so rapid that there is no evidence of it on the plasma concentration–time profile. Thus, after an intravenous injection of a drug, plasma concentrations appear to be influenced only by first-order elimination, and the plasma concentration–time profile presents as a smooth monoexponential fall on a linear scale, and as a straight line on a semilogarithmic scale (Figure 7.1).

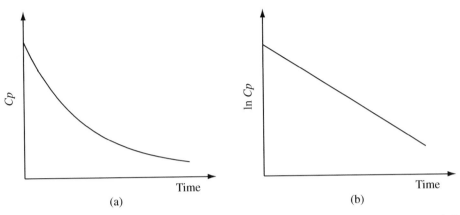

FIGURE 7.1   Linear (a) and semilogarithmic (b) plots of Cp against time after intravenous administration in the one-compartment model.

When a drug is administered ($t = 0$), the initial amount of drug in the body (Ab_0) is equal to the effective dose ($S \cdot F \cdot D$). Drug distribution from the plasma to the tissues is essentially instantaneous, and the initial plasma concentration (Cp_0) is equal to Ab_0 /Vd, or $S \cdot F \cdot D/Vd$. The body is represented by a single imaginary compartment. By definition, the compartment is homogeneous, and at any given time the drug concentration throughout is exactly the same. By definition, the concentration of drug in the compartment is equal to the plasma concentration (Cp). The amount of drug in the compartment (A_1) is equal to the amount of drug in the body (Ab). The volume of the compartment (V_1) is equal to

$$V_1 = \frac{A_1}{C_1} = \frac{Ab}{Cp}$$

But by definition,

$$\frac{Ab}{Cp} = Vd$$

Thus, for a one-compartment model,

$$V_1 = Vd$$

To help understand how compartments are used in pharmacokinetics, it is useful to bear in mind how the compartmental characteristics are related to true body characteristics. These relationships are summarized in Table 7.1.

TABLE 7.1   Comparison of True Body Characteristics and Those of the Single Compartment

Characteristic	Body	Compartment
Ab	Amount of drug in the body	Amount of drug in the compartment
Cp	Plasma concentration	Compartment concentration
Drug concentration	Varies from tissue to tissue	Constant throughout
Vd	Ratio: Ab/Cp	Volume of the compartment

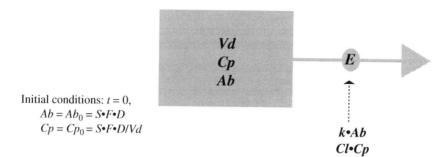

Initial conditions: $t = 0$,
$Ab = Ab_0 = S \bullet F \bullet D$
$Cp = Cp_0 = S \bullet F \bullet D / Vd$

FIGURE 7.2   Model for intravenous injection in a one-compartment model. S is the salt factor, F is the bioavailability, D is the dose, Ab is the amount of drug in the body, Cp is the plasma concentration, Vd is the apparent volume of distribution (Ab/Cp), Cl is the clearance, and k is the overall elimination rate constant. Note that $F = 1$ after intravenous administration.

7.3   PHARMACOKINETIC EQUATIONS

7.3.1   Basic Equation

The basic model for an intravenous injection is shown in Figure 7.2. This model can be used to write expressions for how the amount of drug in the body changes over time. Once an expression for amount of drug in the body has been derived, it can be converted to an expression for the plasma concentrations using the drug's volume of distribution ($Cp = Ab/Vd$). Thus, the starting point,

$$\frac{dAb}{dt} = \text{rate of inputs} - \text{rate of outputs}$$

$$\frac{dAb}{dt} = 0 - k \cdot Ab \tag{7.1}$$

Integrate equation (7.1) from zero to infinity:

$$Ab = Ab_0 \cdot e^{-kt} \tag{7.2}$$

Recall that the function e^{-kt} decays from 1 to zero over time (see Appendix A). During this period, Ab decays from Ab_0 to zero. The speed of decay is governed by k. The larger the value of k, the faster is the decay. Recall $Ab_0 = S \cdot F \cdot D$, thus,

$$Ab = S \cdot F \cdot D \cdot e^{-kt} \tag{7.3}$$

and $Cp = Ab/Vd$, thus,

$$\boxed{Cp = \frac{S \cdot F \cdot D}{Vd} \cdot e^{-kt} \text{ or } Cp = Cp_0 \cdot e^{-kt}} \tag{7.4}$$

where $Cp_0 = S \cdot F \cdot D / Vd$.

TABLE 7.2   Number of Half-Lives to Eliminate a Certain Fraction of the Original Dose

Fraction of Dose Eliminated	Number of Half-Lives
0.10	$\sim \frac{1}{6}$ [a]
0.20	$\sim \frac{1}{3}$ [a]
0.50	1
0.90	3.3
0.95	4.4
0.99	6.6

[a] Approximate values.

Also, since $k = Cl/Vd$ [see equation (5.21)], all of the above equations could be rewritten substituting Cl/Vd for k. For example,

$$Cp = \frac{S \cdot F \cdot D}{Vd} \cdot e^{-(Cl/Vd) \cdot t} \qquad (7.5)$$

In summary, after an intravenous injection in a one-compartment model, Cp and Ab, which are always directly proportional to each other, decay from their initial values in a first-order manner:

- Ab decays over time from $S \cdot F \cdot D$ to zero.
- Cp decays from $S \cdot F \cdot D/Vd$ to zero.
- The rate of decay is controlled by k; the larger the k is, the more rapid is the decay.

7.3.2 Half-Life

The *half-life* is the time required for the plasma concentration or the amount of drug in the body to fall by 50%. Elimination is a first-order process, and as shown in Appendix B,

$$t_{1/2} = \frac{0.693}{k}$$

7.3.3 Time to Eliminate a Dose

The plasma concentration and the amount of drug in the body are affected only by elimination, which is a first-order process. As a result, the number of half-lives required to eliminate any fraction of the original dose is the same as those needed to complete any fraction of a first-order process (see Appendix B). These are shown in Table 7.2.

7.4 SIMULATION EXERCISE:
http://web.uri.edu/pharmacy/research/rosenbaum/sims

Open simulation model 4, IV Bolus Injection 1-Compartment Model, which can be found at, which can be found at http://web.uri.edu/pharmacy/research/rosenbaum/sims/Model4.

Default settings for the model are dose = 100 mg; Cl = 4.6 L/h, and Vd = 20 L.

1. *Review the objectives and the "Model Summary" page.*
2. *Explore the model.*
3. *Go to the "Cp–Time Profile" page. Perform a simulation using a default dose of 100 mg and observe the shape of the Cp–time profile on the linear and semilogarithmic scales.*
    Observe:
    - *The Cp falls monoexponentially. It is influenced only by first-order elimination: $Cp = Cp_0 \cdot e{-}kt$.*
    - *A linear relationship exists between $\ln Cp$ and time: $\ln Cp = \ln Cp_0 - kt$. These plots are observed for drugs that distribute in a very rapid, essentially instantaneous manner.*
    - *Note: $Cp_0 = 5\,mg/L = \frac{100\,mg}{20\,L} = \frac{S \cdot F \cdot D}{Vd}$, Cp_0 is inversely proportional to Vd, $t_{1/2} = 3\,h$, and $k = 0.693/t_{1/2} = 0.231\,h^{-1}$.*
4. *Go to the "Effect of Dose" page. Use doses of 50, 100, and 200 mg to observe how dose influences Cp_0, Cp at any time, the slope of the fall in Cp, and $t_{1/2}$. Summarize the answers in Table SE7.4.*

TABLE SE7.4   Summary of the Effects of Dose, Clearance, and Volume of Distribution on the Plasma Concentration–Time Profile

	Cp_0	Cp	Slope	Half-Life
Effect of dose				
Effect of Cl				
Effect of Vd				

Observe:
- *Cp_0 is proportional to the dose and Cp at any time is proportional to the dose. The slope and $t_{1/2}$ are not influenced by the dose.*
5. *Go to the "Effect of Clearance" page. Use Cl values of 2.3, 4.6, and 9.2 L/h to observe how clearance influences Cp_0, Cp at any time, the slope of fall in Cp, and $t_{1/2}$. Summarize the answers in Table SE7.4.*
    Observe:
- *Cl does not influence Cp_0, but as Cl increases the slope of the fall in Cp becomes steeper (k increases and $t_{1/2}$ decreases). Thus, increases in clearance result in lower plasma concentrations at all times, apart from that at time zero.*
- *Clearance is a constant for a particular drug, assuming normal healthy function. It should be noted, however, that as a biological parameter it will vary somewhat within the population. The values reported in textbooks and in the literature represent population average values. Beyond normal biological variability, clearance will change if the function of one or both of the major organs of elimination changes. Thus, clearance is often changed in renal and/or hepatic disease. Concomitant medications can also alter the clearance of some drugs by inhibiting or inducing the enzymes involved in their metabolism. Changes in the activity of uptake and/or efflux transporters in the liver and kidney can also alter clearance.*

6. *Go to the "Effect of Volume of Distribution" page. Use Vd values of 10, 20, and 40 L to observe how the volume of distribution influences Cp$_0$, Cp at any time, the slope of the fall in Cp, and t$_{1/2}$. Summarize the answers in Table SE7.4.*
   Observe:
   - *As Vd increases, Cp$_0$ gets smaller and the slope gets less steep (k decreases and t$_{1/2}$ increases; t$_{1/2}$ is proportional to Vd). Essentially, increases in Vd compress the Cp-time profile and result in much less change or fluctuation in Cp.*
   - *Again, the volume of distribution is a constant for a drug but in common with other biological parameters, its value will vary somewhat within the population. Beyond the normal variability, the volume of distribution can be altered by factors that change either body volumes or alter tissue/plasma protein binding. These include, hydration, dehydration, diseases such as congestive heart failure, hepatic disease, and renal disease, and concomitant medications that displace drugs from their binding sites volume of distribution.*

7.5 APPLICATION OF THE MODEL

7.5.1 Predicting Plasma Concentrations

If a drug's pharmacokinetic parameters are known, the plasma concentration can be estimated at any time after any intravenous dose.

Example 7.1   A 20-mg dose of a drug ($S = 1$) was administered as an intravenous bolus injection. The drug has the following pharmacokinetic parameters: $k = 0.1 \text{ h}^{-1}$ and $Vd = 20$ L.

(a) Calculate Cp_0:

$$Cp_0 = \frac{S \cdot F \cdot D}{Vd} \quad S = 1 \text{ (given) and } F = 1 \text{ for IV administration}$$
$$= \frac{20}{20}$$
$$= 1 \text{ mg/L}$$

(b) Calculate the plasma concentration at 3 h.

Solution Note that half-life is very useful for getting rough estimates of the answers to pharmacokinetic calculations and for checking calculations and should be calculated as soon as possible.

$$t_{1/2} = \frac{0.693}{k}$$
$$= \frac{0.693}{0.1 \text{ h}^{-1}}$$
$$= 6.93 \text{ h}$$

Thus, plasma concentrations will fall by 50% every 6.9 h. At 3 h, Cp should be about 75% its initial value, or about 0.75 mg/L:

$$
\begin{aligned}
Cp &= \frac{S \cdot F \cdot D}{Vd} \cdot e^{-kt} \\
&= \frac{20}{20}\,\text{mg/L} \cdot e^{-0.13} \\
&= 1 \times 0.74 \\
&= 0.74\,\text{mg/L}
\end{aligned}
$$

7.5.2 Duration of Action

The duration of action of a drug may be considered to be the length of time the plasma concentration spends above the MEC. Its determination is best illustrated by example.

Example 7.2 Continuing with the drug used in Example 7.1, if the therapeutic range is between 5 and 0.3 mg/L, how long are the plasma concentrations in the therapeutic range?

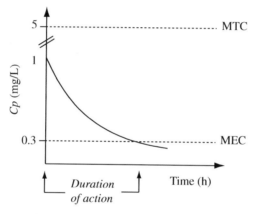

FIGURE E7.2 Therapeutic range superimposed over the plasma concentration–time profile.

Solution A small diagram is useful for this type of problem (Figure E7.2). $Cp_0 = 1$ mg/L. Thus, at time zero, the plasma concentration is in the therapeutic range. The plasma concentration will remain therapeutic until it falls to the MEC (0.3 mg/L). At what time does this occur?

$$
\begin{aligned}
Cp &= Cp_0 \cdot e^{-kt} \\
0.3 &= 1 \cdot e^{-0.1t} \\
\ln 0.3 &= -0.1\,t \\
-1.204 &= -0.1\,t \\
t &= 12.04\,h
\end{aligned}
$$

Thus, the drug is in therapeutic range for 12 h. (Use the drug's $t_{1/2}$ value to check the answer: after $1t_{1/2}$ (7h), Cp will fall to 0.5 mg/L; after $2t_{1/2}$ (14h), Cp will fall to 0.25 mg/L.)

7.5.3 Value of a Dose to Give a Desired Initial Plasma Concentration

The equation for the initial plasma concentration can be used to determine the value of a dose to give a certain desired plasma concentration (Cp_{des}).

Example 7.3   The initial Cp of 1 mg/L is unsatisfactory. Calculate a dose to provide an initial plasma concentration of 5 mg/L.
Solution

$$Cp_0 = \frac{S \cdot F \cdot D}{Vd}$$

Let $Cp_0 = Cp_{des}$ and rearrange:

$$\text{dose} = Cp_{des} \cdot \frac{Vd}{S \cdot F}$$
$$= \frac{5 \times 20}{1 \times 1} = 100\,\text{mg} \tag{7.6}$$

7.5.4 Intravenous Loading Dose

Most patients receive long-term treatment with a drug rather than a single isolated dose. Figure 7.3 shows the typical average plasma concentration observed over extended drug therapy. This profile is typical of that of an intravenous infusion, where no fluctuation in the plasma concentration is observed. It can be seen that the plasma concentration gradually increases during the course of therapy and eventually reaches a plateau. The plateau is known as the *steady state*, and the plasma concentration at this time is known as the *steady-state plasma concentration* (Cp_{ss}). Dosing regimens are designed so that the plasma concentration at steady state is therapeutic. Often, the plasma concentrations leading up to steady state are subtherapeutic, and drug only becomes effective once steady state is achieved. In Chapter 9, we show that it takes about 3–5 elimination half-lives to get to steady state. If a drug has a very long half-life and/or if it is clinically important to achieve therapeutic plasma concentrations immediately, it may be necessary to administer a loading dose that will achieve the steady state immediately.

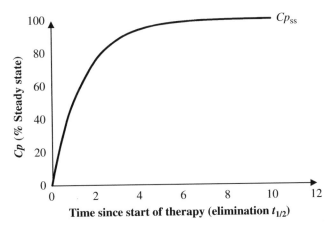

FIGURE 7.3   Graph of typical plasma concentration–time profile associated with extended drug administration.

Equation (7.6) can be used to calculate the value of the loading dose. The value of Cp_{ss} is equal to Cp_{des}. The general expression of the formula to calculate a loading dose, D_L is

$$\boxed{D_L = Cp_{ss} \cdot \frac{Vd}{S \cdot F}} \tag{7.7}$$

Note that formula (7.7) contains the bioavailability factor even though $F = 1$ for intravenous administration. This formula is frequently used for other routes of administration, and by always including the bioavailability factor in the formula, there is less chance that it will be ignored when it is needed.

Example 7.4   Calculate the value of an intravenous loading dose of phenytoin sodium ($S = 0.92$) for an 80-kg patient. A plasma concentration of 12 mg/L phenytoin is desired. The volume of distribution of phenytoin is 0.65 L/kg.

Solution

$$Vd = 0.65 \, \text{L/kg} \times 80 \, \text{kg} = 52 \, \text{L}$$
$$D_L = Cp_{ss} \cdot \frac{Vd}{S \cdot F} = \frac{12 \times 52}{0.92} = 678 \, \text{mg}$$

7.6 DETERMINATION OF PHARMACOKINETIC PARAMETERS EXPERIMENTALLY

The expression of an intravenous injection in a one-compartment model consists essentially of two pharmacokinetic parameters: the primary parameter for elimination (Cl) and the primary parameter for distribution (Vd). From these, an additional parameter for the rate of drug elimination is derived (k or its reciprocal form, $t_{1/2}$). All the parameters of the model can be determined either from the two primary parameters or from one primary and one secondary parameter. For example, k and $t_{1/2}$ can be determined if Cl and Vd are known. Also, Cl can be determined if Vd and k are known. The pharmacokinetic parameters are determined by fitting plasma concentration–time data to the pharmacokinetic model.

7.6.1 Study Design for the Determination of Parameters

The plasma concentration–time data needed to model a drug's pharmacokinetics must be obtained from human subjects. The protocol or procedure for any study that involves humans must be approved by the institutional review board of the institution where the study is to be conducted and/or where the scientists conducting the study are employed. Additionally, anyone who volunteers to participate in a clinical study must sign an informed consent form. The specific structure of the study will depend on the goal of the study and on the pharmacokinetic characteristics of the drug predicted for the population under study. The study will take the following general form:

1. An intravenous dose is administered to about 10–12 volunteers.
2. Plasma samples (10–20) are collected at various times after the dose for a period of at least three elimination half-lives (at this time, 90% of the dose will have been eliminated).

3. Plasma samples are prepared and frozen until they can be analyzed to obtain the concentration of parent drug. The concentration of metabolites may also be measured if the pharmacokinetics of metabolites are to be studied.

4. The plasma concentration–time data from each person are subject to pharmacokinetic analysis as described below. The parameters are determined.

5. The individual parameters for each subject are combined to determine the mean values for the study population and to determine their variability (variance or standard deviation).

7.6.2 Pharmacokinetic Analysis

All the mathematical expressions that relate a drug's pharmacokinetic parameters to the plasma concentration are nonlinear [see equations (7.4) and (7.5)]. Computer software is now readily available that can perform nonlinear regression analysis and fit the plasma concentrations directly to pharmacokinetic models. However, prior to the availability of this software, it was necessary to linearize the expression for the plasma concentration so that ordinary linear regression analysis could be used to determine the parameter values. The latter procedure is presented here. In order to focus on the procedure itself, most data used in this book for these examples and problems are "perfect" rather than "real." Thus, the data should fit the models perfectly. In this book, we do not discuss statistical procedures such as least-squares regression analysis for obtaining the best fit for real data that are scattered around the model-predicted data. These procedures can be found in any basic textbook on statistics.

1. The plasma concentration–time data are *observed* on linear and semilogarithmic plots to ensure that the data fit the model and that there are no data points that appear to be vastly different from the others (outliers).

2. The elimination rate constant (k) is determined from the *slope* of the plot of ln Cp and time (Figure 7.4). Recall from equation (7.4) that

$$Cp = Cp_0 \cdot e^{-kt}$$

Taking the natural logarithm gives

$$\ln Cp = \ln Cp_0 - kt \tag{7.8}$$

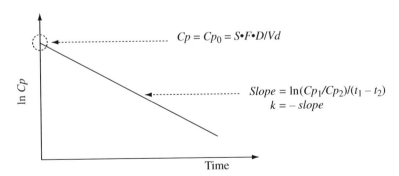

FIGURE 7.4 Determination of k and Vd from semilog plot of plasma concentration against time.

This is the equation of a straight line (Figure 7.4):

$$\text{slope} = \frac{ln(Cp_1/Cp_2)}{t_1 - t_2}$$
$$k = -\text{slope}$$
$$= \frac{ln(Cp_1/Cp_2)}{t_2 - t_1}$$

(7.9)

3. The *half-life* is determined:

$$t_{1/2} = 0.693/k$$

4. The *volume of distribution* (*Vd*) is determined from the relationship

$$Vd = \frac{Ab}{Cp}$$

The only time the amount of drug in the body (*Ab*) is known is at time zero, when *Ab* is equal to the effective dose ($S \cdot F \cdot D$). Thus,

$$Vd = \frac{S \cdot F \cdot D}{Cp_0}$$

The value of Cp_0 is obtained from the intercept of the ln *Cp*–time plot (Figure 7.4).
5. The *clearance* can be determined in several ways:
   (a) It can be calculated from *k* and *Vd*:

$$Cl = k \cdot Vd$$

   (b) It can be determined from the area under the curve (AUC). It was shown previously (see Chapter 5) that

$$Cl = \frac{D_{IV}}{AUC}$$

(7.10)

The AUC can be determined using the trapezoidal rule, but more simply for the intravenous injection in a one-compartment model, the AUC can be calculated as:

$$AUC = \int_0^\infty Cp \cdot dt = \int_0^\infty Cp_0 \cdot e^{-kt} \cdot dt = \frac{Cp_0}{k}$$

(7.11)

Substituting for AUC in equation (7.10) yields

$$Cl = \frac{D_{IV}}{AUC} = \frac{D_{IV} \cdot k}{Cp_0}$$

(7.12)

Example 7.5   A single intravenous bolus injection of a drug (50 mg) was administered to 10 normal subjects. Plasma samples were taken at various intervals and were analyzed for unchanged drug. The data from one subject are listed in Table E7.5. Determine the drug's clearance, volume of distribution, and elimination half-life.

TABLE E7.5   Plasma Concentrations of Drug in a Subject at Various Times After an Intravenous Dose of 50 mg

Time (h)	Cp (mg/L)	Time (h)	Cp (mg/L)
0.1	2.45	3	1.37
0.2	2.40	5	0.92
0.5	2.26	7	0.61
1	2.04	10	0.33
1.5	1.85	12	0.22
2	1.67	15	0.12

This problem can be solved either by hand using semilogarithmic graph paper or by creating a special Excel worksheet for the analysis. Instructions to create an Excel worksheet to conduct the analysis of the data are given in Appendix C.

Solution   Create a worksheet as described in Appendix C.

1. Plot Cp against time on both the linear and semilogarithmic scales to visualize the data and to ensure that the data appear to fit the one-compartmental model (Figure E7.5).
2. Calculate the elimination rate constant. The slope function in Excel is applied to the ln Cp–time data. All the data should be used to determine the slope in Excel.

$$\text{Slope} = -0.20\,\text{h}^{-1}$$
$$k = -\text{slope}$$
$$= 0.20\,\text{h}^{-1}$$

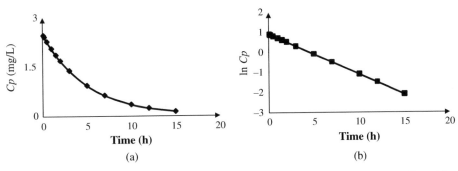

FIGURE E7.5   Plots of plasma concentration against time on the linear (a) and semilogarithmic scales (b).

3. Half-life:

$$t_{1/2} = \frac{0.693}{k}$$
$$= \frac{0.693}{0.2}$$
$$= 3.47\,\text{h}$$

4. Volume of distribution: Cp_0 is found using the intercept function in Excel:

$$\text{intercept} = \text{In}\,Cp_0 = 0.916$$
$$Cp_0 = e^{0.916} = 2.5\,\text{mg/L}$$
$$Vd = \frac{\text{dose}}{Cp_0}$$
$$= \frac{50\,\text{mg}}{2.5\,\text{mg/L}}$$
$$= 20\,\text{L}$$

5. Clearance:

$$Cl = k \cdot Vd$$
$$= 0.2 \times 20 = 4\,\text{L/h}$$

or

$$Cl = \frac{\text{dose}_{\text{IV}}}{\text{AUC}}$$

$\text{AUC} = Cp_0/k$, so

$$Cl = \frac{\text{dose}_{\text{IV}}}{Cp_0/k}$$
$$= \frac{50 \times 0.2}{2.5} = 4\,\text{L/h}$$

6. The plasma concentration 6 h after a 100-mg IV dose of this drug is found as

$$Cp = \frac{D}{Vd} \cdot e^{-kt}$$
$$= \frac{100}{20} \cdot e^{-0.2 \times 6} = 1.51\,\text{mg/L}$$

7. The plasma concentration 10 h after this, that is, 16 h after the dose, is determined using

$$Cp = Cp_0 \cdot e^{-kt}$$

where $Cp_0 = 1.51$ mg/L, $t = 10$ h or $Cp_0 = \frac{100}{20}$ mg/L, $t = 16$ h
$Cp = 0.204$ mg/L

7.7 PHARMACOKINETIC ANALYSIS IN CLINICAL PRACTICE

As discussed earlier, the primary pharmacokinetic parameters (and by extension the secondary parameters) are considered to be constants for a drug. However, as biological parameters, they will display some person-to-person, or *interindividual, variability*. Furthermore, within a person, some day-to-day *intraindividual variability* in the parameters will be observed. Intraindividual variability is usually much smaller than interindividual variability. Population average values of the parameters can be obtained from the literature. Since the pharmacokinetics parameters control the dose–plasma concentration relationship, interindividual variability in the pharmacokinetic parameters will result in interindividual variability in the plasma concentrations produced by a standard dose. For many drugs, the margin of safety is large enough that interindividual variability is not associated with adverse clinical effects. However, for drugs that have narrow therapeutic ranges, interindividual variability can result in the standard dose producing subtherapeutic plasma concentrations in some patients, toxic concentrations in others, and therapeutic plasma concentrations only in some patients. Drugs that have both wide interindividual variability in their pharmacokinetic parameters and narrow therapeutic ranges include digoxin, lithium, warfarin, phenytoin, the aminoglycosides, and the immunosuppressants (i.e., cyclosporine and tacrolimus). When standard doses of these drugs are used, the plasma concentrations should be assessed in individual patients. If plasma concentrations are not therapeutic, doses must be individualized, based ideally on a patient's individual pharmacokinetic parameters. In a clinical setting, it is not possible to collect a large number of blood samples for pharmacokinetic analysis. Instead, a patient's pharmacokinetic parameters must frequently be determined from only two plasma concentrations.

Example 7.6   A patient is to be given an 80-mg IV dose of gentamicin every 8 h. A peak and a trough of 6 and 0.5 mg/L, respectively, are desired after the first dose. Two plasma concentrations obtained after the first dose are shown in Table E7.6. Determine if the peak and trough after this dose meet the goal. If not, suggest a more appropriate dose.

Solution

$$k = \frac{\text{Ln}(4.5/1.1)}{4} = 0.352\,\text{h}^{-1}$$
$$t_{1/2} = \frac{0.693}{0.352} = 1.97\,\text{h}$$

A peak and a trough from the dose occur at $t = 0$ and 8 h, respectively:

$$Cp = Cp_0 \cdot e^{-kt}$$

TABLE E7.6 Plasma Concentrations of Gentamicin After an 80-mg Intravenous Dose

Time After Dose (h)	Cp (mg/L)
2	4.5
6	1.1

(a) Cp_0:

$$1.1 = Cp_0 \cdot e^{-0.352 \times 6}$$
$$Cp_0 = 9.1 \, \text{mg/L}$$

(b) Cp at 8 h and Cp_8:

$$Cp = 9.1 e^{-0.352 \times 8}$$
$$Cp_8 = 0.54 \, \text{mg/L}$$

The volume of distribution:

$$Vd = \frac{\text{dose}}{Cp_0} = \frac{80 \, \text{mg}}{9 \, \text{mg/L}}$$
$$= 8.8 \, \text{L}$$

Thus, the dose did not achieve the therapeutic goal. A more appropriate dose must be calculated.

We want $Cp_0 = 6$ mg/L:

$$Cp_0 = \frac{S \cdot F \cdot D}{Vd}$$
$$S \cdot F \cdot D = Cp_0 \cdot Vd$$
$$= 6 \, \text{mg/L} \times 8.8 \, \text{L}$$
$$= 52.8 \, \text{mg}$$

A trough of 0.5 mg/L is required. Thus, the time when Cp falls to 0.5 mg/L will be the dosing interval, or the time when the next dose should be given.

$$Cp = Cp_0 \cdot e^{-kt}$$
$$0.5 = 6 e^{-0.352 t}$$
$$t = 7.1 \, \text{h}$$

PROBLEMS

7.1 A drug ($S = 1$) has the therapeutic range 3.5–1.0 mg/L. It has a Vd of 120 L and a Cl of 20 L/h.

(a) Recommend an intravenous dose of the free base to give an initial plasma concentration of 3 mg/L.

(b) How long do plasma concentrations remain in the therapeutic range?

(c) If the lower plasma concentration must not to fall below 1.5 mg/L, when should the second dose be administered?

(d) If the drug was given to a patient suffering from malnutrition in whom the Vd is estimated to be 160 L, what changes in the drug's pharmacokinetic profile would you expect?

7.2   A 35-year-old female patient (weight 60 kg), who has been taking theophylline for several years, is being treated in the emergency room for an asthma attack. Her theophylline plasma concentration is found to be 5 mg/L. Calculate the value of an intravenous loading dose of aminophylline ($S = 0.8$) that will bring the plasma concentration up to 15 mg/L. In this patient, theophylline's pharmacokinetic parameters are estimated to be as follows: $Cl = 0.04$ L/h/kg and $Vd = 0.5$ L/kg.

7.3   Procainamide is an antiarrhythmic used in the treatment of ventricular tachyarrhythmias. Determine the value of an intravenous loading dose of procainamide hydrochloride ($S = 0.87$) that would achieve immediate plasma concentrations of 6 mg/L in a 70-kg man. Procainamide's Vd is 2 L/kg.

7.4   A loading dose of digoxin is to be administered to a 55-kg woman who has a creatinine clearance (Cl_{CR}) of 75 mL/min. Digoxin's volume of distribution is dependent on renal function. Specifically,

$$Vd(L) = 3.8 \times \text{weight(kg)} + 3.1 Cl_{CR}(\text{mL}/\text{min})$$

Determine the value of an oral loading dose for digoxin ($F = 0.7$) that will achieve a desired serum digoxin of 0.8 µg/L. Use the equations for an intravenous bolus injection.

7.5   A loading dose of phenobarbital sodium ($S = 0.9$) was administered to a 60-kg female patient. The initial plasma concentration was estimated to be 20 mg/L. The clearance and volume of distribution of phenobarbital are 4 mL/h/kg and 0.6 L/kg, respectively. How long will it take for the plasma concentration to fall to 15 mg/L?

7.6   A patient with pneumonia due to *Klebsiella pneumonia* is being treated with gentamicin. Therapeutic drug monitoring is being performed in order to have peaks and troughs of 20 and <0.5 mg/L, respectively, after the first dose. An initial regimen of 400 mg every 24 h was selected. The first intravenous dose was administered and plasma samples taken 1 and 7 h later had a gentamicin concentration of 12.5 and 1.51 mg/L, respectively. Assume that the dose was given by intravenous bolus injection.

(a) Calculate the peak and trough plasma concentrations after this first dose. Are the troughs and peaks acceptable?

(b) If not, what dose would have produced a peak of 20 mg/L? Would this dose have produced an acceptable trough?

7.7   After the intravenous administration of a new drug (dose = 100 mg, $S = 1$), plasma concentrations of 8 and 3 mg/L were found at 1 and 7 h after the dose, respectively.

(a) Estimate the drug's elimination rate constant.

(b) Estimate the drug's half-life.

(c) Estimate the AUC from zero to infinity.

(d) Estimate the drug's clearance.

(e) Estimate the drug's volume of distribution.

7.8   An IV bolus injection of an antibiotic is to be administered to an 80-year-old patient. It is suspected that her pharmacokinetics will be markedly different from normal. The team intends to administer 250 mg every 8 h. The first dose produces the following plasma concentrations:

Time (h)	Cp (mg/L)
1	15
6	2.03

(a) What is the peak plasma concentration after this dose?

(b) What is the patient's Vd?

(c) Assuming that the therapeutic range of this drug is 25–1.5 mg/L, what is the duration of action after this dose?

7.9 The problem set in Table P5.7 (Chapter 5) provided plasma concentration–time data for lipoamide, nosolatol, and disolvprazole after an intravenous bolus injection. The data are repeated in Table P7.8.

TABLE P7.8   Plasma Concentrations of Lipoamide, Nosolatol, and Disolvprazole After Intravenous Doses

Lipoamide		Nosolatol		Disolvprazole	
T (h)	Cp (μg/L)	T (h)	Cp (μg/L)	T (h)	Cp (μg/L)
0	23.8	0	476	0	286
0.5	22.1	0.5	462	0.2	266
1	20.5	1	448	0.4	249
1.5	19	1.5	435	0.8	216
2	17.6	2	422	1	202
3	15.2	2.5	409	1.2	188
5	11.3	5	352	1.6	163
7.5	7.82	8	294	2	142
10	5.39	12	231	3	100
15	2.57	15	193	5	50
20	1.22	20	143	8	18
24	0.68	24	112	12	4

Doses administered: 10, 100, and 10 mg for lipoamide, nosolatol, and disolvprazole, respectively. Create an Excel worksheet using the directions provided in Appendix C and analyze the data given to determine the following pharmacokinetic parameters for each drug: elimination rate constant, volume of distribution, clearance, and elimination half-life.

SUGGESTED READING

1. Winter, M. E. (2010) *Basic Clinical Pharmacokinetics*, 5th ed., Lippincott Williams & Wilkins, Baltimore.

8

PHARMACOKINETICS OF AN INTRAVENOUS BOLUS INJECTION IN A TWO-COMPARTMENT MODEL

Sara E. Rosenbaum

Objectives

The material in this chapter will enable the reader to:

1. Understand the physiological basis for the two-compartment model and the characteristics of the Cp versus time profile after intravenous administration
2. Identify the various ways in which the model can be parameterized
3. Identify and understand the difference between the three volumes of distribution of the model
4. Understand the relationships among the various parameters
5. Use feathering to estimate the model parameters
6. Understand how the model is applied clinically to determine an elimination half-life, estimate loading doses, and evaluate drug therapy

8.1   INTRODUCTION

The distribution of many drugs follows two-compartment pharmacokinetics. This is apparent because a steep fall in the plasma concentration is observed in the early period after the administration of an intravenous dose (Figure 8.1a). As a result, the plasma concentration–time curve is biphasic, a feature that is most apparent on the semilogarithmic scale (Figure 8.1b). The simple one-compartment model, in which plasma concentration falls monoexponentially under the sole influence of first-order elimination, cannot be used to predict this behavior. Two-compartment characteristics are the result of a slower distribution of the drug to some tissues in the body. This distribution pattern is presented below, and it is followed by a discussion of how it is represented in the two-compartment model.

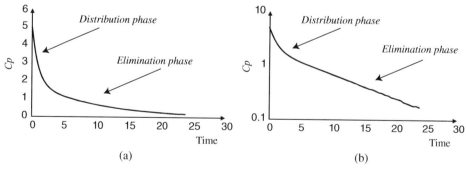

FIGURE 8.1   Graph of plasma concentration against time on a linear (a) and a semilogarithmic scale (b) for a drug that displays two-compartmental characteristics after an intravenous bolus injection.

8.2 TISSUE AND COMPARTMENTAL DISTRIBUTION OF A DRUG

8.2.1 Drug Distribution to the Tissues

For drugs that display two-compartmental pharmacokinetics, there appear to be two types of tissues with respect to their rate of uptake of drug. One group of tissues, like those of the one-compartment model, take up the drug extremely quickly. The uptake is so rapid that there is no evidence of the distribution based on blood samples taken during the early period after injection. The tissues where this occurs are usually the well-perfused tissues, and the tissue–plasma ratio in these tissues achieves its equilibrium value extremely rapidly and remains constant. Distribution to some other tissues, usually the poorly perfused tissues, occurs more gradually. It is the distribution of the drug to these tissues that is associated with the pronounced initial fall in the plasma concentration. This period is known as the *distribution phase* (Figure 8.1). Note that drug elimination also occurs during this phase, but it is drug distribution that dominates the fall in the plasma concentration.

In these tissues, where distribution proceeds more slowly, the tissue–plasma concentration ratio increases throughout the distribution phase. Eventually, a type of equilibrium is achieved between the plasma and the poorly perfused tissues. At this time, the distribution phase is complete and the tissue/plasma concentration ratio remains constant. First-order drug elimination then drives the fall in plasma concentration, which as a result falls in a smooth monoexponential manner. This period is known as the *elimination* or *postdistribution phase*. Figure 8.2 shows how drug concentrations change in hypothetical tissues in both the central and peripheral compartments relative to the plasma concentration. Note that the concentration of drug in both groups of tissues will vary from tissue to tissue. The concentration of drug in a tissue in either compartment could be greater than, less than, or equal to the plasma concentration, depending on factors such as binding and drug transporters.

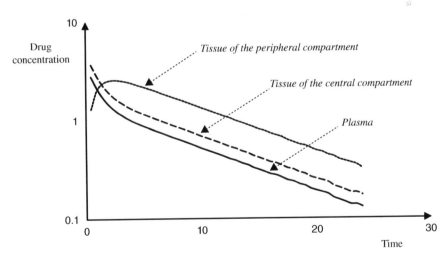

FIGURE 8.2   Time course of drug concentrations in the plasma and two hypothetical tissues. Note that drug distribution to the tissue of the central compartment (dashed line) appears to be instantaneous and is not visible on the graph. Distribution to the tissue of the peripheral compartment (dotted line) proceeds more slowly and is associated with a sharp fall in concentrations in the plasma (solid line) and tissue of the central compartment.

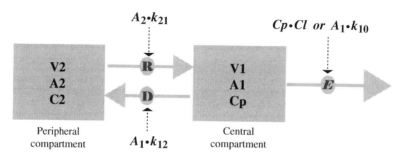

Initial Condition: t = 0
A1=SFD, A2 = 0

FIGURE 8.3   Two-compartment model with intravenous bolus injection. Ab, A_1, and A_2 are the amounts of drug in the body, the central compartment, and the peripheral compartment, respectively; Cp is the plasma concentration of the drug and the concentration in the central compartment; C_2 is the drug concentration in the peripheral compartment; V_1 and V_2 are the respective volumes of the central and peripheral compartments; k_{10} is the first-order elimination (E) rate constant; k_{12} and k_{21} are the rate constants for distribution (D) and redistribution (R), respectively; Cl is the clearance; and the effective dose is given by the product of S (salt factor), F (bioavailability factor), and D (the dose administered). Note that for intravenous administration, $F = 1$.

8.2.2   Compartmental Distribution of a Drug

According to the pharmacokinetic model, the body is assumed to consist of two hypothetical compartments (Figure 8.3). The central compartment consists of the plasma and those tissues where drug distribution proceeds very rapidly. By definition, the concentration throughout this compartment is equal to the plasma concentration (see Chapter 6). Drug elimination is usually assumed to occur from the central compartment because the organs of elimination are well perfused and are usually part of the central compartment. The second, peripheral compartment consists of those tissues where distribution proceeds more slowly. By definition, it is homogeneous and the drug concentration throughout is uniform at all times. Movement between the compartments is assumed to be first order driven by the amount of drug in a compartment. The movement of drug from the central to the peripheral compartment is referred to as *distribution* (rate constant k_{12}) and the movement of drug back from the peripheral to the central compartment is referred to as *redistribution* (rate constant k_{21}). When an intravenous dose is administered, the drug is assumed to undergo instantaneous distribution throughout the central compartment. At this time, the entire dose is present in the central compartment and is distributed throughout the compartment in a completely uniform manner; that is, at any time, the drug concentration throughout is the same (Figure 8.4). At time zero, no drug is present in the peripheral compartment. The concentration gradient between compartments then causes a net movement of drug into the peripheral compartment. The concentration in the peripheral compartment increases and the concentration in the central compartment decreases (due to distribution and elimination) (Figure 8.4). Eventually, an equilibrium (pseudo) is achieved, at which time the concentration in the central compartment equals that of the peripheral compartment (Figure 8.4). At this time, the concentration in the central compartment decreases due to elimination. As the concentration in the central compartment falls, there is a net movement of drug from the peripheral compartment back into the central compartment. The concentration of drug in the peripheral compartment does not correspond to the concentration of

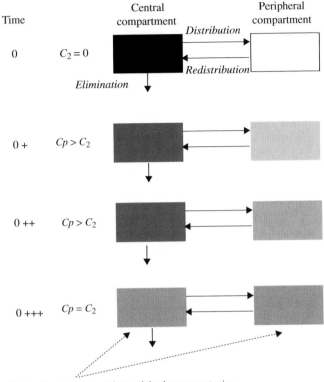

Distribution phase is complete and the drug concentration
in the compartments is the same. It is not a true equilibrium
because it is continuously destroyed by elimination.

FIGURE 8.4   Relative concentrations of drug in the central (Cp) and peripheral (C_2) compartments
at different times after intravenous injection in a two-compartment model.

drug in any particular tissue that is part of the peripheral compartment. Instead, it represents
an averaged concentration of all the tissues that comprise the peripheral compartment. The
time course of the distribution process for the two compartments is demonstrated in the
simulation model, Model 5, Single Injection in a 2-Compartment Model, which can be
found at http://web.uri.edu/pharmacy/research/rosenbaum/sims/Model5.

8.3 BASIC EQUATION

Based on the model shown in Figure 8.3, it is possible to write equations for the rate of
change of the amount of drug in the two compartments: rate of change of the amount of
drug in any compartment = rate of inputs − rate of outputs

For the central compartment,

$$\frac{dA_1}{dt} = k_{21}A_2 - k_{12}A_1 - k_{10}A_1 \tag{8.1}$$

For the peripheral compartment,

$$\frac{dA_2}{dt} = k_{12}A_1 - k_{21}A_2 \tag{8.2}$$

When these equations are integrated and solved for Cp, the following biexponential solution is obtained:

$$Cp = A \cdot e^{-\alpha t} + B \cdot e^{-\beta t} \qquad (8.3)$$

where α is the hybrid rate constant for distribution, β is the hybrid rate constant for elimination, and A and B are the intercepts of the two exponential functions. Thus, according to equation (8.3), the plasma concentration–time profile consists of two exponential terms, $A \cdot e^{-\alpha t}$ and $B \cdot e^{-\beta t}$. According to convention, α is always larger than β, and in the vast majority of situations, $A \cdot e^{-\alpha t}$ represents drug distribution and $B \cdot e^{-\beta t}$, drug elimination.

8.3.1   Distribution: A, α, and the Distribution $t_{1/2}$

The function $A \cdot e^{-\alpha t}$ describes the distribution characteristics of a drug during the distribution phase. Note the parameter A, which is an intercept, is dependent on the dose as well as a drug's pharmacokinetic parameters. The rate constant α is the *hybrid* rate constant for distribution because although it expresses distribution, it is neither k_{12} nor k_{21}. It is referred to as a *macro rate constant*, as it is a complex function of all three of the first-order rate constants (k_{10}, k_{12}, and k_{21}) [see equation (8.13)]. The latter first-order rate constants are referred to as the *micro rate constants*. The half-life determined from α is known as the *distribution half-life*:

$$t_{1/2,\alpha} = \frac{0.693}{\alpha} \qquad (8.4)$$

As distribution is a first-order process, it takes 1 $t_{1/2,\alpha}$ for distribution to go to 50% completion and around 3–5 $t_{1/2,\alpha}$ for the distribution phase to go to completion.

8.3.2   Elimination: B, β, and the β $t_{1/2}$

The function $B \cdot e^{-\beta t}$ describes the characteristics of the plasma concentration–time profile in the elimination phase. The parameter B, like A, is an intercept that is dependent on the dose as well as a drug's pharmacokinetic parameters. The rate constant β is the hybrid rate constant for elimination and is distinct from the true elimination rate constant k_{10}. It expresses the manner in which the plasma concentration and the amount of drug in the body fall due to drug elimination during the elimination phase. It is also a macro rate constant that is dependent on all three of the micro rate constants (k_{10}, k_{12}, and k_{21}) [see equation (8.14)].

The half-life determined from β is referred to as the *elimination, biological,* or *disposition half-life*:

$$t_{1/2,\beta} = \frac{0.693}{\beta} \qquad (8.5)$$

Once the distribution phase is complete, the β half-life is used to determine how long it will take to eliminate a drug from the body. Since elimination is a first-order process, it will take 1 $t_{1/2,\beta}$ to eliminate 50% of a dose and around 3–5 $t_{1/2,\beta}$ to eliminate the dose.

Clinically, β or, more specifically, $t_{1/2,\beta}$ is an important parameter and may be measured in individual patients to optimize therapy. In contrast, α is rarely determined clinically, but it is important to know its approximate value so that the approximate duration of the distribution phase can be determined. This is because when blood samples are collected to determine the $t_{1/2,\beta}$, it is important to avoid taking samples in the distribution phase. For example, the elimination half-lives of aminoglycosides such as tobramycin are often measured in patients. These drugs have an $t_{1/2,\alpha}$ of about 5 min. Thus, it is important to wait at least 20 min after an injection before taking blood samples to estimate the $t_{1/2,\beta}$. In case of digoxin, which also displays two-compartment pharmacokinetics, the $t_{1/2,\alpha}$ is about 1.5 h. Thus, the distribution phase for digoxin lasts about 6 h.

8.4 RELATIONSHIP BETWEEN MACRO AND MICRO RATE CONSTANTS

The macro rate constants (α and β) and intercepts (A and B) are complex functions of the first-order micro rate constants (k_{10}, k_{12}, and k_{10}). The relationship between these parameters is as follows:

$$\alpha + \beta = k_{12} + k_{21} + k_{10} \tag{8.6}$$

$$\alpha \cdot \beta = k_{21} \cdot k_{10} \tag{8.7}$$

$$A = \frac{S \cdot D_{IV} \cdot (\alpha - k_{21})}{V_1 \cdot (\alpha - \beta)} \tag{8.8}$$

$$B = \frac{S \cdot D_{IV} \cdot (k_{21} - \beta)}{V_1 \cdot (\alpha - \beta)} \tag{8.9}$$

where S is the salt factor, and D_{IV} is the value of the intravenous dose. It can be seen in equations (8.8) and (8.9) that A and B are directly proportional to the dose. When the parameters of the two-compartment model are determined experimentally, A, B, α, and β are determined first. These are then used to determine the value of the micro rate constants using the computational formula based on equations (8.6)–(8.9):

$$k_{21} = \frac{A \cdot \beta + B \cdot \alpha}{A + B} \tag{8.10}$$

$$k_{10} = \frac{\alpha \cdot \beta}{k_{21}} \tag{8.11}$$

$$k_{12} = \alpha + \beta - k_{10} - k_{21} \tag{8.12}$$

Explicit equations for α and β have also been derived, which allow α and β to be calculated from the micro rate constants:

$$\alpha = 0.5 \left[(k_{10} + k_{12} + k_{21}) + \sqrt{(k_{12} + k_{21} + k_{10})^2 - (4 \times k_{21} \times k_{10})} \right] \tag{8.13}$$

$$\beta = 0.5 \left[(k_{10} + k_{12} + k_{21}) - \sqrt{(k_{12} + k_{21} + k_{10})^2 - (4 \times k_{21} \times k_{10})} \right] \tag{8.14}$$

8.5 PRIMARY PHARMACOKINETIC PARAMETERS

The pharmacokinetic parameters of the model shown in Figure 8.3 consist of first-order rate constants (k_{10}, k_{12}, and k_{21}) and volumes (V_1 and V_2). As was the case for the one-compartment model, the rate constants are derived, or dependent pharmacokinetic parameters with little direct physiological meaning. The two-compartment model has a total of four primary pharmacokinetic parameters: clearance (Cl), distribution clearance (Cld), volume of the central compartment (V_1), and volume of the peripheral compartment (V_2). A description of these primary parameters and their relationship to the volume of distribution and the dependent parameters (k_{10}, k_{12}, and k_{21}) is presented below.

8.5.1 Clearance

Clearance is consistent with previous definitions: It is a measure of the ability of the organs of elimination to remove drug from the plasma, and it is a constant of proportionality between the rate of elimination at any time and the corresponding plasma concentration. The rate of elimination of a drug can be expressed using either the elimination rate constant (k_{10}) or clearance:

$$-\frac{dAb}{dt} = k_{10} \cdot A_1 \tag{8.15}$$

$$-\frac{dAb}{dt} = Cl \cdot Cp \tag{8.16}$$

Equating equations (8.15) and (8.16), and given that $Cp = A_1/V_1$, the equation can be rearranged to yield

$$k_{10} = \frac{Cl}{V_1} \tag{8.17}$$

Clearance can be determined in the usual way from the area under the curve (AUC):

$$Cl = \frac{S \cdot F \cdot D}{\text{AUC}} \tag{8.18}$$

For the two-compartment model, the AUC can be calculated as:

$$\text{AUC} = \int_0^\infty Cp \cdot dt = \int_0^\infty A \cdot e^{-\alpha t} + B \cdot e^{-\beta t} \cdot dt \tag{8.19}$$

$$\text{AUC} = \frac{A}{\alpha} + \frac{B}{\beta} \tag{8.20}$$

8.5.2 Distribution Clearance

The *Distribution clearance* (Cld) is a measure of the ability of a drug to pass into and out of the tissues of the peripheral compartment. It is determined by the permeability of the drug across the membranes of these tissues as well as the blood flow to the tissues. It can be shown that

$$Cld = Q_b(1 - e^{-P/Q_b}) \tag{8.21}$$

where P is the permeability, and Q_b is the blood flow. It can be seen in equation (8.21) that as the permeability increases, the distribution clearance becomes limited by blood flow. Thus, when a drug is able to diffuse across a membrane with ease, as is the case for most small lipophilic drugs, the distribution clearance will be dependent on the blood flow to a tissue and will be high in those tissues with large blood flows. The distribution clearance is the constant of proportionality between the rates of distribution and redistribution and the concentration driving each process.

Drug distribution from the central compartment to the peripheral compartment can be expressed using either the first-order rate constant for distribution (k_{12}) or the distribution clearance:

$$\text{rate of distribution} = A_1 \cdot k_{12}$$
$$\text{rate of distribution} = Cld \cdot Cp$$
$$(8.22)$$

Equating the two expressions in equation (8.22), and substituting for Cp ($Cp = A_1/V_1$), it can be written as:

$$k_{12} = \frac{Cld}{V_1} \qquad (8.23)$$

The rate constant for distribution to the peripheral compartment is derived from the two primary parameters: distribution clearance and the volume of the central compartment.

Drug redistribution from the peripheral compartment back into the central compartment can also be expressed using either distribution clearance or the rate constant for redistribution:

$$\text{rate of redistribution} = Cld \cdot C_2$$
$$\text{rate of redistribution} = A_2 \cdot k_{21}$$
$$(8.24)$$

Equating the two expressions in equation (8.24) and substituting for C_2 ($C_2 = A_2/V_2$), it can be shown as:

$$k_{21} = \frac{Cld}{V_2} \qquad (8.25)$$

The rate constant for redistribution from the peripheral compartment is derived from the two primary parameters of distribution: distribution clearance and the volume of the peripheral compartment. Thus, distribution clearance is a primary pharmacokinetic parameter that determines the values of the rate constants for distribution and redistribution. The rate constants for distribution and redistribution are also determined by V_1 and V_2, respectively.

When there is equilibrium between the two compartments, the rate of distribution = the rate of redistribution. Thus,

$$A_1 \cdot k_{12} = A_2 \cdot k_{21}$$
$$\frac{k_{12}}{k_{21}} = \frac{A_2}{A_1}$$
$$(8.26)$$

Substituting for k_{12} and k_{21} from equations (8.23) and (8.25) yields

$$\frac{V_2}{V_1} = \frac{A_2}{A_1} \qquad (8.27)$$

Thus, both the ratio k_{12}/k_{21} [equation (8.26)] and the ratio V_2/V_1 [equation (8.27)] are measures of the relative distribution of the drug between the two compartments. A large ratio indicates that a large fraction of the drug in the body resides in the peripheral compartment.

8.5.3 Volume of Distribution

The two-compartment model contains two volume terms (V_1 and V_2), but it is not clear how these volumes are related to the volume of distribution. Recall that the *volume of distribution* of a drug is a ratio of the amount of drug in the body at any time to the plasma concentration at that time. In a two-compartment model, the volume of distribution changes after the administration of a dose, and at different times one of three volumes of distribution may hold: V_1, V_β, and Vd_{ss}. The definition and characteristics of these three volumes are discussed below.

8.5.3.1 Volume of the Central Compartment

The volume of the central compartment (V_1) is the volume of distribution at time zero immediately after intravenous administration of a drug. At this time, the entire dose is contained within the central compartment: $A_1 =$ dose; $A_2 = 0$. Thus,

$$Vd = \frac{Ab}{Cp} = \frac{A_1}{Cp} = V_1 \tag{8.28}$$

The plasma concentration at $t = 0$ (Cp_0) can be expressed as

$$Cp_0 = A \cdot e^{-\alpha t} + B \cdot e^{-\beta t} = A + B \tag{8.29}$$

Thus, V_1 may be determined:

$$V_1 = \frac{\text{dose}_{IV}}{Cp_0} = \frac{\text{dose}_{IV}}{A + B} \tag{8.30}$$

8.5.3.2 Volume of Distribution in the Distribution Phase

At time zero, the entire dose is contained within the central compartment and $Vd = V_1$. The drug then gradually distributes to the peripheral compartment. As the physical volume through which the drug distributes increases, the volume of distribution increases. This can be appreciated by considering the relative rates of fall of the plasma concentration and the total amount of drug in the body during the distribution period. During this period, the plasma concentration falls as a result of distribution and elimination. But distribution dominates and as a result the relative fall in the plasma concentration (Cp) is greater than the relative fall in the amount of drug in the body (Ab). Consequently, the volume of distribution ($Vd = Ab/Cp$) increases (Figure 8.5). Once the distribution phase has been completed, the plasma concentration and the amount of drug in the body fall in parallel, the volume of distribution is constant and is called V_β. Thus, V_β represents the volume of distribution in the postdistribution or elimination phase.

The disadvantage of V_β is that it is dependent on elimination and as a result is not a true primary, independent parameter. In the postdistribution or elimination phase, true equilibrium between the two compartments does not exist. A momentary equilibrium is established and then destroyed continuously by drug elimination. If true equilibrium was established,

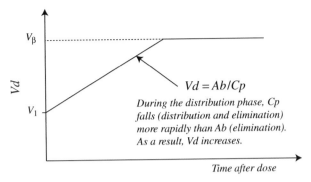

$$Vd = Ab/Cp$$

During the distribution phase, Cp falls (distribution and elimination) more rapidly than Ab (elimination). As a result, Vd increases.

FIGURE 8.5   Graph showing how the volume of distribution changes with time after an intravenous injection in a two-compartment model.

Vd would equal the sum of V_1 and V_2. Because elimination occurs from the central compartment only, the drug concentration in the central compartment (Cp) falls to a greater extent than the amount of drug in the body (Ab). As a result, V_β (Ab/Cp) is larger than $V_1 + V_2$. Furthermore, the greater the extent of elimination, the greater is the difference between V_β and $V_1 + V_2$. When elimination tends towards zero, the system tends toward true equilibrium, and V_β tends toward $V_1 + V_2$. A true equilibrium between the two compartments can also be established if drug elimination from the central compartment is matched exactly by drug administration into the central compartment (Figure 8.6).

The value of V_β is usually close to the value of $V_1 + V_2$. It is easily calculated and is a useful volume of distribution, but its dependence on elimination can limit its use. For example, it would not be an appropriate parameter to use in a clinical study designed to evaluate if distribution was altered in a situation in which clearance may be altered. It would not be possible to determine if any changes in V_β were due to altered clearance or altered distribution.

Determination of V_β   During the elimination phase, $Vd = V_\beta$ and the rate of drug elimination can be expressed as:

$$\text{rate of elimination} = \beta \cdot Ab \qquad (8.31)$$

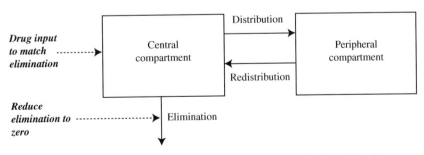

FIGURE 8.6   Ways to establish true equilibrium between the central and peripheral compartments. True equilibrium between compartments can be obtained either by exactly matching the rate of elimination with drug input or by reducing elimination to zero.

But, elimination can also be expressed in terms of clearance:

$$\text{rate of elimination} = Cl \cdot Cp \tag{8.32}$$

equating equations (8.31) and (8.32). Substituting Ab/V_β for Cp, and substituting $S \cdot F \cdot D/\text{AUC}$ for Cl, the equation can be rearranged as:

$$V_\beta = \frac{S \cdot F \cdot D}{\beta \cdot \text{AUC}} \tag{8.33}$$

The AUC is calculated as described previously in equation (8.20).

8.5.3.3   Volume of Distribution at Steady State

At steady state, the loss of drug from elimination is matched exactly by the gain of drug from administration. True equilibrium exists between the compartments, and the volume of distribution is equal to $V_1 + V_2$. This volume of distribution is known as the *volume of distribution at steady state* (Vd_{ss}). It is a true primary pharmacokinetic parameter that reflects only distribution and is not influenced by elimination.

At steady state, rate of distribution = rate of redistribution:

$$A_1 \cdot k_{12} = A_2 \cdot k_{21} \tag{8.34}$$

Thus,

$$A_2 = \frac{A_1 \cdot k_{12}}{k_{21}} \tag{8.35}$$

$$Vd_{ss} = \frac{Ab}{Cp} = \frac{A_1 + A_2}{Cp} = \frac{A_1 + A_2}{A_1/V_1} \tag{8.36}$$

Substituting A_2 from equation (8.35) into equation (8.36) yields

$$Vd_{ss} = V_1 \cdot \frac{k_{12} + k_{21}}{k_{21}} \tag{8.37}$$

In summary, the model for an intravenous injection in a two-compartment model has four primary parameters: clearance, distribution clearance, volume of the central compartment, and volume of the peripheral compartment (or Vd_{ss}, which is equal to $V_1 + V_2$). This model can be parameterized in terms of these primary pharmacokinetic parameters. Alternatively, the model can be described using the derived parameters or micro rate constants: k_{10}, k_{12}, k_{21}, and the volumes. The various ways of parameterizing the model are summarized in Table 8.1, which for comparison include the parameterization of the one-compartment model.

8.6   SIMULATION EXERCISE:
http://web.uri.edu/pharmacy/research/rosenbaum/sims

Open simulation model 5, Single Injection in a 2-Compartment Model, which can be found at http://web.uri.edu/pharmacy/research/rosenbaum/sims/Model5.

TABLE 8.1   Various Ways of Parameterizing One- and Two-Compartment Models

	Rate Constants	Physiological Parameters
Intravenous		
One-compartment	k and Vd	Cl and Vd
Two-compartment	k_{10}, k_{12}, k_{21}, V_1, and V_2^a	Cl, Cld, V_1, and V_2^b

^{a}Since one of these parameters can be calculated if the other four are known, this parameterization consists of four, not five, parameters.
$^b Vd_{ss} = V_1 + V_2$.

The default parameters of the model are dose = 1000 mg, S = 1, Cl = 4 L/h, Cld = 30 L/h, V_1 = 10 L, and V_2 = 40 L.

1. *Review the objectives and model summary.*

2. *Explore the model and the various pharmacokinetic parameters.*

3. Exercise 1: Cp–time profile. *The left graph shows the drug concentration in plasma and in the hypothetical peripheral compartment on a linear scale. The right graph shows a plasma concentration–time profile on the semilogarithmic scale. Choose a dose.*

   Observe:

   • *The nature of the Cp–time profile is biphasic.*

   • *The steep initial fall corresponds to the distribution of drug to the peripheral compartment (distribution phase). When it is over, the fall of ln Cp with time is linear.*

   • *The peak concentration in the peripheral compartment corresponds to the end of the distribution phase.*

   • *In the postdistribution or elimination phase, the drug concentration in the hypothetical peripheral compartment is equal to the plasma concentration.*

   • *In the elimination phase, the peripheral compartment concentration and the plasma concentration fall in parallel as drug is eliminated from the body.*

4. Exercise 2: Effect of dose. *Graphs of plasma concentration against time are shown on the linear and semilogarithmic scales. The $t_{1/2,\beta}$ is also shown in a display window. Without clearing the graphs between doses, give doses of 50, 100, and 150 mg.*

   Observe:

   • *Drag the mouse along the curves of the plots to display the values of Cp and time. It can be seen that Cp at any time is proportional to the dose.*

   • *From the plot of ln Cp against time, it can be seen that the slope of the terminal linear portion of the graph does not change with dose. The elimination half-life does not change with dose.*

5. Prominence of two-compartment characteristics. *The distribution of many drugs to some of the tissues in the body, particularly the poorly perfused tissues, is not instantaneous. Yet, a two-compartment model is not always needed for these drugs. Sometimes, the simpler one-compartment model will provide an acceptable degree of accuracy. The prominence of two-compartmental pharmacokinetics, and the error that would result if a one-compartmental model was used, depends on a number of factors. First, the amount of drug involved in the slower distribution is important. If this distribution involves only a relatively small amount of the total drug in the body, it*

will have little impact on the initial plasma concentrations. The amount of elimination that occurs during the distribution phase is another important factor. In contrast to the one-compartment model, where distribution is instantaneous, some elimination will occur during distribution to the peripheral compartment. The greater the amount of drug elimination during the distribution phase, the greater the prominence of two-compartmental characteristics.

Exercise 3: Elimination during the distribution phase. *During the early period after an injection, distribution to the peripheral compartment and elimination compete for the drug in the central compartment. The rate of distribution is controlled by k_{12}, which is equal to Cld/V_1. The rate of elimination is controlled by k_{10}, which is equal to Cl/V_1. Thus, the relative values of Cld and Cl control whether distribution or elimination is the dominant process. As Cl increases relative to Cld, the amount of drug eliminated during the distribution phase increases, and the prominence of the two-compartmental characteristics increases.*

Go to the "Elimination, Cl and Cld" interface page. The graph on the left is a plot of Ln(Cp) against time, and can be used to evaluate the duration of the distribution period. The graph on the right shows the percentage of the dose (1000 mg) eliminated at any time. The values of α and β are also displayed:

- *With the default value of Cld (30 L/h), simulate with Cl values of 10, 20, and 40 L/h. Comment on how Cl effects the two-compartmental characteristics, the amount of drug eliminated during the distribution phase, β and α.*

- *Clear the graphs. With Cl set to 4 L/h, simulate with values of Cld of 30, 15, and 7 L/h. Comment on the effects on the two-compartmental characteristics, the amount of drug eliminated during the distribution phase, β and α.*

- *Clear the graphs. Now, make Cld very low (1 L/h) and observe the effects of Cl values of 10, 20, and 40 L/h. Note as above, the prominence of the two-compartmental characteristics increases as Cl increases, but note the changes are associated with minimal change in β and instead bring about almost proportional changes in α. This is because in the early period after the dose, the rate of elimination is greater than the rate of distribution and dominates the fall in the plasma concentrations. At later times, when most of the dose has been eliminated, the gentler fall in the plasma concentration is due to drug redistributing from the peripheral compartment. This is known as a flip-flop model because the normal arrangement of the phases is reversed: A and α reflect elimination, and B and β reflect distribution. This situation is much less common in a two-compartment model but is observed in a three-compartment model (Section 6.3.3) where a deep tissue compartment is incorporated into the model. The pharmacokinetics of both gentamicin and digoxin are most accurately modeled using a three-compartment model. The tissues of the central compartment take up the drug in an essentially instantaneous manner; the tissues of the peripheral compartment take up the drug more slowly, and this distribution is associated with a steep initial decline in plasma concentrations; the tissues of the deep tissue compartment take up the drug extremely slowly. This distribution is slower than elimination, and at later times redistribution from the deep tissue compartment controls the terminal slope of the LnCp versus time plot (Figure 6.3b). In the case of gentamicin, this latter phase is only apparent many hours after a dose when plasma concentrations are very low.*

6. Exercise 4: The fraction of the drug that distributes to the peripheral compartment. *Observe how the amount of drug that distributes to the peripheral compartment*

influences the prominence of two-compartmental characteristics. Note, the fraction of the overall drug that distributes to the peripheral compartment is reflected by the relative values of V_1 and V_2, and recall that k_{12} is Cld/V_1, and k_{21} is Cld/V_2. Thus, V_2/V_1 is equal to k_{12}/k_{21}.

- *Simulate with values of V_2 of 10, 40, 80, and 160 L. Comment on the effects on the difference between the initial Cp, and Cp at the beginning of the postdistribution phase. Also comment on the effects on β.*

8.7 DETERMINATION OF THE PHARMACOKINETIC PARAMETERS OF THE TWO-COMPARTMENT MODEL

The parameters of the two-compartment model are determined using a study protocol similar to the one discussed for a one-compartment model. Thus, an intravenous dose is administered to subjects, and plasma concentrations of the drug obtained at various times after the dose are subject to pharmacokinetic analysis. In the case of a two-compartment model, it is important to obtain sufficient blood samples during the distribution phase to characterize the two-compartmental characteristics.

The plot of plasma concentration against time for a two-compartment model is described by a biexponential equation and cannot be converted to a straight line by converting plasma concentrations to the logarithmic domain. Thus, simple linear regression cannot be used to estimate the parameters of the two-compartment model. Today, a wide variety of commercial software packages, such as WinNonlin (Pharsight, Mountain View, California, USA), are available that can perform nonlinear regression analysis. These products use nonlinear regression analysis to model the plasma concentration–time data directly to obtain estimates of the pharmacokinetic parameters (i.e., they do not need the plasma concentrations to be converted to the logarithmic domain). Prior to the general availability of nonlinear regression software, the plasma concentration–time data had to be linearized using a process called *curve stripping* (also known as the *method of residuals* or *feathering*). This method is still useful today when initial estimates of the parameters are needed for computer analysis. The process takes the basic equation for the two-compartment model:

$$Cp = A \cdot e^{-\alpha t} + B \cdot e^{-\beta t}$$

and isolates the two-component exponential functions to allow A and α and B and β to be determined from straight lines obtained from semilogarithmic plots. The micro rate constants and the primary pharmacokinetic parameters are then calculated from these four parameters. This method is described in detail below.

8.7.1 Determination of Intercepts and Macro Rate Constants

8.7.1.1 Determination of B and β

The equation for the overall plasma concentration–time is given as:

$$Cp = A \cdot e^{-\alpha t} + B \cdot e^{-\beta t} \tag{8.38}$$

Recall that the hybrid rate constant for distribution (α) is almost always larger than the hybrid rate constant for elimination (β). As a result, $e^{-\alpha t}$ decays to zero (at about 3–5 α $t_{1/2,\alpha}$) before $e^{-\beta t}$. At this point, the equation becomes monoexponential:

$$Cp = B \cdot e^{-\beta t} \tag{8.39}$$

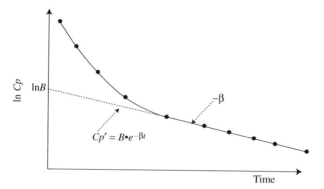

FIGURE 8.7   Determination of B and β from a semilogarithmic plot of plasma concentration against time. During the elimination phase, $Cp' = Cp$, but during the distribution phase, $Cp' < Cp$. Estimates of B and β can be determined from the intercept and slope, respectively, of a semilogarithmic plot of Cp' against time (Figure 8.7).

Taking logarithms of equation (8.39) converts it into the equation of a straight line. Let Cp all along this line (from time zero to infinity) $= Cp'$:

$$Cp' = B \cdot e^{-\beta t} \tag{8.40}$$
$$\ln Cp' = \ln B - \beta \cdot t \tag{8.41}$$

Thus, a plot $\ln Cp'$ versus time yields a straight line of slope $(-\beta)$ and intercept $\ln B$ (Figure 8.7). The drug's half-life during the elimination phase can be calculated as:

$$t_{1/2,\beta} = \frac{0.693}{\beta} \tag{8.42}$$

8.7.1.2   *Determination of A and α*
Parameters A and α are determined using curve stripping to separate the two exponential components of equation (8.38). Recall that during the distribution phase, $Cp' < Cp$. If during this period, Cp' is subtracted from Cp, we obtain

$$Cp - Cp' = A \cdot e^{-\alpha t} - B \cdot e^{-\beta t} - B \cdot e^{-\beta t} \tag{8.43}$$

or

$$Cp - Cp' = A \cdot e^{-\alpha t} \tag{8.44}$$

Thus, $A \cdot e^{-\alpha t}$ is isolated, and taking logarithms yields

$$\ln(Cp - Cp') = \ln A - \alpha \cdot t \tag{8.45}$$

Thus, a plot of $\ln(Cp - Cp')$ yields a straight line of slope $(-\alpha)$ and intercept $\ln A$. The plot of $\ln(Cp - Cp')$ is constructed as follows:

1. The times of the observed data points in the distribution phase are noted.
2. From the back-extrapolated part of the plot of $\ln Cp'$ against time, the corresponding Cp' values of these times are noted. Alternatively they can calculated from $Cp' = Be^{-\beta t}$.

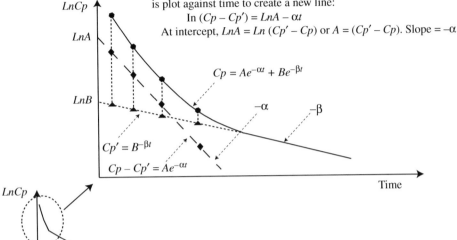

1. Plot ln Cp against time. Note the linear terminal linear portion
2. Let Cp along this line and its back extrapolated portion = Cp':
$$LnCp' = LnB - \beta t$$
   At intercept, $LnB = LnCp'$, or $B = Cp'$. Slope = $-\beta$
2. Values of Cp' (▲) that correspond to the time of given data (●) are read off the line or calculated
3. Values of $Cp - Cp'$ (● – ▲ = ◆) are calculated and $Ln(Cp - Cp')$ is plot against time to create a new line:
$$\text{In}(Cp - Cp') = LnA - \alpha t$$
   At intercept, $LnA = Ln(Cp' - Cp)$ or $A = (Cp' - Cp)$. Slope = $-\alpha$

$$Cp = Ae^{-\alpha t} + Be^{-\beta t}$$

$Cp' = B^{-\beta t}$

$Cp - Cp' = Ae^{-\alpha t}$

FIGURE 8.8   Method of residuals to determine A and α.

3. These values of Cp' are subtracted from their corresponding given data points to obtain the values of $Cp - Cp'$.
4. $Cp - Cp'$ is plotted against time on a semilogarithmic scale.

The process is summarized in Figure 8.8.

8.7.2 Determination of the Micro Rate Constants: k_{12}, k_{21}, and k_{10}

The micro rate constants k_{10}, k_{21}, and k_{12} can be calculated from the formulas presented earlier (8.10)–(8.12).

8.7.3 Determination of the Primary Pharmacokinetic Parameters

The primary pharmacokinetic parameters of the two-compartment model can be determined using formulas presented previously:

1. V_1 from equation (8.30)
2. V_β from equation (8.33)
3. Vd_{ss} from equation (8.37)

4. Clearance from equation (8.18)

5. Distribution clearance from equation (8.23) or (8.25)

Example 8.1   The data in Table E8.1 were simulated for a 100-mg intravenous bolus injection in a two-compartment model. Analyze the data to determine:

(a) The intercepts and macro rate constants: A, B, α, and β
(b) The micro rate constants: k_{10}, k_{12}, and k_{21}
(c) The primary pharmacokinetic parameters: Cl, Cld, V_1, V_β, and Vd_{ss}

TABLE E8.1   Plasma Concentrations at Various Times After a 100-mg Intravenous Dose

Time (h)	Cp (mg/L)	Time (h)	Cp (mg/L)
0.1	7.95	2	1.07
0.2	6.38	3	0.89
0.4	4.25	4	0.76
0.7	8.57	6	0.56
1	1.79	8	0.42
1.5	1.27	12	0.23

Solution   A complete Excel worksheet created for this analysis is shown in Appendix C (Figure C.6). The answers are as follows:

(a) $A = 8.47$ mg/L; $B = 1.38$ mg/L; $\alpha = 2.62$ h^{-1}; $\beta = 0.149$ h^{-1}
(b) $k_{10} = 0.789$ h^{-1}; $k_{12} = 1.49$ h^{-1}; $k_{21} = 0.495$ h^{-1}
(c) $Cl = 8.02$ L/h; $Cld = 15.1$ L/h; $V_1 = 10.2$ L; $V_\beta = 53.8$ L; $Vd_{ss} = 40.7$ L

8.8 CLINICAL APPLICATION OF THE TWO-COMPARTMENT MODEL

When pharmacokinetics is used to optimize drug therapy in individual patients, it is rarely possible to obtain enough plasma samples to be able to use the two-compartment model, and as a result, the simpler one-compartment model is frequently used. It has been found that provided that certain precautions are taken, the one-compartment model provides an acceptable degree of accuracy when applied to drugs that display two-compartmental pharmacokinetics.

8.8.1 Measurement of the Elimination Half-Life in the Postdistribution Phase

For drugs that display wide interpatient variability in clearance and/or the volume of distribution, it is often necessary to determine the drug's elimination half-life in individual patients. Usually, the half-life is determined from only two blood samples, and if a drug displays two-compartmental pharmacokinetics, it is important to wait until the conclusion of the distribution phase before taking blood samples to measure the elimination half-life. If sample(s) are taken in the distribution phase, the estimate of the half-life will be biased (Figure 8.9).

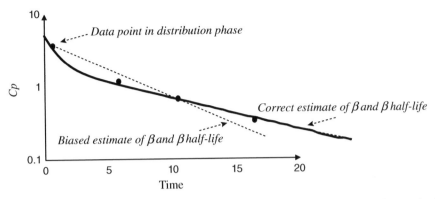

FIGURE 8.9   Data points used to estimate the β elimination half-life. Biased results are obtained when plasma concentrations in the distribution phase are used to calculate $t_{1/2,\beta}$.

For example, the half-life of the aminoglycoside antibiotics is frequently determined in individual patients because these antibiotics display wide interindividual variability in their clearance. These drugs are administered as short infusions over a period of about 30 min–1 h to treat very serious, often life-threatening conditions. They can also produce very serious toxicity, including renal toxicity, which is usually reversible, and ototoxicity, which often is not reversible and may leave the patient with residual hearing loss and/or vestibular damage. To maximize the therapeutic response of the drugs, and to minimize toxicity, aminoglycoside levels are usually monitored in individual patients, and the patient's individual half-life is determined to help guide therapy. Because the aminoglycosides display two-compartmental characteristics, and one-compartmental pharmacokinetics are used to guide dosage adjustment, it is important to avoid the distribution phase when sampling for determination of the half-life. It is usual to wait about 30 min after the end of a 30-min infusion before taking blood samples.

8.8.2   Determination of the Loading Dose

As discussed in Chapter 7, the volume of distribution is used to determine loading doses. The two-compartment model has three volumes of distribution, each of which applies at different times. V_1 is the smallest and applies only at time zero, when the entire dose is in the central compartment. Vd_{ss} (Vd at steady state) and V_β (Vd in the postdistribution phase) are similar in value and can be considered to provide equivalent loading doses, which are however much larger than loading doses based on V_1.

When V_1 is used to calculate a loading dose, the plasma concentration at time zero will achieve the desired concentration, but it will fall rapidly as drug distributes to the peripheral compartment (Figure 8.10). When either of the other two volumes are used, the initial plasma concentration will overshoot the desired concentration but will quickly approach the target, depending on the duration of the distribution phase (Figure 8.10).

The compartmental location of the site of action or toxicity is an important factor in determining which volume it is appropriate to use. If the site of action or toxicity is in the peripheral compartment, the high initial plasma concentrations associated with using Vd_{ss} or V_β should not, within reason, lead to adverse effects. If, on the other hand, the site of action or toxicity is in the central compartment, the high initial concentration could cause toxicity. In this case, a loading dose based on V_1 could be used. But as the drug distributes

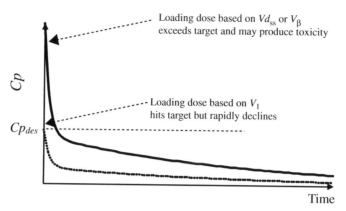

FIGURE 8.10   Plasma concentrations produced by different loading doses. Loading doses calculated using V_1 achieve the desired plasma concentration (Cp_{des}) immediately, but rapidly decline (dotted line). The initial concentration produced by a loading dose calculated using Vd_{ss} or V_β exceeds the target and may produce toxicity (solid line).

to the peripheral compartment, plasma concentrations will rapidly become subtherapeutic. Alternatively, a total loading dose based on Vd_{ss} or V_β could be estimated and split into a few smaller units that could be administered in several minute intervals, depending on the speed of drug distribution and the patient's response. Lidocaine and procainamide are examples of drugs with sites of action/toxicity in the central compartment.

Example 8.2   Lidocaine is an antiarrhythmic drug that is used in the treatment of premature ventricular contractions. A 70-kg male patient is to receive an intravenous infusion of lidocaine to maintain a plasma concentration of 2 mg/L. Calculate a loading dose of lidocaine hydrochloride ($S = 0.87$) to achieve this plasma concentration immediately. Lidocaine has the following volumes: $V_1 = 0.5$ L/kg and $Vd_{ss} = 1.3$ L/kg.

Solution   The site of action or toxicity of lidocaine is in the central compartment, and the initial loading dose is often based on the volume of the central compartment (V_1):

$$D_L = Cp_{SS} \cdot \frac{Vd}{S \cdot F}$$
$$D_L = \frac{2\ \text{mg/L} \times 0.5\ \text{L/kg} \times 70\ \text{kg}}{0.87 \times 1}$$
$$= 80\ \text{mg}$$

To avoid toxicity, the loading dose would be administered over a period of about 2–3 min. The plasma concentration will fall rapidly as the drug distributes throughout the tissues of the peripheral compartment. To maintain the plasma concentration at a therapeutic level, it is often necessary to give additional injections which are usually about half the initial loading dose.

Digoxin's site of action and toxicity is in the peripheral compartment, and loading doses of digoxin are based on the larger Vd_{ss} or V_β. However, because digoxin has a narrow therapeutic range, the total dose is still split into smaller units, which are given in 6-h intervals. The patient is monitored between the units, and subsequent doses are withheld if necessary.

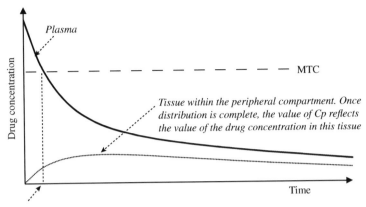

FIGURE 8.11   Time course of drug concentrations in the plasma (*Cp*) and a hypothetical tissue of the peripheral compartment after an intravenous dose. At time zero, *Cp* is at its maximum value and the concentration in the tissue is zero. During the distribution phase, *Cp* decreases and the tissue concentration increases. During this period, *Cp* is not reflective of the concentration in the peripheral compartment. Once distribution is complete, the ratio of the two concentrations remains constant. It is only at this time that the *Cp* reflects drug concentration in the peripheral compartment. For drugs whose site of action is in the peripheral compartment, it is only at this time that the therapeutic range holds and *Cp* can be used to predict the effect of the drug.

8.8.3 Evaluation of a Dose: Monitoring Plasma Concentrations and Patient Response

In the two-compartment model, the tissues of the central compartment are always in equilibrium with the plasma. This is not the case for the tissues of the peripheral compartment. Immediately after an intravenous dose, the plasma concentration is at its highest and the peripheral compartment concentration is zero. During the course of the distribution phase, the concentration in the tissues of the peripheral compartment increase and approache equilibrium with the plasma (Figure 8.11). If the site of action of the drug is in the peripheral compartment, the plasma concentration will reflect concentrations at the site of action only during the postdistribution phase, and the therapeutic range of these drugs will apply only at this time. This concept is particularly important for digoxin because it has an exceptionally long distribution phase (over 4 h after an intravenous dose and over 6 h after an oral dose) and its site of action is in the peripheral compartment. Because digoxin has a narrow therapeutic range and variable pharmacokinetics, serum levels are monitored to check the adequacy of the dose. It is important that digoxin's serum levels be evaluated only at least 6 h after an intravenous dose and about 8 h after an oral dose, as it is only at these times that the plasma concentration (serum concentration) reflects the concentration at the site of action.

PROBLEMS

8.1   Plasma concentration–time data collected after the intravenous administration of a dose (100 mg) of a drug ($S = 1$) were best fit by a two-compartment model. The following equation was obtained:

$$C_p = 8.47e^{-2.62t} + 1.38e^{-0.15t}$$

where Cp is in mg/L and time is in hours. Calculate the following parameters for this drug: k_{10}, k_{12}, k_{21}, V_1, V_β, Vd_{ss}, Cl, and Cld.

8.2 How long would the distribution phase last for the drug presented in Problem 8.1?

8.3 If a 50-mg dose of the drug discussed in Problem 8.1 was administered, estimate:
(a) Cp at 0.5 h
(b) Cp at 6 h

8.4 The drug discussed in Problem 8.1 was administered to a patient who was suspected to have altered clearance. Three plasma samples were collected after the administration of a 100-mg IV dose. The samples were analyzed for unchanged drug, and the data are shown in Table P8.4.

TABLE P8.4   Plasma Concentrations at Different Times After a 100-mg Intravenous Dose

T (h)	Cp (mg/L)
0.5	2.20
2.0	0.82
12	0.19

Calculate $t_{1/2,\beta}$.

8.5 A study was conducted to see how renal impairment might affect a drug's disposition ($fe = 0.95$). The drug's pharmacokinetic parameters were estimated in a group of patients with normal renal function and in a group that had impaired renal function. Table P8.5 summarizes the results. From this information:

TABLE P8.5   Pharmacokinetic Parameters of a Drug in Normal Patients and Patients with Impaired Renal Function

Parameter	Renal Function	
	Normal	Less Than 20% Normal
Cl (L/h)	16.8 ± 0.87	2.2 ± 1.2^b
V_β (L)	46 ± 5.6	36 ± 6.3^b
Vd_{ss} (L)	37 ± 5.5	34 ± 6.3
$t_{1/2,\beta}$ (h)	1.80 ± 0.65	9.67 ± 2.7^b

[a]Mean parameter values ± the standard deviation.
[b]Of statistical significance.
Cl is the clearance, V_β is the volume of distribution in the postdistribution phase, Vd_{ss} is the steady-state volume of distribution, and $t_{1/2,\beta}$ is the elimination half-life.

(a) Do you conclude that renal impairment affects this drug's elimination?
(b) Do you conclude that renal impairment affects this drug's elimination distribution?
(c) Discuss how renal impairment affects each parameter.

8.6 A 72-year-old female patient with congestive heart failure has been taking digoxin 250 μg for several years. On a routine visit to the community health center, she discusses her medication with her health team. She says she finds it easy to remember to take her digoxin, as it is a once-daily regimen and she always takes it with her breakfast at 8:00 A.M. Her physician would like to maintain her serum digoxin in the range 0.5–1.5 µg/L. A blood sample is taken just before she leaves at 9:30 A.M. The following day, the results come back from the laboratory and reveal a serum digoxin level of 2.6 µg/L. Is this patient at risk for digoxin toxicity?

8.7 A 100-mg dose of a drug was administered intravenously. Plasma samples were taken at various times after the dose and analyzed for unchanged drug. The data are listed in Table P8.7. The data indicate that the drug follows two-compartmental pharmacokinetics. Set up an Excel worksheet and:

(a) Plot Cp against time on the linear and semilogarithmic scales.

(b) Determine the intercepts and macro rate constants: A, B, α, and β.

(c) Determine the micro rate constants: k_{10}, k_{12}, and k_{21}.

(d) Determine the primary pharmacokinetic parameters: Cl, Cld, V_1, V_β, and Vd_{ss} (use the formula $Vd_{ss} = V_1 (k_{12} + k_{21})/k_{21}$).

TABLE P8.7   Plasma Concentrations at Various Times After a 100-mg Intravenous Dose

Time (h)	Cp (mg/L)	Time (h)	Cp (mg/L)
0.1	7.12	1.5	0.88
0.2	5.15	2	0.84
0.4	2.88	3	0.8
0.5	2.24	5	0.74
0.7	1.51	7	0.68
1	1.07	12	0.56

SUGGESTED READINGS

1. Wagner, J. (1993) *Pharmacokinetics for the Pharmaceutical Scientist*, Technomic, Lancaster, PA.
2. Jambhekar, S. S., and Breen, P. J. (2009) *Basic Pharmacokinetics*, Pharmaceutical Press, London.

9

PHARMACOKINETICS OF EXTRAVASCULAR DRUG ADMINISTRATION

Dr. Steven C. Sutton

Basic Pharmacokinetics and Pharmacodynamics: An Integrated Textbook and Computer Simulations,
Second Edition. Edited by Sara E. Rosenbaum.
© 2017 John Wiley & Sons, Inc. Published 2017 by John Wiley & Sons, Inc.

Objectives

The material in this chapter will enable the reader to:

1. Apply a pharmacokinetic model to understand the derivation of a general equation that describes plasma concentration of a drug at any time after the administration of an oral dose
2. Understand the meaning and significance of the absorption parameters
3. Understand the factors that control the time it takes to achieve therapeutic plasma concentrations
4. Understand the factors that control the value of the peak plasma concentration
5. Apply the model to determine the major pharmacokinetic parameters from plasma concentration–time data obtained after the oral administration of a drug
6. Define absolute and relative bioavailability
7. Understand how bioavailability is assessed
8. Understand how an *in vitro-in vivo* correlation is assessed and utilized

9.1   INTRODUCTION

Extravascular drug administration refers to any route of drug administration where the drug is not administered directly into the systemic circulation. Generally, drugs administered by extravascular routes rely on the systemic circulation to deliver them to their site of action. Thus, access of the drug to the systemic circulation, or absorption, is a critical pharmacokinetic characteristic of extravascular administration. The typical plasma concentration–time profile observed after extravascular drug administration is shown in Figure 9.1. After drug administration, the plasma concentration increases gradually as a result of absorption, a peak is achieved, and then plasma concentrations fall. The pharmacokinetics of absorption are presented in this chapter, with the major emphasis being placed on oral drug administration. However, almost all of the general principles discussed in this chapter apply equally to other forms of extravascular drug absorption.

The administration of drugs by the oral route is noninvasive and very convenient for patients. As a result, it is the most common, and in most situations, the preferred route of drug administration. Several oral dosage forms are available to accommodate the needs of a variety of patients. Solid dosage forms, such as tablets and capsules, are the most common, but liquid dosage forms, including syrups, suspensions, and emulsions, are available to groups of patients, such as children and the elderly, who may have difficulty in swallowing

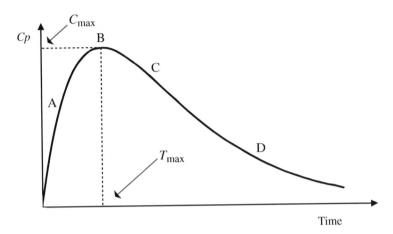

FIGURE 9.1 Typical plasma concentration–time profile after extravascular drug administration. The curve can be considered to have four areas: A, B, C and D. These will be discussed in the text. Point B corresponds to the peak plasma concentration. The value of the peak is C_{max} and the time of the peak is T_{max}.

solid dosage forms. Despite the popularity of oral dosage forms, they cannot be used in all situations. Some of the major reasons that preclude the oral route include the destruction of a drug by components of the gastrointestinal fluid and/or its inability to pass through the intestinal membrane; extensive presystemic extraction; an immediate drug action is required; the dose must be administered with great accuracy; or the patient is unconscious, uncooperative, or nauseous.

In view of the widespread use of the oral route, it is important to appreciate the unique pharmacokinetic characteristics of oral administration and understand how these may affect drug response. The absorption process brings two additional parameters into the pharmacokinetic model: the bioavailability factor (F) and a parameter for the rate of drug absorption, the first-order absorption rate constant (k_a). Unlike clearance and volume of distribution, the absorption parameters (F and k_a) are properties not only of the drug itself but also of the dosage form, and can vary from one brand of a drug to another.

In this chapter, we focus on presenting a pharmacokinetic model for orally administered drugs and discuss how the various model parameters affect the plasma concentration–time profile. The determination of the model parameters and the assessment of bioavailability are addressed. In clinical practice, the absorption parameters (k_a and F) cannot be determined from the limited (1–2) samples available from patients. Consequently, the equations for oral administration are not frequently used clinically to individualize doses for patients.

9.2 FIRST-ORDER ABSORPTION IN A ONE-COMPARTMENT MODEL

9.2.1 Model and Equations

As discussed in Chapter 2, the absorption of drugs from the gastrointestinal tract (GIT) often follows first-order kinetics. As a result, the pharmacokinetic model can be created simply by adding first-order absorption into the central compartment of the one-compartment model (Figure 9.2). The gastrointestinal tract is represented by a compartment in Figure 9.2.

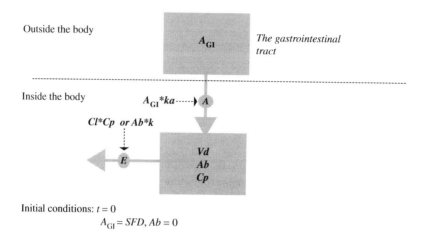

Initial conditions: $t = 0$
$A_{GI} = SFD, Ab = 0$

FIGURE 9.2 Pharmacokinetic model for first-order absorption in a one-compartment model. Ab and A_{GI} are the amounts of drug in the body and gastrointestinal tract, respectively; k and k_a are the first-order rate constants for elimination (E) and absorption (A), respectively; Cp is the plasma concentration and the concentration of drug in the compartment. The compartment has a volume of Vd, the drug's volume of distribution; Cl is the clearance; and the effective dose is the product of S (salt factor), F (bioavailability factor), and D (the dose administered).

However, since the GIT compartment is outside the body, the body is still modeled as a single compartment. The amount of drug in the GIT compartment is influenced only by first-order drug absorption:

$$\frac{dA_{GI}}{dt} = -k_a \cdot A_{GI} \tag{9.1}$$

where A_{GI} is the amount of drug in the GIT tract, and k_a is the first-order absorption rate constant. Integrating, we have

$$A_{GI} = A_{GI,0} \cdot e^{-k_a t} \tag{9.2}$$

where $A_{GI,0}$ is the initial amount of drug in the GIT tract, and is equal to the effective dose ($S \cdot F \cdot D$):

$$A_{GI} = S \cdot F \cdot D \cdot e^{-k_a t} \tag{9.3}$$

Equation (9.3) shows that the amount of drug in the GIT tract starts off at $S \cdot F \cdot D$ and decays to zero by infinity. The speed of the decay is dependent on the first-order rate constant for absorption.

The amount of drug in the body at any time will depend on the relative rates of drug absorption and elimination:

rate of change of the amount of drug in the body = rate of inputs − rate of outputs

$$\frac{dAb}{dt} = k_a \cdot A_{GI} - k \cdot Ab \tag{9.4}$$

Consideration of equation (9.4) provides an explanation for the shape of the plasma concentration–time curve (Figure 9.1). Immediately after drug administration (area A), plasma concentrations increase because the rate of absorption is greater than the rate of elimination. The amount of drug in the GIT tract is at its maximum, so the rate of absorption is also maximum. In contrast, initially, the amount of drug in the body is small, so the rate of elimination is low. As the absorption process continues, drug is depleted from the GIT tract, so the rate of absorption decreases. At the same time, the amount of drug in the body increases, so the rate of elimination increases. At the peak (B), the rate of absorption is momentarily equal to the rate of elimination. After this time, the rate of elimination exceeds the rate of absorption and plasma concentrations fall (area C). Eventually, all the drug is depleted from the GIT tract and drug absorption stops. At this time (area D), the plasma concentration is influenced only by elimination.

Equation (9.3) can be substituted into equation (9.4), which can then be integrated to yield

$$Ab = \frac{S \cdot F \cdot D \cdot k_a}{k_a - k} \cdot (e^{-kt} - e^{-k_a t}) \tag{9.5}$$

But $Cp = Ab/Vd$:

$$Cp = \frac{S \cdot F \cdot D \cdot k_a}{Vd \cdot (k_a - k)} \cdot (e^{-kt} - e^{-k_a t}) \tag{9.6}$$

Thus, for the 1 compartment model described in Figure 9.2, the plasma concentration at any time after an oral dose is described by a biexponential equation.

9.2.2 Parameter Determination

The pharmacokinetic model for extravascular administration has four fundamental parameters. Two of the parameters, clearance and volume of distribution, are disposition (elimination and distribution) parameters that are not dependent on the nature of the extravascular dosage form and drug absorption. The other two parameters, the bioavailability factor (F) and the first-order rate constant for absorption (k_a) are functions of both the drug and dosage form. Thus, these parameters can vary from one type and brand of dosage form to another. As always, the one-compartment model has the derived parameter for the rate of elimination (the elimination rate constant and the half-life).

Experimentally, the parameters of the model are determined by following a protocol similar to those presented in earlier chapters. Oral doses are administered to a group of individuals, and plasma concentrations are determined at various times after the dose. It is important to obtain several plasma concentration samples around the peak in order to characterize this feature adequately. Data from each person are subject to pharmacokinetic analysis to determine the pharmacokinetic parameters. Each parameter is then averaged across the group to calculate the mean and standard deviation. The basic equation for oral absorption [equation (9.6)] is biexponential and cannot be made linear by transforming the data to the logarithm scale. Generally, pharmacokinetic analysis is conducted using computer software that can perform nonlinear regression analysis to find the model parameters that will most closely match the data observed. However, as was the case with the two-compartment model, the parameters can be obtained by linearizing the data through curve stripping. A discussion of this method helps to demonstrate the importance and influence of each parameter of the model. Additionally, it is a useful procedure to employ if initial estimates of the parameters are needed for computer analysis.

9.2.2.1 First-Order Elimination Rate Constant

At some time after drug administration, the entire dose will have been absorbed and the plasma concentration will decline in a monoexponential manner, due only to first-order drug elimination. Mathematically:

- For extravascular administration, k_a is usually greater than k.
- As a result, $e^{-k_a t}$ becomes equal to zero before e^{-kt}.
- When this occurs, the equation for the plasma concentration (9.6) reduces to

$$Cp = \frac{S \cdot F \cdot D \cdot k_a}{Vd \cdot (k_a - k)} \cdot (e^{-kt} - 0)$$

$$Cp = \frac{S \cdot F \cdot D \cdot k_a}{Vd \cdot (k_a - k)} \cdot e^{-kt}$$

(9.7)

Taking logarithms gives

$$\ln Cp = \ln \frac{S \cdot F \cdot D \cdot k_a}{Vd \cdot (k_a - k)} - kt$$

(9.8)

This is the equation of a straight line. Thus, at later times, the plot of $\ln(Cp)$ against time becomes straight with a slope of the equal to the negative value elimination rate constant $(-k)$ and an intercept of $\ln[S \cdot F \cdot D \cdot k_a/Vd\,(k_a - k)]$ (Figure 9.3). This period is referred to as the *terminal elimination phase*.

9.2.2.2 Elimination Half-Life

As always, the elimination half-life is calculated from the elimination rate constant:

$$t_{1/2} = \frac{0.693}{k}$$

(9.9)

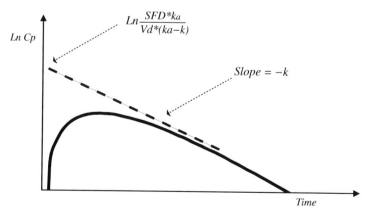

FIGURE 9.3   Plot of logarithm of plasma concentration against time. At later times, a linear relationship is observed. The slope of the line is $-k$ and the intercept is $\ln S \cdot F \cdot D \cdot k_a/[Vd\,(k_a - k)]$.

9.2.2.3 *First-Order Absorption Rate Constant*

The period before the elimination phase is referred to as the *absorption phase*. During this period, the plasma concentration is under the influence of both absorption and elimination, and the equation is biexponential. Curve stripping is used to separate the two exponential functions during this phase.

To make the equations less cumbersome, let

$$I = \frac{S \cdot F \cdot D \cdot k_a}{Vd \cdot (k_a - k)} \tag{9.10}$$

The full expression for Cp [equation (9.6)] is given by

$$Cp = I \cdot (e^{-kt} - e^{-k_a t}) \tag{9.11}$$

Let the plasma concentration during the elimination phase and its back-extrapolated component be Cp'. Thus,

$$Cp = I \cdot e^{-kt} \tag{9.12}$$

In the elimination phase, $Cp' = Cp$, but in the absorption phase, $Cp' > Cp$. Subtracting equation (9.11) from equation (9.12) yields

$$\begin{aligned} Cp' - Cp &= I \cdot e^{-kt} - I \cdot (e^{-kt} - e^{-k_a t}) \\ Cp' - Cp &= I \cdot e^{-k_a t} \end{aligned} \tag{9.13}$$

Taking logarithms gives us

$$\ln(Cp' - Cp) = \ln I - k_a \cdot t \tag{9.14}$$

This is the equation of a straight line of slope $(-k_a)$ and intercept $\ln I$. It is referred to as the *feathered line*.

The plot of $\ln(Cp' - Cp)$ is constructed as follows:

1. Note the time of the given data points in the absorption phase (open circles in Figure 9.4).
2. From the back-extrapolated part of the plot of $\ln Cp'$ against time, read off the corresponding values of Cp' at these times (solid circles in Figure 9.4). Alternatively, the values of Cp' can be calculated.
3. Subtract the given data points from these values of Cp' to obtain the values of $Cp' - Cp$.
4. Plot $Cp' - Cp$ against time on the semilogarithmic scale (diamonds in Figure 9.4).
5. Note that the two straight lines intercept at the same place on the Cp-axis.

This procedure is performed most conveniently using either semilogarithmic (base 10 logarithms) graph paper or using an Excel worksheet. The creation of an Excel worksheet is described in Appendix C.

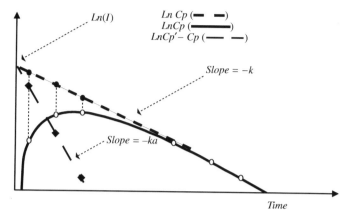

FIGURE 9.4 Plot of logarithm of Cp (solid line), Cp' (upper dashed line), and $Cp' - Cp$ (broad dashed line) against time. The values of Cp' (closed circles) that correspond to the time of the given values of Cp (open circles) are noted. $\ln(Cp' - Cp)$ (diamonds) is plotted against time to obtain a straight line of slope $-k_a$ and intercept $\ln I$, where I is $S \cdot F \cdot D \cdot k_a/[Vd\,(k_a - k)]$.

The absorption half-life can be determined from the first-order rate constant for absorption:

$$t_{1/2,\text{absorption}} = \frac{0.693}{k_a} \tag{9.15}$$

This parameter is useful to determine the approximate time for absorption to be completed (3–5 absorption $t_{1/2}$ values).

9.2.2.4 Volume of Distribution

The absolute values of the primary pharmacokinetic parameters, volume of distribution, and clearance cannot be determined from oral data alone because the bioavailability factor (F) is unknown. The volume of distribution relative to F (Vd/F) can, however, be determined from the intercept of the plots of $\ln Cp'$ and $\ln(Cp' - Cp)$ against time (Figure 9.4). The intercept is $\ln I$, where

$$I = \frac{S \cdot F \cdot D \cdot k_a}{Vd \cdot (k_a - k)} \tag{9.16}$$

Thus,

$$\frac{Vd}{F} = \frac{S \cdot D \cdot k_a}{I \cdot (k_a - k)} \tag{9.17}$$

9.2.2.5 Clearance

Clearance may be calculated from the first-order rate constant and the volume of distribution. If only oral data are available, F cannot be determined and only clearance relative to the bioavailability (Cl/F) can be estimated. This clearance (Cl/F) is called *apparent clearance* or *oral clearance*, and can be calculated from k and Vd/F:

$$\frac{Cl}{F} = k \cdot \frac{Vd}{F} \tag{9.18}$$

Oral clearance can also be calculated from the area under the plasma concentration–time curve (AUC) from zero to infinity:

$$\frac{Cl}{F} = \frac{S \cdot D}{\text{AUC}} \tag{9.19}$$

Then, AUC can be calculated:

$$\text{AUC} = \int_0^\infty Cp \cdot dt = \frac{S \cdot F \cdot D \cdot k_a}{Vd \cdot (k_a - k)} \cdot \left(\frac{1}{k} - \frac{1}{k_a} \right) = I \cdot \left(\frac{1}{k} - \frac{1}{k_a} \right) \tag{9.20}$$

Alternatively, the AUC can be estimated from the trapezoidal rule.

Example 9.1   Parameter Determination from Plasma Concentration–Time Data. The plasma concentration–time data in Table E9.1A were obtained after the administration of a 100-mg oral dose to a healthy volunteer. Analyze the data and determine (a) k, (b) k_a, (c) Vd/F, and (d) Cl/F by creating an Excel worksheet as described in Appendix C. Assume that $S = 1$.

TABLE E9.1A   Plasma Concentrations of a Drug at Various Times After the Administration of a 100-mg Oral Dose

Time (h)	Cp (mg/L)	Time (h)	Cp (mg/L)
0	0	2	3.43
0.6	2.74	2.6	3.12
0.8	3.13	3	2.89
1	3.37	4	2.33
1.4	3.55	7	1.17
1.8	3.5	12	0.37

Solution A detailed solution and associated plots are shown in Appendix C, Figure C.8.

(a) From the straight line from the last three data points on the semilogarithmic scale:

$$\text{slope} = -0.23 \text{ h}^{-1}$$
$$k = 0.23 \text{ h}^{-1}$$
$$\ln I = 1.77$$
$$I = 5.85 \text{ mg/L} \quad \text{where} \quad I = \frac{S \cdot F \cdot D \cdot k_a}{Vd \cdot (k_a - k)}$$

(b) The earlier values along the back-extrapolated portion of this terminal elimination line are calculated using

$$Cp' = I \cdot e^{-kt}$$

where at later times, $Cp = Cp'$, but at earlier times, $Cp' > Cp$. The values of Cp' at the times of the early given data points are calculated in Table E9.1B. The values of $Cp' - Cp$ are determined and the values of k_a and the intercept are determined from the line of $\ln(Cp' - Cp)$ against time (Figure 9.4):

$$\text{slope} = -1.57 \text{ h}^{-1}$$
$$k_a = 1.57 \text{ h}^{-1}$$
$$\ln I = 1.80$$
$$I = 6.07 \text{ mg/L} = \frac{S \cdot F \cdot D \cdot k_a}{Vd \cdot (k_a - k)}$$

TABLE E9.1B   Values of Cp, Cp', and ($Cp' - Cp$) at Various Times

T (h)	Cp (mg/L): Given Values	Cp' (mg/L) $= 5.85e^{-0.23t}$	$Cp' - Cp$
0	0	5.85	5.85
0.6	2.74	5.10	2.36
0.8	3.13	4.87	1.74
1	3.37	4.65	1.28
1.4	3.5	4.24	0.69
1.8	3.55	3.87	0.37
2	3.43	3.69	0.26
2.6	3.12	3.22	0.10

(c) The value of Vd is determined. Since intravenous data are not available for this drug, pure Vd cannot be determined, only Vd/F:

$$S = 1 \qquad \frac{Vd}{F} = \frac{D \cdot k_a}{I \cdot (k_a - k)}$$
$$= 20.0 \text{ L}$$

(d) Cl/F can be calculated as follows:
 1. From k and Vd/F:

$$\frac{Cl}{F} = \frac{Vd \cdot k}{F} = 20.0 \times 0.23$$
$$= 4.61 \text{ L/h}$$

 2. From the AUC:

$$\text{AUC} = \frac{S \cdot F \cdot D \cdot k_a}{Vd \cdot (k_a - k)} \cdot \left(\frac{1}{k} - \frac{1}{k_a} \right) = 21.71 \text{ mg} \cdot \text{h/L}$$
$$\frac{Cl}{F} = \frac{D}{\text{AUC}} = 4.61 \text{ L/h}$$

9.2.3 Absorption Lag Time

The absorption of a drug from the oral route may not occur immediately. Absorption can be delayed by several factors, including slow disintegration, poor dissolution, delayed stomach emptying, or a coating that delays drug release. Some controlled-release dosage forms are designed specifically to incorporate a delay in absorption. In all these cases, an absorption lag time or delay can be incorporated into the pharmacokinetic model. Experimentally, the

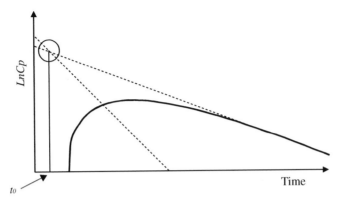

FIGURE 9.5 Semilogarithmic plot of plasma concentration against time. The terminal linear line and the feathered line do not intercept at the y-axis. Their point of intersection corresponds to the absorption lag time (t_0).

absorption lag time is apparent in clinical data if the back-extrapolated terminal elimination line and the feathered absorption line intercept at a point to the right of the y-axis. The time at which they intercept corresponds to the absorption lag time (Figure 9.5). The absorption lag time simply shifts the curve to the right and is accommodated in equations by subtracting the lag time from the absolute time in the basic equation (9.6):

$$Cp = \frac{S \cdot F \cdot D \cdot k_a}{Vd \cdot (k_a - k)} \cdot (e^{-k(t-t_0)} - e^{-k_a(t-t_0)}) \tag{9.21}$$

where t_0 is the absorption lag time.

You will recall that in Chapter 3, pregnancy had an apparent effect on the gastric emptying of acetaminophen (Figure 3.11). The effect of food on gastric emptying was specifically seen for the plasma concentration after the administration of sildenafil in humans (Figure 9.6). Food slowed the onset, and extent of the absorption of sildenafil [1]. The food effect in this case probably had a clinically significant effect on the onset of action. If the extent of drug absorption is not impacted, a delayed absorption due to food may not be of clinical significance for some drugs, such as atorvastatin [2].

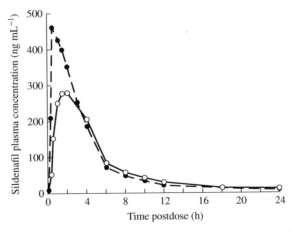

FIGURE 9.6 The effect of food on the rate and extent of sildenafil absorption in humans. *Source:* Nichols *et al.* 2002, pp. 5S–12S [1]. Reproduced with permission of John Wiley & Sons, Inc.

9.2.4   Flip-Flop Model and Sustained-Release Preparations

Recall the mathematical procedure to separate the two exponential components of the full equation for the plasma concentration (9.6) assumed that the rate constant for absorption was greater than the rate constant for elimination. As a result,

$$e^{-k_a t} \rightarrow 0 \text{ before } e^{-kt}$$

This is not always the case.

Drugs that have large elimination rate constants (short half-lives) are eliminated rapidly and often need to be administered very frequently to maintain therapeutic plasma concentrations. To improve patient adherence, these drugs are commonly formulated into prolonged-release products that slow down absorption and permit less frequent dosing. The formulation modification made to reduce the rate of absorption results in a reduction in the absorption rate constant (k_a). Under these conditions, the elimination rate constant may become greater than the absorption rate constant. As a result,

$$e^{-kt} \rightarrow 0 \text{ before } e^{-k_a t}$$

Under these conditions, the basic formula for Cp (9.6) at later times reduces to

$$Cp = \frac{S \cdot F \cdot D \cdot k_a}{Vd \cdot (k_a - k)} \cdot (0 - e^{-k_a t})$$

$$Cp = -\frac{S \cdot F \cdot D \cdot k_a}{Vd \cdot (k_a - k)} \cdot e^{-k_a t} \qquad (9.22)$$

$$Cp = \frac{S \cdot F \cdot D \cdot k_a}{Vd \cdot (k - k_a)} \cdot e^{-k_a t}$$

Taking logarithms yields

$$\ln Cp = \ln \frac{S \cdot F \cdot D \cdot k_a}{Vd \cdot (k - k_a)} - k_a t \qquad (9.23)$$

In this situation, the terminal fall in Cp is controlled not by k but by k_a. The slope of the corresponding feathered line is controlled by elimination and equal to $-k$ (Figure 9.7).

This is referred to as a *flip-flop model* and is frequently the case for sustained-release preparations where drugs have very large values of k and are formulated in a manner to create small values of k_a. A flip-flop model may be identified by comparing the value of the elimination rate constant or half-life to values obtained after intravenous administration. A flip-flop model can also be identified if the dosage form is administered to patients with altered clearance. The altered clearance will be apparent in changes of the slope of the feathered line and not the terminal line.

9.2.5   Determinants of T_{max} and C_{max}

The presence of a peak in the plasma concentration–time profile is characteristic of extravascular administration (Figure 9.1). The peak can be summarized by the value of the peak plasma concentration (C_{max}) and the time at which it occurs (T_{max}) (Figure 9.1). These two metrics can have an important influence on drug response. The time of the peak can

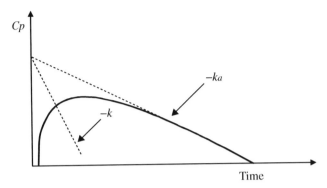

FIGURE 9.7 Semilogarithmic plot of plasma concentration against time for the flip-flop model. When the elimination rate constant (k) is greater than the absorption rate constant (k_a), the negative slope of the terminal line is k_a and the negative slope of the feathered line is k.

control the onset of action of the drug, and C_{max} may determine if a dose is subtherapeutic, therapeutic, or toxic. The values of C_{max} and T_{max} can also easily be measured directly from the data, and they frequently play an important role in evaluating the results of clinical pharmacokinetic studies, including bioavailability studies and drug–drug interaction (DDI) studies. To understand the factors that control C_{max} and T_{max}, equations must be derived for these two parameters.

9.2.5.1 $\mathbf{T}_{max}$

When the plasma concentration reaches its peak, $t = T_{max}$. At the peak,

$$\frac{dCp}{dt} = 0$$

The basic equation for Cp [equation (9.6)] is differentiated and set to zero. Time in the equation is set to T_{max}. The equation is rearranged to yield

$$T_{max} = \frac{\ln(k_a/k)}{k_a - k} \tag{9.24}$$

From equation (9.24), it can be seen that the value of T_{max} is a function of the first-order elimination rate constant and the first-order absorption rate constant.

Under conditions where elimination remains constant, T_{max} becomes a function of only the absorption rate constant (k_a). Bioavailability studies are performed to evaluate a drug's absorption properties among different formulations. These studies are designed to minimize variability in elimination, and under these conditions T_{max} can be used to assess the rate of drug absorption. Because k_a is present in both the numerator and denominator of equation (9.24), it is difficult to predict how k_a will affect T_{max}. Figure 9.8b shows that as k_a increases, T_{max} decreases. This is in keeping with common sense: If k_a increases, the rate of absorption increases and it will take less time to reach the peak (T_{max} decreases).

Under conditions where elimination does not remain constant, T_{max} will change if either the rate of absorption and/or the rate of elimination changes. Figure 9.8a shows the relationship between k and T_{max}. It can be seen that as k increases, T_{max} decreases. This also makes sense based on the knowledge that after a dose, the rate of absorption decreases and the rate of elimination increases, and the peak occurs when the rate of elimination equals the rate of absorption. This will occur fastest when the elimination rate constant is high.

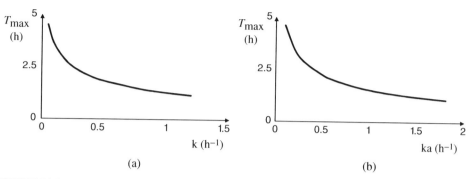

FIGURE 9.8   Dependency of time of peak plasma concentration (T_{max}) on the elimination rate constant (k) (a) and the absorption rate constant (k_a) (b). T_{max} was calculated for values of k from 0.05 to 1.2 h^{-1} with k_a fixed to 0.6 h^{-1}. T_{max} was also calculated for values of k_a from 0.1 to 1.8 h^{-1} with k fixed at 0.4 h^{-1}.

9.2.5.2 C_{max}

The peak plasma concentration (C_{max}) is the plasma concentration at time T_{max}. Thus, an expression for C_{max} may be obtained by substituting the expression for T_{max} [equation (9.24)] into equation (9.6) and rearranging to solve for C_{max}:

$$C_{max} = \frac{S \cdot F \cdot D}{Vd} \cdot e^{-kT_{max}} \tag{9.25}$$

Equation (9.25) demonstrates that C_{max} is dependent on all the pharmacokinetic parameters of a drug. It is directly proportional to the effective dose, dependent on the volume of distribution, and through its dependency on T_{max}, the rate of absorption and elimination.

Bioavailability studies are designed to minimize variability in the disposition parameters (clearance, volume of distribution, and the elimination rate constant). Under these conditions, C_{max} will only be a function of F and k_a. It is directly proportional to F: If F doubles, C_{max} doubles. This is also in keeping with common sense: If F increases, the effective dose of the drug increases and thus C_{max} increases. An inverse relationship exists between C_{max} and T_{max}. For example, if the rate of absorption increases, absorption is more rapid, the time to peak decreases, and the value of the peak increases.

The value of C_{max} is frequently evaluated in DDI studies. In these studies, the clearance of a drug and/or the volume of distribution of a drug may vary between the control and test conditions. Under these circumstances, changes in C_{max} may be brought about by changes in the clearance, volume of distribution, the rate of drug absorption, and/or the extent of absorption.

9.3   MODIFIED RELEASE AND GASTRIC RETENTION FORMULATIONS

9.3.1   Impact of the Stomach

The stomach functions as a grinding and storage organ that happens to predigest some types of food. For certain drugs with a fast rate of absorption and a dose not limited by their solubility, the onset of absorption and subsequently, their T_{max} depends on gastric emptying. In Chapter 3, we reviewed the effects of food on gastric emptying. For decades, pharmaceutical scientists have tried to develop a dosage form that would have a delayed gastric emptying in the fasted state. They have all tried—and failed—with swelling, buoyant, or unfolding dosage forms [3].

9.3.2 Moisture in the Gastrointestinal Tract

According to one text, the saliva, gastric juice, bile, pancreatic enzymes, and bicarbonate contribute 1.5, 2.5, 0.5, and 1.5 L, totaling 6 L of fluid each day. And all of this fluid is reabsorbed in the small intestine [4], such that in the fasted state there is only about 100 mL fluid in the entire small intestine [5]. While there is even less water in the colon, there is a 100% relative humidity. The humidity is important for osmotic dosage forms to function.

9.4 BIOAVAILABILITY

The *bioavailability* of a dosage form is the rate, and extent to which, the drug reaches the systemic circulation. It is a very important characteristic of an oral dosage form: The rate of absorption controls the speed with which therapeutic plasma concentrations are achieved; and more important, the extent of drug absorption controls the effective dose of a drug. As discussed previously, bioavailability is a property not only of the drug but also of the dosage form. It is important that it remains constant among different batches of a product. It is also important that it be constant among a drug's brand name product and generic equivalents, as these products may be used interchangeably in patients.

9.4.1 Bioavailability Parameters

9.4.1.1 Rate of Drug Absorption

From a consideration of the pharmacokinetic model and equations associated with oral absorption, the most obvious way to assess the rate of absorption would appear to be the measurement of the first-order rate constant for absorption (k_a). However, it is frequently very difficult to obtain precise estimates of this parameter. Many drugs display two-compartment characteristics, and early after drug administration, drug absorption, distribution, and elimination occur simultaneously, and it can be very difficult to separate these processes to measure the absorption rate constant. Additionally, the measurement of k_a assumes that absorption is a single first-order process. But the absorption of some drugs may be more complex and may involve multiple first- and/or zero-order processes. As a result, two other metrics are used to assess the rate of absorption: T_{max} [equation (9.24)] and C_{max} [equation (9.25)]. It was shown previously that when a drug is administered under conditions where disposition (distribution and elimination) is unlikely to vary, T_{max} and C_{max} are measures of the rate of drug absorption. These metrics are obtained directly from the plasma concentration–time data. Thus, C_{max} and T_{max} are simply the highest recorded plasma concentration and its corresponding time.

9.4.1.2 Extent of Drug Absorption

The extent of drug absorption is evaluated through assessment of the bioavailability factor (F) and C_{max}, which is directly proportional to F [equation (9.25)] and can be read directly from the data. The *bioavailability factor* is the fraction of the dose that is able to gain access to the systemic circulation. It is assessed by means of the AUC, which is a measure of the body's exposure to a drug. Recall that

$$AUC = \frac{S \cdot F \cdot D}{Cl} \tag{9.26}$$

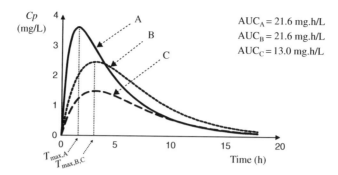

FIGURE 9.9   Plasma concentration–time profile of three different formulations of equal doses of a drug. The rate of absorption from formulation B is the same as from formulation C. The rate of absorption from A is greater than that from B and C. The extents of absorption of A and B are the same and greater than that from formulation C.

Equation (9.26) demonstrates that the AUC is directly proportional to the effective dose of drug and inversely proportional to its clearance. The AUC is a measure of drug exposure, and for a given drug (clearance is constant) the AUC is directly proportional to the effective dose:

$$\text{AUC} \propto F \cdot D \tag{9.27}$$

or

$$\frac{\text{AUC}}{D} \propto F \tag{9.28}$$

Assuming a constant value of S, the AUC per unit dose of a drug is directly proportional to F. As a result of this relationship, the AUC is used to assess the extent of drug absorption.

In summary, bioavailability is assessed by measuring AUC, C_{max}, and T_{max}. AUC and C_{max} are measures of the extent of drug absorption (F), and C_{max} and T_{max} are measures of the rate of drug absorption. Figure 9.9 shows the plasma concentration–time profile of three formulations of equal doses of a drug. The relative bioavailability characteristics of the three formulations are summarized as:

$$F_A = F_B > F_C$$
$$k_{aA} > k_{aB} = k_{aC}$$

Thus,

$$\text{AUC}_A = \text{AUC}_B > \text{AUC}_C \quad \text{(Figure 9.9)}$$

$$T_{max,A} < T_{max,B} = T_{max,C} \quad \text{(Figure 9.9)}$$

$$C_{max,A} > C_{max,B} > C_{max,C} \quad \text{(Figure 9.9)}$$

9.4.2 Absolute Bioavailability

The actual value of F is referred to as the *absolute bioavailability*. It can only be determined by comparing the AUC from an oral dosage form (PO) to the AUC after intravenous administration (IV):

$$\frac{F_{PO}}{F_{IV}} = \frac{AUC_{PO}/D_{PO}}{AUC_{IV}/D_{IV}} \tag{9.29}$$

But $F_{IV} = 1$,

$$F_{PO} = \frac{AUC_{PO}/D_{PO}}{AUC_{IV}/D_{IV}} \tag{9.30}$$

Thus, F for an oral dosage form is the AUC per unit dose divided by the AUC per unit dose when the drug is given IV. A more computationally friendly version of equation (9.30) is

$$F_{PO} = \frac{AUC_{PO} \cdot D_{IV}}{AUC_{IV} \cdot D_{PO}} \tag{9.31}$$

9.4.3 Relative Bioavailability

The bioavailability of an oral dosage form may also be assessed through comparison to a standard oral preparation. This may be an oral solution, which as it is further along in the absorption process, often has the highest bioavailability of all the oral dosage forms of a drug. Alternatively, the bioavailability may be compared to a standard oral preparation or to one that has optimal bioavailability characteristics. These are examples of *relative bioavailability*. The relative bioavailability of a test product is

$$\frac{F_T}{F_S} = \frac{AUC_T/D_T}{AUC_S/D_S} \quad \text{or} \quad \frac{AUC_T \cdot D_S}{AUC_S \cdot D_T}$$

where the subscript S stands for standard and T for test.

9.4.4 Bioequivalence

Bioequivalence is a special type of relative bioavailability. Two or more products are classified as *bioequivalent* if a clinical study has demonstrated that the products have essentially the same bioavailability. A thorough account of the assessment bioequivalence and the analysis of the data may be found in the literature [6]. To demonstrate the bioequivalence of two oral products, their AUC and C_{max} ratios are calculated for each subject in a crossover study. The ratios are calculated on log transformed data. The log transformed AUC and C_{max} ratios for the group are then calculated. The 90% confidence interval (CI) of the average ratios of "test versus reference" for the group must lie within the range 80–125%. This range is not symmetrical because for bioequivalence, the pharmacokinetic parameter of the test formulation cannot be less than 80% of the pharmacokinetic parameter for the reference formulation. In addition, the pharmacokinetic parameter of the *reference* formulation cannot be less

TABLE 9.1   Example Data From a Bioequivalence Study

Subject	Test AUC ng/mL.h	Ref AUC ng/mL.h	Ln Test AUC	Ln Ref AUC	AUC Ratio: LnTest-Ln Ref
1	2560	4020	7.85	8.3	−0.45
2	118	211	4.77	5.35	−0.58
3	905	572	6.81	6.35	0.46
4	764	815	6.64	6.7	−0.06
5	729	715	6.59	6.57	0.02
6	2460	1940	7.81	6.57	0.24
7	3180	1750	8.07	7.47	0.6
8	2740	2720	7.92	7.91	0.01
9	3260	4670	8.09	8.45	−0.36
10	1220	1930	7.11	7.57	−0.46
11	2340	2240	7.76	7.72	0.04
12	1050	1010	6.95	6.91	0.04
				Mean	−0.0427
				SD	0.368
				90% CI	0.79−1.16

Source: Data from Reference [6].

than 80% of the pharmacokinetic parameter for the *test* formulation. Since all data must be expressed as "test over reference," the latter becomes 100/80 or 125%. In the logarithmic domain, this range is symmetrical: The value of log 0.8 = −0.09691, and of log 1.25 = +0.09691. The analysis of the data is best understood by example. Data from a crossover study described in the paper cited above are shown in Table 9.1. The values of AUC for 12 subjects administered Test and Reference formulations are shown. The logarithms of the values for each subject are calculated, and the ratios of the Test to Reference AUC are determined by subtracting the Reference LnAUC from the Test LnAUC. The mean and the standard deviation of the ratios in the Ln domain (−0.0427, 0.37), and the test statistic are used to calculate the 90% CI. The test statistic is from a table of Student's t-distribution, for an $\alpha = 0.1$, and $(n - 1)$ degrees of freedom (1.796). Why is $\alpha = 0.1$? Remember that this is a two one-sided t-test, the value of $\alpha = 0.05$ for each t-test (this test keeps the consumer risk at 5%), and the total of both tails is 10%.

In this data set, the 90% CI is 0.79–1.16. Based on the AUC alone, the products would not be considered bioequivalent since the lower bound is less than 0.8.

The value of T_{max} is compared between groups, but this parameter cannot be subject to statistical analysis noted above because unlike AUC and C_{max} which are continuous variables, T_{max} is a categorical variable that can only take on values selected by the plasma concentrations sampling scheme. Bioequivalence studies must be performed during drug development to demonstrate the equivalency of the various batches and trial formulations that are used in clinical studies. Drug companies must perform bioequivalence studies whenever major formulation changes are made. Bioequivalence studies are also conducted routinely by drug manufacturers who wish to market a generic form of an innovator or brand-name product. In addition to the demonstration of bioequivalence, generic products must also be pharmaceutical equivalents of the innovator product. That is, they must be the same type of dosage form (tablets, capsules, etc.), they must contain the same dose of the drug(s), and they must have the same chemical form (e.g., salt). Pharmaceutical equivalents that are also shown to be bioequivalent may be classified as therapeutic equivalents.

9.4.5 Single-Dose Crossover Parallel and Steady-State Study Designs

In support of bioequivalence, different statistical designs are utilized for clinical studies depending on whether they are for single dose or multiple dose studies. The so-called *test article* may be any number of different formulations; for example, placebo versus an active formulation, or two active formulations with certain manufacturing or formulation differences, or they could be the innovator versus the generic products with the same active drug. For most single-dose studies, a crossover design is used; here, half of the subjects are randomly selected to receive test article 1, while the other half receive test article 2. Drug concentrations are measured by a specific assay of plasma or serum harvested from blood samples collected at specific times following drug administration. After a suitable period of time, during which essentially all of the drugs have been eliminated from the body (i.e., the *wash-out period*), the two groups switch; those who were administered the article 1, are next administered article 2, and vice versa. For studies where a crossover is not feasible (e.g., if the wash-out period is too long, or the effects of one test article will have an effect on the performance of the second test article), a parallel study design is implemented. In this case, the overall group of subjects is separated into two groups. Every attempt is made to match all demographics of the two groups, and then one test article is given to one group, and a second test article is given to the other group. They do not undergo a crossover. In both of these study designs, a pharmacokinetic analysis of the drug concentrations is completed, and the AUC, C_{max}, and T_{max} are compared.

In some instances, a multiple dose administration is desirable. For example, in a clinical study using patients afflicted with a chronic disease, the test article might be expected to be taken for the duration of the patients' lives; or, the absorption and bioavailability of the active drug may depend on the severity of the disease. In these cases, the study could span months of daily administration. After a specified period of dosing, the patients are subjected to blood collection, and the drug analysis and pharmacokinetics are completed as described for the single-dose study.

9.4.6 Example Bioavailability Analysis

An example of a bioavailability analysis can be found in the problems at the end of Chapter 10.

9.5 *IN VITRO-IN VIVO* CORRELATION

9.5.1 Definitions

An *in vitro-in vivo* correlation (IVIVC) is a statistical relationship between a parameter measured *in vitro* (commonly dissolution) and a parameter measured *in vivo* (e.g., absorption). The *in vitro* dissolution is usually determined with United States Pharmacopeia dissolution apparatus I ("basket") or apparatus II ("paddle"). The basket apparatus contains a steel basket containing the dosage form, and is rotated by an overhead motor (e.g., 50 revolutions per minute, rpm). For the paddle apparatus, the dosage form is simply dropped into the beaker, and the paddle is similarly rotated. Both methods use a beaker, the contents of which are warmed to 37°C. Typically, the dissolution media consists of 900 mL buffer, with the pH adjusted to a specified pH between 1.5 and 7.5. At specified times after adding the media, samples of the buffer are taken and analyzed for drug. The amount of drug dissolved at a specific time is calculated and compared to the eventual total amount dissolved. This becomes the *in vitro* dissolution—time—profile.

The amount of drug absorbed versus time profile can also be constructed from the drug concentration versus time data provided by a clinical study. If for each time that blood was collected, an interpolated value from the dissolution profile is matched, then in some cases a point-to-point correlation can be made between the amount of drug dissolved *in vitro* and the amount of drug absorbed *in vivo*. This is called a Level A IVIVC.

9.5.2 Assumptions

Implicit in this analysis is that the process rate—limiting appearance of drug in the blood is also the rate-limiting process responsible for the drug dissolution *in vitro*. For example, if a drug has a biopharmaceutics classification system (BCS) II designation, it is likely that the appearance of the drug in the blood (i.e., drug absorption) depends on its dissolution in the gastrointestinal tract fluids. That is, it is solubility—rate-limited. If one drug product formulation dissolves slowly *in vitro* (a slow dissolution rate), then it is expected to dissolve slowly *in vivo*, and produce a slower rate of absorption than a fast-dissolving drug product.

The media employed in most *in vitro* dissolution methods is a simple buffer. This is because most of the time the method is a so-called Quality Control test. The introduction of bile salts, surfactant, and lipids—while more physiologic, in that it more closely mimics the *in vivo* milieu—may also greatly complicate the analytical method. Furthermore, mixing in the stomach and small intestine probably is not as intense or as regular as the 50–150 rpm stirring often found in the dissolution method. Therefore, assumptions are made that the results using the simplified *in vitro* dissolution media approximate the *in vivo* dissolution.

9.5.3 Utility

The ultimate use of a validated IVIVC is to show what effect (if any) a change (e.g., in formulation, process, location, and NOT dosage form) would have on the *in vitro* dissolution of the drug product, which is then used to predict the *in vivo* absorption of the drug after administration of the drug product. From the *in vivo* absorption, a statistical and pharmacokinetic analysis is completed to produce simulated drug concentration versus time profiles (Figure 9.10). Using these profiles, the pharmaceutical scientist predicts the ultimate effect of the change on certain pharmacokinetic parameters (e.g., C_{max}, T_{max}, and AUC). In this manner, the sponsoring company can petition the Food and Drug Administration (FDA) for a waiver of a clinical study. Since these studies take months to years and millions of dollars, the use of IVIVC represents a highly sought after alternative.

9.5.4 Immediate Release IVIVC

The biowaivers granted by the FDA for BCS Class I, rapidly dissolving dosage forms, utilize a form of IVIVC in lieu of a clinical study for certain qualifying changes in manufacturing processes and for generic formulation comparisons. Since BCS Class I drugs are not likely to have dissolution as a rate-limiting process in their absorption, an IVIVC is unlikely. However, since a poorly made dosage form that results in a slowed dissolution would be expected to have a reduced absorption, the relationship still has value. As discussed above (see Section 9.5.2), an IVIVC is likely for BCS Class II compounds. Would BCS Class IV compounds to be good candidates for an IVIVC? As for Class II, Class IV drugs have poor solubility. However, they also have poor permeability. If the rate-limiting

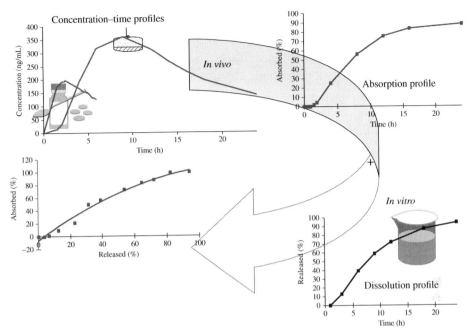

FIGURE 9.10   The IVIVC is illustrated here for a modified release dosage form. The plot in the lower right corner contains the *in vitro* dissolution versus time profile. The plot in the upper left corner contains the *in vivo* plasma concentration versus time profiles for an immediate release and the modified release formulations. The absorption versus time profile is derived from the *in vivo* data through a statistical pharmacokinetic analysis (upper right plot). The absorption data and the dissolution data are related in the IVIVC (lower left plot). By reversing the steps of this validated IVIVC, a different formulation with a different dissolution profile is used as the input for a pharmacokinetic simulation that predicts the *in vivo* concentration—time—profile. *(For a color version of this figure, see the color plate section.)*

process is solubility, then it is possible for an IVIVC. Would BCS Class III compounds be good candidates for an IVIVC?

9.5.5   Modified Release IVIVC

The FDA expects that a Level A IVIVC is attempted on the target formulation before it can be approved for marketing. Often the manufacturer will internally use a Level A IVIVC during the dosage form development stage. If validated, then the clinical study of these formulations may be shortened or eliminated. For particularly complicated formulations (e.g., solubility enabling formulations, i.e., amorphous form of a poorly soluble drug), some of the underlying assumptions are violated. In this case, a Level A IVIVC is not possible, but a Level C IVIVC is sometimes used. The Level C IVIVC does not use all of the dissolution or absorption versus time data; it may define the time by which a specified amount of drug dissolves/releases (e.g., t_{50} is the time at which 50% of the drug is released). In Figure 9.11 is shown the effect of including varying amounts of an excipient (poloxamer or polyoxamer) in various formulation batches during the development of the single-dose azithromycin formulation [7]. As a surrogate for the total amount absorbed, the AUC at 4 h was used as the *in vivo* parameter. This made sense, since azithromycin permeability in the colon is much less than in the small intestine.

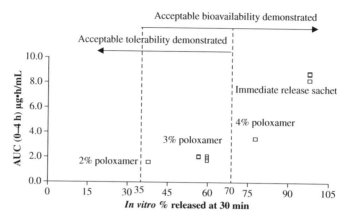

FIGURE 9.11   Relationship between AUC (0–4 h) and *in vitro* release of azithromycin. *Source:* Lo *et al.* 2009, pp. 1522–1529 [7]. Reproduced with permission of Taylor & Francis Ltd.

For poloxamer levels that resulted in less than 70% azithromycin released *in vitro* at 30 min, the formulation was found to be well tolerated, and for levels that resulted in at least 35% azithromycin released *in vitro* at 30 min, acceptable bioavailability was demonstrated. Using this Level C IVIVC, the pharmaceutical scientists predicted that a 3% level of poloxamer would produce a drug product that would be bioequivalent with the marketed formulation, and have acceptable tolerability [7].

9.6   SIMULATION EXERCISE:
http://web.uri.edu/pharmacy/research/rosenbaum/sims

Open simulation model 6, First-Order Absorption in a One-Compartment Model, which can be found at http://web.uri.edu/pharmacy/research/rosenbaum/sims/Model6.

   Default settings for the model are dose = 100 mg, Cl = 4.6 L/h, Vd = 20 L, F = 1, and $k_a = 0.6 \ h^{-1}$.

1. *Review the objectives, the "Model Summary" page, and explore the model.*
2. *Go to the "Transfer of Drug" page. Give a dose (100 mg) and observe how the amount of drug changes over time in the compartments representing the gastrointestinal tract, the body, and the drug eliminated. Based on the amount of drug that has been eliminated at the end of the simulation, it is possible to obtain a minimum value of bioavailability (F). By 12 h, 90 mg of drug has been eliminated, so F must be at least 0.9. Since drug is still present in the body at 12 h, the actual value of F will be greater than 0.9.*
3. *Go to the "Cp–Time Profile" page. Give the default dose (100 mg) and observe the plasma concentration on the regular linear scale and the semilogarithmic scale. Note that at later times on the semilogarithmic scale, a straight-line relationship is observed between ln Cp and time.*
4. *Compare the profiles after doses of 50, 100, and 200 mg. Note:*
   - *Cp at any time is proportional to dose.*
   - *T_{max} is independent of dose.*

- *AUC increases in proportion with dose.*
- *The slope of the linear terminal slope of the plot of ln Cp is constant with dose—each line is parallel.*
- *The $t_{1/2}$ remains constant as the dose changes.*

5. *Go to the "Influence of k_a and F" page.*
6. *Observe the effects of increases in k_a:*
   - *T_{max} gets smaller as k_a increases.*
   - *C_{max} increases as k_a increases.*
   - *AUC is not affected.*
7. *Observe the effects of increases in F:*
   - *T_{max} is not affected.*
   - *C_{max} increases in proportion with increases in F.*
   - *AUC increases in proportion with increases in F.*
8. *Go to the "Flip-Flop Model" page. With the slow release (SR) switch off (down), give doses with different values of clearance. Note that the terminal slope of the plot of ln Cp versus time changes. Flip the SR switch on (up: green) and repeat the exercise. Note that in this case, the terminal slope of the plot of ln Cp versus time does not change with clearance. The lines are all parallel. This is because the slope of this line is controlled by k_a, and not by k.*

PROBLEMS

9.1 A 75-mg dose of a drug was administered as an oral solution to nine healthy volunteers. Plasma samples were collected at various times after administration and were analyzed for the parent drug. After at least 10 elimination half-lives, the study was repeated but on these occasions the drug (75 mg) was administered as an oral tablet. The results from one of the subjects are given in Table P9.1. Analyze the data using a one-compartment model with first-order absorption. Determine Cl/F, Vd/F, k, $t_{1/2}$, and k_a for each formulation. Comment on any differences between the two formulations.

TABLE P9.1   Plasma Concentrations at Different Times After the Administration of a Drug (75 mg) as a Tablet and an Oral Solution

Solution Time (h)	Cp (mg/L)	Tablet Time (h)	Cp (mg/L)
0	0	0	0
1	0.78	1	0.46
2	1.21	2	0.75
3	1.42	3	0.91
4	1.5	4	1
5	1.49	5	1.03
6	1.43	6	1.02
7	1.35	7	0.98
9	1.14	10	0.8
12	0.84	16	0.45
18	0.43	18	0.36
24	0.21	24	0.18

9.2 The bioavailability of four different formulations (A, B, C, and D) of a drug is being compared. The results of a bioavailability study are provided in Table P9.2. How do the rate and extent of drug absorption compare among the formulations?

TABLE P9.2 Bioavailability Metrics for Four Different Formulations of a Drug

Formulation	AUC (mg · h/L)	C_{max} (mg/L)	T_{max} (h)
A	21.4	1.68	3.4
B	21.4	1.37	5.3
C	16.1	1.26	3.2
D	10.7	0.69	5.2

REFERENCES

1. Nichols, D. J., Muirhead, G. J., and Harness, J. A. (2002) Pharmacokinetics of sildenafil after single oral doses in healthy male subjects: absolute bioavailability, food effects and dose proportionality, *Br J Clin Pharmacol, 53*, 5S–12S.

2. Radulovic, L. L., Cilla, D. D., Posvar, E. L., Sedman, A. J., and Whitfield, L. R. (1995) Effect of food on the bioavailability of atorvastatin, an HMG-CoA reductase inhibitor, *J Clin Pharmacol, 35*, 990–994.

3. Waterman, K. C. (2007) A critical review of gastric retentive controlled drug delivery, *Pharm Dev Technol, 12*, 1–10.

4. Thiagarajah, J., and Verkman, A. (2012) Water transport in the gastrointestinal tract, in *Physiology of the Gastrointestinal Tract*. (Johnson, L., Ed.), Elsevier, Boston, 2, 1757–1780.

5. Sutton, S. (2009) Role of physiological intestinal water in oral absorption, *AAPS J, 11*, 277–285.

6. Balthasar, J. P. (1999) Bioequivalence and bioequivalency testing, *Am J Pharm Educ, 63*, 194–198.

7. Lo, J. B., Appel, L. E., Herbig, S. M., McCray, S. B., and Thombre, A. G. (2009) Formulation design and pharmaceutical development of a novel controlled release form of azithromycin for single-dose therapy, *Drug Dev Ind Pharm, 35*, 1522–1529.

10

INTRODUCTION TO NONCOMPARTMENTAL ANALYSIS

SARA E. ROSENBAUM

Objectives

The material in this chapter will enable the reader to:

1. Understand how the simpler approach of noncompartmental analysis can be used to estimate a drug's pharmacokinetic parameters

2. Use noncompartmental analysis to determine the mean residence time after intravenous administration

3. Use noncompartmental analysis to evaluate the results of a clinical study

10.1   INTRODUCTION

Clinical pharmacokinetic studies performed during drug development, and after a drug has been marketed, are frequently designed to study how specific conditions or patient characteristics may affect a drug's pharmacokinetics. The purpose of these studies is usually to try to identify special populations that may have altered dose requirements. The pharmacokinetic parameters of a drug are assessed in a special population. Any changes found in one or more of the parameters are then used to develop more appropriate dosing for

Basic Pharmacokinetics and Pharmacodynamics: An Integrated Textbook and Computer Simulations,
Second Edition. Edited by Sara E. Rosenbaum.

this group of people. For example, if food is found to reduce a drug's bioavailability, the labeling may be modified to recommend that the drug be taken on an empty stomach. If a perpetrator drug is found to reduce the clearance of a victim drug, the labeling of the victim drug may be modified to contraindicate the concomitant administration of the two drugs. Alternatively, the labeling may recommend a dosage reduction for the victim drug if it is taken with the perpetrator drug. Other common focuses of these studies include, how a drug's pharmacokinetics may be influenced by: renal disease and/or hepatic disease; age; genetic polymorphism in drug metabolizing enzymes or transporters; and transporter-based drug-drug interactions.

Typically these studies are conducted using orally administered drugs, and their focus is to compare a drug's pharmacokinetic parameters (clearance, volume of distribution, bioavailability, and half-life) in a normal and a special population. Rather than determining the pharmacokinetic parameters by trying to fit the data to compartmental models, a simpler approach known as *noncompartmental analysis* (NCA) is used. NCA offers several benefits over compartmental analysis. These include:

1. Fewer plasma samples may be required than in compartmental analysis.
2. The timing of the samples is not as critical as it is for compartmental analysis.
3. The modeling process is more straightforward and requires less experience and skill on the part of the modeler.
4. It avoids a problem frequently encountered with the compartmental approach, where a drug displays one-compartmental properties in some study participants, and multi (two or even three)-compartmental properties in others.

Although NCA can get quite complex, its application to the types of studies discussed above is very straightforward. The starting point of the discussion on NCA is the mean residence time of a drug.

10.2 MEAN RESIDENCE TIME

After an intravenous dose of a drug, the time that an individual drug molecule spends in the body will vary enormously: Some drug molecules will be eliminated almost instantaneously, whereas others may reside in the body much longer. A few molecules may still be in the body several weeks after the dose. The *mean residence time* (MRT) is defined as the average time spent in the body by a drug molecule. The determination of the MRT requires no assumptions about the number of compartments involved in the drug's disposition, and the derivation of its formula is best understood by using an example of a situation that may be encountered in everyday life.

Example 10.1   Suppose that a hotel is interested in determining the average length of stay of guests who attend a professional meeting at the hotel. Over the 6 days of the meeting, they track 20 guests. The results are shown in Table E10.1.

Four guests stayed for 1 day. This group provided a total of 4 days' stay.
Five guests stayed for 2 days. This group provided a total of 10 days' stay.
Six guests stayed for 3 days. This group provided a total of 18 days' stay.
Two guests stayed for 4 days. This group provided a total of 8 days' stay.

TABLE E10.1   Length of Stay of 20 Guests in a Hotel

Duration of Stay (days) (a)	Number of Guests (b)	Total Length of Stay of Group (days) (a · b)
1	4	$1 \times 4 = 4$
2	5	$2 \times 5 = 10$
3	6	$3 \times 6 = 18$
4	2	$4 \times 2 = 8$
5	2	$5 \times 2 = 10$
6	1	$6 \times 1 = 6$
Overall	20	56

Two guests stayed for 5 days. This group provided a total of 10 days' stay.
One guest stayed for 6 days. This group provided a total of 6 days' stay.

Overall, the 20 guests stayed a total of $(4 + 10 + 18 + 8 + 10 + 6) = 56$ days. The MRT is the total number of days spent divided by the total number of guests: $56/20 = 2.8$ days.

A drug's MRT, which can be considered to be the mean time spent in the body by a small mass of drug, is determined in the same way. A drug is administered intravenously. Assuming first-order elimination, the amount of drug eliminated per unit time is

$$\frac{dAe}{dt} = k \cdot Ab \tag{10.1}$$

where Ae is the amount of drug eliminated, k is the elimination rate constant, and Ab is the amount of drug in the body.

During the period dt, the small mass or amount of drug eliminated is given by

$$dAe = k \cdot Ab \cdot dt \tag{10.2}$$

During the period dt, the amount of drug eliminated is equal to $k \cdot Ab \cdot dt$ (equivalent to b in Table E10.1). This amount of drug has a residence time of t (equivalent to a in Table E10.1). The total amount having this residence time is $(a \cdot b)$, or

$$k \cdot Ab \cdot dt \cdot t \tag{10.3}$$

The sum of all the residence times from the time of administration $(t = 0)$ until all the drug has been eliminated $(t = \infty)$ is

$$\sum_{0}^{\infty} k \cdot Ab \cdot dt \cdot t \tag{10.4}$$

or

$$k \sum_{0}^{\infty} Ab \cdot dt \cdot t \tag{10.5}$$

The MRT is the sum of all the residence times divided by the total amount of drug originally present in the body, the effective dose ($S \cdot F \cdot D$):

$$MRT = \frac{k \sum_0^\infty Ab \cdot dt \cdot t}{S \cdot F \cdot D} \tag{10.6}$$

Assuming that Cp and Ab are always proportional and $Ab = Cp \cdot Vd$, we have

$$MRT = \frac{k \sum_0^\infty Cp \cdot Vd \cdot dt \cdot t}{S \cdot F \cdot D} \tag{10.7}$$

Rearranging yields

$$MRT = \frac{\sum_0^\infty Cp \cdot t \cdot dt}{S \cdot F \cdot D / k \cdot Vd} \tag{10.8}$$

But $Cl = k \cdot Vd$, so

$$MRT = \frac{\sum_0^\infty Cp \cdot t \cdot dt}{S \cdot F \cdot D / Cl} \tag{10.9}$$

But $S \cdot F \cdot D / Cl = AUC$, so

$$MRT = \frac{\sum_0^\infty Cp \cdot t \cdot dt}{AUC} \tag{10.10}$$

The denominator in equation (10.10) is the area under the plasma concentration–time curve from time zero to infinity (AUC) (Figure 10.1a). The numerator is the area under the curve of the plot of $Cp \cdot t$ versus time from zero to infinity (Figure 10.1b). This is referred to as the *area under the first moment curve* (AUMC):

$$MRT = \frac{AUMC}{AUC} \tag{10.11}$$

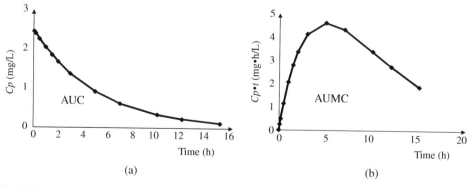

FIGURE 10.1 Graphs of plasma concentration (Cp) against time (t) (a) and Cp^*t against time (b). The AUC is the area under the Cp versus time curve and the AUMC is the area under the $Cp \cdot t$ versus time curve.

Thus, MRT is calculated from the area under the curve (from time zero to ∞) for the plot of plasma concentration (Cp) against time (t) (Figure 10.1) (AUC), and the area under the curve (from time 0 to ∞) for the plot of Cp^*t against time (AUMC) (Figure 10.1). Both the AUC and the AUMC can be determined using the trapezoidal rule (see Appendix C). Note that in NCA, the terminal elimination rate constant is given by the symbol λ. Recall that for the AUC calculation, the area from the last data point to infinity is Cp_{last}/λ. Note that for the AUMC, the area from the last data point to infinity is $(Cp_{last} \cdot t_{last}/\lambda) + (Cp_{last}/\lambda^2)$. Thus, the MRT can be determined without subjecting the data to compartmental analysis.

10.3   DETERMINATION OF OTHER IMPORTANT PHARMACOKINETIC PARAMETERS

The other important pharmacokinetic parameters, including the mean elimination rate constant, the mean elimination half-life, and the volume of distribution at steady state, can be determined as follows. The mean elimination rate constant

$$k = \frac{1}{MRT} \tag{10.12}$$

the elimination half-life

$$t_{1/2} = \frac{0.693}{k} \tag{10.13}$$

the clearance

$$Cl = \frac{S \cdot F \cdot D}{AUC} \tag{10.14}$$

and the volume of distribution at steady state,

$$Vd_{ss} = \frac{Cl}{k} = \frac{S \cdot F \cdot D/AUC}{1/MRT} = \frac{S \cdot F \cdot D \cdot MRT}{AUC} \tag{10.15}$$

Substituting for MRT from equation (10.12) yields

$$Vd_{ss} = \frac{S \cdot F \cdot D \cdot AUMC}{AUC^2} \tag{10.16}$$

Example 10.2   In Chapter 7, a data set was presented and subject to compartmental analysis using the model for an intravenous injection on a one-compartment model. The data are shown in Table E10.2A and will now be subjected to NCA.

Solution   The parameters are determined using NCA as follows:

1. Terminal elimination rate constant (λ). This is determined from the slope of ln Cp versus time for the last three data points:

$$\lambda = 0.20\,h^{-1}$$

TABLE E10.2A   Plasma Concentration–Time Data Simulated After a 50-mg Intravenous Dose in a One-Compartment Model

Time (h)	Cp (mg/L)	Time (h)	Cp (mg/L)
0	2.5	3	1.37
0.1	2.45	5	0.92
0.2	2.40	7	0.62
0.5	2.26	10	0.34
1	2.05	12	0.23
1.5	1.85	15	0.124
2	1.68		

2. Terminal elimination half-life ($t_{1/2,\lambda}$)

$$t_{1/2,\lambda} = \frac{0.693}{0.2} = 3.46\,\text{h}$$

3. Determination of AUC_0^∞. This is calculated using the trapezoidal rule (Appendix C) as outlined in Table E10.2B.

$$\text{AUC}_0^{15} = 12.00\,\text{mg} \cdot \text{h/L}$$
$$\text{AUC}_{15}^\infty = \frac{0.124}{0.2} = 0.62\,\text{mg} \cdot \text{h/L}$$
$$\text{AUC}_0^\infty = 12.62\,\text{mg} \cdot \text{h/L}$$

TABLE E10.2B   Determination of the AUC and the AUMC

AUC Calculation			AUMC Calculation		
Time (h)	Cp (mg/L)	AUC Segment[a] (mg · h/L)	Time (h)	$Cp \cdot t$ (mg · h/L)	AUMC Segment[a] (mg · h^2/L)
0	2.50	0.25	0	0.00	0.01
0.1	2.45	0.24	0.1	0.25	0.04
0.2	2.40	0.70	0.2	0.48	0.24
0.5	2.26	1.08	0.5	1.13	0.79
1	2.05	0.97	1	2.05	1.21
1.5	1.85	0.88	1.5	2.78	1.53
2	1.68	1.52	2	3.35	3.73
3	1.37	2.29	3	4.12	8.72
5	0.92	1.54	5	4.60	8.91
7	0.62	1.43	7	4.31	11.54
10	0.34	0.57	10	3.38	6.10
12	0.23	0.53	12	2.72	6.88
15	0.124		15	1.86	

[a]The area of each segment was determined using the trapezoidal rule as described in Appendix C.

4. Determination of $AUMC_0^\infty$. This is calculated using the trapezoidal rule as outlined in Table E10.2B.

$$AUMC_0^{15} = 49.70\,mg \cdot h^2/L$$

$$AUMC_{15}^\infty = \frac{1.86}{0.2} + \frac{0.124}{0.04} = 12.4\,mg \cdot h^2/L$$

$$AUMC_0^\infty = 62.1\,mg \cdot h^2/L$$

5. Determination of MRT

$$MRT = \frac{AUMC}{AUC} = \frac{62.1}{12.6} = 4.92\,h$$

6. Determination of mean elimination rate constant

$$k = \frac{1}{MRT} = \frac{1}{4.92} = 0.2\,h^{-1}$$

Note that in this example, because Cp falls in a monoexponentially the mean elimination rate constant is the same as the terminal elimination rate constant (λ).

7. Determination of clearance

$$Cl = \frac{S \cdot F \cdot D}{AUC} = \frac{50}{12.6} = 3.97\,L/h$$

8. Determination of steady-state volume of distribution

$$Vd_{ss} = \frac{S \cdot F \cdot D \cdot AUMC}{AUC^2} = \frac{50 \times 62.1}{12.6^2} = 19.47\,L$$

10.4 DIFFERENT ROUTES OF ADMINISTRATION

With a route of drug administration that does not involve drug absorption, such as an intravenous bolus injection, the MRT reflects the average time it takes for a drug molecule to pass through the body. When drug input is noninstantaneous, such as oral administration, the drug molecule's journey is extended by the absorption process. In this situation, the time (after administration) it takes a drug molecule to pass through the body is the sum of the absorption time and the residence time. This overall time is known as the *transit time*. The *mean transit time* (MTT) is the sum of mean absorption time (MAT) and the MRT:

$$MTT = MRT + MAT$$

For noninstantaneous routes,

$$MTT = \frac{AUMC}{AUC} \tag{10.17}$$

MAT is the difference between the MRT obtained after intravenous administration and the MTT after oral administration and reflects the mean time for absorption.

The dependency of MTT after oral administration on both absorption and elimination limits its use in NCA. The focus of many clinical studies, such as drug interaction studies, is to observe how clearance and the rate of elimination (terminal elimination rate constant and $t_{1/2}$) may be affected. In many cases, intravenous data are not available, which makes it impossible to determine the MRT from the MTT. As a result, the volume of distribution at steady state cannot be determined [see equation (10.15)]. These studies generally calculate the volume of distribution based on the terminal elimination rate constant. This volume is equivalent to V_β in the two-compartment model.

10.5 APPLICATION OF NONCOMPARTMENTAL ANALYSIS TO CLINICAL STUDIES

As discussed in the introduction, NCA is often used to analyze the results of clinical studies designed to quantify the effects, if any, of specific conditions on the drug's pharmacokinetics. Clinically significant changes will be translated into dosage recommendations or contraindication warnings in the drug's labeling. Typically, the crossover design is used for these clinical studies. Thus, in one leg of the study, the drug is administered to a subject in the absence of the factor (control leg). Plasma concentration–time data are collected and NCA is used to estimate the pharmacokinetic parameters. In the other leg of the study, the drug is administered to the same subject in the presence of the factor (test leg). The sequencing of the legs is usually randomized among participants. Thus, half of the group members participate in the control leg first, while the other half participate in the test leg first. The two legs are separated by a suitable washout period (over seven elimination half-lives). Any changes in the pharmacokinetic parameters are assessed. The study must be performed in several subjects to provide the statistical power needed to perform tests of statistical significance. Typically, somewhere between 10 and 20 subjects are required, depending on the variability of the pharmacokinetic parameters and the magnitude of any expected changes.

Example 10.3   Drug–Drug Interaction Study During the course of this book, the pharmacokinetic characteristics of the fictitious drug lipoamide have evolved. Lipoamide is cleared almost exclusively by metabolism by cytochrome 2C9 (CYP 2C9). It is a high-extraction drug and undergoes nonrestrictive hepatic clearance. Fluconazole is a strong inhibitor of CYP2C9 and alters the pharmacokinetics of several CYP2C9 substrates, including phenytoin warfarin and losartan. The results of a hypothetical drug–drug interaction study conducted to evaluate the effects of fluconazole on lipoamide are presented. A randomized crossover study with a 2-week interval between the phases was conducted in 12 healthy volunteers. In each phase, the subjects received 200 mg of either fluconazole (test leg) or placebo (control leg) once daily for 5 days. On day 5, each subject received 120 mg of lipoamide before breakfast. Blood samples were taken at various times and analyzed for unchanged lipoamide. The results from one subject are presented in Table E10.3A.

Directions to create an Excel worksheet to analyze these data using NCA are provided in Appendix C Section 5. Note that the purpose of this exercise is to provide experience with NCA. As a result, the analysis will be performed on the data from one subject. Conclusions about altered pharmacokinetics cannot be based on the results of one subject. Assume that the analysis of data from the other subjects demonstrated that the effects observed on C_{max} and AUC are statistically significant.

TABLE E10.3A   Plasma Concentration–Time Data Obtained After the Oral Administration of Lipoamide (120 mg) to a Healthy Volunteer Concurrently with Placebo (Control) and Fluconazole (Test)

Time (h)	Control Cp (μg/L)	Test Cp (μg/L)	Time (h)	Control Cp (μg/L)	Test Cp (μg/L)
0.0	0.0	0.0	1.2	52.0	160.9
0.2	38.1	117.8	2.0	46.3	143.2
0.4	50.6	156.7	4.0	34.4	106.4
0.6	54.1	167.4	10.0	14.1	43.6
0.8	54.3	168.0	15.0	6.7	20.7
1.0	53.3	165.0	24.0	1.8	5.4

Plots of plasma concentration against time for the two phases are shown in Figure E10.3, where it can be seen that coadministration of fluconazole resulted in higher plasma concentrations of lipoamide. A summary of lipoamide's pharmacokinetic parameters in the absence and presence of fluconazole is provided in Table E10.3B.

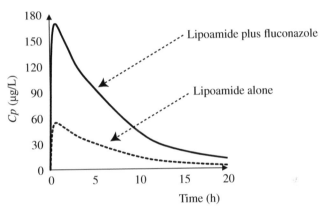

FIGURE E10.3   Plasma concentration of lipoamide administered with placebo (dashed line) and with fluconazole (solid line).

TABLE E10.3B   Summary of the Effect of Fluconazole on the Pharmacokinetics of Lipoamide

Parameter	Control (Placebo)	Test (Fluconazole)
Cl/F (L/h)	284	91.8[a]
λ (h^{-1})	0.15	0.15
$t_{1/2,\lambda}$ (h)	4.67	4.66
C_{max} (μg/L)	54.3	168[a]
T_{max} (h)	0.8	0.8

[a]Statistically significant when combined with the results from the other subjects.

The data show that lipoamide's oral clearance decreases and C_{max} increases with concomitant fluconazole. The decrease in oral clearance (Cl/F) could result from either a decrease in clearance (Cl) or an increase in the bioavailability (F). Any changes in the clearance would alter the drug's half-life. Since the half-life of lipoamide was not affected, one can assume that the reduction in oral clearance is primarily the result of increased bioavailability. In keeping with this theory, the C_{max} of lipoamide increased with concomitant fluconazole. Furthermore, the increase in C_{max} (about threefold) was about the same magnitude as the decrease in oral clearance (about threefold). It is likely that fluconazole reduces the presystemic hepatic extraction of lipoamide. As lipoamide is a high-extraction drug, it is likely that its hepatic clearance is fairly insensitive to changes in intrinsic clearance brought about by modifiers of the CYP2C9 enzyme system.

In conclusion, the results demonstrate that the pharmacokinetics of lipoamide are altered by fluconazole and suggest that decreased first-pass hepatic extraction may be the cause of the interaction. Based on these results, the combination of lipoamide and fluconazole should either be avoided or the dose of lipoamide should be reduced by about one-third.

PROBLEMS

10.1 Oral tablets of lipoamide (120 mg), nosolatol (250 mg), and disolvprazole (50 mg) were all subject to a relative bioavailability study to determine if food altered the bioavailability of these drugs. The design of the three studies was similar, and each consisted of a randomized crossover study involving 20 healthy volunteers. In one leg of the study, the subjects took the drug with water after an overnight fast (fast leg). On the other occasion, the participants took the drug in the morning of the study after a standard US Food and Drug Administration breakfast consisting of two eggs, bacon, hash browns, two slices of toast, and an 8-oz serving of milk (fed study). The two legs were separated by a period of 2 weeks. Example data from one participant from each of the studies are presented in Table 10.1.

TABLE P10.1   Results of Three Separate Relative Bioavailability Studies Designed to Probe the Effect of Food on the Bioavailability of Lipoamide, Nosolatol, and Disolvprazole

Lipoamide			Nosolatol			Disolvprazole		
Time (h)	Fast Cp (µg/L)	Fed Cp (µg/L)	Time (h)	Fast Cp (µg/L)	Fed Cp (µg/L)	Time (h)	Fast Cp (µg/L)	Fed Cp (µg/L)
0	0	0	0	0	0	0	0	0
0.2	35.0	20.4	0.2	299	274	0.2	252	93.3
0.4	48.3	33.2	1	717	822	0.6	473	213
0.6	52.7	41.0	1.6	756	949	1	516	271
0.8	53.6	45.5	2	752	978	1.6	469	294
1	53.0	48.0	2.6	732	982	2.6	345	258
1.2	51.9	49.1	3	716	972	3.2	282	223
2	46.3	47.2	4	675	928	4	213	177
4	34.4	35.8	8	531	733	6	106	92.4
10	14.2	14.7	12	417	576	8	52.9	46.5
15	6.75	7.02	24	203	280	10	26.3	23.2
24	1.78	1.85	48	47.8	68.0	12	13.1	11.6

Use NCA to analyze the results and determine how food affects the bioavailability of these drugs. Assume that any differences that you find achieve statistical significance when combined with the results from the other participants.

10.2 A study was conducted on 10 healthy volunteers to determine if itraconazole alters the pharmacokinetics of nosolatol. A sequential two-treatment design was used. On day 1 of the study, participants received an oral dose of nosolatol (250 mg) after an overnight fast. Blood samples were taken at various times after the dose, and the plasma concentration of the drug was determined. At the conclusion of the first part of the study, participants returned home and were instructed to take 200 mg of oral itraconazole twice daily. On day 6, the subjects returned to the clinic and received another dose of nosolatol (250 mg). Blood samples were withdrawn and analyzed for nosolatol. The data from a single subject are presented in (Table 10.2).

TABLE P10.2   Plasma Concentrations of Nosolatol at Various Times After an Oral Dose in the Absence and Presence of Itraconazole

	Cp (µg/L)			Cp (µg/L)	
Time (h)	Nosolatol Alone	Nosolatol Plus Itraconazole	Time (h)	Nosolatol Alone	Nosolatol Plus Itraconazole
0	0	0	3	716	1033
0.2	299	406	4	675	998
1	717	987	8	531	865
1.6	756	1055	12	417	750
2	752	1059	24	203	488
2.6	732	1046	48	47.8	207

Use NCA to analyze the results and comment on the effect of itraconazole. Assume that any differences you find achieve statistical significance when combined with the results from the other participants. Interpret the results based on nosolatol's pharmacokinetic properties summarized in Appendix E.

10.3   A randomized crossover study was conducted on 15 healthy volunteers to determine if probenecid alters the pharmacokinetics of disolvprazole. In one phase of the study, subjects received an oral dose of disolvprazole after an overnight fast. In the second phase, subjects received disolvprazole (50 mg) in combination with probenecid (1 g). In both phases, blood samples were withdrawn over a 12-h period and the plasma was analyzed for unchanged drug. The two phases were separated by a washout period of 1 week. The data are shown in Table 10.3. Use NCA to analyze the results and comment on the effect, if any, of probenecid. Assume that any differences you find achieve statistical significance when combined with the results from the other participants. Interpret the results based on disolvprazole's pharmacokinetic properties summarized in Appendix E.

TABLE P10.3   Plasma Concentrations of Disolvprazole at Various Times After an Oral Dose in the Absence and Presence of Probenecid

	Cp (µg/L)			Cp (µg/L)	
Time (h)	Disolvprazole Alone	Disolvprazole Plus Probenecid	Time (h)	Disolvprazole Alone	Disolvprazole Plus Probenecid
0	0	0	3.2	282	485
0.2	252	255	4	213	433
0.6	473	504	6	106	324
1	516	584	8	52.9	243
1.6	469	589	10	26.3	182
2.6	345	527	12	13.1	137

11

PHARMACOKINETICS OF INTRAVENOUS INFUSION IN A ONE-COMPARTMENT MODEL

Sara E. Rosenbaum

Basic Pharmacokinetics and Pharmacodynamics: An Integrated Textbook and Computer Simulations,
Second Edition. Edited by Sara E. Rosenbaum.
© 2017 John Wiley & Sons, Inc. Published 2017 by John Wiley & Sons, Inc.

Objectives

The material in this chapter will enable the reader to:

1. Have an understanding of the pharmacokinetics of continuous drug administration
2. Appreciate the determinants of steady-state plasma concentrations, particularly the influence of clearance and the rate of drug administration
3. Understand the factors that control the time to reach steady state
4. Develop an appropriate drug administration regimen based on population average pharmacokinetic parameter values
5. Individualize a dosing regimen for a patient based on the patient's steady-state plasma concentration

11.1 INTRODUCTION

In previous chapters, we addressed the pharmacokinetics of single doses. Clinically, the administration of isolated single doses is limited to only a few situations, such as over-the-counter analgesics and cough and cold remedies. Most drugs used in the treatment of diseases are taken over a course of at least several days and sometimes a lifetime. For long-term drug treatment, drugs may be administered in many different ways, including intravenous infusions, multiple intravenous doses, skin patches, and multiple oral doses.

An understanding of the pharmacokinetics and pharmacodynamics of continued drug administration is needed to design optimum dosing regimens. For example, in Chapter 7, we demonstrated how a drug's pharmacokinetic characteristics could be used to determine the value of single doses to achieve certain target plasma concentrations. But if a drug's primary pharmacokinetics parameters (*Cl* and *Vd*) and therapeutic range are known, how can a dosing regimen be developed to maintain plasma concentrations in the therapeutic range over an extended period? The answer to this question requires an understanding of the pharmacokinetics of extended drug administration. Extended or chronic drug administration involves two phenomena that have not been addressed previously: accumulation and fluctuation.

Accumulation refers to a gradual buildup of drug concentrations with successive doses. It occurs whenever a dose is administered at a time when drug from a previous dose is still in the body. It is important to understand the properties of accumulation. For example, does accumulation continue for as long as the therapy continues? Alternatively, does accumulation gradually attenuate and eventually stop?

Multiple doses are administered in a quantum or pulse-like fashion; doses are given at regular intervals (e.g., 10 mg every 8, 12, or 24 h) over the course of therapy. This pulse-like administration is associated with *fluctuation*, the rise and fall in plasma concentration during a dosing interval. A peak concentration is usually seen at the time of, or slightly after, the administration of a dose. Trough concentrations usually occur at the time the next dose is given. However, in the case of orally administered drugs, the trough may occur slightly later if there is an absorption lag time.

The simplest way to initially study the pharmacokinetics of chronic drug administration is to consider the characteristics of constant (zero order) continuous drug input into the body. Under these circumstances, no fluctuation in the plasma concentration will be observed. The most common example of zero-order drug administration is the intravenous infusion, where drug is administered directly into a patient's vein at a constant continuous rate using a drip or electronic infusion pump. Intravenous infusions offer several advantages: They provide a very accurate means of administering drugs; they can be very convenient if the patient has an existing indwelling catheter; they eliminate fluctuation and provide a constant plasma concentration, which can be targeted to the middle of the therapeutic range; and the absence of fluctuation reduces the tendency of the peak and trough plasma concentrations to venture into toxic and subtherapeutic areas, respectively. Pharmaceutical scientists strive to develop controlled release oral dosage forms that provide constant, continuous drug input. The elementary infusion pump or Oros system is an example of an oral dosage form that appears to provide a zero-order input.

11.2 MODEL AND EQUATIONS

In the one-compartment model, the body is represented by a single imaginary compartment. Recall from Chapter 7 that the drug concentration in the compartment is assumed to be equal to the plasma concentration, and the volume of the imaginary compartment is equal to the drug's volume of distribution (Vd). Like the distribution of drug throughout the body, the distribution of drug throughout the compartment is assumed to occur extremely rapidly, in an essentially instantaneous manner. The compartment is homogeneous and at any time, the concentration of drug throughout is constant. As always, elimination is first order and can be described using clearance (Cl) or the overall elimination rate constant (k), where $k = Cl/Vd$. Drug administration into the body or compartment occurs at a constant continuous rate (zero-order process). The rate (k_0) has units of amount per unit time (e.g., mg/h). In the event that the salt of a drug is used or the equations are applied to extravascular administration, the rate of administration is qualified by the salt factor and bioavailability, respectively. The model is shown in Figure 11.1.

11.2.1 Basic Equation

The starting point for the development of the basic equation is to consider how the amount of drug in the body changes with time:

rate of change of the amount of drug in the body = rate of inputs − rate of outputs

$$\frac{dAb}{dt} = S \cdot F \cdot k_0 - k \cdot Ab \tag{11.1}$$

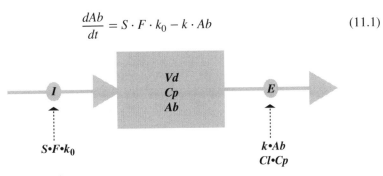

Initial conditions: $t = 0$,
$Ab = Ab_0 = 0$

FIGURE 11.1 Intravenous infusion in a one-compartment model. Drug input (I) into the body is constant and equal to the product of the infusion rate (k_0), the salt factor (S), and the bioavailability (F). For intravenous administration, $F = 1$. Ab is the amount of drug in the body, Vd is the drug's volume of distribution, and Cp is the plasma concentration. Elimination (E) is a first-order process and can be expressed using clearance (Cl) or the elimination rate constant (k).

where S is the salt factor, F is the bioavailability, and k_0 is the constant rate of drug administration. Equation (11.1) is integrated from zero to infinity:

$$Ab = \frac{S \cdot F \cdot k_0}{k} \cdot (1 - e^{-kt}) \qquad (11.2)$$

with $Cp = Ab/Vd$,

$$Cp = \frac{S \cdot F \cdot k_0}{Vd \cdot k} \cdot (1 - e^{-kt}) \qquad (11.3)$$

and with $Cl = Vd \cdot k$,

$$Cp = \frac{S \cdot F \cdot k_0}{Cl} \cdot (1 - e^{-kt}) \qquad (11.4)$$

Analysis of the Equation

- Recall (see Appendix A) that $1 - e^{-kt}$ is the growth factor that starts at zero when $t = 0$ and grows to 1 at infinity.
- Thus, plasma concentrations start at zero and grow to the value of $S \cdot F \cdot k_0 /Cl$ at infinity.
- The speed of growth is determined by the value of k ($t_{1/2}$).
- The equation allows the plasma concentration to be estimated at any time during zero-order drug input.
- The shape of the plasma concentration–time profile corresponding to equation (11.4) is shown in Figure 11.2.

Note in Figure 11.2 that after the start of the infusion, the drug accumulates in the body and the plasma concentration increases. The rate of increase in the plasma concentration and the accumulation become less and less as therapy continues. Eventually, the plasma concentration becomes constant and drug accumulation ceases. The latter period is

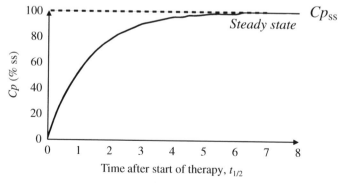

FIGURE 11.2 Plasma concentration–time profile during an intravenous infusion. When the plasma concentration remains constant, steady state has been achieved. The plasma concentration at steady-state plasma concentration is Cp_{ss}. Note that the unit of time is the elimination half-life.

known as a steady state, and the corresponding plasma concentration is referred to as the steady-state plasma concentration (Cp_{ss}). It can be concluded that during a constant intravenous infusion, drug accumulation is a self-limiting process that eventually stops at steady state.

11.2.2 Application of the Basic Equation

The basic equation (11.4) enables the plasma concentration to be calculated at any time during continuous zero drug input (e.g., from an infusion or an oral preparation that delivers drug at a constant continuous rate).

Example 11.1   A drug ($S = 1$, $Cl = 2$ L/h, and $Vd = 50$ L) is administered as an intravenous infusion at a rate of 10 mg/h. Calculate the plasma concentration 4 h into the infusion.

Solution $Cl = 2$ L/h, $Vd = 50$ L, $k = Cl/Vd = 2/50 = 0.04$ h^{-1}, and $t_{1/2} = 0.693/k = 17.3$ h.

$$
\begin{aligned}
Cp &= \frac{S \cdot F \cdot k_0}{Cl} \cdot (1 - e^{-kt}) \\
&= \frac{10}{2}(1 - e^{-0.04 \times 4}) \\
&= 0.74 \text{ mg/L}
\end{aligned}
$$

11.2.3 Simulation Exercise: Part 1: http://web.uri.edu/pharmacy/research/rosenbaum/sims

Open model 7, Constant Continuous Drug Administration, which can be found at http://web.uri.edu/pharmacy/research/rosenbaum/sims/Model7
   The default model parameters are $S = 1$, $F = 1$, infusion rate $= 10$ mg/h, $Cl = 5$ L/h, and $Vd = 20$ L.

 1. *Review the objectives, explore the model, and review the "Model Summary" page.*
 2. *Go to the "Cp–time Profile" page. Perform a simulation with the default rate of administration and observe the Cp–time profile.*
    (a) Simulate using infusion rates of 5, 10, and 20 mg/L. Hold the mouse over each line to note the values of the steady-state plasma concentration. Add these to Table SE11.1.
    (b) Describe the relationship between Cp_{ss} and the infusion rate.
    (c) Determine an infusion rate to give a Cp_{ss} of 6 mg/L.

TABLE SE11.1   Infusion Rates and the Corresponding Cp_{ss}

Simulation	Infusion Rate	Cp_{ss}
1	5 mg/h	
2	10 mg/h	
3	20 mg/h	
4		6 mg/L

11.3 STEADY-STATE PLASMA CONCENTRATION

At steady state, the plasma concentration becomes constant and independent of time (Figure 11.2). The value of the steady-state plasma concentration is a very important focus of drug treatment. Usually, it is desirable to have a steady-state plasma concentration in the middle of the therapeutic range. To plan this, it is necessary to understand the factors that control the steady-state plasma concentration.

11.3.1 Equation for Steady-State Plasma Concentrations

There are two ways to derive the equation for the steady-state plasma concentration.

Derivation 1   Before steady state, the plasma concentration is given by equation (11.4). As t increases, the exponential growth function, $1 - e^{-kt}$, tends to 1, and Cp tends to Cp_{ss}:

$$\boxed{Cp_{ss} = \frac{S \cdot F \cdot k_0}{Cl}} \tag{11.5}$$

The box around equation (11.5) signifies that it is an important equation, as we demonstrate in Section 11.3.4.

Derivation 2   At steady state, the plasma concentration is constant. Thus, the rate of drug administration must equal the rate of drug elimination:

$$S \cdot F \cdot k_0 = Cl \cdot Cp_{ss} \tag{11.6}$$

Equation (11.6) can be rearranged to yield equation (11.5).

11.3.2 Application of the Equation

Next, we look at two examples that illustrate an application of the steady-state plasma concentration equation.

Example 11.2   The same drug as that described in Example 11.1 is administered as an intravenous infusion at a rate of 10 mg/h. Calculate the steady-state plasma concentration. Recall that $Cl = 2$ L/h, $Vd = 50$ L, $S = 1$, $k = Cl/Vd = 2/50 = 0.04$ h^{-1}, and $t_{1/2} = 0.693/k = 17.3$ h.

Solution

$$Cp_{ss} = \frac{S \cdot F \cdot k_0}{Cl} = \frac{10}{2} = 5 \text{ mg/L}$$

Example 11.3   A drug ($S = 0.9$, $F = 0.94$, $Cl = 1.44$ L/h, and $Vd = 0.65$ L/kg) has a therapeutic range of 10–20 mg/L. It is formulated into an oral elementary osmotic pump, which delivers the drug at a constant rate of 12 mg/h. The preparation is designed for administration every 12 h and is available in units of 250, 300, and 400 mg. Determine a suitable dose to achieve a steady-state plasma concentration of 15 mg/L in a 60-kg woman.

Solution

$$Cp_{ss} = \frac{S \cdot F \cdot k_0}{Cl}$$

$$k_0 = \frac{Cl \cdot Cp_{ss}}{S \cdot F} = \frac{1.44 \times 15}{0.9 \times 0.94}$$

$$= 25.5 \text{ mg/h}$$

The unit dosage forms are designed to administer the dose at a constant rate over a 12-h period. If a rate of 25.5 mg/h is required, the unit dose must contain $25.5 \times 12 = 306$ mg. Thus, the 300-mg unit should be given twice daily.

11.3.3 Basic Formula Revisited

The expression for the steady-state plasma concentration given in equation (11.5) may be substituted into the basic equation for the plasma concentration before steady state, as given in equation (11.4):

$$Cp = Cp_{ss} \cdot (1 - e^{-kt}) \tag{11.7}$$

This equation shows that the plasma concentration grows from zero at time zero $(1 - e^{-kt} = 0)$ to the steady-state plasma concentration at time infinity $(1 - e^{-kt} = 1)$.

11.3.4 Factors Controlling Steady-State Plasma Concentration

Equation (11.5), which shows the factors that control the steady-state plasma concentration, is reproduced below.

$$\boxed{Cp_{ss} = \frac{S \cdot F \cdot k_0}{Cl}}$$

The box surrounding it designates that it is an important equation. This equation, probably the most important and useful of all pharmacokinetic equations, shows that the terminal plasma concentration achieved by a given rate of drug administration is dependent only on the effective rate of drug administration and clearance. It also provides insight into when it may be prudent to modify the usual rate of drug administration.

Specifically, the equation shows the following points:

1. Cp_{ss} is directly proportional to the infusion rate (k_0). If the infusion rate is doubled, Cp_{ss} will double. For example, if a drug is administered at a rate of 5 mg/h and achieves a steady-state plasma concentration of 2 mg/L, doubling the infusion rate to 10 mg/h would double the steady-state plasma concentration to 4 mg/L.

2. Cp_{ss} is directly proportional to the drug's bioavailability (F).

3. Cp_{ss} is inversely proportional to the drug's clearance (Cl). For example, consider a drug normally administered at a rate of 10 mg/h to achieve a desired steady-state plasma concentration of 2 mg/L. The same rate of administration in an elderly patient, who has a clearance of half the normal value, would result in a steady-state plasma concentration twice the desired value—4 mg/L.

4. Cp_{ss} is independent of the volume of distribution (Vd). The volume of distribution is absent from the basic formula for the steady-state plasma concentration. Variability in Vd will not influence the steady-state plasma concentration. In the next section, we demonstrate that volume of distribution, through its influence on the half-life, influences the *time* it takes to get to steady state.

5. The equation can be used to estimate a rate of drug administration to achieve a desired steady-state plasma concentration and to estimate a steady-state plasma concentration from a given rate of administration.

6. The equation demonstrates that it may be necessary to modify the usual rate of drug administration in patients who have altered clearance or bioavailability.

11.3.5 Time to Steady State

The basic equation for the plasma concentration during constant continuous drug administration is given by equation (11.7). It can be rearranged as:

$$\frac{Cp}{Cp_{ss}} = 1 - e^{-kt} \tag{11.8}$$

The left-hand side of equation (11.8) is the fraction of steady state achieved at any time. Thus, $1 - e^{-kt}$ represents the fraction of steady state achieved at any time. It was shown in Appendix B that the time it takes for $1 - e^{-kt}$ to grow from zero at time zero to 1 at time infinity, is controlled the first order elimination rate constant (k) or the half-life. The number of half-lives to achieve various fractional growths were calculated in Appendix B and are reproduced here (Table 11.1).) to show the number of half-lives it takes to achieve various fractions of steady state during a zero order drug input.

The time to achieve various fractions of steady state can also be proven through calculation.

TABLE 11.1   Time (Half-Lives) to Achieve Certain Fractions of Steady State

Time ($t_{1/2}$)	$1 - e^{-kt}$	Fraction of Steady State (%)
$\frac{1}{6}a$	0.1	10
$\frac{1}{3}a$	0.2	20
1	0.5	50
3.3	0.9	90
4.3	0.95	95
6.6	0.99	99

^{a}Approximate value.

Example 11.4   How many half-lives does it take to get to 95% steady state?

Solution   At 95% of steady state, $Cp = 0.95\ Cp_{ss}$. Let $k = 0.693/t_{1/2}$. Substituting into equation (11.8) for Cp and k gives us

$$\frac{0.95Cp_{ss}}{Cp_{ss}} = 1 - e^{-(0.693/t_{1/2})\cdot t}$$

$$e^{-(0.693/t_{1/2})\cdot t} = 0.05$$

$$\frac{0.693t}{t_{1/2}} = -\ln 0.05 = 3.0$$

$$t = 4.33 t_{1/2}$$

In summary, the time to get to steady state is determined by a drug's half-life. Clinically, it is usual to consider that it takes 3–5 half-lives to achieve steady state. It can be seen in Figure 11.2 (the units of time are elimination half-lives) that steady state is achieved by about five half-lives. Recall that the half-life is a secondary pharmacokinetic parameter, determined by a drug's clearance and volume of distribution. Thus, changes in either of these primary parameters will alter the time to steady state by virtue of their influence on the half-life. For example, increases in the volume of distribution and decreases in clearance will increase the time it takes to get to steady state.

11.3.6 Simulation Exercise: Part 2: http://web.uri.edu/pharmacy/research/rosenbaum/sims

Open simulation model 7, Constant Continuous Drug Administration, which can be found at, http://web.uri.edu/pharmacy/research/rosenbaum/sims/Model7
  Go to the "Effect of Cl and Vd" page.

1. *Record the value of Cp_{ss} for the three values of Cl (2.5, 5, and 10 L/h) in Table SE11.2 and summarize the relationship between Cl and Cp_{ss}.*
2. *Describe how Cl affects the time to reach steady state.*
3. *Clear the graph and record the value of Cp_{ss} for the three values of Vd (10, 20, and 40 L) in Table SE11.2 and summarize the relationship between Vd and Cp_{ss}.*
4. *Describe how Vd affects the time to reach steady state.*
5. *Would you recommend dosage adjustments in patients with (a) altered Cl; (b) altered Vd?*
6. *List three situations where a patient may present with an altered Cl, and three situations where a patient may present with an altered Vd.*

TABLE SE11.2   Influence of Changes in Clearance and Volume of Distribution on the Value of the Steady-State Plasma Concentration and the Time to Get to Steady State

Simulation	Clearance	Volume of Distribution	Cp_{ss}
1	2.5 L/h	20 L (default)	
2	5 L/h	20 L (default)	
3	10 L/h	20 L (default)	
4	5 L/h (default)	10 L	
5	5 L/h (default)	20 L	
6	5 L/h (default)	40 L	

11.4 LOADING DOSE

If a drug has a long half-life and/or if it is necessary to achieve therapeutic plasma concentrations immediately, a loading dose may be given to achieve steady state immediately.

11.4.1 Loading-Dose Equation

A loading dose may be calculated using equation (7.9) with Cp_{ss} as the target plasma concentration at time zero:

$$D_L = \frac{Cp_{ss} \cdot Vd}{S \cdot F} \tag{11.9}$$

If the loading dose is administered simultaneously with the start of the infusion, the net drug in the body at any time is the sum of that remaining from the bolus loading dose and that gained from the infusion:

$$Cp_{net} = Cp_{D_L} + Cp_{inf} \tag{11.10}$$

where Cp_{D_L} is the plasma concentration from the loading dose, and Cp_{inf} is that from the infusion; and can be calculated from equations (7.4) and (11.4), respectively,

$$Cp_{D_L} = \frac{S \cdot F \cdot D_L}{Vd} \cdot e^{-kt}$$

$$Cp_{inf} = \frac{S \cdot F \cdot k_0}{Cl} \cdot (1 - e^{-kt})$$

Substituting for the expressions above into equation (11.10) yields

$$Cp = \frac{S \cdot F \cdot D_L}{Vd} \cdot e^{-kt} + \frac{S \cdot F \cdot k_0}{Cl} \cdot (1 - e^{-kt}) \tag{11.11}$$

But

$$\frac{S \cdot F \cdot D_L}{Vd} = Cp_{ss}$$

and

$$\frac{S \cdot F \cdot k_0}{Cl} = Cp_{ss}$$

Thus,

$$Cp = Cp_{ss} \cdot e^{-kt} + Cp_{ss} \cdot (1 - e^{-kt})$$
$$= Cp_{ss} \tag{11.12}$$

In other words, the loss of drug from the bolus is exactly matched by the gain of drug from the infusion (Figure 11.3).

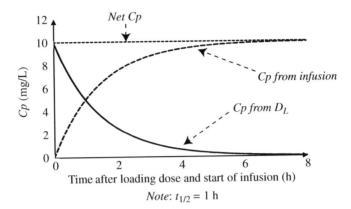

Note: $t_{1/2} = 1$ h

FIGURE 11.3 Net plasma concentration of drug from an intravenous infusion and a bolus loading dose. The rate of the infusion is $Cp_{ss} \cdot Cl/S \cdot F$ and the loading dose is $Cp_{ss} \cdot Vd$. Note that the $t_{1/2}$ value of this drug is 1 h. It can be seen that by about 6 h, the loading dose is almost completely eliminated and the infusion is at steady state.

Example 11.5 A drug ($Cl = 6$ L/h, $Vd = 150$ L, and $S = 1$) is to be administered as an intravenous infusion. A steady-state plasma concentration of 1.2 mg/L is desired. Calculate:

(a) A suitable infusion rate.
(b) The time it would take to achieve steady-state plasma concentrations.
(c) The value of a loading dose that would immediately achieve the desired steady-state plasma concentration of 1.2 mg/L.

Solution As with all pharmacokinetic calculations, the half-life should be calculated as soon as possible because it can be used to check calculations and make sure that they are in the correct range. The elimination rate constant should also be calculated, as that is used frequently in calculations.

$$t_{1/2} = 0.693 Vd/Cl = 17.3 \text{ h} \quad k = 0.04 \text{ h}^{-1}$$

(a) The rate of the infusion is found using equation (11.5); $Cp_{ss} = 1.2$ mg/L:

$$k_0 \frac{1.2 \text{ mg/L} \times 6 \text{ L/h}}{1 \times 1} = 7.2 \text{ mg/h}$$

(b) Time to steady state
It takes 3–5 $t_{1/2}$ to get to steady state. Thus, it takes $(3 \times 17) - (5 \times 17) = 51$–85 h.

(c) Loading dose, using equation (11.9), we have

$$D_L = \frac{1.2 \text{ mg/L} \times 150}{1 \times 1} = 180 \text{ mg}$$

The need for a loading depends on two factors:

1. The drug's half-life and how long it takes to get to steady state
2. How quickly a therapeutic response is required in a given clinical situation

For example, it takes over a week to get to steady state when therapy with digoxin is started. But it is not critical to achieve therapeutic plasma concentration immediately, and a loading dose is not frequently administered. In contrast, it takes only about 6–8 h to reach steady state with lidocaine. However, this drug is used to treat serious life-threatening ventricular arrhythmias, and as a result it is important to achieve therapeutic plasma concentrations quickly, and a loading dose is usually administered.

11.4.2 Simulation Exercise: Part 3

Open simulation model 7, Constant Continuous Drug Administration, which can be found at, http://web.uri.edu/pharmacy/research/rosenbaum/sims/Model7
   Go to the "Loading Dose" page.

   1. Note the value of Cp_{ss} achieved using the default settings.
   2. Calculate a loading dose to achieve this Cp immediately.
   3. Simulate Cp when a loading dose is given.
   4. Note the Cp–time profile.

11.5 TERMINATION OF INFUSION

11.5.1 Equations for Termination Before and After Steady State

At some time, the infusion will be stopped or terminated. At this time, there will be no ongoing inputs into the body, and first-order elimination becomes the only process that affects the plasma concentration. Thus, after termination, the plasma concentration will decay monoexponentially from its value at the time of termination:

$$Cp = Cp_T \cdot e^{-kt'} \tag{11.13}$$

where Cp_T is Cp when the infusion is terminated at time T, and t' is the time elapsed since termination.

Termination After Steady State   When the infusion is stopped after steady state has been achieved, the plasma concentration at termination is Cp_{ss}, and after termination,

$$Cp = Cp_{ss} \cdot e^{-kt'} \tag{11.14}$$

where t' is the time elapsed since termination.

Termination Before Steady State   When the infusion is stopped before steady state has been achieved, the basic equation (11.4) for an infusion has to be used to calculate the plasma concentration at the time of termination:

$$Cp_T = \frac{S \cdot F \cdot k_0}{Cl} \cdot (1 - e^{-kT}) \tag{11.15}$$

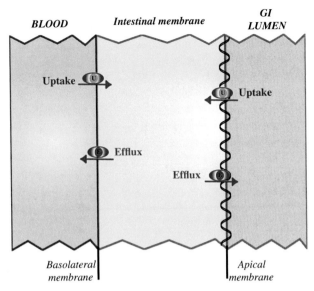

FIGURE 2.5 Theoretical placements of uptake and efflux transporters in an epithelial cell membrane such as the intestinal membrane. E represents an efflux transporter such as permeability glycoprotein (P-gp) or breast cancer-resistance protein (BCRP); U represents an uptake transporter such as organic anion transporting polypeptide (OATP) or organic cation transporter (OCT). Uptake transporters on the apical membrane and efflux transporters on the basolateral side promote the retention of drugs in the body. Uptake transporters on the basolateral side of the membrane and efflux transporters on the apical side promote the removal of drug from the body. Courtesy of Linnea E. Anderson.

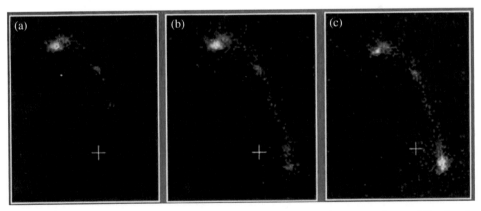

FIGURE 3.4 A series of γ scintigraphs showing the transit in the human esophagus following the administered of a liquid [4]. Courtesy of Clive Wilson, D.o.P.S., Strathclyde Institute for Biomedical Sciences.

Basic Pharmacokinetics and Pharmacodynamics: An Integrated Textbook and Computer Simulations,
Second Edition. Edited by Sara E. Rosenbaum.
© 2017 John Wiley & Sons, Inc. Published 2017 by John Wiley & Sons, Inc.

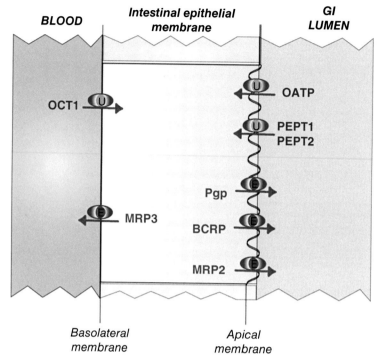

FIGURE 3.10   Transporters in the intestinal epithelia.

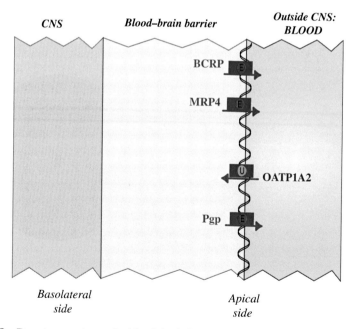

FIGURE 4.8   Drug transporters at the blood–brain barrier. Efflux transporters such as BCRP, P-gp, and MRP4 are expressed on the apical side and reduce the CNS exposure of their substrates. The OATP1A2 uptake transporter is also expressed on the apical side and increases the CNS exposure of its substrates.

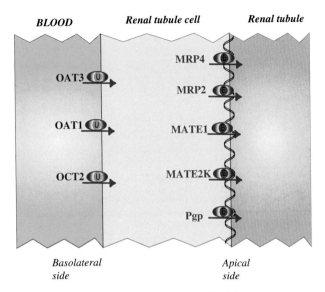

FIGURE 5.5 Drug transporters in the human renal tubule. The uptake transporters (U) organic cation transporter (OCT2) and organic anion transporters (OAT1 and OAT3) are found on the basolateral side of the renal tubular membrane. These transporters promote excretion by transporting drugs from the blood into the tubular cells. The efflux transporters (E), permeability glycoprotein (P-gp), multidrug resistance-associated protein family (MRP2 and MRP4), and multidrug and toxin extrusion protein (MATE) can conclude the process by transporting drugs from the tubular cells into the tubule.

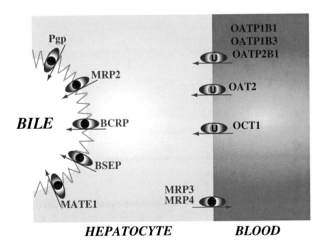

FIGURE 5.8 Drug transporters in the liver. The diagram shows a hepatocyte. The uptake transporters (U), organic anion transporting polypeptide (OATP), organic cation transporter (OCT), and organic anion transporter (OAT) are found on the basolateral side of the hepatocyte. The efflux transporters (E), permeability glycoprotein (P-gp), multidrug resistance-associated protein family (MRP), breast cancer-resistance protein (BCRP), bile salt export pump (BSEP), and multidrug and toxin extrusion protein (MATE) are found mainly on the canalicular membrane. Two efflux transporters (MRP3 and MRP4) are found on the basolateral membrane.

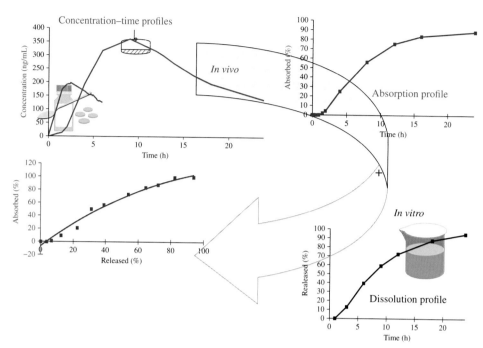

FIGURE 9.10 The IVIVC is illustrated here for a modified release dosage form. The plot in the lower right corner contains the *in vitro* dissolution versus time profile. The plot in the upper left corner contains the *in vivo* plasma concentration versus time profiles for an immediate release and the modified release formulations. The absorption versus time profile is derived from the *in vivo* data through a statistical pharmacokinetic analysis (upper right plot). The absorption data and the dissolution data are related in the IVIVC (lower left plot). By reversing the steps of this validated IVIVC, a different formulation with a different dissolution profile is used as the input for a pharmacokinetic simulation that predicts the *in vivo* concentration—time—profile.

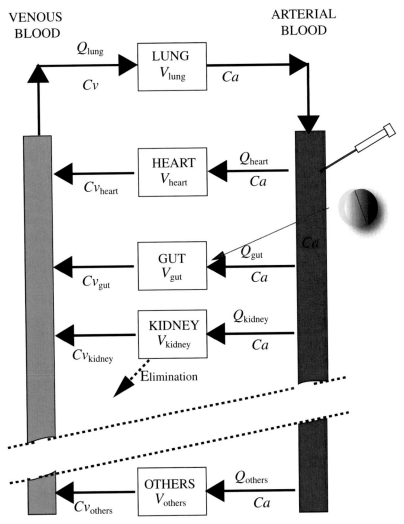

FIGURE 18.1 An abbreviated PBPK model. The tissues of the model are linked by the systemic circulation. Arterial blood delivers drug to the tissues and the venous blood leaving the tissue is then returned to the systemic circulation. The concentration in arterial blood is Ca and that in the venous blood leaving a tissue Cv_t. Drug elimination may occur as the blood flows through the kidney (shown) and liver. The physiological parameters used in the model are tissue blood flow (Q_t) and tissue volume (V_t). This model shows only the lungs, heart, and the kidney. A typical model may consist of around 7–15 tissues. The model shows intravenous drug input directly into the venous blood and oral administration where absorption occurs into the gut.

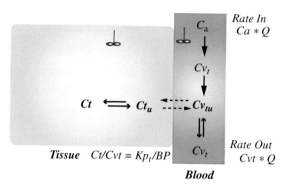

FIGURE 18.2 Perfusion-controlled distribution. The tissue is viewed as a well-stirred single compartment. Drug is delivered to the tissue in arterial blood: Q is the blood flow to the tissue and Ca is the drug concentration in arterial blood. The rate of drug delivery is $Q * Ca$. Drug may bind to proteins and macromolecules in the blood and tissue. The unbound fraction in blood, plasma, and the tissue are fu_b, fu, and fu_t, respectively. The unbound drug concentration in the tissue (Ct_u), venous blood (Cv_{ut}), and plasma (Cp_u) are all equal. The ratio of the total drug concentration in the tissue (Ct) and the concentration in venous blood (Cv_t) can be expressed in terms of the tissue:plasma partition coefficient (Kp_t) and the drugs blood:plasma concentration ratio (BP). The rate the drug leaves the tissue is $Q * Cv_t$.

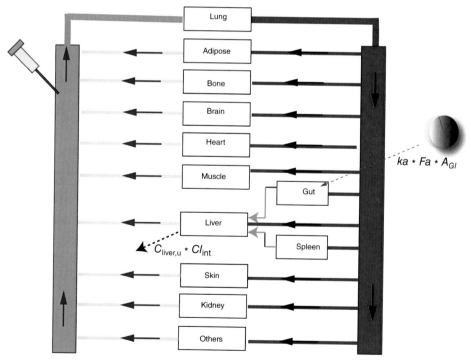

FIGURE 18.4 A full PBPK model. This model consists of 11 specific tissues and the remaining tissues grouped as "Others." In this model, elimination is modeled from the liver with a rate equal to the product of the unbound drug concentration and the drug's intrinsic metabolic clearance (Cl_{int}). It is assumed that there is no renal elimination. Oral absorption is modeled as a first-order process controlled by the absorption rate constant (ka), the fraction of the dose absorbed into the GI membrane (Fa), and the amount of drug in the GI tract (A_{GI}).

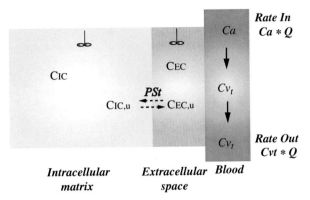

FIGURE 18.5 Permeability-limited distribution. The tissue is compartmentalized into two units, the extracellular compartment (tissue blood and extracellular space) and the intracellular tissue compartment. Drug is delivered by arterial blood, concentration Ca (blood flow Q). Distribution between the blood and the extracellular fluid is perfusion controlled. It occurs rapidly and the drug concentrations in the venous blood (Cv_t) and the extracellular space (C_{EC}) are equal. The movement of unbound drug back and forth across the cell membrane is controlled by the drug's permeability surface area product (PS_t) and the concentration gradient of the unbound drug in the extracellular ($C_{EC,u}$) and intracellular ($C_{IC,u}$) spaces.

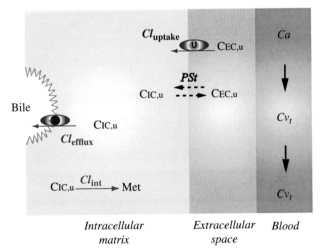

FIGURE 18.6 Liver model incorporating the action of transporters. Transporters are usually added to permeability-limited distribution models. In this model for hepatic elimination, the drug's elimination incorporates an uptake transporter on the basolateral membrane and an efflux transporter on the canalicular side of the hepatocyte membrane. Drug may pass into the hepatocyte by passive diffusion (permeability surface area product, PS_t) and/or through the action of the uptake transporter (intrinsic clearance, Cl_{uptake}). Once inside the cell, the drug may diffuse passively back into the blood; undergo metabolism (intrinsic clearance, Cl_{int}); and/or be subject to efflux into the bile (intrinsic clearance, Cl_{efflux}). See Figure 18.5 for the definition of other symbols.

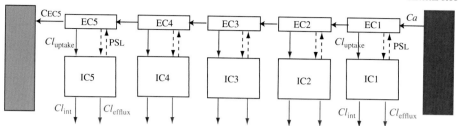

FIGURE 18.7 Transit through the liver modeled using five compartments. The model is essentially the same as the previous model (Figure 18.6) but in this case, the extracellular and intracellular spaces of the liver are divided into five units. EC represents the extracellular space and IC the intracellular space. Black dashed lines indicate passive diffusion (liver permeability surface area product (PS_L)); blue lines indicate transporter-mediated uptake (clearance, Cl_{uptake}); purple lines indicate hepatic metabolism (intrinsic clearance, Cl_{int}); and red lines indicate transporter-mediated efflux into the bile (clearance, Cl_{efflux}).

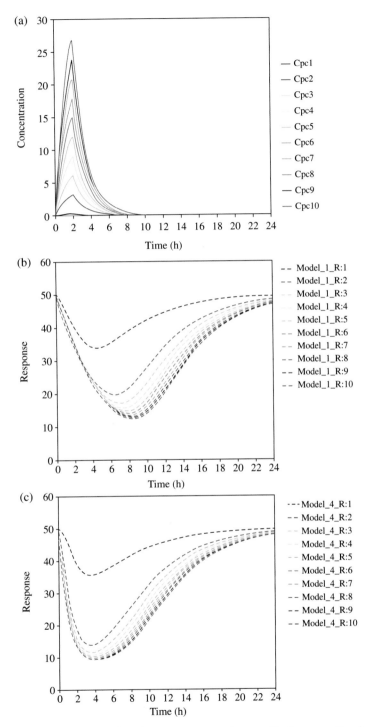

FIGURE 20.15 Effect of changing dose on response–time profile for competing indirect effect models. The pharmacokinetic profile (a) Model 1 (b) and Model 4 (c). Parameter values for the models are those given in the legend of Table 20.1.

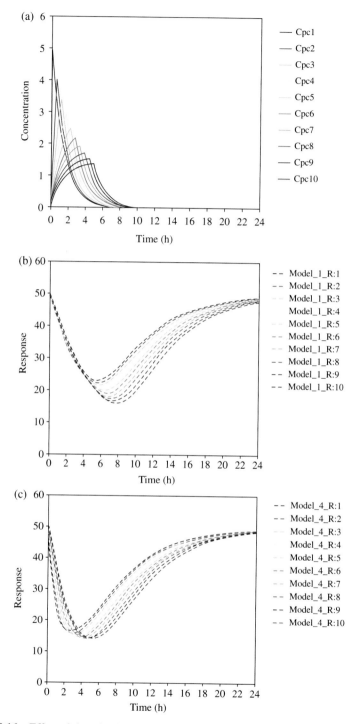

FIGURE 20.16 Effect of changing input rate on response–time profile for competing indirect effect models. The pharmacokinetic profile (a) Model 1 (b) and Model 4 (c). Parameter values for the models are those given in the legend of Table 20.1.

where T is the time of termination. After termination, Cp will decay monoexponentially from this value:

$$Cp = \frac{S \cdot F \cdot k_0}{Cl} \cdot (1 - e^{-kT}) \cdot e^{-kt'} \tag{11.16}$$

where t' is the time elapsed since termination.

11.5.2 Simulation Exercise: Part 4

Open simulation model 7, Constant Continuous Drug Administration, which can be found at, http://web.uri.edu/pharmacy/research/rosenbaum/sims/Model7
Go to the "Termination" page.

1. *Simulate Cp without terminating the infusion.*
2. *Perform several simulations when the infusion is terminated at various times both before and after the achievement of steady state.*
3. *Comment on the Cp–time profile after termination for both linear and semilog plots.*
4. *Write an equation for the plasma concentration after termination (Cp') using Cp_T for the plasma concentration at the time of termination and t' for the time since termination.*

11.6 INDIVIDUALIZATION OF DOSING REGIMENS

11.6.1 Initial Doses

Infusion rates or rates at which drugs are administered are designed to achieve steady-state plasma concentrations in the middle of the therapeutic range. Typical infusion rates are based on average values of clearance, which, as can be seen from equation (11.5), is the only parameter (assuming intravenous administration and $F = 1$) that affects the dose. If a drug has both a narrow therapeutic range and displays a lot of variability in its clearance in the population, it may be necessary to either modify an initial dose, based on a suspected altered clearance, and/or to monitor steady-state plasma concentrations to ensure that they are therapeutic. If they are found to be outside the therapeutic range, it will be necessary to alter the dose and individualize it for the patient.

Patient's Clearance   For drugs that have narrow therapeutic ranges, it is important to evaluate patients before therapy is started to determine if they possess any characteristics that are known to alter a specific drug's clearance. If as a result of this evaluation they are suspected to have altered clearance, the dose of the drug can be modified accordingly. For example, if the patient is taking a concomitant medication known to induce the enzymes involved in elimination of the drug, their clearance may be higher than normal, and a higher than normal rate of drug administration may be required. Conversely, if a patient is taking a drug that inhibits the metabolism of the subject drug, or if the patient has a disease (e.g., hepatic disease, renal disease and congestive heart failure) that is known to reduce a patient's clearance, their clearance may be lower than normal and it may be appropriate to use a dose that is lower than normal.

In many situations, there is often no information about a patient's individual pharmacokinetic parameters, including clearance. Thus, the population average value of clearance is assumed, and the typical population average infusion rate is used. Alternatively, equation (11.5) can be used to calculate an infusion rate to achieve the desired plasma concentration, based on the population average clearance.

11.6.2 Monitoring and Individualizing Therapy

It is most convenient to wait 3–5 elimination half-lives after the start of therapy and monitor when steady state has been achieved.

11.6.2.1 *Proportional Changes in the Rate of Administration*
It can be seen from equation (11.5) that the steady-state plasma concentration is directly proportional to the infusion rate. This allows proportional changes to the infusion rate to be made to achieve different steady-state plasma concentrations.

Example 11.6   A 70-kg patient is receiving an infusion of lidocaine hydrochloride ($S = 0.87$) (1 mg/min) to achieve a desired steady-state plasma concentration of 4 mg/L. His steady-state plasma concentration is found to be 3 mg/L. Recommend a new infusion rate.

Solution   Using proportions, we have

$$\frac{4 \text{ mg/L}}{3 \text{ mg/L}} = \frac{k_0 \text{mg/min}}{1\text{mg/min}}$$
$$k_0 = 1.33 \text{ mg/min}$$

11.6.2.2 *Estimation of Patient's Clearance*
Alternatively, a steady-state plasma concentration from a known rate of drug administration can be used to calculate a patient's clearance. The calculated clearance can then be used in equation (11.5) to determine a new rate of drug administration. This method involves an extra step compared to the proportional method presented above, but it provides a little more pharmacokinetic information, and the clearance calculated can be used in conjunction with a population average volume of distribution to estimate the patient's elimination half-life.

Example 11.7   Use the information from Example 11.6 and substitute in equation (11.5):

$$3.0 \text{ mg/L} = \frac{0.87 \times 1 \times 1 \text{ mg/min}}{Cl}$$
$$Cl = 0.29 \text{ L/min}$$

Use the patient's clearance and the population average volume of distribution (0.88 L/kg) to calculate the half-life:

$$t_{1/2} = \frac{0.693 \times 0.88 \times 70}{0.29} = 147 \text{ min}$$

Estimate a new infusion rate by again using equation (11.5):

$$4 \text{ mg/L} = \frac{0.87 \times 1 \times k_0}{0.29 \text{ L/min}}$$
$$k_0 = 1.33 \text{ mg/min}$$

An infusion of 1.33 mg/min should provide a steady-state plasma concentration of 4 mg/L.

Example 11.8   A drug ($S = 1$) has the population average parameters $Cl = 10.3$ L/h and $Vd = 75$ L. The therapeutic range is 0.5–1.25 mg/L. An elderly patient is to be treated with the drug.

  (a) Calculate a suitable intravenous infusion rate to achieve a Cp_{ss} value of 1 mg/L.
  (b) What is the earliest time that a plasma sample could be withdrawn to ensure that the steady-state plasma concentration is on target?
  (c) Forty-eight hours after the start of an infusion of 10.3 mg/h, a plasma concentration is measured and found to be 1.5 mg/L. Suggest a more appropriate infusion regimen.

Solution

  (a) At this point, there is only information on the population average parameters. These will be used to estimate the initial infusion rate:

$$k = \frac{Cl}{Vd} = \frac{10.3}{75} = 0.1371 \text{ h}^{-1} \quad t_{1/2} = \frac{0.693}{0.137} = 5.05 \text{ h}$$

Rearrange equation (11.5) to solve for the infusion rate:

$$k_0 = \frac{Cl \cdot Cp_{ss}}{S \cdot F}$$
$$k_0 = \frac{10.3 \text{ L/h} \times 1\text{mg/L}}{1 \times 1} = 10.3 \text{ mg/h}$$

  (b) It will take about 15–25 h to get to steady state in a person with a normal half-life. An elderly patient may have an increased half-life, so it may take a little longer. Thus, it would be wise to wait until at least 24 h before checking.

  (c) The plasma concentration was obtained at 48 h, which is equivalent to approximately 10 (48/5) half-lives of the drug in a normal patient. It is therefore likely that steady state has been achieved at this time, even in a patient who has a reduced clearance and a correspondingly increased half-life. Thus, it can be assumed that in this patient, an infusion rate of 10.3 mg/h results in a steady-state plasma concentration of 1.5 mg/L. The patient's individual clearance can be calculated from these data:

$$Cl = \frac{S \cdot F \cdot k_0}{Cp_{ss}}$$
$$= \frac{10.3}{1.5} = 6.87 \text{ L/h}$$

The patient's half-life can be estimated using the population average Vd:

$$t_{1/2} = \frac{0.693 \times 75}{6.87} = 7.6 \text{ h}$$

In this patient, who has reduced clearance, the half-life is 7.6 h. It would be estimated to take 23–38 h to achieve steady state. So the plasma concentration sampled at 48 h would be expected to be in steady state.

The patient's clearance can be used to determine a more appropriate infusion rate to achieve the desired steady-state plasma concentration (1 mg/L):

$$k_0 = \frac{Cp_{ss} \cdot Cl}{S \cdot F}$$
$$= 1 \text{ mg/L} \times 6.87 \text{ L/h} = 6.87 \text{ mg/h}$$

PROBLEMS

11.1 A drug ($Cl = 100$ mL/min, $Vd = 0.7$ L/kg, and $S = 1$) is administered by intravenous infusion at a rate of 5 mg/h to a 70-kg man.

(a) Calculate the plasma concentration 6 h after the start of the infusion.

(b) What is the steady-state plasma concentration?

(c) Calculate the plasma concentration 4 h after termination when the infusion is terminated 3 h after the start.

(d) Calculate the plasma concentration 4 h after infusion is terminated 30 h after the start.

11.2 Vancomycin is administered as in IV infusion at a rate of 500 mg/h. The infusion is terminated after 1 h. A plasma concentration taken 2 h after the start of the infusion is 20 mg/L. A second plasma concentration taken 10 h after the start of the infusion is 7 mg/L. What is vancomycin's half-life in this patient?

11.3 A drug company has developed an elementary osmotic pump formulation of the hydrochloride salt ($S = 0.85$) of their β-blocker. The formulation, which is designed to be taken twice daily, contains 96 mg of drug which is released in zero-order fashion over a 12-h period. The entire dose is released and absorbed across the gastrointestinal membrane and undergoes no significant intestinal extraction. It is susceptible to first-pass hepatic extraction ($E = 0.8$). The drug has the following pharmacokinetic parameters: $Cl = 1080$ mL/min, $Vd = 250$ L, and $f_e < 0.01$. Calculate the steady-state plasma concentration achieved by this dosage form.

11.4 A 70-kg male patient with premature ventricular contractions is to receive treatment with lidocaine hydrochloride ($S = 0.87$). Calculate a loading dose and the rate of an intravenous infusion that would achieve a desired plasma concentration of 2 mg/L. Lidocaine has the following population average parameters: $Cl = 6$ mL/kg $\cdot$ min, $V_1 = 0.5$ L/kg, and $Vd_{ss} = 1.3$ L/kg.

11.5 Phenobarbital sodium ($S = 0.90$) is to be administered to a 70-kg male who is experiencing seizures as a result of head trauma. A desired steady-state plasma concentration of 30 mg/L is desired. Phenobarbital's clearance and volume of distribution are 0.1 L/kg/day and 0.7 L/kg, respectively.

(a) Use the infusion equations to determine an appropriate oral daily dose ($F = 1$).

(b) How long will it take to achieve, 50%, 90%, and 95% steady state.

(c) After 2 weeks, therapy is stopped and a second drug is to be administered which adversely interacts with phenobarbital. How long will it take to eliminate 90% and 95% of the phenobarbital in the body at the time therapy is stopped?

11.6 Recommend suitable rates for administration of the fictitious drugs lipoamide, nosolatol, and disolvprazole by intravenous infusion to target steady-state plasma concentrations of 50, 1250, and 400 μg/L, respectively. Their relevant pharmacokinetic parameters are summarized in Table P11.5.

TABLE P11.5 Summary of the Important Pharmacokinetic Parameters of Lipoamide, Nosolatol, and Disolvprazole

	Lipoamide	Nosolatol	Disolvprazole
Cl (L/h)	62	12.6	12
Vd (L/70 kg)	420	210	35
S	1	1	1

11.7 Theophylline is a broncodilator used in the treatment of bronchial asthma and other respiratory diseases. Chemically, it is a xanthene (1,3-dimethylxanthine) bearing a close structural similarity to caffeine (1,3,7-trimethylxanthine). About 6% of a dose of theophylline is metabolized to caffeine, which is subsequently metabolized to uric acid derivatives. Theophylline is eliminated primarily by metabolism ($fe = 0.1–0.2$). Owing to a wide interpatient variability in pharmacokinetic parameters of theophylline (particularly clearance), there is a wide interpatient variation in the blood levels achieved by a given dose. Furthermore, since theophylline has a very narrow therapeutic range (5–15 mg/L), a given dose may produce toxic plasma concentrations in some patients and subtherapeutic levels in others. Thus, it is frequently necessary to individualize a person's dose of theophylline. An initial estimate of theophylline's clearance in a patient can be obtained based on some demographic characteristics, such as the presence of certain diseases, concomitant medications, and age. This, in turn, allows an initial infusion rate to be estimated. However, since both the clearance and the infusion rate are only estimates, it is important that the steady-state plasma concentration be monitored and the infusion rate adjusted if necessary.

A.M. is an 80-kg, 5 foot 11 inch, 50-year-old male who is to be treated with theophylline for an asthmatic attack. Theophylline's clearance in A.M. is estimated to be 1.64 L/h based on his demographic features: severe obstructive pulmonary disease, congestive heart failure, and smoking a pack of cigarettes a day. The population average volume of distribution of theophylline is 0.5 L/kg.

(a) Advise on a suitable infusion rate of aminophylline ($S = 0.8$) to achieve a plasma concentration of 15 mg/L theophylline.

(b) Determine a suitable intravenous loading dose of aminophylline.

(c) What is the earliest time that a plasma sample can be taken to determine if the steady-state plasma concentration is in the therapeutic range?

(d) An infusion of 30.75 mg/h is used. A steady-state plasma sample is obtained and reveals a theophylline *Cp* value of 25 mg/L (A.M.'s clearance was only *estimated*). Recommend a more suitable infusion rate based on this information.

(e) Assume that the new infusion rate is used and that steady state is achieved. The infusion is terminated. How long would it take plasma concentrations to fall to 3.5 mg/L?

(f) Comment on how steady-state plasma concentrations of theophylline may be affected by:

(1) Compounds such as cimetidine and the quinolone antibiotics that inhibit theophylline's intrinsic clearance

(2) Compounds that alter hepatic blood flow

(3) Phenytoin, which induces theophylline's metabolism

11.8 Treat the patient described in the "Infusion Challenge", simulation model 8 (http://web.uri.edu/pharmacy/research/rosenbaum/sims), which can be found at http://web.uri.edu/pharmacy/research/rosenbaum/sims/Model8

12

MULTIPLE INTRAVENOUS BOLUS INJECTIONS IN THE ONE-COMPARTMENT MODEL

Sara E. Rosenbaum

Basic Pharmacokinetics and Pharmacodynamics: An Integrated Textbook and Computer Simulations,
Second Edition. Edited by Sara E. Rosenbaum.
© 2017 John Wiley & Sons, Inc. Published 2017 by John Wiley & Sons, Inc.

Objectives

The material presented in this chapter will enable the reader to:

1. Identify the characteristics of the plasma concentration profile after multiple intravenous doses
2. Understand the derivation of an expression for the plasma concentration at any time during therapy with multiple intravenous doses
3. Understand the factors controlling the average steady-state plasma concentration and the time to steady state
4. Understand the factors controlling fluctuation
5. Understand the factors controlling accumulation
6. Design dosage regimens based on pharmacokinetic principles

12.1 INTRODUCTION

In Chapter 11, we introduced the pharmacokinetics of continuous drug administration and demonstrated that once therapy begins, drug concentrations build up gradually until steady state is achieved. At steady state, plasma concentrations remain constant. The value of the steady-state plasma concentration is controlled by the rate of drug administration and the drug's clearance. The time it takes to get to steady state is dependent on the drug's half-life.

Most drugs are not administered in a constant and continuous fashion, but as multiple discrete doses. Generally, the dose is administered in a pulse-like fashion one, two, three, or four times daily. From the perspective of patient convenience—and by extension, adherence—once daily dosing is most desirable, followed in order of decreasing desirability by two, three, or four times daily. Most commonly, the goal of therapy is to achieve a sustained therapeutic response, and the choice of dosing frequency is dependent on the drug's pharmacokinetic and pharmacodynamic properties. The pharmacokinetics of multiple intravenous doses are presented in this chapter. Although the oral route is most frequently used for multiple-dose administration, the pharmacokinetics of this route are complicated by the absorption process. Consequently, the characteristics of multiple-dose pharmacokinetics are initially studied most conveniently by removing the absorption process and considering intravenous doses.

The typical plasma concentration–time profile observed after multiple intravenous doses is shown in Figure 12.1. The units of time are the drug's elimination half-life, which is also the dosing interval or frequency of drug administration. The profile has some notable characteristics:

- *Fluctuation.* The profile appears as a series of peaks and troughs, known as fluctuation. The peaks occur at the time a dose is given, and the troughs occur immediately before the next dose.
- *Accumulation.* It can be seen in Figure 12.1 that the troughs and peaks increase with each dose, known as accumulation. This occurs when a dose is given at a time when drug from a previous dose is still in the body. Note that there is less accumulation with each successive dose.
- *Steady state.* Eventually, accumulation between doses stops altogether. At this time, the peaks and troughs with successive doses are the same; that is, steady state has been achieved.

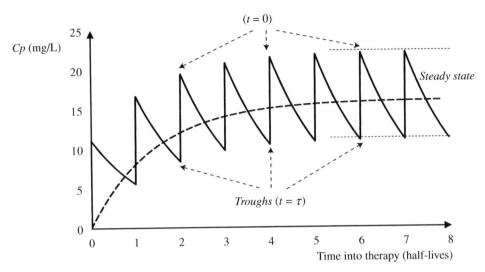

FIGURE 12.1 Plasma concentration–time profile observed with multiple intravenous injections (solid line) in a one-compartment model. The data were simulated using the following parameters: dose = 64 mg, $Cl = 4$ L/$t_{1/2}$, $Vd = 5.77$ L, and the dosing interval (τ) = 1 $t_{1/2}$ Fluctuation is observed in the profile. A peak occurs at the time a dose is given ($t = 0$), and a trough occurs immediately before the next dose ($t = \tau$). Note that the value of the peaks and troughs increases with each successive dose. This is because of accumulation. The amount of accumulation gets smaller and smaller with each dose. At steady state, there is no further accumulation. The steady-state peaks and troughs are exactly the same. It takes about five half-lives to reach steady state. The average plasma concentration (dashed line) has the same profile as that of a continuous intravenous infusion.

- *Average Cp*. Note that the average plasma concentration throughout therapy (indicated by the dashed line in Figure 12.1) has the same shape as the plasma concentration–time profile of a continuous constant infusion.

The goal of drug therapy is to devise a dosing regimen that will maintain therapeutic steady-state plasma concentrations. A multiple-dosing regimen consists of two parts: (1) the dose and (2) the dosing interval, or the frequency with which the doses are repeated. For example, in Chapter 11, it was found that a constant continuous infusion of 3.1 mg/h of the fictitious drug lipoamide would provide a therapeutic plasma concentration of 50 µg/L (see Problem 11.5). It has been found that plasma concentrations of lipoamide greater than 90 µg/L are associated with a high frequency of side effects. Plasma concentrations below 25 µg/L are subtherapeutic. If multiple discrete doses of lipoamide are to be given, what dose and what dosing interval should be used to ensure that plasma concentrations are therapeutic and nontoxic at all times? The material presented in this chapter is directed at answering this question.

12.2 TERMS AND SYMBOLS USED IN MULTIPLE-DOSING EQUATIONS

The formulas for multiple-dosing pharmacokinetics introduce some new symbols. These are shown in Figure 12.2 and described below.

- n is the number of the last dose administered.
- τ (the lowercase Greek letter tau) is the dosing interval. If 50 mg is administered every 8 h, τ is 8 h.

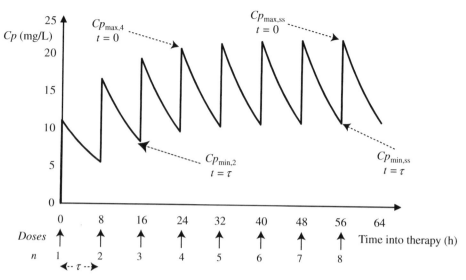

FIGURE 12.2   Symbols used in multiple-dose pharmacokinetics. In this example, the dose is administered every 8 h. n is the number of the last dose administered, τ is the dosing interval (8 h), and t is the time since the last dose (in this regimen, t will vary continuously from 0 through 8 h). $Cp_{\min,n}$ and $Cp_{\min,ss}$ are the trough plasma concentrations ($t = \tau$) before and after steady state, respectively; $Cp_{\max,n}$ and $Cp_{\max,ss}$ are the peak plasma concentrations ($t = 0$) before and after steady state, respectively.

- t is the time since the last dose. During therapy, t varies continuously from 0 at the beginning of a dosing interval to τ at the end. When the next dose is given, t once more becomes 0.

- Time into therapy can be calculated from the product of $n \cdot \tau$. Specifically, time into therapy $= [(n - 1) \cdot \tau] + t$. For example, let $\tau = 12$; then:

  3 h after the first dose, $t = (0 \times 12) + 3 = 3$ h

  3 h after the second dose, $t = (1 \times 12) + 3 = 15$ h

  At the end of the fourth dosing interval, $t = (3 \times 12) + 12 = 48$ h

  6 h after the tenth dose, $t = (9 \times 12) + 6 = 114$ h

- Peak plasma concentrations, which occur when $t = 0$, have the symbol $Cp_{\max}$. Before steady state, $Cp_{\max}$ is dependent on the number of the last dose, so it has the symbol $Cp_{\max,n}$. After steady state, the peak is independent of the number of the last dose and has the symbol $Cp_{\max,ss}$.

- Trough plasma concentrations, which occur when $t = \tau$, have the symbol $Cp_{\min}$. Before steady state, $Cp_{\min}$ is dependent on the number of the last dose and has the symbol, $Cp_{\min,n}$. After steady state, the peak is independent of the number of the last dose and has the symbol $Cp_{\min,ss}$.

- The symbols, Cp_n and Cp_{ss}, are used to represent the plasma concentration at any other time during a nonsteady state and a steady-state dosing interval, respectively.

The derivation of the equations for multiple doses involves a number of assumptions, which include:

1. With the possible exception of the first dose (loading dose), the dose and the dosing interval are constant throughout the duration of therapy. The dose may be referred to as the maintenance dose.

2. The drug's pharmacokinetic parameters remain constant throughout the entire duration of therapy. This assumes that the drug displays linear pharmacokinetics.

Thus, these equations can only be applied to situations where the assumptions hold. For example, the equations should not be used for drugs that display nonlinear pharmacokinetics, such as phenytoin (Chapter 15).

12.3 MONOEXPONENTIAL DECAY DURING A DOSING INTERVAL

When a dose is administered, it is assumed that the entire dose enters the systemic circulation at time zero, even though in reality an injection may be given gradually over a period of 1 min or more. For the one-compartment model, the drug is assumed to distribute in a rapid, essentially instantaneous manner. Thus, the peak plasma concentration is assumed to occur at time zero. During a dosing interval, t increases from zero at the time of the dose up to its maximum value of τ just before the next dose. During this period, the plasma concentration is under the influence of only one process: first-order elimination (Figure 12.3). During a dosing interval, the plasma concentration decays monoexponentially from the peak (Cp_{max}) to the trough (Cp_{min}).

Before steady state, during a dosing interval,

$$Cp_n = Cp_{max,n} \cdot e^{-kt} \tag{12.1}$$

and at the trough,

$$Cp_{min,n} = Cp_{max,n} \cdot e^{-k\tau} \tag{12.2}$$

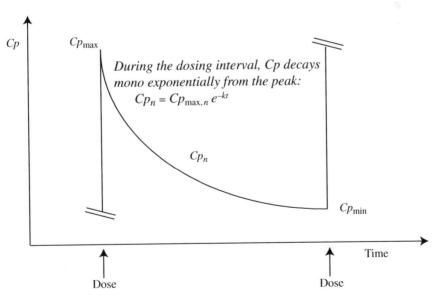

FIGURE 12.3 Monoexponential decay during a dosing interval. During a dosing interval, plasma concentrations are influenced only by first-order elimination. As a result, they decay monoexponentially from the peak. The first-order decay equation can be used to express the plasma concentration during the interval as a function of the peak concentration and the time after the dose.

At steady state, during a dosing interval,

$$Cp_{ss} = Cp_{max,ss} \cdot e^{-kt} \tag{12.3}$$

and at the trough,

$$Cp_{min,ss} = Cp_{max,ss} \cdot e^{-k\tau} \tag{12.4}$$

This basic relationship between the plasma concentration and time during a dosing interval permits the simple derivation of an important equation that is used to calculate dosing intervals needed to achieve certain peak and trough plasma concentrations.

12.3.1   Calculation of Dosing Interval to Give Specific Steady-State Peaks and Troughs

Knowing that the fall in the plasma concentration between doses is simple monoexponential decay makes it possible to calculate the value of a dosing interval to give specific peaks and troughs. This is best addressed through an example.

Example 12.1   Assume that a new drug is under development. It has a very narrow therapeutic range (12–25 mg/L). However, since it is being used to treat a serious life-threatening condition for which few other treatments are available, development of this drug is being pursued. The goal is to design a dosing regimen that will result in a steady-state peak and trough of 20 and 14 mg/L, respectively. The drug's elimination rate constant has a population average value of 0.043 h^{-1}. What dosing interval is needed to provide the desired steady-state peaks and troughs?

Solution   The relationship between the steady-state peak and trough is given in equation (12.4). Substituting the desired steady-state trough and peak into this equation gives us

$$14 = 20e^{-0.043\tau}$$
$$\ln \frac{14}{20} = -0.043\tau$$
$$\tau = \frac{0.357}{0.043} = 8.3\,\text{h}$$

A more useful arrangement of equation (12.4) for use in calculating a dosing interval is

$$\boxed{\tau = -\frac{1}{k} \ln \frac{Cp_{min,ss}}{Cp_{max,ss}}} \tag{12.5}$$

The box around equation (12.5) indicates that it is an important equation that is frequently used clinically.

12.4   BASIC PHARMACOKINETIC EQUATIONS FOR MULTIPLE DOSES

12.4.1   Principle of Superposition

When a dose of a drug is administered at a time when drug from a previous dose(s) is still in the body, it is assumed that the total amount of drug in the body is equal to the

TABLE 12.1   Maximum (Ab_{max}) and Minimum (Ab_{min}) Amounts of Drug in the Body and Accumulation After Successive Doses of 64 mg are Given Every Half-Life

Dose	AB_{max} (mg)	AB_{min} (mg)	Accumulation Between Peaks
1	64	32	
2	96	48	32
3	112	56	16
4	120	60	8
5	124	62	4
6	126	63	2
7	127	63.5	1
$\vdots$			
Steady state			
N	128	64	0
$N+1$	128	64	0

amount provided by the new dose, plus the drug remaining from previous dose(s). This is known as the *principle of superposition*. This is illustrated in Table 12.1 for a drug that is administered as a 64-mg dose every half-life. At the end of the first dosing interval, half (32 mg) of the first dose remains. So the peak amount after the second dose is the dose (64 mg) plus that remaining from the first dose (32 mg), or 96 mg. The same process can be used to calculate the next trough amount and the peaks and troughs after successive doses as shown in Table 12.1. Note that after the first dose, the body accumulates 32 mg, but with each successive dose the amount of accumulation between doses decreases. For example, in Table 12.1, it can be seen that only 2 mg is accumulated between the fifth and sixth doses. Eventually, no further accumulation occurs, and steady state is achieved. At steady state, an entire dose (64 mg) is lost during a dosing interval, only to be replaced exactly by the next dose.

12.4.2 Equations that Apply Before Steady State

The equations for multiple intravenous bolus injections are derived using exactly the same process as that described above; the full derivation appears in Appendix D. The basic equation that can be used to determine the plasma concentration at any time during multiple-dose therapy is

$$Cp_n = \frac{S \cdot F \cdot D \cdot (1 - e^{-nk\tau})}{Vd \cdot (1 - e^{-k\tau})} \cdot e^{-kt} \qquad (12.6)$$

Recall that t is the time that has elapsed since the last dose, n is the number of the last dose, and τ is the dosing interval. When $t = 0$, a peak plasma concentration is observed:

$$Cp_{n,max} = \frac{S \cdot F \cdot D \cdot (1 - e^{-nk\tau})}{Vd \cdot (1 - e^{-k\tau})} \qquad (12.7)$$

When $t = \tau$, a trough is observed:

$$Cp_{n,min} = \frac{S \cdot F \cdot D \cdot (1 - e^{-nk\tau})}{Vd \cdot (1 - e^{-k\tau})} \cdot e^{-k\tau} \qquad (12.8)$$

Alternatively, the trough may be expressed as:

$$Cp_{n,min} = Cp_{n,max} \cdot e^{-k\tau} \tag{12.9}$$

Example 12.2 Multiple intravenous bolus injections (250 mg) of a drug are administered every 8 h. The drug has the following parameters: $S = 1$, $Vd = 30$ L, $k = 0.1$ h^{-1}, and $\tau = 8$ h. Calculate:

(a) The plasma concentration 3 h after the second dose.
(b) The peak and trough plasma concentrations during this second dosing interval.

Solution

(a) Substituting into equation (12.6) yields

$$Cp_n = \frac{250(1 - e^{-2\times0.1\times8})}{30(1 - e^{-0.1\times8})} \cdot e^{-0.1\times3}$$
$$= 8.96 \, \text{mg/L}$$

(b) $Cp_{max,2}$ can be calculated when $t = 0$ [equation (12.7)]:

$$Cp_{max,2} = \frac{250(1 - e^{-2\times0.1\times8})}{30(1 - e^{-0.1\times8})}$$
$$= 12.1 \, \text{mg/L}$$

$Cp_{min,2}$ can be determined when $t = \tau$ [equation (12.8) or (12.9)]. Using the latter yields

$$Cp_{min,2} = 12.1e^{-0.1\times8}$$
$$= 5.4 \, \text{mg/L}$$

During the second dosing interval, the plasma concentrations at the peak, 3 h into the dosing interval, and at the trough are 12.1, 8.96, and 5.4 mg/L, respectively.

12.5 STEADY STATE

Usually, steady state is the focus of drug therapy and the goal is to achieve steady-state plasma concentrations that are in the therapeutic range. Consequently, the equations associated with steady state are very important and are more commonly used clinically than the equations that apply prior to steady state. The specific aspects of steady state that are of most interest are the determinants of:

- The steady-state peak and trough plasma concentrations.
- The average plasma concentration during a steady-state dosing interval.
- The factors that control the amount of fluctuation observed at steady state ($Cp_{max,ss}$ versus $Cp_{min,ss}$).
- The degree of accumulation that ultimately occurs at steady state.
- The time to reach steady state.

12.5.1 Steady-State Equations

At steady state, the plasma concentration–time profile is exactly the same for all dosing intervals (i.e., the plasma concentrations become independent of n, the number of the last dose). Recall the basic equation that applies before steady state:

$$Cp_n = \frac{S \cdot F \cdot D \cdot (1 - e^{-nk\tau})}{Vd \cdot (1 - e^{-k\tau})} \cdot e^{-kt} \tag{12.10}$$

During therapy, n increases with each successive dose. As a result, as therapy progresses and steady state is approached, $e^{-nk\tau}$ tends to zero, and $1 - e^{-nk\tau}$ becomes 1 and disappears from the equation. Thus, the basic equation for steady state is expressed as:

$$Cp_n = \frac{S \cdot F \cdot D}{Vd \cdot (1 - e^{-k\tau})} \cdot e^{-kt} \tag{12.11}$$

The corresponding equation for the peak and trough may be expressed by letting $t = 0$ and τ, respectively:

$$Cp_{\max,\,ss} = \frac{S \cdot F \cdot D}{Vd \cdot (1 - e^{-k\tau})} \tag{12.12}$$

$$Cp_{\min,ss} = \frac{S \cdot F \cdot D}{Vd \cdot (1 - e^{-k\tau})} \cdot e^{-k\tau} \tag{12.13}$$

or

$$Cp_{\min,ss} = Cp_{\max,ss} \cdot e^{-k\tau} \tag{12.14}$$

Example 12.3   Next continuing with our example of a drug ($Vd = 30$ L, $k = 0.1$ h^{-1}) that is administered intravenously as a 250 mg dose every 8 h. Recall that after the second dose,

$$Cp_{\max} = 12.1 \, \text{mg/L}$$
$$Cp_{3h} = 8.96 \, \text{mg/L}$$
$$Cp_{\min} = 5.4 \, \text{mg/L}$$

Calculate the maximum and minimum steady-state plasma concentrations achieved by the regimen.

Solution

$$Cp_{\max,ss} = \frac{250}{30(1 - e^{-0.1\times8})} = 15.1 \, \text{mg/L}$$

$$Cp_{\min,ss} = \frac{250}{30(1 - e^{-0.1\times8})} \cdot e^{-0.1\times8} = 6.8 \, \text{mg/L}$$

The steady-state peaks and troughs are 15.1 and 8.8 mg/L, respectively.

These equations can also be used in the reverse direction to determine a dose to produce a desired steady-state peak and/or trough.

Example 12.4 Recall that it was determined earlier (Example 12.1) that a dosing interval of 8.3 h (approximately 8 h) was needed for a drug ($Vd = 50$ L, $k = 0.043$ h^{-1}) to achieve steady-state troughs and peaks of 14 and 20 mg/L, respectively. What dose should be used?

Solution Either the formula for $Cp_{max,ss}$ or that for $Cp_{min,ss}$ can be used. The only unknown in either case is the dose:

$$Cp_{max,ss} = \frac{S \cdot F \cdot D}{Vd \cdot (1 - e^{-k\tau})} \quad \text{where} \quad Cp_{max,ss} = 20\,\text{mg/L}$$

or

$$Cp_{min,ss} = \frac{S \cdot F \cdot D}{Vd \cdot (1 - e^{-k\tau})} \cdot e^{-k\tau} \quad \text{where} \quad Cp_{min,ss} = 14\,\text{mg/L}$$

Using the $Cp_{max,ss}$ of 20 mg/L and assuming that $S = 1$, $F = 1$,

$$20 = \frac{S \cdot F \cdot D}{50(1 - e^{-0.043 \times 8})}$$
$$D = 290\,\text{mg}$$

The intravenous injection of 290 mg of this drug every 8 h should result in a steady-state peak and trough of 20 and 14 mg/L, respectively.

12.5.2 Average Plasma Concentration at Steady State

Frequently, rather than concentrating on the peaks and troughs, the emphasis of multiple-dosing therapy is to achieve a desired therapeutic average steady-state plasma concentration. For example, digoxin has a very long half-life, and plasma concentrations remain fairly consistent during a dosing interval. It is often necessary to determine the dose needed to achieve an average plasma concentration of 1 μg/L. It would be useful to have an expression that relates the average steady-state plasma concentration to the dose and dosing interval.

Because the fall in Cp during a dosing interval is monoexponential and not linear, the average steady-state plasma concentration is not the arithmetic mean of the troughs and peaks [$(Cp_{max,ss} + Cp_{min,ss})/2$]. In Figure 12.4, it can be seen that the arithmetic mean of the peak and the trough is not representative of the average concentration during the dosing interval. The plasma concentration is above this value for a much shorter time than it is below it. The average plasma concentration during the interval is calculated as the area under the steady-state dosing interval divided by the dosing interval:

$$Cp_{av,ss} = \frac{\int_0^T Cp \cdot dt}{\tau} = \frac{\text{AUC}_0^\tau}{\tau} \tag{12.15}$$

$\text{AUC}_0^\tau = S \cdot F \cdot D/Cl.$

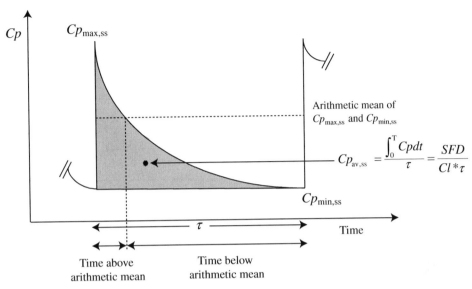

FIGURE 12.4 Average steady-state plasma concentration. Plasma concentrations fall monoexponentially during a dosing interval. As a result, the arithmetic mean of the peak and trough is not representative of the average plasma concentration. The average steady state plasma concentration is the area under the curve during a steady-state dosing interval divided by τ.

Note that the AUC during a steady-state dosing interval is the same as the AUC from zero to infinity after a single dose. Substituting for AUC_0^{τ} into equation (12.15) yields

$$Cp_{\text{av, ss}} = \frac{S \cdot F \cdot D}{Cl \cdot \tau} \tag{12.16}$$

It can be observed by rearranging formula (12.16) that the average steady-state plasma concentration occurs at the time when the rate of drug administration $(S \cdot F \cdot D/\tau)$ is equal to the rate of drug elimination $(Cp \cdot Cl)$.

Note that D/T represents the average rate of drug administration over the dosing interval (e.g., 160 mg every 8 h represents an average of 20 mg/h). Equation (12.16) can also be written using R_a:

$$Cp_{\text{av, ss}} = \frac{S \cdot F \cdot R_a}{Cl} \tag{12.17}$$

where $R_a = D/\tau$ and represents the average rate of drug administration.

If equation (12.17) is compared to the equation for the steady-state plasma concentration that results from a constant, continuous infusion (12.18), it can be seen that they are equivalent:

$$Cp_{\text{ss}} = \frac{S \cdot F \cdot k_0}{Cl} \tag{12.18}$$

A general equation for chronic drug administration may be written as equation (12.17), where R_a may be either a continuous constant administration rate (as for an infusion) or an average rate of administration (D/τ) achieved by individual discrete doses during multiple-dose therapy:

$$Cp_{ss} = \frac{S \cdot F \cdot R_a}{Cl} \qquad (12.19)$$

Some important points were made from a consideration of this equation in Chapter 11. Owing to the importance of these points, they will be reiterated here. When a drug is administered over an extended period, either at a constant continuous rate or as individual discrete doses, the average steady-state plasma concentration is:

1. Directly proportional to the effective rate of drug administration, $S \cdot F \cdot R_a$ (this is a characteristic of linear pharmacokinetics)
2. Inversely proportional to clearance
3. Independent of the volume of distribution

Equation (12.19) also provides a handle to use to calculate dosing regimens to achieve the desired steady-state plasma concentrations. It is very frequently used clinically for this purpose.

Example 12.5   Doses of digoxin are usually administered every 24 h. Calculate an appropriate dose of digoxin to achieve a concentration of 1 μg/L in a patient whose digoxin clearance is estimated to be 123 L/day.

Solution   Substituting into equation (12.19), assuming intravenous doses $(F = 1)$ and $S = 1$, we obtain

$$1\,\mu g/L = \frac{R_a}{123\,\text{L/day}}$$
$$R_a = 123\ \mu g/\text{day}$$

A daily dose of 123 μg, rounded to 125 μg, is recommended.

Example 12.6   An average steady-state plasma concentration of 50 μg/L is required from the administration of multiple intravenous bolus injections of the fictitious drug lipoamide. $Vd = 420$ L and $Cl = 62$ L/h. What rate of drug administration should be used?

Solution   Substituting into equation (12.19) and rearranging yield

$$R_a = \frac{62\,\text{L/h} \times 50\,\mu g/L}{1 \times 1} = 3.1\,\text{mg/h}$$

Any combination of dose and τ that gives a rate of administration of 3.1 mg/h will achieve an average steady-state plasma concentration of 50 μg/L. The following regimens could be used:

3.1 mg/h—infusion	no fluctuation
3.1 mg every hour	little fluctuation
24.8 mg every 8 h	more fluctuation
37.2 mg every 12 h	even greater fluctuation
74.4 mg every 24 h	large amount of fluctuation

12.5.3 Fluctuation

Fluctuation refers to the difference between the peak and the trough plasma concentrations within a dosing interval. As such, it reflects the amount of drug that is eliminated during a dosing interval. As the amount eliminated increases, the amount of fluctuation will increase. The amount of elimination during a dosing interval is dependent on a drug's rate of elimination ($t_{1/2}$ or k) and the length of the dosing interval.

Elimination, and by extension fluctuation, will obviously be greatest when the dosing interval is long and the drug's $t_{1/2}$ short. This can be shown mathematically by considering the ratio of $Cp_{max,ss}$ to $Cp_{min,ss}$ [see equation (12.14)]:

$$\frac{Cp_{max,ss}}{Cp_{min,ss}} = \frac{1}{e^{-k\tau}} \tag{12.20}$$

The value of the ratio is a measure of fluctuation, and equation (12.20) demonstrates that it is dependent only on k (or the half-life) and τ. The value of $e^{-k\tau}$ will be smallest, and the fluctuation greatest, when τ and k are large ($t_{1/2}$ short). Thus, short half-lives and long dosing intervals promote large fluctuation. Conversely, long half-lives and short dosing intervals promote little fluctuation. Since the half-life is a constant for a given drug (assuming normal conditions and health), the length of the dosing interval controls fluctuation.

12.5.4 Accumulation

Accumulation is the increase in drug concentrations that occur with each additional dose (Figure 12.1). It occurs whenever a dose is given when drug from a previous dose is still in the body. With each successive dose, the accumulation between doses decreases more and more and eventually stops altogether when steady state is achieved. The ultimate amount of accumulation that occurs at steady state can be quantified by comparing a steady-state plasma concentration to the equivalent concentration after the first dose. For example, the steady-state peak could be compared to the peak after the first dose, the troughs could be compared, the average plasma concentrations during the intervals could be compared, and so on (Figure 12.5). The ratio of these values is known as the *accumulation ratio, r*:

$$r = \frac{Cp_{ss}}{Cp_1} \quad \text{at equivalent times in the dosing interval} \tag{12.21}$$

Comparing the peaks gives us

$$r = \frac{Cp_{max,ss}}{Cp_{max,1}} = \frac{(S \cdot F \cdot D/Vd) \cdot 1//(1 - e^{-k\tau})}{S \cdot F \cdot D/Vd} \tag{12.22}$$

$$r = \frac{1}{1 - e^{-k\tau}} \tag{12.23}$$

Note the expression for r demonstrates that, like fluctuation, accumulation is controlled by the elimination half-life and the dosing interval. But accumulation and fluctuation run counter to each other. If little drug is eliminated during a dosing interval (small τ and long $t_{1/2}$), fluctuation will be small, but the buildup of drug from one dose to the next will be large, and accumulation will be large.

r = ratio of Cp at steady state to Cp at same time after the first a dose

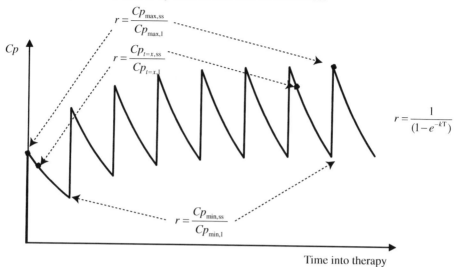

FIGURE 12.5   Assessment of accumulation. Accumulation can be assessed using the accumulation ratio (r), which is the ratio of a plasma concentration at steady state and the equivalent concentration after the first dose.

Example. Let $t_{1/2}$ = 12 h and tau = 12 h.

$$r = \frac{1}{1 - e^{-0.693/12*12}} = 2$$

This demonstrates that when a drug is administered every half-life, the plasma concentration at any time during multiple-dosing therapy will be twice the value of the equivalent Cp after the same single dose.

If tau was changed to 6 h: r = 3.4: Steady-state plasma concentrations would be 3.4 times greater than the equivalent after a single dose.

If tau was changed to 24 h: r = 1.3. This regimen, with a long dosing interval would be associated with large fluctuation but small accumulation. Steady-state plasma concentrations would only be 1.3 times greater than the equivalent after a single dose

The accumulation ratio can also be calculated from observed data if there is some uncertainty associated with the estimate of a drug's elimination rate constant or half-life. This method involves comparing plasma concentrations measured at the same time after a single dose, and after a dose at steady state, for example, ($Cp_{max,ss}/Cp_{max,1}$). A discrepancy between values calculated by both methods can be indicative of a poorly estimated half-life.

Accumulation can also be expressed by comparing the average amount of drug in the body at steady state ($Ab_{av,ss}$) to the dose:

$$\frac{Ab_{as,ss}}{S \cdot F \cdot D} = \frac{C_{av,ss} \cdot Vd}{S \cdot F \cdot D} = \frac{(S \cdot F \cdot D/Cl \cdot \tau) \cdot Vd}{S \cdot F \cdot D} \tag{12.24}$$

Given that $t_{1/2} = 0.693 Vd/Cl$,

$$\frac{Ab_{av,ss}}{S \cdot F \cdot D} = 1.44 \frac{t_{1/2}}{\tau} \tag{12.25}$$

Like equation (12.23), equation (12.25) demonstrates that accumulation is controlled by the elimination half-life and the dosing interval.

Example. Let $t_{1/2} = 12$ h and tau $= 12$ h.

$$\text{Accumulation can be expressed } \frac{Ab_{av,ss}}{S \cdot F \cdot D} = 1.44 \frac{12}{12} = 1.44$$

When a drug is administered every half-life, the average amount of drug in the body at steady state is 1.44 times the value of the dose.

If tau was changed to 6 h, the average amount of drug in the body at steady state would be 2.88 times the value of the dose.

If tau was changed to 24 h, the average amount of drug in the body at steady state would be 0.72 times the value of the dose. This latter regimen would be associated with large fluctuation and minimal accumulation.

In summary, the plasma concentration during a steady-state dosing interval is r times higher than the corresponding plasma concentration after a single dose [equations (12.21) and (12.23)]. Accumulation will be most apparent when the dosing interval is short and the drug's half-life long. If a drug is administered every half-life, on average the amount of drug in the body at steady state will be 1.44 times greater than the value of the dose [equation (12.25)].

Clinically, accumulation may become an important consideration in patients who have impaired clearance, which in turn will result in an increased half-life. If the normal dosing interval is used in these patients, a greater degree of accumulation will occur. If the drug has a narrow therapeutic range, this accumulation may be associated with toxicity. For example, the elimination half-life of methadone, which is being used increasingly to treat severe pain, displays wide variability in the population. It has been found that the accumulation of the drug in patients with long half-lives can cause accumulation and potentially life-threatening toxicity. Accumulation is also a problem with environmental pollutants that have long half-lives. Continuous exposure to only small amounts of these compounds can result in their significant buildup in the body.

12.5.5 Time to Reach Steady State

Recall that $n \cdot \tau$ represents time into therapy. As n increases with each dose, $1 - e^{-nk\tau}$ gets closer and closer to 1. When $1 - e^{-nk\tau}$ reaches 1, steady state is achieved and the plasma concentration does not increase further with each dose. If an equation that applies before steady state is compared to the equivalent steady-state equation [e.g., compare $Cp_{max,n}$ in equation (12.7) to $Cp_{max,ss}$ in equation (12.12)], it can be observed that the equation before steady state can be expressed as:

$$Cp_{max,n} = Cp_{max,ss} \cdot (1 - e^{-nk\tau}) \tag{12.26}$$

Thus, $1 - e^{-nk\tau}$ represents the fraction of steady state achieved at any time:

$$\text{fraction of steady state} = 1 - e^{-nk\tau} \tag{12.27}$$

In common with intravenous infusions, the time $n \cdot \tau$ to achieve steady state is dependent only on k or $t_{1/2}$. The number of half-lives necessary to achieve a certain fraction of steady state is shown in Table 12.2. Clinically, it is usually considered to take 3–5 half-lives to achieve steady state.

TABLE 12.2 Fraction of Steady State Achieved at Various Times in Terms of Half-Life

Time Into Therapy ($t_{1/2}$)	Fraction of Steady State (%)
1	50
3.3	90
4.4	95
6.6	99

12.5.6 Loading Dose

If it is necessary to achieve steady-state plasma concentrations immediately, a loading dose may be administered. The purpose of the loading dose is to provide all the drug that ultimately accumulates at steady state in an initial single dose. At steady state, there is r times more drug in the body than after a single dose. Thus, the loading dose will need to be r times greater than the usual maintenance dose.

$$D_L = r \cdot D_M$$

$$\boxed{D_L = \frac{D_M}{1 - e^{-k\tau}}}$$

(12.28)

Note that if a drug is administered every half-life, the loading dose is double the maintenance dose.

12.6 BASIC FORMULA REVISITED

The phenomenon of accumulation differentiates single and multiple doses. During the course of this chapter, expressions have been presented to describe:

- The ultimate amount of accumulation that occurs at steady state
- The fraction of steady state achieved at any time during therapy

These expressions for accumulation (Figure 12.6) can be used to construct the basic equation for multiple doses. Figure 12.6 shows that the plasma concentration at any time after a dose during multiple doses is equal to:

- the plasma concentration at the same time after a single dose, multiplied by
- the fraction of steady state achieved at this point in the therapy, multiplied by
- the ultimate accumulation that occurs at steady state

Breaking down the basic equation in this way should help demystify the equation and promote better understanding.

12.7 PHARMACOKINETIC-GUIDED DOSING REGIMEN DESIGN

12.7.1 General Considerations for Selection of the Dosing Interval

Dosing regimens must be determined for new drugs as they progress through the development process. Clinically, dosing regimens may be determined for established drugs in

| Cp Multiple doses | = | Cp Single dose | * | Fraction of steady state achieved at any time | * | Ultimate accumulation at steady state |

| Cp Multiple doses | = | $Cp = \dfrac{SFD}{Vd}e^{-kt}$ | * | $(1 - e^{-nk\tau})$ | * | $r = \dfrac{1}{(1 - e^{-k\tau})}$ |

FIGURE 12.6   Component parts of the multiple-dosing equation. The basic equation for multiple doses consists of three parts: the equation for a single dose, the fraction of steady state achieved at any time, and the ultimate accumulation that occurs at steady state.

individual patients if it is thought that the patient may experience suboptimal concentrations from a standard dose. The dose is chosen to achieve therapeutic concentrations that produce minimal side effects or toxicity. The specific value of the dose is based on a drug's pharmacokinetic and pharmacodynamic properties. The value of the dosing interval is selected to ensure that the therapeutic response is maintained between doses. In many cases, a drug's pharmacokinetic properties, specifically the elimination half-life, dictate the value of the dosing interval. However, as will be demonstrated in subsequent chapters, a drug's pharmacodynamic properties can affect, and in some cases control, the optimum dosing interval.

Once-daily dosing, which is associated with the greatest patient convenience and adherence, is generally regarded as the preferred dosing interval. However, if a drug has a short elimination half-life, daily dosing may result in excessive fluctuation, which may be associated with toxic and/or subtherapeutic plasma concentrations. As a result, dosing intervals of 12, 8, or 6 h may have to be used.

Many therapeutic drugs have half-lives within the range 24–8 h, and they are frequently administered approximately every half-life. As a result, plasma concentrations will fall by about 50% during a dosing interval, the trough will be about half the peak, and the loading dose will be about twice the maintenance dose. For drugs that have short half-lives (6 h or less), from a perspective of patient convenience, it is desirable to use a dosing interval greater than the half-life. But this will result in a large fluctuation, and the therapeutic range will dictate whether or not the fluctuation will be tolerated. If the range is wide, such as for the penicllins, large fluctuations in the plasma concentrations will be tolerated, and dosing intervals of several half-lives can be used. If, however, a drug's therapeutic range is narrow, it may not be possible to use a dosing interval greater than the half-life. For example, theophylline has a very narrow therapeutic range (5–15 mg/L), and it also has a short half-life. As a result, short dosing intervals may be necessary. For example, the elimination half-life in smokers and in children can be less than 6 h, and the regular or rapid release preparations of theophylline may have to be administered every 6 h.

The inconvenience of short dosing intervals usually results in the development of prolonged-release preparations. Several of these are available for theophylline, and they can be administered twice daily to patients who have very short half-lives and once daily in other patients. A very short half-life may limit the marketability of a drug if it is dosed on pharmacokinetics principles. It is interesting to note that several therapeutic drugs that have very short half-lives have long dosing intervals because their pharmacodynamic properties, not their pharmacokinetics, control the dosing interval. For example, both aspirin (antiplatelet action) and proton pump inhibitors such as omeprazole have very short half-lives (<1 h), and both are eliminated from the body within a few hours of the dose. But both act by irreversibly destroying their target receptor. So, their duration of action is dependent not on their continued presence in the body but on the regeneration or synthesis of their target receptor. For both drugs, this takes over 24 h so that both can be administered daily.

In theory, extended dosing intervals of greater than 24 h could be used for drugs that have very long half-lives (greater than 24 h). However, for patient adherence, dosing intervals are frequently limited to 24 h. For example, phenobarbital ($t_{1/2} \sim 5$ days) and digoxin ($t_{1/2} \sim 2$ days) are both given daily. Weekly or monthly dosing may be used for a small number of drugs that have very long half-lives. For example, the antimalarial drug chloroquine ($t_{1/2} = 10$–24 days) is administered weekly, and alendronate, which binds to bone, from which it is released only very slowly ($t_{1/2} \sim 10$ years), is also administered weekly. If a drug has a long half-life, it will take a long time to reach steady state and a loading dose may be necessary. The long half-lives will produce a large accumulation, which will require loading doses that are much greater than the maintenance doses.

12.7.2 Protocols for Pharmacokinetic-Guided Dosing Regimens

Clinically, it may be necessary to apply pharmacokinetic principles to determine dosing regimens for individual patients when one or more of the following criteria are met:

1. A drug has a narrow therapeutic range, and plasma concentrations are outside the range are associated with serious clinical consequences.
2. A drug displays wide interpatient variability in its pharmacokinetic parameters.
3. A patient possesses a characteristic that is frequently associated with altered pharmacokinetics. This may include renal disease, hepatic disease, altered activity of the drug metabolizing enzymes or transporters as a result of genetic polymorphism or concomitant medications.

Drugs that are commonly subject to pharmacokinetic-based dosage individualization include aminoglycosides, phenytoin, lithium, immunosuppressants, and digoxin. Warfarin is also a very important example of a drug whose dose must be individualized for each patient. However, since the response to warfarin is easily measured (clotting time or international normalized ratio), dosage adjustments to warfarin are based on the response itself rather than on plasma concentrations and pharmacokinetics.

Several approaches are available to determine dosing regimens based on pharmacokinetic principles. The most appropriate approach will depend on the goal of the therapy. Two approaches are presented below. In protocol I, the goal of the therapy is to produce a desired average steady-state plasma concentration. In protocol II, the regimen is based on the attainment of specific desired peaks and troughs.

12.7.2.1 Protocol I: Targeting the Average Steady-State Plasma Concentration

Step 1.

Note the drug's therapeutic range.

Step 2.

Note the patient's estimated pharmacokinetic parameters (Cl, $t_{1/2}$, and Vd). In the absence of any specific information about the patient's pharmacokinetic parameters, population average values must be assumed. Even then, any patient characteristics that are known to affect any of the pharmacokinetic parameters should be considered. For example, in the absence of any other information, the clearance of theophylline in a smoker should be considered to be 1.6 times the value of a non-smoker, and its clearance for a patient on concomitant fluvoxamine should be considered to be 30% of the normal value [1].

Step 3.

Select a suitable $Cp_{av,ss}$ value from the middle of the therapeutic range.

Step 4.

Calculate the rate of drug administration necessary to achieve the average steady-state plasma concentration desired (similar to determination of the infusion rate):

$$S \cdot F \cdot R_a = Cp_{av,ss} \cdot Cl \qquad (12.29)$$

Step 5.

Determine the dosing interval based on the drug's therapeutic range, the drug's half-life, and patient convenience. If the therapeutic range is narrow, a suitable interval can be calculated using equation (12.5):

$$\tau = -\frac{1}{k} \ln \frac{Cp_{min,ss}}{Cp_{max,ss}} \qquad (12.30)$$

Step 6.

Calculate the specific dose:

$$D = \frac{R_a \cdot \tau}{S \cdot F} \qquad (12.31)$$

Step 7.

If the therapeutic range is narrow, the estimated steady-state peaks and troughs can be calculated to ensure that they are within the range.

Example 12.7   Following a severe blow to the head, an 80-kg man (L.K.) developed seizures. Recommend a suitable dosing regimen for phenobarbital sodium. Even though the drug will be administered orally, use the equations associated with intravenous bolus injections for your calculations. Would you recommend a loading dose? If so, calculate one. TR = 10–30 mg/L, $F = 0.9$, $S = 0.9$, $Vd = 0.7$ L/kg, and $Cl = 4.0$ mL/h · kg.

Solution   The half-life is a very important parameter for these calculations and it is important to calculate it as soon as possible:

$$t_{1/2} = \frac{0.693 Vd}{Cl} = \frac{0.693 \times 0.7 \times 80\,\text{L}}{(4 \times 80)/1000\,\text{L/h}} = 121.3\,\text{h} = 5.05\,\text{days}$$

Phenobarbital has a very long half-life of 5 days.

A goal for the average plasma concentration is chosen in the middle of the therapeutic range: 20 mg/L. The rate of administration necessary to achieve 20 mg/L is determined from (12.29):

$$\frac{S \cdot F \cdot D}{\tau} = 20\,\text{mg/L} \times (4 \times 80)/1000\,\text{L/h} = 6.4\,\text{mg/h}$$

The dosing interval is selected. The $t_{1/2}$ is over 5 days, which will permit the optimum dosing interval of 24 h to be used. This represents only $\frac{1}{5}$ or 20% of the half-life. So, during a 24-h period, the plasma concentration will easily remain within the therapeutic range. $\tau = 24$ h. The dose is now calculated.

$$\frac{S \cdot F \cdot D}{\tau} = 6.4\,\text{mg/L}$$

$$D = \frac{6.4 \cdot \tau}{S.F} = \frac{6.4 \times 24}{0.9 \times 0.9} = 190\,\text{mg of phenobarbital sodium per day}$$

It will take about 15–25 days to reach steady state, so a loading dose may be advantageous. Using equation (12.28) yields

$$D_L = \frac{190}{1 - e^{-1 \times 0.693/5.05}} = 1482\,\text{mg of phenobarbital sodium}$$

The estimated steady-state peaks [equation (12.12)] and troughs [equation (12.13)] may be calculated to ensure that they are within the therapeutic range.

$$Cp_{\text{max,ss}} = 21\,\text{mg/L}$$
$$Cp_{\text{min,ss}} = 18.7\,\text{mg/L}$$

A maintenance dose of 190 mg of phenobarbital sodium daily is recommended, with a loading dose of around 1500 mg. Generally, the loading dose is divided into three or four smaller units that can be administered over a period of several hours.

Example 12.8   It was shown previously that lipoamide ($Cl = 62$ L/h and $Vd = 420$ L) must be administered at a rate of 3.1 mg/h to achieve a desired plasma concentration of 50 µg/L. If peaks and troughs with the range 90–25 µg/L are desired, recommend a suitable dosing regimen.

Solution   The rate of drug administration to achieve a desired steady-state plasma concentration of 50 µg/L was determined for this drug using the infusion formula (Problem 11.5). The same average rate of administration should be maintained to achieve 50 µg/L with multiple doses. Lipoamide's $t_{1/2} = 0.693 \times 420/62 = 4.68$ h. From the perspective of patient convenience, a dosing interval greater than the $t_{1/2}$ of this drug is preferred. Its therapeutic range will permit a fluctuation of greater than 50% [$(Cp_{\text{max,ss}} - Cp_{\text{min,ss}})/Cp_{\text{max,ss}}$] · 100%, so it is possible that a dosing interval greater than the half-life could be used. In this example, the formula to calculate the dosing interval [equation (12.30)] would be useful. Let the desired steady-state peak and trough be 90 and 25 mg/L, respectively:

$$\tau = -\frac{4.68}{0.693} \ln \frac{25}{90} = 8.65\,\text{h}$$

The dosing interval will be rounded off to 8 h and the dose is determined from the calculated rate (3.1 mg/h) and the dosing interval (8 h) with S and $F = 1$:

$$D = 8 \times 3.1 = 24.8 \text{ mg}$$

A dosing regimen of 25 mg of lipoamide administered every 8 h is recommended.

12.7.2.2 *Protocol II: Targeting Specific Steady-State Peaks and Troughs*

Step 1.

Note the therapeutic range of the drug.

Step 2.

Note the patient's estimated pharmacokinetic parameters (Cl, $t_{1/2}$, and Vd). As discussed above, wherever possible the patient's individual characteristics should be considered in estimation of the parameter values.

Step 3.

Note the desired steady-state trough and peak and calculate a dosing interval necessary to achieve the desired trough/peak ratio using equation (12.5):

$$T = -\frac{1}{k} \ln \frac{Cp_{\text{min,ss}}}{Cp_{\text{max,ss}}} \tag{12.32}$$

Step 4.

Calculate the specific dose by substituting into the equation for either $Cp_{\text{max,ss}}$ or $Cp_{\text{min,ss}}$.

Example 12.9 Determine a suitable dose and dosing interval for gentamicin to achieve steady-state peaks and troughs of 8 and 0.5 mg/L in a patient who is estimated to have the following pharmacokinetic parameters: $Vd = 17.5$ L and $t_{1/2} = 2.0$ h.

Solution Note that the aminoglycosides are administered as short intermittent infusions, but this calculation will be performed assuming administration by multiple bolus injections. The doses determined may differ from those used clinically.

The dosing interval to achieve the desired peak and trough is calculated from equation (12.32):

$$\tau = -\frac{2.0}{0.693} \ln \frac{0.5}{8} = 8 \text{ h}$$

The dose can be determined using the equation for either the peak or trough at steady state. Using equation (12.12) for the peak at steady state,

$$8 = \frac{1 \times 1 \times D}{17.5(1 - e^{-8 \times 0.693/2})}$$
$$D = 131 \text{ mg}$$

A dose of around 130 mg of gentamicin administered every 8 h is recommended.

Example 12.10   A drug company is developing a new anticancer drug. Phase I studies have established the population average pharmacokinetic parameters ($Cl = 15$ L/h and $Vd = 2.3$ L/kg). Animal studies indicated that optimum response is obtained with a trough and peak of 0.35 and 0.65 mg/L, respectively. Determine a suitable dosing regimen in an average 70-kg patient.

Solution   The drug's $t_{1/2} = 0.693 \times 70 \times 2.3/15$ h $= 7.44$ h. The dosing interval to achieve the desired peak and trough is calculated from equation (12.32):

$$\tau = -\frac{7.44}{0.693}\ln\frac{0.35}{0.65} = 6.64\,\text{h}$$

The dosing interval would probably be rounded to 6 h and the dose could be calculated from the equation for either the peak or trough at steady state. Using the equation for the peak at steady state, equation (12.12), yields

$$0.65 = \frac{1 \times 1 \times D}{70 \times 2.3(1 - e^{-6\times0.693/7.44})}$$
$$D = 44.8 \text{ or } 45.0\,\text{mg}$$

The recommended dose is 45 mg every 6 h.

12.8   SIMULATION EXERCISE:
http://web.uri.edu/pharmacy/research/rosenbaum/sims

Open model 9, Multiple Bolus Injections, which can be found at http://web.uri.edu/pharmacy/research/rosenbaum/sims/Model9.
  Default settings for the model are dose = 120 mg, $\tau = 6$ h, $Cl = 4$ L/h, and $Vd = 50$ L.

1. *Review the objectives and the "Model Summary" page.*
2. *Go to the "Cp–Time Profile" page. Do a simulation and note that the peaks occur when a dose is given ($t = 0$) and a trough occurs just before the next dose ($t = \tau$). Also note that the plasma concentration at any time during a dosing interval increases with dose. But note that this increase lessens with each dose. Eventually, the accumulation stops. At this time, all the peaks and troughs are exactly the same; steady state has been achieved.*
3. *Go to the "Fluctuation and Accumulation" page to observe how the dosing interval influences fluctuation and accumulation. To maintain the same average plasma concentration, the same rate of drug administration (20 mg/h) must be used throughout these simulations. Thus, when a dosing interval is altered, proportional changes to the dose must be made.*
   (a) *Assess fluctuation, $[(Cp_{\text{max,ss}} - Cp_{\text{min,ss}})/Cp_{\text{max,ss}}] \cdot 100\%$.*
   (b) *Assess accumulation, $Cp_{\text{max,ss}}/Cp_{\text{max,}1}$.*
   (c) *Record in Table SE12.1 how dosing intervals of 2, 6, and 12 h affect fluctuation and accumulation.*

TABLE SE12.1   Effect of the Dosing Interval on Fluctuation and Accumulation

Dosing Interval (h)	Rate of Administration (mg/h)	Dose (mg)	Fluctuation $[(Cp_{max,ss} - Cp_{min,ss})/ Cp_{max,ss}] \cdot 100\%$	Accumulation $(Cp_{max,ss}/Cp_{max,1})$
2	20			
6	20			
12	20			

4. *Go to the "Effect of Clearance" page and conduct simulations with clearance equal to 2, 4, and 12 L/h. Record in Table SE12.2 how clearance affects the parameters.*

TABLE SE12.2   Influence of Clearance on the Cp–Time Profile for Multiple IV Bolus Injections

Cl (L/h)	$Cp_{max,1}$ (mg/L)	$Cp_{av,ss}$ ($\downarrow$, $\uparrow$, or $\leftrightarrow^{a}$)	Time to Steady State ($\downarrow$, $\uparrow$, or $\leftrightarrow^{a}$)	Fluctuation $[(Cp_{max,ss} - Cp_{min,ss})/ Cp_{max,ss}] \cdot 100\%$	Accumulation $(Cp_{max,ss}/Cp_{max,1})$
2		N.A.	N.A.		
4					
12					

^{a}Compare to the first simulation. Use $\uparrow$ for increase, $\downarrow$ for decrease, and $\leftrightarrow$ for no effect.

5. *Go to the "Effect of Volume of Distribution" page and conduct simulations with a volume of distribution equal to 20, 40, and 80 L. Record in Table SE12.3 how the volume of distribution affects the parameters.*

TABLE SE12.3   Influence of Volume of Distribution on the Cp–Time Profile for Multiple IV Bolus Injections

Vd (L)	$Cp_{max,1}$ (mg/L)	$Cp_{av,ss}$ ($\downarrow$, $\uparrow$, or $\leftrightarrow^{a}$)	Time to Steady State ($\downarrow$, $\uparrow$, or $\leftrightarrow^{a}$)	Fluctuation $[(Cp_{max,ss} - Cp_{min,ss})/ Cp_{max,ss}] \cdot 100\%$	Accumulation $(Cp_{max,ss}/Cp_{max,1})$
20		N.A.	N.A.		
40					
80					

^{a}Compare to the first simulation. Use $\uparrow$ for increase, $\downarrow$ for decrease, and $\leftrightarrow$ for no effect.

PROBLEMS

12.1   Recommend a pharmacokinetic-based multiple intravenous bolus dosing regimen for the fictitious drug nosolatol. Single-dose studies indicate that plasma concentrations in the range 1900–750 μg/L are therapeutic. The major pharmacokinetic parameters of nosolatol are $Cl = 12.6$ L/h, $Vd = 210$ L/70 kg, and $S = 1$. Design a dosing regimen that will achieve an average steady-state plasma concentration of 1200 μg/L.

12.2   Recommend a pharmacokinetic-based multiple intravenous bolus dosing regimen for the fictitious drug disolvprazole. Single-dose studies indicate that plasma concentrations in the range 1000–100 µg/L are therapeutic. The major pharmacokinetic parameters of disolvprazole are $Cl = 12$ L/h, $Vd = 35$ L/70 kg, and $S = 1$.

12.3 A synthetic analgesic has the following pharmacokinetic and pharmacodynamic parameters: $Vd = 0.2$ L/kg, $Cl = 0.012$ L/h/kg, and $S = 1$; the therapeutic range is between 0.5 and 1.5 mg/L.

(a) Determine an appropriate dosing regimen for a 75-kg male who has just undergone major orthopedic surgery.

(b) Would you recommend a loading dose? If so, calculate one.

(c) After 10 days of treatment, the patient develops toxicity, and therapy is withdrawn:

(1) How long will it take to eliminate 99% of the drug in the body?

(2) What is the Cp value 24 h after the last dose?

12.4 A 70-kg man is to receive quinidine, an antiarrhymic drug used in the treatment of atrial fibrillation and other cardiac arrhythmias. The pharmacokinetic parameters in this man are estimated to be $Cl = 4$ mL/min/kg and $Vd = 3.0$ L/kg. Use the intravenous bolus formula to devise a dosing regimen for quinidine sulfate tablets ($S = 0.82$ and $F = 0.73$) that will maintain the plasma concentrations in the range 3–1.5 mg/L.

REFERENCE

1. Winter, M. E. (2010) *Basic Clinical Pharmacokinetics*, 5th ed., Lippincott Williams & Wilkins, Baltimore.

13

MULTIPLE INTERMITTENT INFUSIONS

Sara E. Rosenbaum

Objectives

The material presented in this chapter will enable the reader to:

1. Understand the characteristics of the plasma concentration profile after multiple intermittent infusions
2. Understand the derivation of an expression for the steady-state plasma concentrations achieved by intermittent infusions
3. Use two steady-state plasma concentrations to determine a drug's half-life, the steady-state peaks and troughs, and volume of distribution
4. Individualize doses for patients receiving multiple intermittent infusions

13.1 INTRODUCTION

When drugs are administered as bolus injections, typically they are injected over a period of 1 min or more to avoid very high initial concentrations. Even with this approach, the

Basic Pharmacokinetics and Pharmacodynamics: An Integrated Textbook and Computer Simulations,
Second Edition. Edited by Sara E. Rosenbaum.
© 2017 John Wiley & Sons, Inc. Published 2017 by John Wiley & Sons, Inc.

initial plasma concentrations of some drugs may still be high enough to cause toxicity. This can be especially problematic for drugs that display two-compartment pharmacokinetics, where the initial distribution volume is small. These drugs can be administered more safely by extending the administration period and infusing the dose at a constant rate over a period of anywhere from half an hour, up to 2 h or more. The administration is then repeated with the same frequency that it would be for bolus injections. This type of drug administration thus consists of *multiple intermittent infusions* or *multiple short infusions*. The aminoglycoside antibiotics are important examples of drugs administered in this way. These drugs are used to treat serious life-threatening gram-negative infections, and their use is complicated by their potential to cause serious renal impairment and ototoxicity (hearing and vestibular damage). As a result of both wide interindividual variability in their pharmacokinetics and the serious consequences of either subtherapeutic or toxic concentrations, plasma concentrations of these drugs are monitored and doses individualized. A knowledge and understanding of the pharmacokinetics and associated equations of multiple intermittent infusions is necessary to perform this process.

The characteristics and equations for multiple intermittent infusions are very similar to those for multiple bolus injections. Figure 13.1 shows the typical plasma concentration profile associated with this type of administration, which in common with bolus injections, demonstrates fluctuation and an accumulation of drug in the buildup to steady state. Again in common with multiple bolus injections, it takes 3–5 elimination half-lives to achieve steady state. When the plasma concentrations during a dosing interval are studied, some important differences between the two forms of drug administration become apparent (Figure 13.2). Although the trough concentration occurs at the end of the dosing interval, the peak plasma concentrations observed with multiple infusions do not occur at the beginning of the dosing interval but when the infusion is stopped.

The symbols used are the same as those used for bolus injections: t is the time that has elapsed since the dose was administered (start of the infusion), and τ is the dosing interval or time between doses. Tau varies constantly from zero to τ, to zero to τ, and so on. The equations for multiple infusions incorporate an additional time parameter, the duration of the infusion (t_{inf}). The dosing interval can be broken down into two parts: the period from time 0 to t_{inf} when the infusion is running, during which plasma concentrations increase (A in Figure 13.2); and the period from the end of the infusion to the end of the dosing

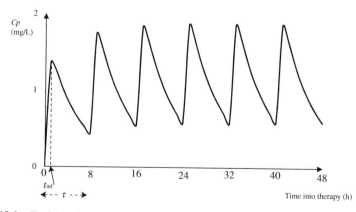

FIGURE 13.1 Typical plasma concentration–time profile observed with multiple intermittent infusions. The duration of the infusion is t_{inf} and the interval between the start of consecutive infusions is τ.

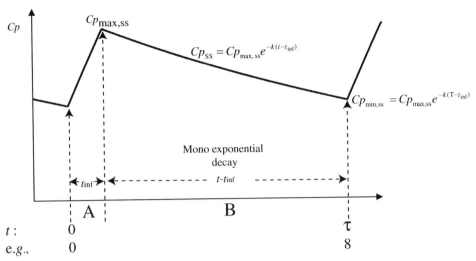

FIGURE 13.2   Multiple intermittent infusions: plasma concentrations during a steady-state dosing interval. Time t is the time after the start of the infusion. The dosing interval can be separated into two periods: A and B. During period A, the infusion is running and plasma concentrations increase. Note that the peak occurs when the infusion stops ($t = t_{inf}$). During period B (from $t = t_{inf}$ to $t = \tau$), there is no ongoing drug input, and plasma concentrations decay monoexponentially.

interval (period t_{inf} to τ) when the infusion is not running. During the latter period, plasma concentrations fall monoexponentially under the influence of first-order elimination (B in Figure 13.2). Note in Figure 13.2 that the peak occurs when $t = t_{inf}$, and a trough is obtained at the end of the dosing interval when $t = \tau$.

In a dosing interval, once the infusion stops, the plasma concentration falls monoexponentially from the peak. As a result, the plasma concentration at any time during this period (B in Figure 13.2) can be expressed in terms of its decay from the peak and the time that has elapsed from the peak ($t - t_{inf}$). For example, at steady state:

$$Cp_{ss} = Cp_{max,ss} \cdot e^{-k(t - t_{inf})} \tag{13.1}$$

where Cp_{ss} is the concentration at any time, t, during a steady state dosing interval and $Cp_{max,ss}$ is the steady-state peak. Cp at the trough during a steady-state dosing interval ($Cp_{min,ss}$) is expressed as:

$$Cp_{min,ss} = Cp_{max,ss} \cdot e^{-k(\tau - t_{inf})} \tag{13.2}$$

13.2   STEADY-STATE EQUATIONS FOR MULTIPLE INTERMITTENT INFUSIONS

In Chapter 12, we demonstrated that an equation for multiple dosing could be constructed as follows (Figure 12.6):

$$Cp_{multiple\ doses} = Cp_{single\ doses} \times \text{fraction of steady state anytime}$$
$$\times \text{final accumulation at steady state}$$

Expressions for the fraction of steady state achieved at any time and the final accumulation at steady state were derived in Chapter 12 [equations (12.27) and (12.23), respectively]. Thus,

$$Cp_{\text{multiple doses}} = Cp_{\text{single doses}} \cdot (1 - e^{-nk\tau}) \cdot \frac{1}{1 - e^{-k\tau}} \tag{13.3}$$

If the equation is to be limited to steady state, the fraction of steady state $(1 - e^{-nk\tau})$ equals 1 and can be removed from the expression:

$$Cp_{\text{multiple doses, ss}} = Cp_{\text{single doses}} \cdot \frac{1}{1 - e^{-k\tau}} \tag{13.4}$$

The equation for the plasma concentration at any time after a single infusion was presented in Chapter 11 [equation (11.16)]:

$$Cp_{\text{single infusion}} = \frac{S \cdot F \cdot k_0 \cdot (1 - e^{-kT})}{Cl} \cdot e^{-kt'} \tag{13.5}$$

where T is the time the infusion was terminated, and t' is the time elapsed since termination. Next, we substitute the time symbols used for multiple infusions: $T = t_{\text{inf}}$ and $t' = t - t_{\text{inf}}$. Substituting these symbols into equation (13.5) and then substituting into equation (13.4) yield

$$Cp_{\text{ss}} = \frac{S \cdot F \cdot k_0 \cdot (1 - e^{-kt_{\text{inf}}})}{Cl \cdot (1 - e^{-k\tau})} \cdot e^{-k(t - t_{\text{inf}})} \tag{13.6}$$

where Cp_{ss} is the plasma concentration at any time during a steady-state dosing interval, k_0 is the infusion rate, S is the salt factor of the drug, F is the bioavailability, k is the elimination rate constant, t_{inf} is the duration of the infusion, t is the time elapsed since the infusion was started, Cl is the clearance, and τ is the dosing interval or time between the start of consecutive infusions.

A peak plasma concentration occurs at the end of the infusion when $t = t_{\text{inf}}$:

$$Cp_{\text{max,ss}} = \frac{S \cdot F \cdot k_0 \cdot (1 - e^{-kt_{\text{inf}}})}{Cl \cdot (1 - e^{-k\tau})} \tag{13.7}$$

A trough plasma concentration occurs at the end of the dosing interval $(t = \tau)$, 0

$$Cp_{\text{min,ss}} = \frac{S \cdot F \cdot k_0 \cdot (1 - e^{-kt_{\text{inf}}})}{Cl \cdot (1 - e^{-k\tau})} \cdot e^{-k(\tau - t_{\text{inf}})} \tag{13.8}$$

Example 13.1   A drug ($Cl = 8.67$ L/h, $Vd = 100$ L, and $S = 1$) was administered as multiple intravenous infusions. The dose (80 mg) was administered over a 1-h period every 8 h. Calculate the estimated plasma concentrations on the third day of therapy, at (a) 1 h, (b) 2 h, (c) 4 h, and (d) 8 h after the start of the first infusion of the day.

Solution   The drug has a $t_{1/2} = 0.693 \times 100/8.67 = 8$ h. A dose of 80 mg is infused over 1 h: $k_0 = 80$ mg/h, $S = 1$, and $F = 1$. The problem is summarized in Figure 13.3. It will take

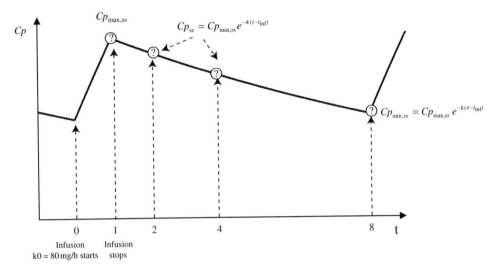

FIGURE 13.3 Example problem using multiple intermittent infusion equations. The drug is administered at a rate of 80 mg/h over a 1-h period. Plasma concentrations at 1, 2, 4, and 8 h must be calculated after the first dose on the third day.

about 24–40 h to get to steady state. By the third day, steady state will have been achieved and the profiles from the three infusions of the day will be exactly the same.

(a) When $t = 1$ h, the infusion has just been terminated, $Cp = Cp_{max,ss}$. Substituting into equation (13.7) yields

$$Cp_{max,ss} = \frac{80(1 - e^{-1 \times 0.693/8})}{8.67(1 - e^{-8 \times 0.693/8})} = 1.53 \text{ mg/L}$$

(b) When $t = 2$ h, it is 1 h after the infusion stops.

$$Cp_{ss,t=2} = \frac{80(1 - e^{-1 \times 0.693/8})}{8.67(1 - e^{-8 \times 0.693/8})} \cdot e^{-(2-1)0.693/8}$$

or

$$Cp_{ss,t=2} = Cp_{max,ss} \cdot e^{-(2-1)0.693/8} = 1.53 e^{-(2-1)0.693/8} = 1.40 \text{ mg/L}$$

(c) When $t = 4$ h, it is halfway through the dosing interval and 3 h after the infusion has stopped:

$$Cp_{ss,t=4} = Cp_{max,ss} \cdot e^{-(4-1)0.693/8} = 1.53 e^{-(4-1)0.693/8} = 1.18 \text{ mg/L}$$

(d) When $t = 8$ h, it is the end of the dosing interval and 7 h from the peak:

$$Cp_{ss,t=8} = Cp_{min,ss} = Cp_{max,ss} \cdot e^{-(8-1)0.693/8} = 1.53 e^{-(8-1)0.693/8} = 0.83 \text{ mg/L}$$

Example 13.2   A 0.5-h infusion is used to administer the dose (80 mg) of the drug described in Example 13.1. Calculate the estimated plasma concentrations on the third day of therapy, at (a) 0.5 h, (b) 1 h, (c) 2 h, and (d) 8 h after the start of the infusion.

Solution   The drug has a $t_{1/2} = 0.693 \times 100/8.67 = 8$ h. A dose of 80 mg is infused over 0.5 h: $k_0 = 160$ mg/h, $S = 1$, and $F = 1$. It will take about 24–40 h to get to steady state. By the third day, steady state will have been achieved. A diagram of the steady-state dosing interval is shown in Figure 13.3 but in this example, $t_{inf} = 0.5$ h.

(a) When $t = 0.5$, the infusion has just been terminated, $Cp = Cp_{max,ss}$. Substituting into equation (13.7), we have

$$Cp_{max,ss} = \frac{160(1 - e^{-0.5 \times 0.693/8})}{8.67(1 - e^{-8 \times 0.693/8})} = 1.58 \text{ mg/L}$$

(b) When $t = 1$, it is 0.5 h after the infusion stops.

$$Cp_{ss,t=1} = Cp_{max,ss} \cdot e^{-(1-0.5)0.693/8} = 1.58 e^{-(1-0.5)0.693/8} = 1.51 \text{ mg/L}$$

(c) When $t = 2$, it is 1.5 h after the infusion stops.

$$Cp_{ss,t=2} = Cp_{max,ss} \cdot e^{-(2-0.5)0.693/8} = 1.58 e^{-(2-0.5)0.693/8} = 1.38 \text{ mg/L}$$

(d) When $t = 8$, it is the end of the dosing interval and 7.5 h from the peak.

$$Cp_{ss,t=8} = Cp_{min,ss} = Cp_{max,ss} \cdot e^{-(8-0.5)0.693/8} = 1.58 e^{-(8-0.5)0.693/8} = 0.82 \text{ mg/L}$$

13.3 MONOEXPONENTIAL DECAY DURING A DOSING INTERVAL: DETERMINATION OF PEAKS, TROUGHS, AND ELIMINATION HALF-LIFE

13.3.1 Determination of Half-Life

A drug's elimination half-life can be determined from two plasma concentrations measured during the period when the infusion is not running (period t_{inf} to τ), when plasma concentrations are falling monoexponentially as a result of first-order elimination. During this period,

$$Cp_n = Cp_{max,n} \cdot e^{-k(t-t_{inf})} \tag{13.9}$$

where $Cp_{max,n}$ and Cp_n are the peak and plasma concentration at time t, respectively, during the nth dosing interval. Taking the logarithmic of equation (13.9) yields

$$\ln Cp_n = \ln Cp_{max,n} - k \cdot (t - t_{inf}) \tag{13.10}$$

Thus, k can be determined:

$$k = \frac{\ln(Cp_1/Cp_2)}{t_2 - t_1} \tag{13.11}$$

and the half-life

$$t_{1/2} = \frac{0.693}{k} \tag{13.12}$$

Example 13.3 A patient is being treated with gentamicin. A 140-mg dose is administered as a short infusion over a 1-h period every 8 h. Plasma concentrations of the drug
were determined during the first dosing interval and are given in Table E13.3. Assume one-
compartmental pharmacokinetics and calculate the drug's half-life.

**TABLE E13.3 Gentamicin Plasma Concentrations Determined
at Two Time Points After the Start of an Infusion**

Time After Start of Infusion (h)	Gentamicin Concentration (mg/L)
1.5	6.1
6	2.2

Solution The problem is summarized in Figure E13.3. The plasma samples were taken
during a period when the infusion was not running. Thus, the only process affecting plasma
concentrations is first-order elimination, and equation (13.11) can be used to determine the
rate constant and half-life.

$$k = \frac{\ln(6.1/2.2)}{6 - 1.5} = 0.227 \text{ h}^{-1}$$

$$t_{1/2} = \frac{0.693}{0.227} = 3.05 \text{ h}$$

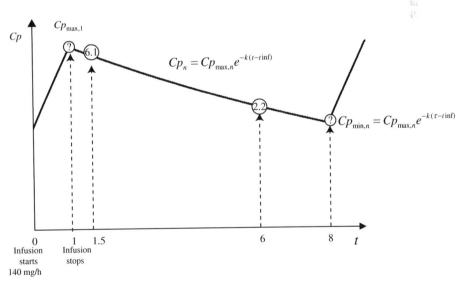

FIGURE E13.3 Calculation of the half-life. If two plasma concentrations are known in the period
when the infusion is not running, the half-life can be calculated. Once the half-life is known, the peaks
and troughs associated with this dosing interval may also be calculated.

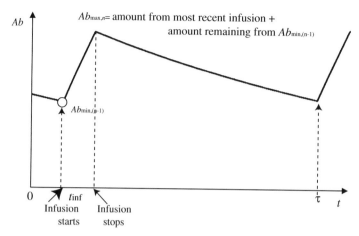

FIGURE 13.4 Determination of the volume of distribution. The derivation of the equation for Vd is based on partitioning the amount of drug in the body at the time of a peak into two components: (1) the amount of drug that came from the most recent infusion and (2) the amount of drug remaining from the previous trough.

13.3.2 Determination of Peaks and Troughs

If a drug's half-life or elimination rate constant is known, and if at least one plasma concentration during the dosing interval is known, the values of the peak and trough associated with the dosing interval can be calculated.

Example 13.4 Continuing with Example 13.3, determine the trough and peak of the dosing interval described above.

Solution The drug's elimination rate constant is $0.227\,\mathrm{h}^{-1}$. Once the infusion is stopped, plasma concentrations decay monoexponentially (Figure 13.4):

$$Cp_n = Cp_{\mathrm{max},n} \cdot e^{-k(t-t_{\mathrm{inf}})} \tag{13.13}$$

$Cp_n = 6.1$ mg/L when $t = 1.5$ h and $t - t_{\mathrm{inf}} = 0.5$ h. Substitute in equation (13.13) to determine the peak:

$$6.1 = Cp_{\mathrm{max},n} \cdot e^{-0.227\times 0.5}$$
$$Cp_{\mathrm{max},n} = 6.83 \text{ mg/L}$$

The trough occurs when $t = \tau$ and $t - t_{\mathrm{inf}} = 7$ h:

$$Cp_{\mathrm{min},n} = Cp_{\mathrm{max},n} \cdot e^{-0.227\times 7}$$

$$= 6.83 e^{-0.27\times 7} = 1.39 \text{ mg/L}$$

13.4 DETERMINATION OF THE VOLUME OF DISTRIBUTION

The volume of distribution can be calculated if a peak plasma concentration and its previous trough are known.

Theory   The equation for the volume of distribution is derived by considering the amount of drug in the body at the time of a peak ($Ab_{max,n}$) (Figure 13.4). The amount of drug in the body at the time of a peak can be partitioned into two parts: drug from the most recent infusion and drug remaining from previous infusions. At the peak:

$$Ab_{max,n} = \text{drug from the most recent infusion} \qquad (13.14)$$
$$+ \text{ the amount remaining from previous infusions}$$

The amount of drug from the most recent infusion is determined by multiplying Vd by the equation for the plasma concentration from a single infusion [see equation (13.5)], with $T = t_{inf}$ and $t' = 0$):

$$Ab_{recent} = Vd \cdot \frac{S \cdot F \cdot k_0}{Cl} \cdot (1 - e^{-kt_{inf}}) \qquad (13.15)$$

As $Cl = k \cdot Vd$,

$$Ab_{recent} = Vd \cdot \frac{S \cdot F \cdot k_0}{k \cdot Vd} \cdot (1 - e^{-kt_{inf}}) \qquad (13.16)$$

The amount remaining from previous infusion(s) is equal to the amount at the time of the previous trough ($Ab_{min,(n-1)}$) minus the amount eliminated during the recent infusion:

$$Ab_{previous} = Ab_{previous\ trough} - \text{elimination during infusion} \qquad (13.17)$$
$$= Vd \cdot Cp_{min,(n-1)} \cdot e^{-kt_{inf}}$$

Substituting the expression of the amount from the most recent infusion (13.15) and the amount from previous infusion(s) [equation (13.17)] into equation (13.14) gives us

$$Ab_{max,n} = Vd \cdot \frac{S \cdot F \cdot k_0}{k \cdot Vd} \cdot (1 - e^{-kt_{inf}}) + Vd \cdot Cp_{min,(n-1)} \cdot e^{-kt_{inf}} \qquad (13.18)$$

Substituting $Cp_{max,n} \cdot Vd$ for $Ab_{max,n}$ results in

$$Vd \cdot Cp_{max,n} = Vd \cdot \frac{S \cdot F \cdot k_0}{k \cdot Vd} \cdot (1 - e^{-kt_{inf}}) + Vd \cdot Cp_{min,(n-1)} \cdot e^{-kt_{inf}}$$
$$Cp_{max,n} = \frac{S \cdot F \cdot k_0}{k \cdot Vd} \cdot (1 - e^{-kt_{inf}}) + Cp_{min,(n-1)} \cdot e^{-kt_{inf}} \qquad (13.19)$$
$$Vd = \frac{S \cdot F \cdot k_0 \cdot (1 - e^{-kt_{inf}})}{k(Cp_{max,n} - Cp_{min,(n-1)} \cdot e^{-kt_{inf}})}$$

Practice   From equation (13.19), it can be seen that the volume of distribution can be calculated if a peak concentration ($Cp_{max,n}$) and a previous trough ($Cp_{min,(n-1)}$) are known. If the therapy is at steady state, any peak and trough may be used because the troughs and peaks are exactly the same at steady state.

Example 13.5   The suitability of a gentamicin regimen (110 mg every 8 h infused over a 1-h period) is being assessed on the third day of treatment. A steady-state trough

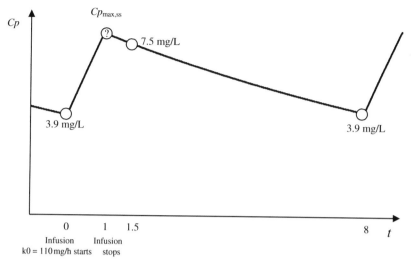

FIGURE 13.5   Example calculation of the volume of distribution. This parameter is determined from a peak plasma concentration and its previous trough. Initially, the half-life must be estimated in order to calculate the peak plasma concentration.

concentration is found to be 3.9 mg/L. The plasma concentration 1.5 h after the start of the most recent infusion is found to be 7.5 mg/L.

(a) Determine the elimination half-life.
(b) Determine the peak plasma concentration after the most recent infusion.
(c) Determine the volume of distribution.

Solution   The infusion is at steady state, so all the peaks and troughs will be the same. The profile associated with this problem is shown in Figure 13.5.
The elimination rate constant may be calculated as:

$$k = \frac{\ln(7.5/3.9)}{8 - 1.5} = 0.101 \text{ h}^{-1}$$

(a) The elimination half-life is determined:

$$t_{1/2} = \frac{0.693}{k} = 6.86 \text{ h}$$

(b) The steady-state peak can be determined:

$$7.5 = Cp_{\text{max},n} \cdot e^{-0.101 \times 0.5}$$
$$Cp_{\text{max},n} = 7.89 \text{ mg/L}$$

(c) The volume of distribution may be calculated from equation (13.19):

$$Vd = \frac{110(1 - e^{-0.101 \times 1})}{0.101(7.89 - 3.9 \times e^{-0.101 \times 1})} = 23.9 \text{ L}$$

13.5 INDIVIDUALIZATION OF DOSING REGIMENS

The methods used to design the dosing regimens discussed in Chapter 12 can be applied to multiple intermittent infusions.

Example 13.6 Continuing with Example 13.5, the trough concentration found in the patient was considered to be too high. Design another regimen that will provide a gentamicin steady-state peak and trough of 8 and 0.5 mg/L, respectively. The pharmacokinetic parameters in this patient were found to be $k = 0.101$ h^{-1}, $Vd = 23.9$ L, and $Cl = k \cdot Vd = 2.41$ L/h.

Solution Here the focus of the regimen is on the achievement of specific peaks and troughs. Recall the equation introduced in Chapter 12 to calculate a dosing interval to provide specific peaks and troughs with multiple intravenous injections:

$$\tau = -\frac{1}{k} \ln \frac{Cp_{min,ss}}{Cp_{max,ss}} \tag{13.20}$$

For multiple infusions, the time between the peak and the trough is $\tau - t_{inf}$ (Figure 13.2) and not τ as it is for multiple bolus injections. Thus, equation (13.20) will have to be modified appropriately:

$$\tau - t_{inf} = -\frac{1}{k} \ln \frac{Cp_{min,ss}}{Cp_{max,ss}} \tag{13.21}$$

Using equation (13.21) to calculate the necessary dosing interval for peaks and troughs of 8 and 0.5 mg/L, respectively, yields

$$\tau - t_{inf} = -\frac{1}{0.101} \ln \frac{0.5}{8} = 27.5 \text{ h}$$

$$\tau = 28.5 \text{ h, which would be rounded to 24 h}$$

The appropriate dose could be calculated using the equation for either the peak (8 mg/L) or the trough (0.5 mg/L). Using the peak equation (13.7), we have

$$Cp_{max,ss} = 8 = \frac{k_0 \cdot (1 - e^{-1 \times 0.101})}{2.41(1 - e^{-24 \times 0.101})}$$

$$k_0 = 183 \text{ mg}$$

To obtain peaks and troughs of 8 and 0.5 mg/L, 183 mg of gentamicin should be infused over a 1-h period every 24 h.

13.6 SIMULATION: http://web.uri.edu/pharmacy/research/rosenbaum/sims

Open model 10, Multiple Intermittent Infusions, which can be found at http://web.uri.edu/ pharmacy/research/rosenbaum/sims/Model10.
  Default settings for the model are dose = 80 mg, $\tau = 8$ h, $t_{inf} = 1$ h, Cl = 8.67 L/h, and Vd = 20 L.

  1. *Review the objectives and the "Model Summary" page.*
  2. *Go to the "Cp–Time Profile" page. Perform a simulation and note that the peaks occur when the infusion stops ($t = t_{inf}$) and a trough occurs just before the next dose*

$(t = \tau)$. *Also note that accumulation occurs with successive doses but stops at steady state.*

3. *Go to the "Influence of Infusion Duration" page. The overall rate of drug administration or the dose administered will remain constant (80 mg every 8 h), but the duration of the infusion will be altered. Since the individual dose will remain constant, the infusion rate will change in inverse proportion to the infusion duration. This adjustment will be made automatically by the software. Observe how the profile changes with infusion of duration 0.5, 2, and 4 h. (The corresponding infusion rates will be 160, 40, and 20 mg/h). As the duration of the infusion increases, the peak gets lower and the trough gets higher; that is, fluctuation decreases.*

4. *Go to the "Determine a Dosing Regimen" page. Use the drugs pharmacokinetic parameters (Cl = 8.67 L/h and Vd = 20 L) and a 1-h infusion to calculate a dose and a dosing interval that will provide a peak and trough of 10 and 1 mg/L, respectively. Check your answers using the model.*

PROBLEMS

13.1 A drug ($Cl = 1.73$ L/h, $Vd = 30$ L, and $S = 1$) was administered as multiple short intravenous infusions. A dose of 40 mg was administered over a 1-h period every 12 h.

   (a) How long will it take to get to steady state?

   (b) Calculate the peak plasma concentration during a steady-state dosing interval.

   (c) Calculate the plasma concentration 6 h into a steady-state dosing interval.

   (d) Calculate the trough plasma concentration during a steady-state dosing interval.

13.2 If the dose of the drug discussed above was infused over a 0.5-h period, calculate the steady-state peak and trough concentrations.

13.3 If the dose of the drug above was infused over a 2-h period, calculate the steady-state peak and trough concentrations.

13.4 A 38-year-old male patient (75 kg) is given gentamicin (120 mg every 8 h infused over a 1-h period). Plasma samples taken after the second dose were analyzed for gentamicin and the results are shown in Table P13.4.

TABLE P13.4   Gentamicin Plasma Concentrations Determined at Two Time Points After the Start of an Infusion

Time After Start of Infusion (h)	Gentamicin Cp (mg/L)
2	3.84
7	1.10

   (a) What is gentamicin's half-life in this patient?

   (b) What is the peak plasma concentration of this dosing interval?

   (c) What is the trough plasma concentration of this dosing interval?

13.5 Tobramycin (120 mg) is being infused over a 1-h period every 8 h. Three days into therapy, at steady state, tobramycin concentrations at 1 and 8 h after the start of an infusion were found to be 7.12 and 0.75 mg/L, respectively. Calculate the drug's half-life and its volume of distribution. Note that because steady state has been achieved, the trough concentration of the previous dosing interval can also be assumed to be 0.75 mg/L.

13.6 Gentamicin (140 mg) is infused over a 1-h period every 8 h. A steady-state peak and trough of 10 and 0.25 mg/L, respectively, are required. At steady state, gentamicin concentrations at 2 and 8 h after the start of an infusion were found to be 5.5 and 0.75 mg/L, respectively. Is this regimen satisfactory? If not, recommend a regimen that would achieve the desired peaks and troughs of gentamicin concentrations.

14

MULTIPLE ORAL DOSES

Sara E. Rosenbaum

Objectives

The material presented in this chapter will enable the reader to:

1. Understand the characteristics of the plasma concentration profile after multiple oral doses
2. Compare the profile to other modes of chronic drug administration
3. Understand how F and k_a influence the plasma concentration profile
4. Identify an appropriate intravenous formula to use to individualize oral doses clinically

14.1 INTRODUCTION

The oral route is the most popular and common form of drug administration. Consequently, it is important for health professions and scientists involved in evaluation of the

Basic Pharmacokinetics and Pharmacodynamics: An Integrated Textbook and Computer Simulations,
Second Edition. Edited by Sara E. Rosenbaum.
© 2017 John Wiley & Sons, Inc. Published 2017 by John Wiley & Sons, Inc.

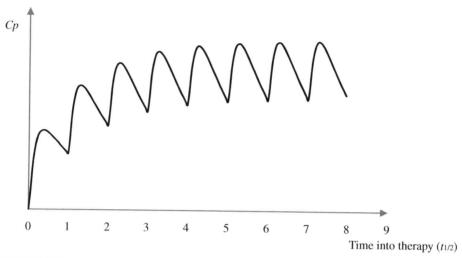

FIGURE 14.1   Typical plasma concentration–time profile observed with multiple oral doses for a drug administered every half-life.

dose–plasma concentration relationship to have good knowledge and understanding of the special pharmacokinetic characteristics of this route. It has the same accumulation properties in the buildup to steady state, and it takes the same time to reach steady state as do other forms of multiple doses (Figure 14.1). Fluctuation also occurs, and in common with the fluctuation observed with multiple short infusions, the peak is seen slightly later than the time at which the dose is administered (Figure 14.1).

The pharmacokinetics of oral drug administration was introduced in Chapter 9, where it was seen that the pharmacokinetic model contains two absorption parameters: F, the fraction of the dose that reaches the systemic circulation and k_a, the first-order rate constant for absorption. It follows that a focus of the discussion on the pharmacokinetics of multiple oral doses should be on how these two special absorption parameters influence the plasma concentration–time profile.

The clearest way to demonstrate the influence of these parameters is, first, through a consideration of the equations for multiple oral doses, and then through computer simulations. In this chapter, we concentrate on steady-state concentrations. It is not uncommon for bioavailability and bioequivalence studies to be carried out at steady state. Thus, an additional and related topic discussed in this chapter is the justification and validation for conducting bioavailability and bioequivalence studies at steady state.

14.2   STEADY-STATE EQUATIONS

As discussed in Chapter 12, steady-state equations for multiple-dosing therapies can be obtained as follows:

$$Cp_{\text{multiple doses, ss}} = Cp_{\text{single doses, ss}} \cdot \text{accumulation ratio}(r)$$

and

$$r = \frac{1}{1 - e^{-k_n \cdot \tau}} \tag{14.1}$$

where k_n is a rate constant in an exponential expression in the single-dose equation.

In the equation for single oral doses,

$$Cp = \frac{S \cdot F \cdot D \cdot k_a}{Vd \cdot (k_a - k)} \cdot (e^{-kt} - e^{-k_a t}) \tag{14.2}$$

it can be seen that it contains two exponential functions. To derive the steady-state equations for multiple doses, each exponential function has to be multiplied by its own accumulation ratio. The steady-state plasma concentration after multiple oral doses may be expressed as:

$$Cp_{ss} = \frac{S \cdot F \cdot D \cdot k_a}{Vd \cdot (k_a - k)} \cdot \left(\frac{e^{-kt}}{1 - e^{-k\tau}} - \frac{e^{-k_a t}}{1 - e^{-k_a \tau}} \right) \tag{14.3}$$

where t is the time since the last dose, and τ is the dosing interval or time between doses.

The typical profile observed after multiple oral doses and the one predicted by equation (14.3) is shown in Figure 14.1, where the typical accumulation of drug up to steady state is present, as is fluctuation. We also see that the peak plasma concentration (C_{max}) does not occur at time zero (i.e., when a dose is given) but later. In common with the symbols used for single oral doses, the time of the peak plasma concentration is T_{max}. After single doses, these parameters are important measures of the rate and extent of drug absorption, and as a result they are used to assess bioavailability. The determinants of C_{max} and T_{max} at steady state are addressed next.

14.2.1 Time to Peak Steady-State Plasma Concentration

At the time of a peak during multiple oral doses, the rate of absorption is momentarily equal to the rate of elimination, and the rate of change of Cp with time is zero. The expression for the time of the maximum steady-state plasma concentration can be obtained by differentiating equation (14.3) and setting $dCp/dt = 0$. Upon rearrangement, the following equation is obtained [1]:

$$T_{max} - T_{max,ss} = \frac{1}{k_a - k} \cdot \ln \frac{1 - e^{-k_a \tau}}{1 - e^{-k\tau}} \tag{14.4}$$

where T_{max} is the time of the peak plasma concentration after a single dose, and $T_{max,ss}$ is the time of the peak during a steady-state dosing interval. Recall from Chapter 9 that

$$T_{max} = \frac{\ln(k_a/k)}{k_a - k}$$

Several important points can be made from a consideration of equation (14.4):

1. The time of the peak steady-state plasma concentration for a given drug (k is constant) is a function only of the absorption rate constant. As a result, in common with its application in single-dose studies, it can be used to assess the rate of drug absorption in multiple-dose bioavailability studies. If the absorption rate constant increases, the time to the peak will decrease, and vice versa.
2. Because the right-hand side of equation (14.4) must always be positive, it can be concluded that it takes less time to reach the peak at steady state than to reach the peak after a single dose. Recall that after a dose, plasma concentrations increase because

the rate of absorption is greater than the rate of elimination. As absorption proceeds after a dose, the rate of absorption decreases as drug is depleted from the gastrointestinal tract and the rate of elimination increases as more drug gets into the body. The peak occurs when the rates of the two processes are momentarily equal. As a result of accumulation, the amount of drug in the body increases with each dose. As a result, with each successive dose, it takes less time for the rate of elimination to equal the rate of absorption, and T_{max} decreases with each dose. At steady state, accumulation stops and $T_{max,ss}$ remains constant.

The determinants of $T_{max,ss}$ are discussed further in Section 14.2.5.

14.2.2 Maximum Steady-State Plasma Concentration

The peak plasma concentration at steady state occurs when the time after the dose is equal to $T_{max,ss}$. Thus, the expression for the peak plasma concentration at steady state is obtained by substituting the expression for $T_{max,ss}$ [equation (14.4)] into the equation for the plasma concentration during a steady-state dosing interval [equation (14.3)] [2].

$$C_{max,ss} = \frac{S \cdot F \cdot D}{Vd} \cdot \frac{1}{1 - e^{-k\tau}} \cdot e^{-kT_{max,ss}} \qquad (14.5)$$

A consideration of equation (14.5) shows that in common with the peak after a single dose, the peak at steady state is directly proportional to bioavailability (F), and through its dependence on $T_{max,ss}$ is also dependent on the rate of drug absorption. If F increases, the value of the peak plasma concentration will increase, and vice versa. If the absorption rate constant increases, $T_{max,ss}$ will decrease and $C_{max,ss}$ will increase. These relationships are discussed further in Section 14.2.5.

14.2.3 Minimum Steady-State Plasma Concentration

Assuming that $k_a > k$ at later times during a dosing interval, $e^{-k_a t}$ in equation (14.3) will tend to zero. Additionally, the trough concentration occurs when $t = \tau$. Thus, equation (14.3) will simplify to

$$C_{min,ss} = \frac{S \cdot F \cdot D \cdot k_a}{Vd \cdot (k_a - k)} \cdot \frac{e^{-k\tau}}{1 - e^{-k\tau}} \qquad (14.6)$$

From equation (14.6), it can be seen that the trough at steady state is equal to the plasma concentration at the same time after a single dose multiplied by the accumulation ratio.

14.2.4 Average Steady-State Plasma Concentration

The average steady-state plasma concentration is equal to the area under the curve during a steady-state dosing interval divided by τ:

$$AUC_0^\tau = \int Cp_{ss} \cdot dt = \frac{S \cdot F \cdot D}{Cl} \qquad (14.7)$$

Note that the area under the curve during a steady-state dosing interval is exactly the same as the area under the plasma concentration time curve from zero to infinity after a single dose (Figure 14.2). Additionally, equation (14.7) shows that for a given drug (*Cl* is

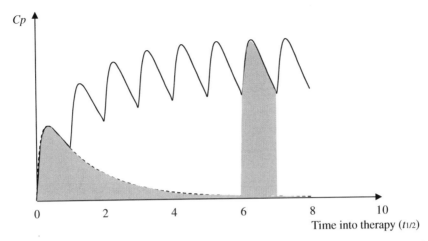

FIGURE 14.2   Area under the curve (AUC) at steady state and after a single dose. The AUC from zero to τ during a steady-state dosing interval is the same as the AUC from zero to infinity after a single dose: $S \cdot F \cdot D / Cl$.

constant), the AUC during a steady-state dosing interval is dependent only on the fraction of the dose absorbed (F) and demonstrates that this area can be used to assess bioavailability.

The expression for the average steady-state plasma concentration can now be obtained:

$$Cp_{\mathrm{av,ss}} = \frac{S \cdot F \cdot D}{Cl \cdot \tau} \tag{14.8}$$

The equation demonstrates the dependency of the average steady-state plasma concentration on clearance and the effective rate of drug administration. It also demonstrates its independence of the volume of distribution and the rate of drug absorption. The equation can be used to determine the rate of drug administration to achieve a desired average concentration. Note that equation (14.8) is exactly the same as that for the average steady-state plasma concentration achieved by multiple intravenous bolus injections. However, with intravenous injections, bioavailability (F) is always equal to 1. In contrast, bioavailability associated with oral doses may be less than 1. This is an important factor to consider when converting an intravenous dosing regimen to an oral dosing regimen. For example, the bioavailability of morphine after oral administration is about 0.3. Thus, for equivalency, the rate of drug administration for oral doses must be about 3.3 times greater than the intravenous rate.

14.2.5   Overall Effect of Absorption Parameters on a Steady-State Dosing Interval

It has been shown that the first-order absorption rate constant influences the $T_{\mathrm{max,ss}}$ and $C_{\mathrm{max,ss}}$ but does not influence either AUC_0^{τ} or $Cp_{\mathrm{av,ss}}$. The fraction of the dose absorbed (F) influences AUC_0^{τ}, $Cp_{\mathrm{av,ss}}$, and $C_{\mathrm{max,ss}}$ but not $T_{\mathrm{max,ss}}$. Figure 14.3 demonstrates these principles and shows the steady-state profile obtained from three different formulations of the same drug. Each formulation contained the same dose and was administered with the same frequency. The formulations differed with respect to the rate and extent of absorption of the drug: $F_A = F_B > F_C$ and $ka_B = ka_C < ka_A$. It can be seen that AUC_0^{τ}, $C_{\mathrm{max,ss}}$, and $Cp_{\mathrm{av,ss}}$ are proportional to F, but F does not affect $T_{\mathrm{max,ss}}$. It can be seen that if k_a increases, $T_{\mathrm{max,ss}}$ decreases and $C_{\mathrm{max,ss}}$ increases, but k_a has no influence on AUC_0^{τ} and $Cp_{\mathrm{av,ss}}$.

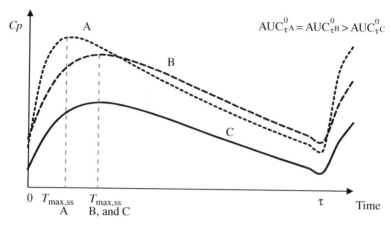

FIGURE 14.3 Steady-state plasma concentrations of three different formulations of a drug. Each formulation has the same dose and is administered with the same frequency. Note that $F_A = F_B > F_C$, and $ka_B = ka_C < ka_A$. As a result of the differences, $AUC_A = AUC_B > AUC_C$; $T_{max,ss,B} = T_{max,ss,C} > T_{max,ss,A}$. The $C_{max,ss}$ values of all three are different because they are influenced by both F and k_a: $Cp_{max,ss,A} > Cp_{max,ss,B} > Cp_{max,ss,C}$. Where AUC is the area under the concentration–time curve during a steady-state dosing interval, $C_{max,ss}$ is the peak plasma concentration at steady state, and $T_{max,ss}$ is the time at which $Cp_{max,ss}$ occurs.

14.3 EQUATIONS USED CLINICALLY TO INDIVIDUALIZE ORAL DOSES

Doses of drugs that have both a narrow therapeutic range and a wide interindividual variability in their pharmacokinetics parameters are frequently individualized for each patient. The individualization process is usually conducted by applying pharmacokinetic principles to the values of one or more plasma concentrations measured in a patient at specific times after a dose(s). Many of these drugs are given orally and include digoxin, theophylline, cyclosporine, lithium, and others. The equations for multiple oral doses are rarely used clinically to individualize doses, as they include the parameter k_a, which is difficult to measure under the best of circumstances and impossible to measure in clinical practice where only one or two plasma concentrations of the drug may be available from a patient. Additionally, the equations are long and cumbersome and mistakes can easily be made if only a handheld calculator is used. It has been found that provided that certain precautions are taken, the simpler equations associated with intravenous administration provide a satisfactory degree of accuracy when applied to orally administered drugs.

Three different types of intravenous drug administrations have been presented in this book: continuous constant infusion, multiple bolus injections, and multiple intermittent infusions. The most appropriate approximation for orally administered drugs depends on a drug's elimination characteristics in a given patient and on the rate of absorption of a specific formulation. A commonly used protocol to select an appropriate equation [3] is provided below.

14.3.1 Protocol to Select an Appropriate Equation

Continuous Input or Multiple Discrete Dose Equations? The degree of fluctuation that occurs during a dosing interval differentiates these two modes of drug administration. No

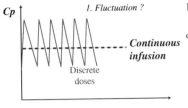

1. Continuous or Discrete Doses: how much fluctuation?

    If absorption is constant and continuous throughout the dosing interval

or If $\tau < 1/3\ t1/2$: Little dose eliminated in a dosing interval

    Minimal fluctuation: Use continuous infusion equations

    If $\tau > 1/3\ t1/2$: Much drug is eliminated in a dosing interval

    Significant flucutation: Use discrete dose equations

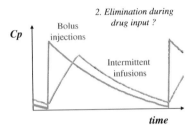

2. IV Bolus or Intermittent Infusion Equations: how much elimination occurs during absorption period?

If absorption period < $1/6\ t1/2$: Little elimination during absorption

Minimal elimination: Use bolus equations

If absorption period > $1/6\ t1/2$: Much elimination during absoprtion

Significant elimination: Use intermittent infusion equations

time

FIGURE 14.4 Contrasting steady-state plasma concentration profiles from continuous drug infusion, multiple bolus injections, and multiple intermittent infusions. The upper panel compares the profiles of continuous drug infusion to multiple discrete doses. The lower panel compares the profile from multiple bolus injections to multiple intermittent infusions. To evaluate which equations would be most accurate to substitute for oral equations, the amount of fluctuation that occurs during the dosing interval is assessed. If little fluctuation occurs, continuous infusion equations may be used. If a significant amount of fluctuation occurs, multiple discrete dose equations must be used. To distinguish between bolus injections and intermittent infusions, the amount of elimination that occurs during the absorption period is evaluated. If little elimination occurs, the bolus equations may be used; otherwise, the intermittent infusion equations will have to be used.

fluctuation is present with continuous infusions, and clear fluctuation is present with the pulse-like administration of discrete doses (Figure 14.4). Multiple oral doses would produce little fluctuation if:

A. The dose is absorbed at a constant rate throughout the entire course of the dosing interval. If this is the case, the equations for a continuous infusion may be used. For example, the continuous infusion model is frequently applied to the slow release and absorption of drugs from sustained-release preparations such as theophylline.

    or

B. If the drug's half-life is much greater than the dosing interval, little of the drug is eliminated during the dosing interval, fluctuation will be minimal, and the continuous infusion equations can be used. Commonly, a cutoff of a 20% loss of drug is used [3]. If less than 20% of the drug in the body is lost during the dosing interval, the continuous infusion model may be used. Recall that 20% of the drug in the body is eliminated in a period equal to $\frac{1}{3}t_{1/2}$ (Appendix B). Thus, if the dosing interval is less than $1/3t_{1/2}$, the continuous infusion equations may be used. For example, the continuous infusion model is often applied to oral digoxin, which has a dosing interval (1 day) of about 20% its half-life (5 days). Thus, if:

- $\tau < 1/3t_{1/2}$: the continuous infusion model may be used.

- $\tau > 1/3t_{1/2}$: much drug is eliminated in the dosing interval and multiple discrete dose equations must be used.

Multiple Bolus Injection or Multiple Intermittent Infusion Equations?   When a drug is administered as a bolus injection, the administration process is very rapid. The entire dose is administered almost instantaneously, and no drug is eliminated during the administration period. In the case of intermittent infusions, the administration period is longer (0.5–2 h) and elimination occurs during this input. To decide whether to use the multiple bolus injection model or the intermittent infusion model for orally administered drugs, it is necessary to assess how much elimination occurs during drug absorption. Commonly, a cutoff of 10% is used [3]. If drug absorption is rapid relative to elimination and less than 10% of the drug in the body is eliminated during absorption, the bolus equations may be used. If not, the intermittent infusion equations must be used. Recall that 10% of the drug in the body is lost in a period of $\frac{1}{6}t_{1/2}$ (Appendix B). For example, bolus equations are usually used for regular-release theophylline and valproic acid, both of which are absorbed very rapidly. Thus, if:

- Duration of absorption phase $< \frac{1}{6}t_{1/2}$, multiple bolus equations may be used.

- Duration of absorption phase $> \frac{1}{6}t_{1/2}$, multiple intermittent infusion equations should be used.

14.4 SIMULATION EXERCISE:
http://web.uri.edu/pharmacy/research/rosenbaum/sims

Open model 11, Multiple Oral Doses, which can be found at http://web.uri.edu/pharmacy/ research/rosenbaum/sims/Model11.

Default settings for the model are: the unit of time is the elimination half-life ($t_{1/2}$), dose = 200 mg, Cl = 34.7 L/$t_{1/2}$, Vd = 50 L, k_a = 8 $t_{1/2}^{-1}$, τ = 1 $t_{1/2}$, F = 1, and S = 1.

1. *Review the objectives and the "Model Summary" Page.*
2. *Go to the "Cp–Time Profile" page. Perform a simulation and note:*
   - *The peaks occur later than the time at which the dose is administered, but the trough occurs just before the next dose (t = τ).*
   - *Accumulation causes the plasma concentration at any time during a dosing interval to increase with dose. The extent of accumulation decreases with each dose and eventually stops at steady state.*
   - *It takes about 5 $t_{1/2}$ to reach steady state.*
   - *Hold the mouse over the first peak and a steady-state peak and note that $T_{max,1}$ and $T_{max,ss}$.*
3. *Go to the "Influence of k_a" page. The influence of k_a on the bioavailability parameters and on fluctuation during a dosing interval will be addressed.*
       Bioavailability parameters. For drugs that have long half-lives, and for drugs that cannot be administered to healthy volunteers, such as anticancer drugs, bioavailability and bioequivalence studies may be conducted during a steady-state dosing interval after multiple doses. Simulate with different values of k_a and note the effects on $T_{max,ss}$, $C_{max,ss}$, and the AUC.
   - *Note that as k_a increases, $T_{max,ss}$ decreases, $C_{max,ss}$ increases, and AUC is unaltered.*
       Fluctuation. The default value of k_a is 8 1/$t_{1/2}$. This compares to a value of k of 0.693 1/$t_{1/2}$. Thus, as is typically observed, $k_a > k$ (in this case, k_a is just over

10 times larger than k). Sustained-release products typically have values of k_a that are substantially less than k.

(a) *Clear the graph and simulate the plasma concentration with a k_a value of 0.3 $1/t_{1/2}$, which is about half the value of k. A more prolonged absorption results and little fluctuation is observed during the dosing interval. This is a flip-flop model (see Chapter 9), where the drug's absorption and not its elimination controls the fall in the plasma concentration at later times. When absorption is prolonged, the equations for continuous infusions can be used clinically to calculate doses.*

(b) *Now, increase k_a to 8 $1/t_{1/2}$. Note that much greater fluctuation is observed and the absorption period which, as shown in the display, is 0.43 $t_{1/2}$ (5 * 0.693/8). Thus, about 25% of a dose will be eliminated during this period and the equations for multiple intermittent infusions will need to be used clinically.*

(c) *Increase k_a to 24 $1/t_{1/2}$. Note that much sharper peaks are obtained and the profile is similar to multiple bolus doses. Note also that the absorption period is equal to $\left(5*\frac{0.693}{24}\right)$ or $0.14t_{1/2}$. Less than 10% of the dose will be eliminated in this period. The equations for multiple bolus injections may be used under these circumstances.*

4. *Go to the "Influence of F" page. Simulate with the different values of F and note the effects on $T_{max,ss}$, $C_{max,ss}$, and AUC (shown in the display window) during a steady-state dosing interval.*

   • *As was the case with a single oral dose, reductions in F result in decreases in $C_{max,ss}$ and AUC, but $T_{max,ss}$ is unaffected.*

5. *Go to the "Influence of τ" page. In these simulations, τ will be altered, and the dose must also be altered proportionally to maintain the default rate of drug administration (200 mg/$t_{1/2}$). In this way, the same average steady-state plasma concentration will be achieved.*

   (a) *Let $\tau = 0.25\ t_{1/2}$. During a dosing interval, slightly less than about 20% of the dose will be eliminated. Note that this value of τ results in minimal fluctuation. When τ is $< \frac{1}{3}t_{1/2}$, the equations for a continuous infusion can be approximated for multiple oral doses.*

   (b) *Let tau $= 2\ t_{1/2}$'s. Note the much greater fluctuation. About 75% of the drug in the body will be lost during a dosing interval. In this situation, equations for multiple discrete doses must be used. As discussed in 14.3.1, the amount of elimination that occurs during the absorption period determines whether multiple bolus or multiple infusion equations would be most appropriate. If a significant portion (>10%) of the dose is lost during absorption, the intermittent infusion equations should be used. Otherwise, the equations for multiple intravenous doses may be used.*

REFERENCES

1. Gibaldi, M., and Perrier, D. (1982) *Pharmacokinetics*, 2nd ed., Marcel Dekker, New York.

2. Jambhekar, S. S., and Breen, P. J. (2009) *Basic Pharmacokinetics*, Pharmaceutical Press, London.

3. Winter, M. E. (2010) *Basic Clinical Pharmacokinetics*, 5th ed., Lippincott Williams & Wilkins, Baltimore.

15

NONLINEAR PHARMACOKINETICS

Sara E. Rosenbaum

Objectives

The material in this chapter will enable the reader to:

1. Differentiate the characteristics of linear and nonlinear pharmacokinetics

2. Understand how nonlinearity can arise in pharmacokinetics

3. Understand thoroughly the pharmacokinetics of single capacity-limited elimination

Basic Pharmacokinetics and Pharmacodynamics: An Integrated Textbook and Computer Simulations,
Second Edition. Edited by Sara E. Rosenbaum.
© 2017 John Wiley & Sons, Inc. Published 2017 by John Wiley & Sons, Inc.

4. Understand how nonlinear pharmacokinetics is handled clinically
5. Gain experience individualizing doses based on estimates of patients' K_m and V_{max} values obtained from one and two plasma concentrations

15.1 LINEAR PHARMACOKINETICS

The vast majority of drugs used clinically follow linear pharmacokinetics. The pharmacokinetics discussed up to this point in the book are all examples of linear pharmacokinetics. The term *linear* clearly cannot refer to the relationship between plasma concentration and time, which is linear only when the plasma concentration is under the sole influence of first-order elimination, and even then, only when the plasma concentration is converted into the logarithm domain. The term *linear* refers to the relationship between the dose and the plasma concentration at any time after drug administration. In linear pharmacokinetics, the plasma concentration at any time after a dose is proportional to the dose. Linearity is a consequence of the fact that all processes in drug disposition are first order and/or that the pharmacokinetic parameters are constant and do not change with dose.

Figure 15.1 shows the outcome of linear pharmacokinetics for single doses. Plasma concentrations at any time after an extravascular or intravenous dose are directly proportional to dose (Figure 15.1a). If plasma concentrations are normalized by dose, the plots from different doses are superimposed (Figure 15.1b). A distinctive characteristic that is often used as a check for linearity is that the area under the plasma concentration–time curve from time zero to infinity (AUC) is directly proportional to dose (Figure 15.1c).

Figure 15.2 shows some important characteristics of linear pharmacokinetics associated with extended drug administration. In Figure 15.2a, it can be seen that plasma concentration doubles with every doubling of the rate of drug administration. Figure 15.2b shows an extremely important characteristic of linear pharmacokinetics: The average steady-state plasma concentration is directly proportional to the rate of drug administration. This relationship is used extensively when measured plasma concentrations are used to make dosage adjustments. For example, if a steady-state plasma concentration is half of its goal value, a doubling of the rate of drug administration (double the dose or halve the dosing frequency) should achieve the goal. If a patient is found to have only one-third of the normal clearance, the usual rate of drug administration would produce three times the usual plasma concentration ($S \cdot F \cdot R_a = Cl \cdot Cp_{ss}$). Thus, for this patient, the normal rate of administration should be reduced by one-third (reduce the dose by one-third or increase the dosing interval threefold).

Linear pharmacokinetics provides the basis of bioavailability and bioequivalence studies. As seen in Chapter 9,

$$\text{AUC} = \frac{F \cdot D}{Cl} \qquad (15.1)$$

In linear pharmacokinetics, clearance is a constant for a given drug:

$$F \propto \frac{\text{AUC}}{D} \qquad (15.2)$$

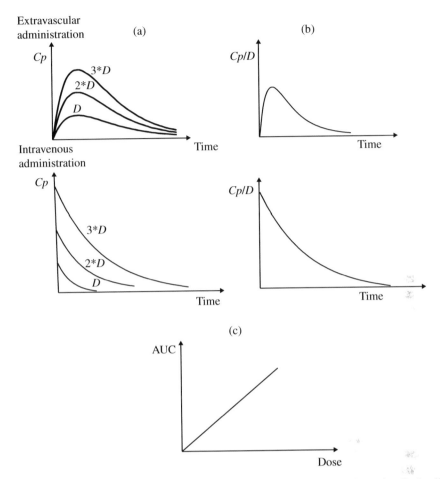

FIGURE 15.1 Characteristics of the plasma concentration–time profile for drugs that display linear pharmacokinetics. Part (a) demonstrates that the plasma concentration is proportional to the dose at any time; (b) shows that dose-normalized plasma concentrations for a drug are superimposed over each other; and (c) demonstrates that the area under the plasma concentration time–curve (AUC) is proportional to the dose.

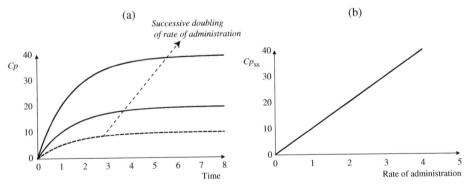

FIGURE 15.2 Relationship between plasma concentration and the rate of drug administration for a drug that displays linear pharmacokinetics. A successive doubling of the rate of administration doubles the plasma concentrations at any time (a). The steady-state plasma concentration (Cp_{ss}) is directly proportional to the rate of drug administration (b).

Thus, the bioavailability (F) of a drug can be assessed from the dose-normalized AUC. Absolute bioavailability of an extravascular dose (F_{PO}) is determined by comparing its dose-normalized AUC to that after intravenous administration ($F_{IV} = 1$).

$$F_{PO} = \frac{AUC_{PO}/D_{PO}}{AUC_{IV}/D_{IV}} \tag{15.3}$$

In bioequivalence studies, where the bioavailability of two different formulations of a drug is compared,

$$\frac{F_T}{F_S} = \frac{AUC_T \cdot D_S}{AUC_S \cdot D_T} \tag{15.4}$$

where the subscripts T and S stand for test and standard, respectively.

If $D_T = D_S$, relative bioavailability can be assessed simply by comparing the AUC values of the two products:

$$\frac{F_T}{F_S} = \frac{AUC_T}{AUC_S} \tag{15.5}$$

Nonlinearity in the pharmacokinetics of a drug greatly complicates drug development, therapeutic drug use, and assessment of bioavailability. Nonlinearity can have a number of different origins but arises when a process in absorption, distribution, metabolism, or excretion (ADME) deviates from a first-order process, and/or when a drug's pharmacokinetic parameters change with dose.

15.2 NONLINEAR PROCESSES IN ABSORPTION, DISTRIBUTION, METABOLISM, AND ELIMINATION

Most commonly, nonlinearity in pharmacokinetics arises when therapeutic drug concentrations are high enough to saturate an enzyme or another protein involved in ADME. Consequently, nonlinear pharmacokinetics has the potential to arise whenever a protein is involved in ADME. Table 15.1 lists processes in ADME that involve proteins and which as a result have the potential to become saturated. The expected outcome of the saturation is also shown.

Some clinical examples of the saturation of the processes listed in Table 15.1 include reduced absorption of riboflavin at higher doses as a result of a saturation of its uptake transporter in the gastrointestinal membrane; reduced presystemic extraction of propranolol with higher doses, resulting in higher bioavailability; dose-dependent protein binding of valproic acid; saturable tissue uptake of methotrexate; and saturation of the metabolism of phenytoin and ethanol at higher doses.

Nonlinearity can also arise through some other mechanisms. For example, drugs such as carbamazepine that induce their own metabolism will display nonlinear pharmacokinetics until the induction process stabilizes, which generally takes about 10–14 days. The bioavailability of drugs that are poorly soluble in gastrointestinal fluid may decrease with increases in dose or changes in pH. For example, the dissolution and bioavailability of ketoconazole change with changes in gastric pH. Nonlinear pharmacokinetics can also arise from pharmacological or toxicological actions of a drug. For example, theophylline

TABLE 15.1   Examples of Processes in ADME That Can Become Saturated

Process	Typical Outcome of Saturation
Absorption	
Uptake transporters	Less absorption at higher doses
Efflux transporters	More absorption at higher doses
Enzymes in enterocytes	More absorption at higher doses
Hepatic first-pass enzymes	More absorption at higher
Distribution	
Plasma proteins	Higher free fractions at higher doses
Uptake transporters	Lower tissue concentrations at higher doses
Efflux transporters	Higher tissues concentrations at higher doses
Metabolism	
Hepatic enzymes	Lower clearance, slower elimination at higher doses
Excretion	
Uptake transporters	Lower clearance, slower elimination at higher doses
Efflux transporters	Lower clearance, slower elimination at higher doses

induces concentration-dependent diuresis, which results in increased renal excretion with dose. Interestingly, theophylline's overall pharmacokinetics tend to be linear because it also displays saturable metabolism, and the increase in renal clearance and decrease in hepatic clearance that occur with higher plasma concentrations tend to offset each other. The clearance of aminoglycosides can decrease with dose as a result of dose-dependent renal toxicity.

The outcome of nonlinearity will depend on the specific process involved. For example, saturation of uptake transporters in the GI membrane or poor dissolution in the GI fluid will result in larger doses producing lower than expected plasma concentrations (Table 15.1). Conversely, with increasing doses, saturation of GI efflux transporters or enzymes in the enterocytes will result in plasma concentrations that are higher than those expected from linear processes (Table 15.1). Nonlinear or capacity-limited metabolism is the most common example of nonlinearity observed clinically, and the remainder of the chapter is devoted to this topic.

15.3 PHARMACOKINETICS OF CAPACITY-LIMITED METABOLISM

The most clinically important type of nonlinear pharmacokinetics is saturable metabolism, which is also referred to as capacity-limited metabolism, biotransformation, or elimination. It arises when therapeutic concentrations of a drug partially or fully saturate an enzyme(s) that plays an important role in elimination of the drug. To understand the factors that control nonlinearity and explain why only a fraction of the drugs that undergo metabolism are subject to nonlinearity, it is necessary to review the kinetics of enzymatic metabolism. This material, which was covered in Chapter 5, is reviewed here.

15.3.1 Kinetics of Enzymatic Processes

The kinetics of hepatic metabolism, like many enzymatic processes often follow Michaelis–Menten kinetics, which provides the following relationship between the rate of metabolism (V) and the unbound drug concentration in the liver (Ch_u):

$$V = \frac{V_{\max} \cdot Ch_u}{K_m + Ch_u} \tag{15.6}$$

where V_{max} is the maximum rate of metabolism that is observed when all the enzyme is saturated with the substrate drug, and K_m is the Michaelis–Menten constant, which is a dissociation constant (as affinity for the enzyme increases, K_m decreases). The units of V are amount per unit time, and the units of K_m are concentration.

If it can be assumed that a drug very rapidly distributes to the liver, the unbound concentration in the plasma will equal to the unbound concentration in the liver. Further, if it is assumed that the fraction unbound does not change over the range of therapeutic plasma concentrations, the Michealis–Menten equation can be expressed using Cp as the driving concentration. This has the advantage of providing K_m in terms of the plasma concentration:

$$V = \frac{V_{max} \cdot Cp}{K_m + Cp} \qquad (15.7)$$

Accordingly, the typical hyperbolic relationship of a capacity-limited system is observed between the rate of metabolism and the plasma concentration (Figure 15.3). Also, as was shown in Chapter 5, the concentration that is associated with half the maximum rate is equal to the drug's K_m value. Two limiting situations exist for the rate of metabolism:

1. At low drug concentrations ($Cp \ll K_m$), there is an excess amount of enzyme present. Under these circumstances, as the concentration of the drug increases, the rate can increase proportionally: The rate is proportional to the plasma concentration, and metabolism is an apparent first-order process (Figure 15.3). Mathematically, $Cp \ll K_m$, $K_m + Cp \approx K_m$, and

$$V = \frac{V_{max} \cdot Cp}{K_m + Cp} = \frac{V_{max} \cdot Cp}{K_m} = \text{constant} \cdot Cp$$

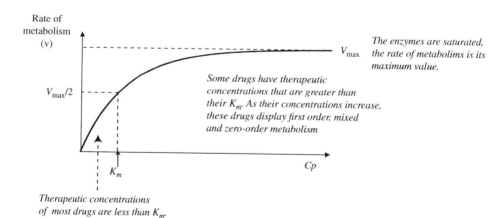

FIGURE 15.3   Michaelis–Menten kinetics. At low drug concentrations, excess enzyme is available to metabolize the drug, and the rate can increase in direct proportion to increases in concentration (first order). As the drug concentration increases, some saturation is seen and the rate of metabolism can no longer keep up with increases in the drug concentration. At high drug concentrations, the enzyme is completely saturated and the maximum rate of metabolism is observed. At this point, increases in drug concentration are not associated with any further increases in the rate of metabolism.

2. When the drug concentration becomes very high, the enzyme is fully saturated and the rate is constant at its maximum value, V_{max}. The rate of metabolism is a zero-order process (Figure 15.3). Mathematically, $Cp \gg K_m$, $K_m + Cp \approx Cp$, and

$$V = \frac{V_{max} \cdot Cp}{K_m + Cp} = \frac{V_{max} \cdot Cp}{Cp} = V_{max}$$

Between these two extremes, metabolism is mixed order and nonlinear.

It is very important to note that the therapeutic concentrations of most drugs are well below their K_m values. As a result, the enzymatic metabolism of the majority of drugs used in clinical practice follow apparent first-order kinetics, and their pharmacokinetics are linear. A small number of drugs, however, have therapeutic plasma concentrations that approach or exceed their K_m value. For example, the average K_m value for phenytoin is 4 mg/L, which compares to a therapeutic range of 10–20 mg/L.

15.3.2   Plasma Concentration–Time Profile

Figure 15.4 shows the fall in the plasma concentration with time on a semilogarithmic scale after a series of intravenous doses of a drug that displays saturable metabolism (Figure 15.4a). The different plots represent a successive doubling of the dose. It can be seen that the profile from the smallest dose resembles that observed with linear pharmacokinetics: a typical straight-line relationship between ln Cp and time. But notice that with the larger doses, the initial fall in the plasma concentration is much less steep than that found with linear pharmacokinetics. At higher concentrations, the initial fall takes on a concave profile. This is the result of a saturation of the enzymes at higher concentrations and the inability of the rate of metabolism to increase in proportion to the increase in concentrations. The rate is less than it would be for a first-order process. As a result, the AUC increases disproportionately with dose (Figure 15.4b). The initial plasma concentration (Cp_0) for drugs that display saturable metabolism is proportional to dose, as it is dependent on the drug's volume of distribution and is independent of its elimination characteristics.

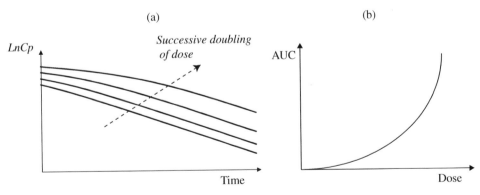

FIGURE 15.4   Impact of nonlinear elimination on the plasma concentration–time profile after single doses. Graph (a) is a semilogarithmic plot of plasma concentration against time after a successive doubling of an intravenous dose. After large doses, the initial fall in the plasma concentration with time is less steep than with linear pharmacokinetics. Graph (b) shows that the area under the plasma concentration–time curve (AUC) increases with dose for drugs that display saturable elimination.

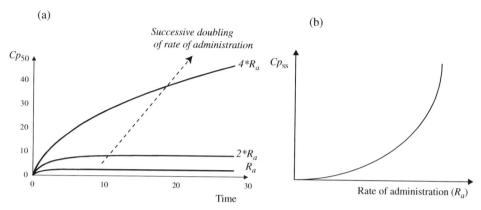

FIGURE 15.5   Impact of nonlinear elimination on the pharmacokinetics of chronic drug administration. Graph (a) shows the plasma concentration–time profile after a successive doubling of the rate of administration from an infusion. After the first doubling, the plasma concentration at any time increases by slightly more than double. After the second doubling, the plasma concentration at any time into therapy increases several folds. Steady state has not been achieved over the observation period, but the steady-state plasma concentration will be over eightfold greater than that from the previous dose. Graph (b) shows that the steady-state plasma concentration (Cp_{ss}) increases disproportionally with the rate of drug administration. At a high rate of administration, the Cp_{ss} tends toward infinity.

The typical plasma concentration profile seen with the extended administration of drugs that display nonlinear metabolism is shown in Figure 15.5a. The profile shows the effect of a successive doubling of the rate of drug administration. Note that the first doubling produces about a three- to fourfold increase in the steady-state plasma concentration. A further doubling results in an over eightfold increase in the plasma concentration. Figure 15.5b shows the relationship between the steady-state plasma concentration and a wide range of rates of drug administration. It can be seen that increases in the rate result in disproportionate increases in the steady-state plasma concentrations. At high rates, the concentration tends toward infinity.

15.4   PHENYTOIN

Phenytoin is an important example of a drug that displays nonlinear pharmacokinetics. Although it has a number of different indications, it is used primarily as an anticonvulsant in the treatment and prophylaxis of seizure disorders. It is very commonly prescribed, and many patients take oral phenytoin over periods of many years. Its widespread use has provided extensive experience handling nonlinear pharmacokinetics clinically. Also, since phenytoin has a narrow therapeutic range, its dose must be individualized, which has resulted in the development of therapeutic monitoring procedures tailored specifically to nonlinear pharmacokinetics. As a result, phenytoin provides an interesting example to use in a discussion of the therapeutic implications of nonlinearity.

There are many interesting aspects to the pharmacokinetics and pharmacodynamics of phenytoin. It has a very narrow therapeutic range (10–20 mg/L), and plasma concentrations outside these values are associated with very serious clinical consequences: Subtherapeutic concentrations place patients at risk for dangerous breakthrough seizures, and concentrations above the maximum tolerated concentration are associated with a number of concentration-dependent conditions. With increasing concentrations of phenytoin, these include nystagmus, ataxia, slurred speech, confusion, and coma. Thus, it is important to maintain plasma concentrations of phenytoin in the therapeutic range.

Phenytoin is eliminated primarily by saturable metabolism, which is described by the Michaelis–Menten equation and parameterized using K_m and V_{max}. The population average value of phenytoin's K_m is around 4 mg/L, which is lower than the therapeutic range and illustrates why nonlinear pharmacokinetics are observed. The population average V_{max} value of phenytoin is about 7 mg/kg/day or about 500 mg/day for the standard 70-kg male.

Phenytoin displays wide interindividual variability in the values of both its K_m and V_{max}. As a result, a standard dose will be subtherpaeutic in some patients, therapeutic in others, and toxic in some. A study demonstrated that a standard dose of 300 mg/day of phenytoin achieved a therapeutic plasma concentration in only about 30% of patients [1]. The remainder had either subtherapeutic or toxic concentrations. The study illustrated the importance of individualizing the dose of phenytoin for each patient. Typically, this is accomplished by measuring a steady-state plasma concentration about 2 weeks after the start of therapy. If the plasma concentration is too low, the dose is increased. Conversely, if the plasma concentration is too high, the dose is decreased. However, nonlinear pharmacokinetics complicate the adjustment process, and proportional adjustments in the dose must not be made. A doubling of the dose in response to a plasma concentration of 6 mg/L could quite possibly produce toxic concentrations and place the patient at risk for the dangerous side effects of this drug.

The extensive and variable plasma protein binding of phenytoin adds another interesting dimension to the evaluation of phenytoin's pharmacokinetics and pharmacodynamics, but this topic is not addressed in this chapter.

15.4.1   Basic Equation for Steady State

The pharmacokinetic model developed for phenytoin must reflect its primary clinical use as an oral preparation that is taken over an extended period of time. The key features of the model are as follows:

- A one-compartmental model can be used to describe the pharmacokinetics of phenytoin after oral doses (Figure 15.6).

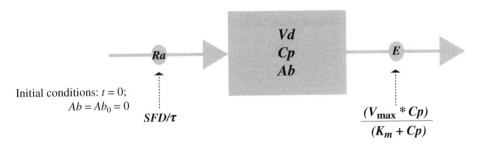

FIGURE 15.6   Pharmacokinetic model for phenytoin consistent with a one-compartment model. The input, the rate of drug administration (R_a), is $S{\cdot}F{\cdot}D/\tau$. Elimination (E) is given by the Michaelis–Menten equation.

- Chronic drug administration is incorporated as the input into the compartment using the rate of drug administration, or dose/dosing interval.

- Phenytoin is eliminated primarily by saturable metabolism ($fe = 0.01–0.05$), mainly by CYP2C9, but CYP2C19 is also involved. Renal excretion is minor and can be ignored, and the various metabolic pathways can be merged into a single capacity-limited process. Thus, elimination is modeled using the Michaelis–Menten equation, which, as discussed earlier, in clinical applications assumes that metabolism is driven by Cp. This is a reasonable assumption for phenytoin and allows K_m to be determined in units of Cp. The rate of elimination is given by:

$$\text{rate of elimination} = \frac{V_{\max} \cdot Cp}{K_m + Cp}$$

$$-\frac{dAb}{dt} = \frac{V_{\max} \cdot Cp}{K_m + Cp} \tag{15.8}$$

- Drug absorption from phenytoin, particularly from the innovator product Dilantin, is very slow, and it can be assumed to occur at a constant rate throughout the entire dosing interval. This enables the infusion model (constant, zero-order drug administration) to be used to derive equations for phenytoin (see Chapter 14). The constant rate of administration of phenytoin is the effective dose divided by the dosing interval, which is typically 0.5 or 1 day. Overall, the rate of change of the amount of drug in the body with time is

$$\frac{dAb}{dt} = \text{rate of inputs} - \text{rate of outputs}$$

$$= \frac{S \cdot F \cdot D}{\tau} - \frac{V_{\max} \cdot Cp}{K_m + Cp} \tag{15.9}$$

where S is the salt factor, F is the bioavailability, D is the administered dose, and τ is the dosing interval.

- Phenytoin's plasma concentrations are monitored primarily at steady state when the equations can be simplified quite considerably. At steady state, the plasma concentration (Cp_{ss}) is constant and the rate of input is equal to the rate of output (Figure 15.7):

$$\text{rate of administration} = \text{rate of elimination}$$

$$\boxed{\frac{S \cdot F \cdot D}{\tau} = \frac{V_{\max} \cdot Cp_{ss}}{K_m + Cp_{ss}}} \tag{15.10}$$

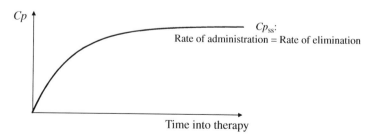

FIGURE 15.7   Predicted plasma concentrations of phenytoin that result from its constant, continuous administration. At steady state, the plasma concentration (Cp_{ss}) remains constant. Thus, the rate of elimination must be equal to the rate of drug administration.

This single equation is used extensively for phenytoin and other drugs that display saturable elimination. Population average values or literature values of the pharmacokinetic parameters can be used in equation (15.10) to estimate plasma concentrations of phenytoin from different doses. It can also be used to estimate doses to achieve desired plasma concentrations. If an individual patient's V_{max} and K_m values are known, patient-specific doses can be determined. Also, as demonstrated in later sections (Sections 15.4.6.1 and 15.4.6.2), this equation is used clinically to estimate a patient's K_m and/or V_{max} values from measured plasma concentrations of phenytoin.

In addition to the arrangement shown above, equation (15.10) has two other useful arrangements. These are provided below.

$$Cp_{ss} = \frac{K_m \cdot S \cdot F \cdot R_a}{V_{max} - S \cdot F \cdot R_a} \tag{15.11}$$

where R_a is the rate of drug administration or D/τ. The denominator in equation (15.11) demonstrates the importance of ensuring that the rate of drug administration does not exceed the drug's V_{max} value. If this happens, the steady-state plasma concentration will tend toward infinity. For example, suppose that a patient who has a V_{max} of phenytoin of 350 mg/day received a dose of 400 mg of phenytoin per day. For every day that the patient took this dose, he or she would accumulate 50 mg phenytoin. Unlike linear pharmacokinetics, the accumulation would not abate but would continue for as long as the patient took 400 mg of phenytoin daily.

$$V_{max} = \frac{S \cdot F \cdot R_a \cdot (K_m + Cp_{ss})}{Cp_{ss}} \tag{15.12}$$

Some example applications of these formulas are presented below.

15.4.2   Estimation of Doses and Plasma Concentrations

Next, we look at the use of the equations to estimate doses and plasma concentrations.

Example 15.1   A patient is to begin taking phenytoin. A steady plasma concentration of 15 mg/L is desired. Assuming a V_{max} of 400 mg/day and a K_m value of 4 mg/L, what rate of administration of phenytoin sodium ($S = 0.92$ and $F = 1$) should be used?

Solution   Using equation (15.10)

$$\frac{0.92 \times 1 \times D}{\tau} = \frac{400 \times 15}{4 + 15}$$

$$\frac{D}{\tau} = 343 \text{ mg per day}$$

Thus, a dose of 350 mg of phenytoin sodium per day would be administered.

Example 15.2   A patient's individual V_{max} and K_m values are found to be 450 mg/day and 5 mg/L, respectively. What are her/his estimated steady-state plasma concentrations from doses of (a) 350 mg/day, (b) 400 mg/day, and (c) 450 mg/day?

Solution

(a) For a rate of administration of 350 mg/day, using equation (15.11), we obtain

$$Cp_{ss} = \frac{5 \times 0.92 \times 350}{450 - 0.92 \times 350} = 12.6 \text{ mg/L}$$

(b) For a rate of administration of 400 mg/day,

$$Cp_{ss} = \frac{5 \times 0.92 \times 400}{450 - 0.92 \times 400} = 22.4 \text{ mg/L}$$

(c) For a rate of administration of 450 mg/day,

$$Cp_{ss} = \frac{5 \times 0.92 \times 450}{450 - 0.92 \times 450} = 57.5 \text{ mg/L}$$

Example 15.2 demonstrates how the steady-state plasma concentration increases disproportionately with increases dose. A 15% increase in the rate of administration from 350 to 400 mg/day increased the steady-state plasma concentration by about 80%. A similar increase from 400 to 450 mg/day increased the steady-state plasma concentration about 150%.

15.4.2.1 Simulation Exercise: http://web.uri.edu/pharmacy/research/rosenbaum/sims
Open model 12, Nonlinear Pharmacokinetics and Phenytoin, which can be found at http://web.uri.edu/pharmacy/research/rosenbaum/sims/Model12.

Default settings for the model are dose = 350 mg, S = 0.92, and F = 1; τ = 1 day; V_{max} = 450 mg/day; K_m = 6 mg/L; and Vd = 45.5 L.

1. *Review the objectives, explore the model, and review the model summary.*

2. *Go to the "Cp–Time Profile" page. Observe the effects of increasing the dose from 350, to 400, and then to 450 mg. Note that, in contrast to linear pharmacokinetics:*

   • *Increases in dose produce disproportionate increases in the steady-state plasma concentration.*

   • *As the dose increases, it takes longer to achieve steady state.*

3. *Observe the effect of doubling the original dose of 350 mg, which achieved a steady-state plasma concentration of about 15 mg/L in about 2–3 weeks. Doubling the dose produces plasma concentrations that exceed the therapeutic range (>20 mg/L) during the third day of treatment and which appear to be heading toward infinity. Note that this rate of administration (700 mg of phenytoin sodium per day or about 650 mg of pure phenytoin per day) exceeds V_{max} (450 mg/day). As therapy continues, the patient will accumulate 200 mg of phenytoin daily.*

15.4.3 Influence of K_m and V_{max} and Factors That Affect These Parameters

For drugs that display nonlinear pharmacokinetics, the relationship between dose and the steady-state plasma concentration is controlled by V_{max} and K_m. Example 15.2 demonstrated the very sensitive nature of this relationship. It is important to understand the role that each parameter plays in the dose–plasma concentration relationship. Additionally, it is important to be aware of any situations where either of the parameters may differ from normal and to know how to plan therapy in the light of any known or suspected changes.

TABLE 15.2   Factors That Can Alter the Value of V_{max} and K_m

Parameter	Factors Affecting Parameter	Direction of Change in Parameter	Outcome
V_{max}	Enzyme induction (e.g., carbamazepine)	↑	↓Cp
	Liver disease (e.g., cirrhosis)	↓	↑Cp
K_m	Reversible, competitive inhibitors (e.g., cimetidine, valproic acid, and fluoxetine)	↑	↑Cp
	Displacement from plasma proteins, valproic acid, and hypoalbinemia	↓	↓Cp

V_{max}, the maximum rate of metabolism, is a function of the amount of enzyme present. Enzyme induction will increase V_{max}, and hepatic diseases such as cirrhosis, which reduces the number of functioning hepatocytes, will decrease V_{max}. K_m is a dissociation constant and is a reciprocal expression of the affinity of the drug for the enzyme. As K_m increases, affinity decreases. Concomitant medications that competitively inhibit enzymes responsible for the elimination of a victim drug will increase its K_m. The displacement of a drug from its plasma protein binding sites will produce an apparent decrease in K_m. This is because displacement increases the unbound fraction, which enables more drug to interact with the enzyme at a given concentration. Thus, based on total plasma concentration, it will appear that affinity has increased (i.e., K_m has decreased).

Table 15.2 shows some factors that can affect phenytoin's V_{max} and K_m. It also shows how the changes affect the plasma concentration. However, the clearest way to appreciate these effects is through simulation.

15.4.3.1   Simulation Exercise

Open model 12, Nonlinear Pharmacokinetics and Phenytoin, which can be found at http://web.uri.edu/pharmacy/research/rosenbaum/sims/Model12.

The default settings for the model are dose = 350 mg, τ = 1 day, V_{max} = 450 mg/day, K_m = 6 mg/L, and Vd = 45.5 L.

Go to the "V_{max} and K_m" page.

1. *While maintaining the default values of K_m (6 mg/L), increase V_{max} from 300 to 400 to 600 mg/day. V_{max} represents the maximum rate of metabolism and is a function of the amount of enzyme present in a system. Note that as V_{max} increases, the plasma concentration at any time decreases. Note also that as V_{max} increases, it takes less time to reach steady state.*

2. *Now maintain the default value of V_{max} (450 mg/day) and increase K_m from 2 to 4 to 8 mg/L. K_m is a dissociation constant, so it is a reciprocal measure of affinity. As K_m increases, the affinity of the drug for the enzyme decreases. Note that as K_m increases (affinity decreases), the Cp at any time increases and it takes more time to get to steady state.*

The simulations have demonstrated that the dose of phenytoin may have to be reduced (increased) in patients with decreased (increased) V_{max} values and/or increased (decreased) K_m values.

15.4.4 Time to Eliminate the Drug

When elimination is not a first-order process, the concept of a half-life does not hold and there is no simple way to estimate the time it takes the plasma concentration to fall by 50% or any other amount. The rate of elimination of phenytoin was presented previously [equation (15.8)]. If there is no ongoing drug input, the drug in the body is only under the influence of elimination:

$$-\frac{dAb}{dt} = \frac{V_{max} \cdot Cp}{K_m + Cp}$$

Substituting for Ab where $Ab = Cp \cdot Vd$, we obtain

$$-\frac{dCp}{dt} = \frac{V_{max} \cdot Cp}{Vd \cdot (K_m + Cp)} \tag{15.13}$$

This equation can be integrated [1] to yield

$$t = \frac{Vd}{V_{max}} \left(Cp_0 - Cp_t + K_m \ln \frac{Cp_0}{Cp_t} \right) \tag{15.14}$$

where Cp_0 is the plasma concentration at $t = 0$, and Cp_t is the plasma concentration at time t. Equation (15.14) can be used to calculate the time for the plasma concentration to fall from one value (Cp_0) to another (Cp_t).

Example 15.3   A patient ($Vd = 45$ L, $V_{max} = 400$ mg/day, and $K_m = 4$ mg/L) presents with a phenytoin concentration of 40 mg/L.

(a) How long will it take for the plasma concentration to reach the therapeutic range (20 mg/L)?

(b) How long will it take for plasma concentrations to fall another 50%, to 10 mg/L?

Solution

(a) Substituting the values into equation (15.14), we have

$$t = \frac{45}{400} \left(40 - 20 + 4 \cdot \ln \frac{40}{20} \right) = 2.56 \text{ days}$$

(b) Substituting into equation (15.14) gives us

$$t = \frac{45}{400} \left(20 - 10 + 4 \times \ln \frac{20}{10} \right) = 1.43 \text{ days}$$

Note that the time for the plasma concentration to fall by 50% is not constant but decreases as the plasma concentration decreases. This is because at higher concentrations, there is a greater degree of saturation of the enzymes and a greater fraction of the drug present cannot be metabolized.

In certain circumstances, it may be necessary to estimate how long it takes a certain amount of drug in the body to fall to a specific amount. Equation (15.14) can be adapted for this:

$$t = \frac{1}{V_{max}} \left(Ab_0 - Ab_t + K_m \cdot \ln \frac{Ab_0}{Ab_t} \right) \tag{15.15}$$

where Ab_0 is the amount in the body at time $t = 0$, Ab_t is the amount at time $= t$, and K_m has units of amount [i.e., K_m (mg/L) $\cdot$ Vd (L)].

15.4.5 Time to Reach Steady State

Once again, because elimination is not a first-order process, there is no simple way to estimate the time it takes to reach steady state. Information on the time to take to get to steady state can be obtained by deriving an equation for the plasma concentration at any time. This is accomplished using the fundamental equation for the model (15.9), which is reproduced here:

$$\frac{dAb}{dt} = \frac{S \cdot F \cdot D}{\tau} - \frac{V_{max} \cdot Cp}{K_m + Cp}$$

This equation is integrated, solved for plasma concentration, and then rearranged to provide an expression for the time it takes to get to 90% steady state ($t_{90\%}$) [2, 3]:

$$t_{90\%} = \frac{K_m \cdot Vd}{(V_{max} - S \cdot F \cdot R_a)^2}(2.3\, V_{max} - 0.9 \cdot S \cdot F \cdot R_a) \tag{15.16}$$

Equation (15.16) demonstrates that the time to steady state, or 90% steady state, is dependent on the pharmacokinetic parameters K_m and V_{max}, and in contrast to linear pharmacokinetics, it is also dependent on the rate of administration. As demonstrated in the simulations, it takes longer to get to steady state with higher rates of administration. More specifically, it is the difference between V_{max} and the rate of drug administration that determines the time to reach steady state. As the rate of administration approaches V_{max} (as complete saturation of the enzyme is approached), the denominator in equation (15.16) gets smaller and it takes longer to get to steady state. As $S \cdot F \cdot R_a$ approaches V_{max}, $t_{90\%}$ tends toward infinity.

Example 15.4   The population average parameters for phenytoin in a standard 70-kg male are: $Vd = 45.5$ L, $V_{max} = 400$ mg/day, and $K_m = 6$ mg/L. How long will it take to get to 90% steady state when the dose is administered at a rate of 300 mg of phenytoin sodium per day?

Solution   Substituting the parameter values into equation (15.16) gives

$$t_{90\%} = \frac{6 \times 45.5}{(400 - 0.92 \times 300)^2}(2.3 \times 400 - 0.9 \times 0.92 \times 300) = 11.9 \text{ days}$$

Note that if the dose is only 250 mg, 90% steady state is reached in about 7 days, but when the dose is increased to 350 mg and approaches V_{max}, the time to reach steady state increases to around 28 days.

15.4.6   Individualization of Doses of Phenytoin

When patients are started on phenytoin therapy, the wide interindividual variability in V_{max} and K_m, combined with phenytoin's narrow therapeutic range, makes it essential to monitor the plasma concentrations and individualize the dose if necessary. When patients start therapy, they are evaluated to determine if any obvious factors are present that would warrant a dose that is different from the standard. Factors to be considered include:

- Concomitant medications that could alter intrinsic clearance or alter plasma protein binding.
- The presence of liver disease, which could reduce intrinsic clearance and/or alter protein binding.
- The presence of renal disease, which could alter protein binding.

Assuming that none of the foregoing factors are present, the patient may be started on a standard dose of about 7 mg/kg/day of phenytoin sodium. Once steady state has been achieved, after about 2 weeks, the phenytoin concentration can be evaluated. If the plasma concentration is in the therapeutic range, the dose will be maintained. If not, the dose will have to be modified, and the process should be based on the patient's history with the drug: that is, the steady-state plasma concentration achieved by the initial rate of drug administration (one $S \cdot F \cdot R_a$–Cp_{ss} data pair).

15.4.6.1   Modification of Dose Based on One Data Pair

The process of individualization involves estimating the patient's individual pharmacokinetic parameters for phenytoin. Recall the basic formula that relates the rate of drug administration to the steady-state plasma concentration:

$$Cp_{ss} = \frac{K_m \cdot S \cdot F \cdot R}{V_{max} - S \cdot F \cdot R}$$

In contrast to linear pharmacokinetics ($Cp_{ss} = S \cdot F \cdot R_a / Cl$), the relationship between Cp_{ss} and $S \cdot F \cdot R_a$ is controlled by two parameters (V_{max} and K_m) rather than one (Cl). With only one Cp_{ss}–$S \cdot F \cdot R$ data pair, it is possible to estimate only *one* of phenytoin's pharmacokinetic parameters. Since it is critical that the drug is not administered at a rate that exceeds V_{max}, this parameter is usually estimated first. The population average value of K_m (4 mg/L) is assumed for the patient.

Recall the arrangement of the basic equation that solves for V_{max}:

$$V_{max} = \frac{S \cdot F \cdot R_a \cdot (K_m + Cp_{ss})}{Cp_{ss}} \tag{15.17}$$

The initial rate of drug administration ($S \cdot F \cdot R_a$) and the steady-state concentration it achieved are substituted in the equation along with the population average K_m of 4 mg/L, and V_{max} is estimated. The V_{max} calculated, the population average K_m (4 mg/L), and the steady-state plasma concentration desired (usually 15 mg/L) are then substituted into the arrangement of the basic equation that solves for $S \cdot F \cdot R_a$:

$$S \cdot F \cdot R_a = \frac{V_{max} \cdot Cp_{ss}}{K_m + Cp_{ss}} \tag{15.18}$$

A new rate of drug administration is then determined based on the patient's previous history with the drug.

Example 15.5   A patient has been taking dilantin 300 mg daily for 2 weeks. At this time, a plasma sample reveals a phenytoin concentration of 8 mg/L. Recommend a new dose to achieve a steady-state concentration of 15 mg/L.

Solution   The population average K_m (4 mg/L) will be assumed. Substituting in equation (15.17) to estimate the patient's V_{max} leads to

$$V_{max} = \frac{0.92 \times 300 \times (4 + 8)}{8} = 414 \text{ mg/day}$$

This estimated V_{max} value and the population average K_m are now used in equation (15.18) to estimate a rate of administration to provide the desired Cp_{ss} of 15 mg/L:

$$R_a = \frac{414 \times 15}{(4 + 15) \times 0.92} = 355 \text{ mg/day}$$

The new rate of drug administration may also be assessed about 2 weeks later when the new steady state would be expected. If this steady-state plasma concentration is not satisfactory, a new rate of drug administration must be determined. If this is the case, two $S \cdot F \cdot R_a$–Cp_{ss} data pairs are now available. These can be used to estimate both the V_{max} and K_m values of the patient.

15.4.6.2 Modification of Dose Based on Two Data Pairs
The method of Ludden is a common mathematical approach used to determine K_m and V_{max} from two or more data pairs. Taking the basic equation that is expressed in terms of Cp_{ss}

$$Cp_{ss} = \frac{K_m \cdot S \cdot F \cdot R_a}{V_{max} - S \cdot F \cdot R_a} \tag{15.19}$$

Rearranging gives us

$$V_{max} - S \cdot F \cdot R_a = \frac{K_m \cdot S \cdot F \cdot R_a}{Cp_{ss}} \tag{15.20}$$

Rearranging again, we obtain

$$S \cdot F \cdot R_a = V_{max} - \frac{K_m \cdot S \cdot F \cdot R_a}{Cp_{ss}} \tag{15.21}$$

A plot of $S \cdot F \cdot R_a$ against $S \cdot F \cdot R_a/Cp_{ss}$ yields a straight line of slope—K_m and intercept V_{max} (Figure 15.8). If more than two data pairs are available, a full plot can be constructed. If only two data pairs are available, they are simply used to calculate the slope of the line $S \cdot F \cdot R_a$ against $S \cdot F \cdot R_a/Cp_{ss}$. This provides a value for K_m. The estimate of V_{max} can be obtained using equation (15.17).

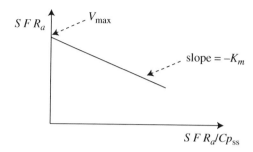

FIGURE 15.8 Method of Ludden to determine K_m and V_{max}. Plot of the effective rate of administration ($S \cdot F \cdot R_a$) against $S \cdot F \cdot R_a$ divided by the steady-state plasma concentration (Cp_{ss}).

Assuming the same F and S values, the slope may be calculated as follows:

$$slope = \frac{R_{a1} - R_{a2}}{R_{a1}/Cp_{ss1} - R_{a2}/Cp_{ss2}}$$
$$K_m = -slope \tag{15.22}$$
$$= \frac{R_{a2} - R_{a1}}{R_{a1}/Cp_{ss1} - R_{a2}/Cp_{ss2}}$$

Example 15.6   Continuing with Example 15.5, recall that an initial dose of 300 mg/day phenytoin sodium provided a steady-state plasma concentration of 8 mg/L. The dose was increased to 350 mg/day. Two weeks later, the second dose was found to provide a steady-state plasma concentration of 11 mg/L. Recommend a dose to provide a steady-state plasma concentration of 15 mg/L.

Solution   The existing history on this patient can be summarized as follows: The first rate of drug administration is

$$R_{a1}(300 \text{ mg/day}) \text{ gave a } Cp_{ss1} \text{ value of 8 mg/L}$$

and the second rate of drug administration is

$$R_{a2}(350 \text{ mg/day}) \text{ gave a } Cp_{ss2} \text{ value of 11 mg/L}$$

The patient's K_m value is estimated first using equation (15.22):

$$K_m = \frac{350 - 300}{300/8 - 350/11} = 8.8 \text{ mg/L} \tag{15.23}$$

V_{max} is calculated, using equation (15.17) and either data pair:

$$V_{max} = \frac{0.92 \times 300 \times (8.8 + 8)}{8} = 579.6 \text{ mg/day}$$

The new dose is calculated using equation (15.18):

$$S \cdot F \cdot R_a = \frac{579.6 \times 15}{8.8 \times 15} = 365$$
$$R_a = 397 \text{ mg}$$

A new dose of 400 mg of phenytoin sodium daily is recommended.

Several other methods are available for estimating phenytoin's V_{max} and K_m values and can be found in clinical pharmacokinetics textbooks [3–5].

PROBLEMS

15.1 C.R. is a 45-year-old 85-kg male (height 180 cm), who experiences simple partial seizures. He has normal liver and renal function and is not taking any other medications. He has started taking 400 mg of extended phenytoin sodium daily. Two weeks later, a plasma concentration, which is assumed to be steady state, is found to be 6.6 mg/L. The patient says that he has taken all the doses as directed. Suggest a dosage regimen to achieve a steady-state phenytoin concentration of 15 mg/L.

15.2 L.M. is a 29-year-old female who has been taking carbamazepine for 7 months to control her epilepsy. She still experiences several seizures each month. It is decided to discontinue carbamazepine and try phenytoin. She is prescribed dilantin (300 mg b.i.d.). Three weeks later, she says that she has not experienced a seizure and feels great. However, about 1 month later, she returns to the physician and complains of feeling unsteady, "out of it," and having difficulty keeping focused on activities. A blood sample is taken and the phenytoin plasma concentration is found to be 28 mg/L. Suggest possible explanations for these observations and recommend a more appropriate dose of phenytoin.

15.3 A patient who is suspected to have reduced intrinsic clearance of phenytoin is started on a dose of 250 mg of phenytoin sodium daily.
  (a) Two weeks after the start of therapy, a steady-state plasma concentration is found to be 4 mg/L. Estimate her V_{max} and recommend a new dose.
  (b) Her dose is increased to 400 mg of phenytoin sodium daily. Two weeks later, a steady-state plasma concentration is found to be 10 mg/L. Determine her K_m and V_{max} values and recommend a new dose.

15.4 A 65-kg 19-year-old male took an overdose of phenytoin. He is admitted to a hospital and a blood sample reveals a phenytoin concentration of 55 mg/L. How long will it take for the plasma concentration to reach the upper limit of the therapeutic range (20 mg/L)? Assume a population average V_{max} of 7 mg/kg/day, a K_m of 4 mg/L, and a Vd of 0.65 L/kg.

15.5 A drug is eliminated by a single metabolic pathway, which has a K_m value of 10 μg/mL and a V_{max} value of 500 mg/day (range 250–1500 mg/day). The therapeutic range of this drug is 10–25 μg/mL.
  (a) Based on the information provided, comment on any special considerations needed when selecting a dosage regimen for this drug.

(b) Calculate the steady-state plasma concentration achieved when 300 mg of the free drug is administered daily to a patient who has the population average parameter values.

(c) Calculate the steady-state plasma concentration if the dose is increased slightly to 350 mg.

(d) Calculate the steady-state plasma concentration if while on the latter dosage the patient develops hepatotoxicity, which causes a decrease in V_{max} to 375 mg.

REFERENCES

1. Koch-Weser, J. (1975) The serum level approach to individualization of drug dosage, *Eur J Clin Pharmacol*, 9, 1–8.

2. Gibaldi, M., and Perrier, D. (1982) *Pharmacokinetics*, 2nd ed., Marcel Dekker, New York.

3. Winter, M. E., and Tozer, T. N. (2006) Phenytoin, in *Applied Pharmacokinetics and Pharmacodyamics*, 4th ed. (Burton, M. E., Shaw, L. M., Schentag, J. J., and Evans, W. E., Eds.), Lippincott Williams & Wilkins, Baltimore.

4. Bauer, L. A. (2008) *Applied Clinical Pharmacokinetics*, 2nd ed., McGraw-Hill, New York.

5. Winter, M. E. (2010) *Basic Clinical Pharmacokinetics*, 5th ed., Lippincott Williams & Wilkins, Baltimore.

16

INTRODUCTION TO PHARMACOGENETICS

Dr. Daniel Brazeau

Objectives

The material in this chapter will enable the reader to:

1. Discuss two critical properties of a drug that need to be present if pharmacogenetics is to play a key role in optimizing patient care for a specific therapeutic agent

Basic Pharmacokinetics and Pharmacodynamics: An Integrated Textbook and Computer Simulations,
Second Edition. Edited by Sara E. Rosenbaum.
© 2017 John Wiley & Sons, Inc. Published 2017 by John Wiley & Sons, Inc.

2. Discuss the nature of pharmacogenetic issues one may expect with a specific drug based upon knowledge of the mechanism of action, metabolic, or transport properties
3. Describe the three basic categories of pharmacogenetic gene–drug interactions

16.1 INTRODUCTION

It has been known for well over 50 years that a significant portion of the variation observed in individual patient response to drugs is genetic. The term "pharmacogenetics" was coined in 1950 in part due to the realization of the commonness of familial patterns in drug response. Many factors are well known to give rise to interpatient drug variability including age, gender, drug interactions, concomitant diseases, or therapies. These factors as well as patient underlying genetics have been recognized to affect the large variation seen in treatment efficacy and/or toxicity of many drugs. Surprisingly, 25–50% of patients fail to respond favorably to the first drug given in the treatment of many diseases [1]. This lack of predictability in patient response results in substantial costs to contemporary health care systems. The field of pharmacogenetics has as its goal the delineation of the variation seen in drug response due to the genes involved in drug action.

Recently, with the advances in molecular genetics and the dramatic development of genomic technologies, it has now become possible to determine a patient's genetic makeup for many thousands of loci and with this information begin to assess the effect a patient's underlying genetic makeup may have on drug response. In fact, advances in next-generation DNA sequencing will soon allow for the entire genome, some three billion base pairs of information, to become a basic component of a patient's medical record. A more recent term, pharmacogenomics, encompasses the application of these genomic technologies in the discovery, development, and understanding of drug action at the molecular level. Pharmacogenomics, like pharmacogenetics, has its ultimate goal of the identification of the underlying genetic factors that play a role in the efficacy or toxicity of all drugs, but pharmacogenomics extends the realm of pharmacogenetics in that it encompasses the actions and interactions of the entire genome influencing drug response. Pharmacogenomics has only recently become possible with the advent of technologies such as high-throughput DNA sequencing, quantitative polymerase chain reaction, and silencing RNA.

As of 2014, the Federal Drug Administration (FDA) has listed over 140 drugs for which there are molecular biomarkers that may aid in providing better therapeutic outcomes for patients carrying these genetic markers. The therapeutic area for which there are the most pharmacogenetic indications (30%) is oncology, largely due to the narrow therapeutic indices typical of most oncology drugs (Figure 16.1). In total, there are presently nearly 20 therapeutic areas with pharmacogenetic indications.

16.2 GENETICS PRIMER

16.2.1 Basic Terminology: Genes, Alleles, Loci, and Polymorphism

The human genome has approximately 23,000 functioning genes. Scattered among these functioning genes are a nearly equal number of nonfunctioning pseudogenes (~20,000). These pseudogenes are the remnants of once functioning genes that through time have acquired debilitating mutations such that they are now entirely nonfunctioning in all humans. Of the functioning genes, 5–10% are RNA genes including ribosomal RNA genes

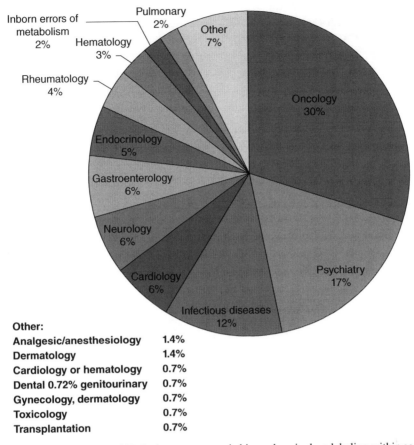

Other:
Analgesic/anesthesiology	**1.4%**
Dermatology	**1.4%**
Cardiology or hematology	**0.7%**
Dental 0.72% genitourinary	**0.7%**
Gynecology, dermatology	**0.7%**
Toxicology	**0.7%**
Transplantation	**0.7%**

FIGURE 16.1   Percentage of FDA pharmacogenomic biomarkers in drug labeling within each therapeutic area. Biomarkers include markers that maybe germline or somatic gene variants, functional deficiencies, expression changes, and chromosomal abnormalities.

(rRNA), transfer RNAs (tRNA), microRNAs, and small nucleolar RNAs (snRNA). For RNA genes, the end product of transcription from the nuclear genome is an RNA construct. The remaining genes are transcribed into mRNAs and translated into polypeptides ultimately building the cell's protein machinery including drug-metabolizing enzymes, and drug transporters and receptors. The average human gene on a chromosome is approximately 27,000 base pairs in length (genomic DNA or gDNA) and this includes exons, the regions which are translated into amino acid sequences (polypeptides) and introns which are almost always much larger regions that are ultimately not included in the mRNA and are spliced out. The average mRNA, the product of the combined exons, is approximately 1/10 in size of the nuclear genomic sequence at an average of 2,600 base pairs in size. Intron sizes range from 0 to 800,000 base pairs. Intergenic regions, the sequence between neighboring genes, average approximately 750,000 base pairs. Thus, within the human genome, the functioning portions of human genes are truly very, very small islands in a very large sea of DNA.

Official human gene names are determined by the Human Genome Organization. Current gene names can be found at http://www.genenames.org/genefamily.html. Gene names are generally short and ideally, though not often enough, convey some information as to

TABLE 16.1   Humans Have 48 Sequenced Genes Belonging to the ATP-Binding Cassette Transporters. ABC Genes are Grouped into Seven Families Based Upon Sequence Similarity. There are Also 19 Pseudogenes in This Superfamily. Alternative or Older Gene Names are Given in Parentheses.

ABCA Family: *ABCA1, ABCA2, ABCA3, ABCA4, ABCA5, ABCA6, ABCA7, ABCA8, ABCA9, ABCA10, ABCA12, ABCA13*

ABCB Family: *ABCB1 (MDR1), ABCB2, ABCB3, ABCB4, ABCB5, ABCB6, ABCB7, ABCB8, ABCB9, ABCB10, ABCB11*

ABCC Family: *ABCC1 (MRP1), ABCC2 (MRP2), ABCC3 (MRP3), ABCC4, ABCC5, ABCC6, ABCC7 (CFTR), ABCC8, ABCC9, ABCC10, ABCC11, ABCC12*

ABCD Family: *ABCD1 (ALD), ABCD2, ABCD3, ABCD4*

ABCE Family: *ABCE1*

ABCF Family: *ABCF1, ABCF2, ABCF3*

ABCG Family: *ABCG1, ABCG2 (BCRP), ABCG4, ABCG5, ABCG8*

gene function. Generally, members of the same gene superfamily share the same root name with Arabic numerals to distinguish individual members of the family (Table 16.1).

Given that among humans the rate of "copying errors" or mutations during meiosis is approximately 2.5 changes in 10^8 sites per generation, there are many variants segregating among human populations. These variants or alleles represent different forms of the gene, and in many cases the copying errors do not affect gene function and are only known from DNA sequencing of the genome. Alleles are designated using the gene name followed by an asterisk and Arabic numeral, for example, *CYP3A4*2* is one allele or variant for the gene encoding cytochrome P450 enzyme, family 3A4. This particular variant is a single nucleotide polymorphism resulting in the substitution of a "T" for a "C" in some individuals. CYP3A4*2 is one of at least 20 alleles identified to date within *CYP3A4*. Allele designations may also include additional information about the specific mutation or its resultant effect. One unique type of allele involves gene duplications, which are "gene duplication mutations" resulting in multiple functioning copies of the gene within an individual. Such gene duplications in the human genome are indicated by the two letter designation "UM." For example, among humans, there are individuals who have 2–16 functioning copies of *CYP2D6* and are ultra-rapid metabolizers. All of the copy number variants have been combined under the designation *CYP2D6 UM*. Allelic designations are often followed by a descriptor providing information about the nature of the mutation. For example, within the gene (*ABCB1*) that encodes the drug efflux pump, P-glycoprotein (P-Gp), a fairly common substitution occurs at the 3,435th nucleotide of the mRNA. Most individuals have a cytosine at this location (wild type), some have a thymine. The allelic designation, *ABCB1 3435 C>T*, thus indicates the location of the substitution with the wild type or reference allele (C) listed first. The variant allele (T) is listed second. Often if the substitution results in an amino acid change in the resultant polypeptide, the allelic designation can indicate that the amino acid has changed. For example, *CYP2C9 144 Arg>Cys* indicates that in the drug-metabolizing enzyme, CYP2C9, the 144th amino acid is different among individuals, again the wild-type variant is listed first (arginine).

16.2.2   Population Genetics: Allele and Genotype Frequencies

While any single individual has only two alleles, one on each chromosome, among individuals in a population there may be many more alleles segregating. Consider a gene for which there are only two alleles, A_1 and A_2, with allele frequencies, p and q. Note that since there are only two alleles, the sum of their frequencies must be equal to 1 ($p + q = 1$). Therefore, the probability of an individual being homozygous for one allele, for example, A_1A_1, is p^2. Similarly, the probability of having two A_2 alleles is q^2. The probability of an individual being heterozygous (A_1A_2 or A_2A_1) is $pq+qp$ or $2pq$. In what had been derisively referred to as "bean-bag genetics," it has been shown that in most cases it is possible to calculate genotype frequencies for a population solely based upon the allele frequencies. Further, two scientists, Hardy and Weinberg, independently demonstrated that these allele and genotype frequencies will remain constant from one generation to the next if four basic assumptions are met:

1. Populations consist of large random mating units. Allele frequencies may change if population sizes are small due to sampling errors.
2. There are no net mutation differences from one allele to another.
3. There is no differential migration of individuals into or out of the population.
4. Selection does not favor one allele over another.

Populations that meet these assumptions are said to be in Hardy–Weinberg (H–W) equilibrium. Calculations of the H–W equilibrium for a study population are often conducted since the equilibrium is robust in the sense that when frequencies are calculated for a given gene, most populations are found to be H–W equilibrium. Given this when a population is found not to be in H–W equilibrium, it is usually an indication that either the method of assessing the genotypes is in error (alleles are miscalled) or one of the above four assumptions has been violated for this population. Generally, if the allele frequencies have been accurately determined, then either the population being studied is not a single randomly interbreeding unit (Assumption #1) or selection is altering allele frequencies (Assumption #4).

16.2.3 Quantitative Genetics and Complex Traits

Most of the well-known genetic disorders that afflict humankind such as sickle-cell anemia, Huntington's disease, Duchene's muscular dystrophy, and cystic fibrosis are familiar to us precisely because they are single gene or monogenic disorders whose underlying patterns of inheritance follow simple Mendelian rules. Unfortunately, most traits and diseases that are of interest are not caused by a single gene and therefore, the genetic basis for these traits is not so easily understood or predicted. In addition, for most human traits, the environment plays a large role in the ultimate display of the trait. Consider height, it is quite clear that humans have been growing taller with each generation; however, it is unlikely that selection is at work here. More likely, better diets (both for the mother during pregnancy and later for the child) and less childhood diseases have resulted in children who are generally taller than their parents. Traits such as height, cognitive abilities, and disease risk display complex patterns of non-Mendelian or multifactorial inheritance, and their study is the basis of quantitative genetics.

The goal of quantitative genetics is to partition the variability seen in a given human trait into those portions which are due to genetic versus environmental factors. Perhaps one of the most straightforward and commonly used methods to assess the genetic component to phenotypic variation is twin studies. Monozygotic twins have the same DNA and therefore, any differences seen in a trait of interest are due to environmental influences or factors. Unfortunately, obtaining enough twins to conduct such studies is very challenging particularly if one is interested in a relatively uncommon disease like most cancers. In these cases,

TABLE 16.2 Heritabilities for Human Traits

Trait	h^2
Height	0.7–0.8
IQ	0.6–0.8
Alcoholism	0.5–0.6
Obesity	0.4–0.7
Type 2 Diabetes	0.2–0.3

family studies are important, particularly families displaying the "extreme phenotypes." For example, extreme phenotypes may include early onset in some cancers or multiple occurrences within the family, or an extreme adverse reaction to a drug. It is thought that such extreme phenotypes are an indication of the presence of many susceptibility alleles in the family.

For quantitate traits, the variance seen in the expression of the trait is given by:

1. Phenotypic Variance (V_P) = Genetic Variance (V_G) + Environmental Variance (V_E)
   The **heritability** of a phenotypic trait is thus defined as
2. Heritability (h^2) = V_G / V_p

That is, h^2 is the relative proportion of total phenotypic variance due to genetic factors. Thus, a trait with high heritability is one in which a large portion of the variation seen in the trait is due to genetics. Conversely, a trait with low heritability is one where most of the variation seen in the trait among individuals is due to environmental causes. Heritabilities for many human traits are available (Table 16.2) and are often misinterpreted.

Specifically, it is important to note that:

• Heritability is not a measure of the proportion of a phenotype due to genetics. Thus, 70–80% of human height is not determined by genes. Heritability is an assessment of the variation seen in a trait that is due to genetic factors relative to total phenotypic variance. Therefore, 70–80% of the variation in human height has a genetic basis.

• Heritability can change in time and among populations—remember that environments are generally not constant and thus, the relative contribution of variation due to genetics may change depending upon environmental factors.

• Heritability is a population concept; it is only valid for a specific population, at a specific time, and in a specific environment.

While the conditional restrictions of the concept of heritability would seem to negate its usefulness, its measurement is important. For example, plant and animal breeders hope that the traits they value (milk production and fruit yields) have high heritabilities. If heritabilities are low, there is very little for breeding programs to select for, better to improve environmental conditions.

16.3 PHARMACOGENETICS

As noted above, there are now many known examples of genes for which there are variants that play a role in drug response or treatment success. The best source for timely information concerning genetic polymorphisms and drug response is the Pharmacogenomics

Knowledge Base (PharmGKB at www.PharmGKB.org). PharmGKB is an integrated database providing clinical, pharmacokinetic, pharmacodynamics, genotypic, and molecular function data for human genetic polymorphisms and drugs. The data within PharmGKB are organized into five basic categories of pharmacogenetic knowledge:

1. Clinical outcome—the role of genetic variation in altering clinical endpoints that aid in determining medical practice or policy.
2. Pharmacodynamics and drug response—the role of genetic variation in differences in the biological or physiological response to drugs. These differences may in some situations be treated as surrogates for clinical responses.
3. Pharmacokinetics—the role of genetic variation in the absorption, distribution, metabolism, or excretion of a drug.
4. Molecular and cellular functional assays—the role of genetic variation in laboratory assays for molecular or cellular responses to drugs.
5. Genotype—data on the type and population structure of genetic polymorphisms relevant to drug action.

The PharmGKB database has been established to allow researchers and health professionals to easily access current data on drugs and genetic variability.

In examining the documented cases of genes that play an important clinical role in drug response, often referred to as "pharmacogenes," there are two fundamental elements common to many. The first element or characteristic is one inherent to the drug or compound itself. Most drugs where pharmacogenetics is clinically relevant have a narrow therapeutic window. The appropriate therapeutic dosage (and blood concentration) range for these drugs is small and thus, slight *genetically based* differences in drug metabolism, absorption, distribution, or clearance may result in adverse effects in the patient. Drugs that have wide therapeutic windows, which show no adverse effects across a wide concentration range, are unlikely to have pharmacogenetic issues since most genetic differences in metabolism, absorption, or distribution will be within the range of the normally administered dose.

The second element common to many pharmacogenes is inherent in the biological pathways involved in the drug's metabolism or transport. Drugs that often have "pharmacogenetic" indications have at least one critical step in the drug response pathway that is controlled principally by a single gene (monogenic). Given a single gene impacting a critical step in the pathway, genetic differences (polymorphisms) among patients in this gene may result in different patient outcomes. For example, for a drug that is metabolized by a single enzyme into an inactive metabolite. Loss of function variants for the gene that encodes the enzyme may result in high concentrations of the active compound. In contrast, drugs for which there are multiple alternate pathways or multiple genes involved are unlikely to elicit varying responses due to polymorphisms in a single gene—the phenotype is said to be polygenic. Thus, most drugs that have pharmacogenetic indications have narrow therapeutic indices and have a critical step in their metabolism or transport controlled by a single gene.

Within pharmacogenetics, there are three broad categories of genes that differ in the role they play drug response. Recognition of these three categories of genes reveals some commonalities in the underlying pharmacogenetics. These categories are:

1. *Drug-metabolizing pharmacogenetics*—involve genes that code for enzymes that are involved in the metabolism of the drug. Genes include those that code for phase I or phase II metabolizing enzymes and may either activate a prodrug into an active agent

or inactivate an active drug into an inactive metabolite. Polymorphisms in genes the code for drug-metabolizing enzymes generally result in differences among patients in the pharmacokinetics of the drug.

2. *Drug transporter pharmacogenetics*—involve genes that code for membrane transporters that move drugs either into or out of cells. Similar to drug-metabolizing genes, polymorphisms in genes that encode drug transporters often result in differences in the pharmacokinetics of the drug.

3. *Drug target pharmacogenetics*—genes that code for the direct target of the drug or code for other proteins that are associated with the biochemical or regulatory pathway of the drug. Unlike the pharmacogenetics of genes involved in drug metabolism or drug transport, drug target pharmacogenetics often results in differences in the pharmacodynamics of the drug. Generally, issues arise concerning reduced efficacy rather than increased toxicity.

16.3.1 Pharmacogenetics of Drug-Metabolizing Enzymes

In order to examine some of the basic issues seen in drug-metabolizing pharmacogenetics, we will consider three classic examples of the pharmacogenetics that will play an important role in explaining variation in patient drug response. All of these examples involve drugs that have narrow therapeutic windows and have drug response phenotypes that are determined by one or two genes. We will use these representative pharmacogenes to elucidate fundamental features of both drugs and genetics that are important in understanding the limitations and complexities of pharmacogenetics in clinical use.

16.3.1.1 *Pharmacogenetics of Codeine*

Codeine is an opioid analgesic used for pain control, cough suppressant, and as an antidiarrheal. Codeine has low affinity for μ-opioid receptors and thus little analgesic effect. It must be converted into morphine and/or morphine-6-glucuronide in the liver in order for patients to experience pain relief (Figure 16.2). This metabolic conversion is carried out by a single enzyme (single gene), the enzyme cytochrome P450 2D6, encoded by the gene *CYP2D6*. Over 100 alleles have been described for this gene in humans. A number of these polymorphisms (alleles *CYP2D6 *4, *5, *6,* for others see PharmGKB.org) result in greatly reduced or no enzyme activity. Patients who carry two copies of these variant alleles (referred to as poor metabolizers) have greatly reduced capacity to convert codeine into morphine and therefore, experience little analgesic effect from taking codeine. Importantly, in this case where the variant alleles result in reduced or loss of function for a prodrug, there is a lack of efficacy but no toxicity. This is in contrast to the case for individuals who carry a variant

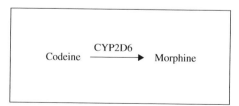

FIGURE 16.2 Codeine pharmacogenetics. Codeine is a prodrug with little analgesic effect. It must be converted to morphine by the enzyme CYP2D6 in the liver for pain relief.

"allele" defined by having more than two copies of this gene, in some cases up to 16 copies. Individuals' carrying this allele on either chromosome exhibit high levels of CYP2D6 activity and are characterized as ultra-rapid metabolizers. These individuals rapidly convert the standard dose of codeine into higher exposure to morphine resulting in a higher risk of toxicity including impaired respiration. Codeine pharmacogenetics provides an excellent example of two basic themes when considering the pharmacogenetics of metabolizing enzymes. An important consideration is whether the drug is an active compound when administered with the assumption that it will be metabolized into inactive (less toxic) metabolites by the enzyme or a prodrug requiring conversion to an active compound for therapeutic benefit. Loss of function mutations result in little or no active CYP2D6 and therefore little metabolism of the *prodrug* resulting in loss of efficacy. However, gain of function mutations (extra copies of *CYP2D6*) in the metabolism of a prodrug often result in toxicity due to increased levels of the active metabolite.

16.3.1.2   *Pharmacogenetics of Thiopurine S-Methyltransferase*

Thiopurines are among the first-line treatments for childhood acute lymphoblastic leukemia, organ transplant recipients, inflammatory bowel disease, and autoimmune diseases. The enzyme, thiopurine S-methyltransferase (TPMT) catalyzes the S-methylation of a number of chemotherapeutic prodrugs such as 6-mercaptopurine (6-MP), 6-thioguanine, and azathioprine (AZA). 6-MP and AZA are converted into thioinosine monophosphate and ultimately to thioguanosine monophosphate (TGMP). TGMP is ultimately converted into cytotoxic nucleotide analogs (TGN) that block DNA and RNA synthesis via inhibition of *de novo* purine synthesis (Figure 16.3). The metabolism of 6-MP and its metabolites by TPMT is a critical step in the inactivation pathways leading to the ultimate clearance of the drug from the body. Loss of function variants for *TPMT* result in high concentrations of the cytotoxic nucleotide analogs (TGN) leading to severe-to-moderate myelosuppression. Specifically, individuals who inherit two copies (homozygous) of the loss of function

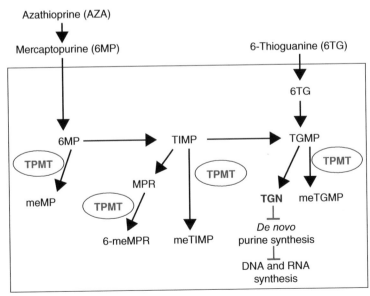

FIGURE 16.3   Pharmacogenetics of thiopurines. Note in each step of this pathway, the enzyme TPMT plays a role in inactivation.

alleles experience severe hematopoietic toxicity. Dosing guidelines (Clinical Pharmacogenetics Implementation Consortium) call for drastically reduced doses, 10-fold or less. Individuals with a single copy of the variant allele and one normal allele (heterozygous) experience moderate concentrations of TGN and are advised to begin treatment with 30–70% of the full dose. Note that this pharmacogenetic example has the opposite outcome compared to the loss of function mutations in the codeine (a prodrug) example. Loss of function mutations in enzymes involved in the inactivation pathways of active drugs often result in toxicity.

16.3.1.3 *Pharmacogenetics of Warfarin*

Warfarin is a commonly prescribed oral anticoagulant for the prevention and treatment of myocardial infarction, ischemic stroke, venous thrombosis, and atrial fibrillation. Warfarin has a narrow therapeutic window with large interpatient variation. Insufficient drug plasma concentrations may prevent thromboembolism, while over dosing may cause risk of bleeding events. Warfarin's mode of action is as a very effective antagonist of the vitamin K epoxide reductase complex (VKORC1), a critical enzyme in the vitamin K-dependent clotting pathway (Figure 16.4). Warfarin is delivered as a racemic mixture of the R and S stereoisomers. The S stereoisomer of warfarin is the more potent inhibitor of VKORC1 and accounts for 60–70% of the anticoagulation response. Importantly, S-warfarin is largely metabolized by a single enzyme (*CYP2C9*). As is the case for many pharmacogenes, there are a large number of variants (>50) of *CYP2C9* segregating in human populations with varying frequencies of these alleles among human ethnic groups. For example, two reduced function alleles (*CYP2C9*2* and **3*) are fairly common among Caucasians ranging from 6% to 20%, but are largely absent in Asian populations and rare in African-American populations with

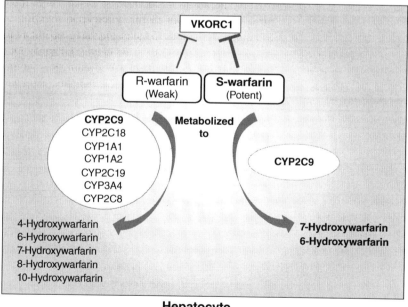

FIGURE 16.4 Warfarin pharmacogenetics. Warfarin is an active agent that inhibits vitamin K reductase. Polymorphisms in the gene responsible for inactivation, CYP2C9, as well the gene that encodes the direct drug target VKORC1 will affect patient outcomes.

frequencies ranging from 1% to 4%. Individuals carrying these reduced function variant alleles metabolize warfarin slowly, thus traditional dosing regimens may lead to bleeding events or longer times to achieve stable drug concentrations. As was the case for the thiopurines, warfarin is an active agent as given. Appropriate and safe plasma concentrations are dependent upon the action of the enzyme (CYP2C9) to inactivate the active compound. Thus, loss or reduced function alleles in the gene involved in the inactivation pathway result in high exposure to the active compound and toxicity.

16.3.2 Pharmacogenetics of Drug Transporters

Drug transporters are fundamental agents in determining drug disposition, tissue penetration, and clearance. Drug transporters mediate hepatobiliary, intestinal, and renal clearance and are the basis of cellular safeguards such as the blood–brain and placental barriers. Variations in the genes that encode these transporters may result in differences among patients in drug disposition and clearance. Unlike the pharmacogenetics of drug-metabolizing enzymes, the genetic variation seen in drug transporters often results in more complicated outcomes in patients since the location of the transporter will affect drug disposition and/or clearance. For example, genetic differences in a transporter for an active drug may have different outcomes depending on whether the transporter is in a hepatocyte, affecting clearance or the blood–brain barrier resulting in possible toxicity. Two well-known pharmacogenes demonstrate this complexity.

16.3.2.1 Pharmacogenetics of Simvastatin

Simvastatin is one of the most commonly prescribed statins in the United States. While simvastatin has a wide therapeutic window, the drugs' wide use has resulted in a large number of adverse drug reactions, most often skeletal muscle toxicity. Simvastatin is a potent inhibitor of a coenzyme A reductase (HMG-COA reductase), the rate-limiting enzyme in cholesterol biosynthesis. One drug transporter plays an important role in mediating hepatic clearance of simvastatin. The membrane-bound sodium independent organic anion transporter protein (OAT1B1) is encoded by the gene (SLCO1B1) that belongs to a family of solute carrier organic anion transporters—family member 1B1. Interestingly, there are other members of this family that are important in the transport of statins (SLCO2B1 and SLCO1B3 for atorvastatin and lovastatin), however, SLCO1B1 is the principal transporter for the hepatic uptake of simvastatin. A number of common variants of the gene have been associated with decreased clearance and linked to simvastatin-induced myopathy particularly patients on high-dose therapy. Note that these same variants in SLCO1B1 have no effects on other statins. In addition, cyclosporine is a strong inhibitor of OAT1B1 (encoded by SLCO1B1) and drug–drug interactions may further increase the severity of the statin-induced muscle damage among individuals already at risk due to genetic factors.

16.3.2.2 Pharmacogenetics of P-Glycoprotein

The drug efflux pump P-gP plays an important role in limiting drug bioavailability by transporting drugs out of the cell at the lumen-facing epithelia of the small intestine and colon, in elimination via biliary excretion and in the proximal tubules in the kidney. P-gP also plays an important protective function as it restricts permeability of drugs and xenobiotics at the blood–brain, placental, and testis barriers. Well over 70 drugs are known to be substrates for P-gp including antiepileptics and antitumor drugs. Variation in the expression of P-gp leads to wide patient variation in resistance to the effects of a variety of drugs. Thus, genetic variation in the gene that encodes P-gp, ABCB1, may result in differing susceptibility to pharmacotherapy. For example, levels of P-gp expression have been correlated to treatment failure in epilepsy, to nonresponse in acute myeloid leukemia, childhood neuroblastoma, and other cancers. Unfortunately, the pharmacogenetic literature concerning the effects of polymorphisms in *ABCB1* while among the most extensive for any pharmacogene is varied in outcomes and often contradictory. This is due in large part to the many roles this transporter plays in the body as well as the many compounds that are known to interact with this transporter (environmental effects). Again unlike the more straightforward outcomes for polymorphisms in drug-metabolizing enzymes, the outcomes for drug transporters are often much more complex.

16.4 GENETICS AND PHARMACODYNAMICS

Much in the same way that the genetic differences in the expression of genes that encode drug-metabolizing enzymes and drug transporters may influence patient response to a drug, genetic differences in the targets of the drug may also affect patient response. Although polymorphisms in drug-metabolizing enzymes and drug transporters generally alter pharmacokinetic parameters, polymorphisms in the targets of drug action generally affect the pharmacodynamics of the drug.

16.4.1 Drug Target Pharmacogenetics

Drug target pharmacogenetics involve genes that encode the direct protein targets of the drug (receptors, enzymes, and transcription factors) as well as genes that encode downstream proteins in drug pathways including signal transduction pathways and proteins involved in disease pathogenesis. As noted earlier, drug target pharmacogenetics often results in differences in the pharmacodynamics of response resulting in loss of efficacy or resistance. We return to an earlier example, warfarin, to examine the role of genetic variation in drug targets and patient response.

16.4.1.1 Pharmacogenetics of Warfarin II
The enzyme, vitamin K reductase catalyzes the conversion of vitamin K-epoxide to vitamin K. This conversion is the rate-limiting step in vitamin K recycling pathway. Vitamin K (in its reduced form) is important for a number of coagulation factors. Inhibition of vitamin K reductase by warfarin gives rise to the drugs' anticoagulant properties (Figure 16.4). The enzyme, vitamin K reductase is encoded by the gene, *VKORC1*. There are at least five important variants as well as numerous less common variants that contribute to interpatient variation in warfarin dosing. The different allelic variants have different outcomes. Individuals with the *VKORC1*2* variant require lower warfarin doses. This variant is common in Asians and Caucasians and rare in African populations. The variants *VKORC1*3* and *VKORC1*4* require a higher warfarin dose. *VKORC1*3* is the most common haplotype in African populations and is also common in Caucasians. Polymorphisms in *VKORC1* account for up to 30% of the variance seen among patients in warfarin dose. Note the importance of genetic variation in *VKORC1* varies among populations. It is highest in individuals of European ancestry and less among patients of Asian or African ancestry. This is likely due to the result of the allelic differences segregating in the populations. Finally, even though *VKORC1* is an enzyme it is also the target of warfarin and thus, polymorphisms in *VKORC1* result in changes in efficacy rather than AUC or disposition as would be the case for drug-metabolizing enzymes or transporters.

16.5 SUMMARY

In summary, the goal of this chapter has been to highlight a number of pharmacogenetic cases as a means of describing some of the complexities that are common to many pharmacogene-drug stories. In all cases, it is important to remain aware of some of basic attributes common to all pharmacogenetics:

- Drugs whose metabolism/transport is affected by multiple genes (polygenic) or multiple pathways do not generally exhibit pharmacogenetic indications.
- Drugs with wide therapeutic indices do not generally exhibit pharmacogenetic indications, though even "safe" drugs may have pharmacogenetic indications if they are widely prescribed.
- Clinically important genes often have many rare allelic variants with similar phenotypes, though not always.
- Variant allele frequencies are often very different among patients due to ancestry. This will often result in differences in the predictability of genetic tests based upon the testing of a limited number of alleles.
- Polymorphisms in drug-metabolizing enzymes of drug transporters generally alter the pharmacokinetic parameters of the drug.
- Polymorphisms in drug targets generally alter the pharmacodynamics of the drug.

REFERENCE

1. Spear, B. B., Heath-Chiozzi, M., and Huff, J. (2001) Clinical application of pharmacogenetics, *Trends Mol Med*, 7, 201–204.

SUGGESTED READINGS

2. Relling, M., and Klein, T. E. (2011) CPIC: clinical pharmacogenetics implementation consortium of the pharmacogenomics research network, *Clin Pharmacol Therap*, 89(3), 464–467.
3. Whirl-Carrillo, M., McDonagh, E. M., Hebert, J. M., Gong, L., Sangkuhl, K., Thorn, C. F., Altman, R. B., and Klein, T. E. (2012) Pharmacogenomics knowledge for personalized medicine, *Clin Pharmacol Therap*, 92(4), 414–417.

17

MODELS USED TO PREDICT DRUG–DRUG INTERACTIONS FOR ORALLY ADMINISTERED DRUGS

Sara E. Rosenbaum

Basic Pharmacokinetics and Pharmacodynamics: An Integrated Textbook and Computer Simulations, Second Edition. Edited by Sara E. Rosenbaum.
© 2017 John Wiley & Sons, Inc. Published 2017 by John Wiley & Sons, Inc.

Objectives

The material presented in this chapter will enable the reader to:

1. Become familiar with the models used to study reversible inhibition, time-dependent inhibition, and the induction of the drug-metabolizing enzymes *in vitro*
2. Become familiar with different surrogate perpetrator concentrations used in predictive models
3. Understand the basis and application of the basic predictive model
4. Understand the basis and application of predictive models that incorporate parallel pathways of elimination
5. Understand how intestinal extraction can be incorporated into predictive models
6. Understand how predictive models can be applied to transporter based drug–drug interactions

17.1 INTRODUCTION

There has been considerable interest over the last 10 years in the development of models that use drug parameters estimated *in vitro* to predict drug–drug interactions (DDIs) *in vivo*. While not perfect at this time, the models have met with some success and are widely used in the pharmaceutical industry to identify potential DDI issues early in the development process and to help prioritize clinical DDI studies. The models are introduced in this chapter.

DDIs occur when one drug, the **perpetrator or precipitant,** alters the pharmacokinetics or the pharmacodynamics of a second, **victim or object** drug, resulting in a clinically significant change in a patient's response to the victim drug. DDIs with a pharmacokinetic basis are the most common and generally occur when the perpetrator brings about changes in the activity of a protein, notably an enzyme or a transporter involved in the absorption, distribution, and/or elimination of the victim drug.

DDIs pose a serious health problem. They are a leading cause of adverse drug reactions, drug-related hospitalizations, and drug-related deaths. The increased awareness of the problem and the use of software in clinical practice to screen for interactions between two coadministered drugs have not been able to eliminate the problem. Further, the increase in polypharmacy associated with an increased prevalence of multiple chronic medical conditions such as diabetes, hypertension, gastroesophageal reflux disease, and hypercholesterolemia in an aging population is likely to increase the risk of DDI problems in the future. This increased risk is also exacerbated when patients receive treatment from several different specialty physicians, each of whom may be unaware of the drugs prescribed by the others. The increased use of herbal drug products and other natural products adds an additional element to DDI risk. The use of these products is largely unregulated and few have undergone thorough evaluation as potential modifiers of either the drug-metabolizing enzymes or transporters. Several products such as St. John's wort have already been identified as important perpetrators of DDIs. As more States legalize the medicinal and recreational use of cannabis, which contains over 100 different components, it is likely that this product will be more frequently combined with medicinal drugs. At the present time, little is known about the ability of the active and inactive ingredients of cannabis to act as perpetrators of DDIs.

Metabolism-based DDIs involving the cytochrome P450 (CYP) enzymes have been responsible for some of the most serious DDIs. In the 5-year period from 1998 to 2003, several drugs were withdrawn from the market because of CYP-based interactions. These included the antihistamines terfenadine and astemizole and the gastrointestinal prokinetic agent cisapride, all of which are inhibitors of the cardiac human ether-a-go-go-related gene (hERG) potassium ion channel that is important for normal electrical activity in the heart. All three of the drugs are also primarily eliminated by CYP3A metabolism, and coadministration with inhibitors of CYP3A, such as ketoconazole, itraconazole, and erythromycin, exposed people to higher concentrations of these hERG inhibitors and predisposed them to life-threatening cardiac arrhythmias and sudden death. The calcium channel blocker mibefradil, which was also withdrawn during this period, is a potent inhibitor of several CYP enzymes, including CYP3A, and had serious interactions with many drugs with which it was frequently coadministered. Although DDIs have not led to the withdrawal of drugs from the market in recent years, many serious DDIs continue to be identified only after a drug has been marketed. For example, simvastatin is primarily eliminated by CYP3A metabolism and several inhibitors of this enzyme have been found to increase simvastatin's concentrations and predispose patients to increased risk of muscle myopathy. As a result, simvastatin is now contraindicated with several potent inhibitors of CYP3A, such as itraconazole and clarithromycin, as well as some other perpetrators affecting other enzymes and transporters involved in the elimination of simvastatin. These include cyclosporine, danzol, and gemfibrozil. Additionally, simvastatin's maximum daily dose has been capped at either 10 or 20 mg when taken with other CYP3A inhibitors, such as diltiazem and amlodipine. These examples demonstrate the need for both continued vigilance identifying new DDIs among marketed drugs and the need to better evaluate the potential of drugs to act as either perpetrator or victims of DDIs before they are released onto the market.

During drug development, pharmaceutical companies are required to fully assess their drug candidate's potential to act as a perpetrator and victim of DDIs. For potential perpetrators, this will mean screening compounds to determine if they inhibit or induce important enzymes. For potential victims, this will involve identifying the major enzymes involved in their elimination. Traditionally, DDIs are evaluated in clinical studies carried *in vivo*, where the area under the curve (*AUC*) of the potential victim is measured in the presence and absence of a perpetrator. On the basis of such studies, clinically significant findings are then incorporated into the product labeling to mitigate the risk. This may include recommending dosage changes, careful monitoring of the victim drug, or contraindicating two or more products. *In vivo* studies are costly and can only be conducted during the later stages of drug development when the lead molecule has already been selected and investment in clinical development has already been made. In order to better identify potential problems early in the development process, models have been developed to predict a drug's likelihood to act as a perpetrator or victim *in vivo* based on parameters obtained from *in vitro* studies carried out early development. The models are useful in:

- Identifying potential DDI issues early in the drug discovery and development process
- Guiding the selection of the lead molecule

- Strategizing the development process
- Eliminating the need for costly *in vivo* studies for compounds found to have little ability to modify enzyme activity
- Strategizing and prioritizing clinical DDI studies.

The use of these *in vitro* models during drug development to aid in the identification of clinically important perpetrators and victims of DDIs is endorsed by the Food and Drug Administration (FDA) [1] and the European Medicines Agency [2]. These predictive models allow drugs to be classified according to the likelihood (likely, possible, remote) that they will be perpetrators (inhibitors and/or inducers) of DDIs. They also enable those drugs identified as unlikely perpetrators to be labeled as noninhibitors or noninducers without the need for *in vivo* studies.

This chapter will begin by presenting the *in vitro* models for inhibitors and inducers of drug metabolism. The next section will discuss the different values of the perpetrator concentrations typically used in the predictive models. The basic and more mechanistic predictive models will then be presented. Finally, the chapter will conclude by examining how the models can be applied to predict transporter-based DDIs.

17.2 MATHEMATICAL MODELS FOR INHIBITORS AND INDUCERS OF DRUG METABOLISM BASED ON *IN VITRO* DATA

Perpetrators of metabolism-based interactions can be broadly classified as either inhibitors or inducers of the drug-metabolizing enzymes. Inhibitors are further classified as reversible or time-dependent inhibitors (TDIs) or mechanism-based inhibitors. The characteristics of all three types of perpetrators were introduced in Chapter 5 (Section 5.4.4), and the *in vitro* models used to describe how the three different perpetrators affect the kinetics of drug metabolism and the intrinsic clearance of victim drugs are presented in detail in Appendix E. In this section, the mathematical model for characterizing *in vitro* data for each type of perpetrator will be provided without derivation. Appendix E also contains several simulation models to help readers understand the meaning and significance of the model parameters.

17.2.1 Reversible Inhibition

A representation of the action of a reversible competitive inhibitor is shown in Figure 17.1.

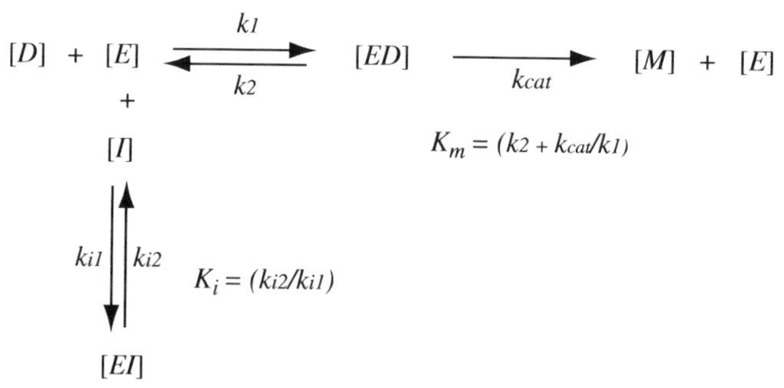

FIGURE 17.1 Effect of a competitive inhibitor on the metabolism of a substrate.

Both the victim drug [D] and the inhibitor [I] bind to and compete for the enzyme [E]. The inhibitor's dissociation constant (K_i) is an inverse measure of the inhibitor's affinity for the enzyme. The inhibitor produces an apparent increase (reduced affinity) in the victim's drug K_m.

The inhibitor competes with the victim drug for the enzyme [E], and in so doing produces an apparent decrease in the victim's affinity for the enzyme. The inhibitor has no effect on the total concentration of enzyme in the system or on the V_{max} of the process. The competition for the enzyme results in an apparent increase in the victim drug's K_m. It was demonstrated in Appendix E that,

$$K_m^I == K_m \left(1 + \frac{[I]}{K_i}\right) \tag{17.1}$$

where, K_m^I and K_m are the victim drug's Michaelis–Menten constants in the presence and absence of an inhibitor, respectively, [I] is the inhibitor's unbound concentration, and K_i is the inhibitor's dissociation constant or potency.

It was shown in Appendix E that the ratio of intrinsic clearance in the absence (Cl_{int}) and the presence (Cl_{int}^I) of an inhibitor is known as R, specifically R_1 for a reversible inhibitor. It was shown that R_1 is given by:

$$R_1 = \frac{Cl_{int}}{Cl_{int}^I} = (1 + [I]/K_i) \tag{17.2}$$

The greater the extent of inhibition, the greater the fall in intrinsic clearance, and the larger the value of R_1. The extent of inhibition is a function of the perpetrator's unbound concentration at the enzyme site and its K_i. Note that when [I] = K_i, intrinsic clearance is reduced by 50%. Small values of K_i are indicative of a high affinity of the inhibitor for the enzyme and high inhibitor potency. Inhibitors' K_i values can be determined *in vitro* using a preparation of active human enzymes, such as hepatocytes, microsomes, or recombinant enzymes. For example, ketoconazole's and fluconazole's reported K_i values for the reversible inhibition of the CYP3A-mediated metabolism of midazolam are 0.006 and 3.4 µM, respectively [3], demonstrating that ketoconazole is the more potent inhibitor. The degree of inhibition is also determined by the unbound concentration of the inhibitor at the enzyme site. The ratio of [I] to K_i is used as a measure of the overall risk posed by an inhibitor. The larger the ratio, the greater the inhibitory effect.

Assuming that an inhibitor's action is completely competitive and that it acts at a single site on the enzyme, its K_i should be constant and independent of the substrate whose metabolism it inhibits. In practice, the inhibitor and the victim drug may bind to multiple sites on the enzyme with cooperativity in these interactions, and the inhibitor may have a noncompetitive component to its inhibition. This is particularly important for CYP3A4 substrates. As a result, a range of K_i values are usually obtained using a number of chemically diverse probe substrates such as testosterone, nifedipine, and midazolam. A conservative approach to DDI risk is taken by using the lowest K_i values in the predicative models.

17.2.2 Time-Dependent Inhibition

Time-dependent inhibition is much more complex than reversible inhibition. It is primarily, though not exclusively, caused by a reactive metabolite intermediate (MI) of the inhibitor that subsequently binds often irreversibly to the enzyme, destroying its activity. The typical

$$[I] \; + \; [E] \; \underset{k_2}{\overset{k_1}{\rightleftharpoons}} \; [EI] \; \xrightarrow{\;\; k_{\text{cat}} \;\;} \; [P] \; + \; [E]$$

$$\downarrow k_{\text{inact}}$$

$$[E.MI]$$

FIGURE 17.2 The interaction of a time-dependent inhibitor with an enzyme. The inhibitor $[I]$ binds to the enzyme $[E]$ to form an inhibitor-enzyme complex (k_1 and k_2 are the rate constants for the forward and backward processes, respectively). The inhibitor-enzyme complex could dissociate to release the drug and the enzyme, undergo catalytic metabolism to form a product $[P]$, or the inhibitor's metabolic intermediate could bind to the enzyme and destroy its activity. The first-order rate constants for the catalytic and inactivation processes are k_{cat} and k_{inact}, respectively.

pathway for TDI is shown in Figure 17.2. The inhibitor binds to the enzyme to produce a complex, which can then proceed in several directions (Figure 17.2) one of which can result in the formation of the MI, which can bind irreversibly to the enzyme and destroy its activity.

The inhibitory activity of TDI perpetrator is described by means of two parameters: K_I and k_{inact}. The K_I is a potency parameter that is a measure of the relationship between the inhibitor's concentration and the amount of MI formed. It is a complex function of several of the rate constants involved in the metabolism of the inhibitor and can be defined as the inhibitor concentration causing half-maximal inactivation [see equation (17.3)]. The smaller the value of an inhibitor's K_I, the greater the potency of the inhibitor. The k_{inact} is the first-order rate constant for the relationship between the concentration of the inhibitor enzyme complex and the rate of inactivation of the enzyme by the MI. It is a measure of the destructive power of the MI. The greater the k_{inact}, the greater the destructive power of the MI. As shown in Appendix E, the inactivation of the enzyme can also be viewed more simply as a first-order process driven by the amount of enzyme and the rate constant k_{obs}. The value of k_{obs} is dependent on K_I, k_{inact}, and $[I]$ (Figure 17.3). This hyperbolic, capacity-limited relationship is expressed mathematically as:

$$k_{\text{obs}} = \frac{k_{\text{inact}} * [I]}{K_I + [I]} \tag{17.3}$$

$$\xrightarrow[\text{Synthesis}]{k_{\text{syn}}} \; [E_t^I] \; \xrightarrow[\text{Degradation}]{k_{\text{degrad}}}$$

$$\downarrow \begin{array}{c} \text{Inactivation} \\ k_{\text{obs}} \end{array}$$

where,
$$k_{\text{obs}} = \frac{k_{\text{inact}} * [I]}{K_I + [I]}$$

FIGURE 17.3 Time-dependent inhibitors can be viewed as adding an additional first-order removal (inactivation) pathway to the total enzyme concentration. The enzyme is synthesized by a zero-order process (rate, k_{syn}) and normally degraded by a first-order process (rate constant, k_{degrad}). In the presence of a TDI, the total enzyme concentration E_t^I undergoes first-order inactivation (rate constant, k_{obs}). k_{obs} is a function of the maximum inactivation rate constant, k_{inact}, the inhibitor concentration $[I]$, and the inhibitor potency, K_I (see Figure 17.4).

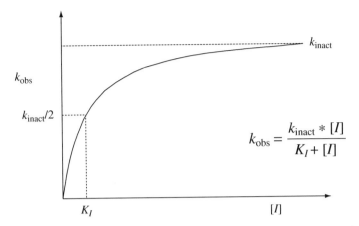

FIGURE 17.4 A hyperbolic, capacity-limited relationship exists between k_{obs} and the inhibitor concentration [*I*]. k_{inact} represents the maximum inactivation rate constant, which is observed at high inhibitor concentrations, and K_I is the inhibitor concentration causing half-maximal inactivation.

The relationship linking k_{obs} to K_i, k_{inact}, and [*I*] (Figure 17.4) enables K_i and k_{inact} to be estimated by measuring k_{obs} at different inhibitor concentrations. The relationship also demonstrates that K_I **is the inhibitor concentration causing half-maximal inactivation** and k_{inact} **is the maximal inactivation rate constant.**

TDIs reduce the concentration of viable enzyme and consequently reduce the V_{max} of other drugs (victims) metabolized by the enzyme. Recovery of enzyme activity after TDI is dependent on the synthesis of new enzyme, which is controlled by a physiological parameter, the first-order degradation constant (k_{degrad}) (see Chapter 20, Section 20.3.2) and will typically take about four k_{degrad} half-lives. Thus, the inhibitory effect may persist well after the perpetrator has been eliminated from the body and can be particularly problematic. Examples of therapeutic drugs that are known TDIs of CYP3A4 include the macrolide antibiotics (clarithromycin and erythromycin), diltiazem, and ritonavir.

The simulation model presented in Appendix E, "DDI 1: Time Dependent Enzyme Inhibition," http://web.uri.edu/pharmacy/research/rosenbaum/sims/Model13 can be used to understand how K_I, k_{inact}, k_{obs}, and the enzymes degradation rate constant (k_{degrad}) affect the magnitude and duration of inhibition.

It was shown in Appendix E that the ratio of intrinsic clearance in the absence and presence of the TDI, which is known as R_2, is given by:

$$R_2 = \frac{Cl_{int}}{Cl'_{int}} = \frac{k_{degrad} + \dfrac{k_{inact} * [I]}{K_I + [I]}}{k_{degrad}} \tag{17.4}$$

Large values of R_2 reflect extensive inhibition. The simulation model in Appendix E illustrates how the inhibitor parameters k_{inact} and K_I and the system parameter k_{degrad} influence the inhibition process. Small values of K_I (potency) and large values of k_{inact} promote most extensive inhibition. But drugs that have large values of k_{inact} can produce significant interactions at low concentration values even if they have high K_I values. Likewise drugs with very small K_I values can produce significant inhibition even if k_{inact} is small. The k_{inact}/K_I is used as a measure of the inactivation efficiency of TDI inhibitors [4]. Some examples of this ratio are shown in Table 17.1 [4].

TABLE 17.1   Examples of the k_{inact}/K_I Ratio for Several TDI Perpetrators

TDI Inhibitor	Enzyme	k_{inact}/K_I (mL/min/µM)
Desmethylamiodarone	CYP3A	4.3
Desmethylamiodarone	CYP 2C9	1.4
Desmethylamiodarone	CYP2D6	1.2
Paroxetine	CYP2A	0.85
Diltiazem	CYP3A	2.7
Erythromycin	CYP3A	3.6
Ritonavir	CYP3A	1200
Verapamil	CYP3A	24

The data indicate that desmethylamiodarone is a more potent inhibitor of CYP3A than CYP2C9, and its inhibition of CYP2D6 is less than that of CYP2C9. It also illustrates that ritonavir is a very powerful inhibitor of CYP3A. However, this ratio per se cannot be used to directly infer clinical DDI consequences as it is purely based on *in vitro* analysis of TDI and does not consider two additional crucial parameters, namely, [I] and k_{degrad}.

Equation (17.4) can be rearranged and expressed as follows:

$$R_2 = \frac{Cl_{int}}{Cl_{int}^I} = 1 + \frac{k_{inact}/k_{degrad}}{1 + (1/[I]/K_I)} \tag{17.5}$$

This arrangement [5] expresses the effect of a TDI in terms of two ratios: the [I]:K_I ratio and the k_{inact}:k_{degrad} ratio, which are measures of the functional inactivation potency and the inactivation rate, respectively. The arrangement illustrates that in common with reversible inhibitors, the degree of inhibition is dependent on the [I]:K_I ratio (the larger the [I]:K_I ratio, the greater the inhibition). The equation also illustrates the importance of the k_{inact}:k_{degrad} ratio (the larger this ratio, the greater the inhibition). If this ratio is very large, a highly clinically significant DDI could be observed from inhibitors with very low inactivation potencies. For example, based on the low value of the [I]/K_I ratio alone, paroxetine and erythromycin would not be predicted to produce clinically significant interactions from their respective inactivation of CYP2D6 and CYP3A. Yet, both cause clinically significant DDIs *in vivo* because the k_{inact}:k_{degrad} ratio is large [5].

The inhibitor's parameters are determined *in vitro*. The k_{obs} is determined directly, and K_I and k_{inact} are estimated from k_{obs} values at different inhibitor concentrations using equation (17.3). The degradation rate constant of the enzyme is a physiological parameter. It cannot be measured *in vivo* and is difficult to estimate *in vitro*. Consequently, the values of k_{degrad} for each of the enzymes published in the literature display wide variability, which can add some uncertainty to accuracy of the model. Some of the values of k_{degrad} reported in the literature are shown in Table 17.2.

TABLE 17.2   Literature Values for the Different CYP Enzymes

CYP Enzyme	k_{degrad} (h^{-1})
CYP1A2	0.0178[a]
CYP2D6	0.0136[a]
CYP3A	0.0289[a]; 0.0192[b]

[a]From [4].
[b]From [3].

17.2.3 Induction

Inducers of drug metabolism, such as rifampin, phenobarbital, and carbamazepine, increase the metabolism and clearance of their victim drugs. This can result in therapeutic failure and/or increased adverse effects if a metabolite is toxic. Rifampin, for example, which induces several of the CYP enzymes, decreases the *AUC* of oral midazolam to 2–4% of control values [6]. Inducers do not interfere with the binding of the drug to the enzyme but alter the regulation of the gene encoding the enzyme, which results in increased production and larger amounts of enzyme. Most commonly inducers activate the pregnane X receptor, which results in increased expression of several enzymes including CYP3A, CYP2C, and CYP2B. Over the years, clinical practice has identified far fewer inducers compared to inhibitors. As a result, induction-based DDIs have not received as much attention as inhibitor-based interactions. However, the *in vitro* screening studies that are now being used to identify inducers are finding that a large number of compounds are capable of inducing the CYP enzymes. It is possible that historically induction-based DDIs may have been underestimated, because the clinical effects associated with the subtherapeutic drug concentrations most commonly associated with induction are more subtle and more difficult to recognize in clinical practice.

In Appendix E, it was shown that the ratio of intrinsic clearance in the absence and presence of the inducer (R_3) is given by:

$$R_3 = \frac{Cl_{int}}{Cl_{int}^{Ind}} = \frac{1}{1 + \dfrac{E_{max} * [I]}{EC50 + [I]}} \tag{17.6}$$

where Cl_{int}^{Ind} is the victim drug's intrinsic clearance in the presence of an inducer, E_{max} is the maximum induction, and EC50 is the inducer concentration that brings about 50% induction.

The values of E_{max} and EC50 are determined *in vitro*. For example, Table 17.3 presents several E_{max} and EC50 values estimated from human hepatocytes for the induction of CYP3A. The data indicate that rifampin is capable of producing the greatest induction of CYP3A and that troglitazone is the most potent.

17.3 SURROGATE *IN VIVO* VALUES FOR THE UNBOUND CONCENTRATION OF THE PERPETRATOR AT THE SITE OF ACTION

The models used to predict *in vivo* DDIs apply the *in vitro* models described above to *in vivo* setting. Each of the three models above is driven by the unbound concentration [I] of the inhibitor at the enzyme or inducer at its receptor. Consequently, when applying these formulas *in vivo*, a relevant perpetrator concentration is needed. *In vivo* metabolism-based

TABLE 17.3 Example of the E_{max} and EC50 Values for the Induction of CYP3A by Several Inducers of Drug Metabolism

Inducer	E_{max} (fold increase)	EC50 (μM)
Rifampin	12.3	0.847
Omeprazole	2.36	0.225
Troglitazone	6.86	0.002
Phenobarbital	7.62	58.4

Source: Data from Reference [7].

DDIs primarily occur in the liver and intestine, where the relevant concentrations are $[I_h]$, the unbound concentration of perpetrator in the hepatocyte, and $[I_g]$, the unbound concentration in the enterocyte. Neither of these concentrations can be measured *in vivo*. Furthermore, they will change continuously over time after the administration of the perpetrator as it is absorbed into, and eliminated from the body. "Static" predictive models simplify the effect of a perpetrator by assuming a single, constant concentration. Generally, a conservative approach is taken and the highest concentration experienced at each site is selected for the values of $[I_h]$ and $[I_g]$.

17.3.1 Surrogate Measures of Hepatic Inhibitor and Inducer Concentrations

Several different concentrations have been proposed for the surrogate value for the unbound perpetrator concentration at the hepatic enzyme site. These include (see [8]):

- The maximum observed plasma concentration: C_{max} or $[I]_{max}$
- The maximum unbound plasma concentration: C_{maxu} or $[I]_{max,u}$
- The average plasma concentration after multiple oral doses
- The maximum unbound concentration in the portal vein or maximum unbound hepatic inlet concentration $C_{maxhi,u}$ or $[I]_{u,hi,max}$ [9]

$$[I]_{u,hi,max} = fu_b * \left(C_{maxb} + \frac{Dose * ka * Fa}{Q_h} \right) \tag{17.7}$$

where fu_b is the unbound fraction in the blood (see Chapter 5: $fu_b = fu/BP$); C_{maxb} is the maximal blood concentration), ka is the first-order absorption rate constant, Fa is the fraction of the dose absorbed into the apical side of the membrane, and Q_h is the hepatic blood flow (88.2 L/h). In the absence of a known value of Fa, 1 is often assumed. When ka is unknown, values of either 6.0 h^{-1} [1] or 1.8 h^{-1} [10] have been recommended.

At this time, a consensus has not been reached on which of the above values may be optimum and there is some empirical support to suggest it may depend on the type of perpetrator: $[I]_{u,hi,max}$ may work best for reversible inhibitors; and C_{maxu} for TDI and inducers [3].

17.3.2 Surrogate Measures of Intestinal Inhibitor and Inducer Concentrations

Similarly, conservative approaches have been taken for surrogate measures of the unbound concentration of the perpetrator in the enterocyte $[I_g]$. The concentrations used include (see [8]):

- maximal perpetrator concentration in the intestinal lumen after an oral dose:

$$[I_g] = \frac{Dose}{250 \text{ mL}} \tag{17.8}$$

In the above formula, it is assumed that 250 mL is the volume in which the entire dose dissolves and that dissolution is instantaneous. It also assumes that the entire dose becomes available to the intestinal enzymes. As such, it provides a high estimate of $[I_g]$.

• the estimated concentration of the perpetrator in the enterocyte during absorption

$$[I_g] = \frac{Dose * Fa * ka}{Q_{ent}}$$ (17.9)

where *Fa* is the fraction of the dose of the perpetrator entering the apical side of the gastrointestinal membrane, *ka* is the perpetrator's first-order rate constant, and Q_{ent} is the blood flow to the enterocytes (248 mL/min see [11]). In the absence of values for *Fa* and *ka*, default values are used as discussed above.

Dynamic models that use physiologically based pharmacokinetic (PBPK) modeling (see Chapter 18) to simulate the constantly changing concentrations of the perpetrators are being used increasingly in this field. In addition to more closely replicating the true time course of perpetrator concentrations, they are also able to simulate concentrations in the liver and intestine, which in theory should provide more meaningful estimates of $[I_h]$ and $[I_g]$.

17.4 MODELS USED TO PREDICT DDIs *IN VIVO*

17.4.1 Introduction

In vivo, DDIs are assessed by noting the changes in the *AUC* in the presence of a potential perpetrator of DDIs. The predictive models use the change in intrinsic clearance estimated from the *in vitro* models described above to estimate the ratio of the *AUC* in the presence and absence of the perpetrator *in vivo*. The *AUC* ratio is referred to as *AUCR*.

Recall for orally administered drugs:

$$AUC = \frac{Dose * F}{Cl}$$ (17.10)

Separating out the components of *F*

$$AUC = Dose * Fa * Fg * \frac{Fh}{Cl}$$ (17.11)

But as shown in Chapter 5 [equation (5.67)]

$$\frac{Fh}{Cl_h} = \frac{1}{Cl_{int} * fu}$$ (17.12)

where Cl_{int} and *fu* are intrinsic clearance and the fraction unbound in the plasma, respectively. Substituting into equation (17.11)

$$AUC = Dose * Fa * Fg * \left(\frac{1}{Cl_{int} * fu} \right)$$ (17.13)

In the presence of a perpetrator of a hepatic metabolism-based DDI, only Cl_{int} will be affected. From equation (17.13), the *AUC* ratio is expressed as:

$$\frac{AUC^P}{AUC} = \frac{Cl_{int}}{Cl_{int}^P}$$ (17.14)

where, AUC^P and Cl_{int}^P are the *AUC* and Cl_{int} in the presence of a perpetrator, respectively.

17.4.2 Basic Predictive Models: *R* Values

The basic predictive models assume that the victim drug is completely eliminated along the affected pathway. By ignoring other pathways of elimination that may be unaffected by the perpetrator, it constitutes the worst-case scenario. Although this basic model is expected to produce a large number of false positive results, its simplicity and conservative approach make it a valuable initial screen for perpetrators.

Thus, in the basic model, the ratio of the *AUC* in the absence and presence of the perpetrator is simply the *R* value for each type of perpetrator as shown in equations (17.2), (17.4), and (17.6), which are reproduced below:

$$\text{Reversible inhibition: } \frac{AUC^I}{AUC} = R_1 = \frac{Cl_{\text{int}}}{Cl_{\text{int}}^I} = (1 + [I]/Ki)$$

$$\text{Time-dependent inhibition: } \frac{AUC^I}{AUC} = R_2 = \frac{Cl_{\text{int}}}{Cl_{\text{int}}^I} = \frac{k_{\text{degrad}} + \dfrac{k_{\text{inact}} * [I]}{K_I + [I]}}{k_{\text{degrad}}}$$

$$\text{Induction [see equation (17.6)]: } \frac{AUC^{Ind}}{AUC} = R_3 = \frac{Cl_{\text{int}}}{Cl_{\text{int}}^{Ind}} = \frac{1}{1 + \dfrac{E_{\max} * [I]}{EC50 + [I]}}$$

Where the superscripts *I* and *Ind* represent inhibitor and inducer, respectively.

According to the FDA guidance [1], if the calculated *R* value for an inhibitor is less than 1.1, it can be concluded that the drug under evaluation is not a perpetrator of DDIs. Accordingly, no additional studies are required by the FDA. Likewise if the calculated *R* value for an inducer is greater than 0.9, according to the FDA guidance the drug may be labeled as a noninducer based on the *in vitro* data. If these criteria are not met (R_1 and $R_2 >$ 1.1 or $R_3 < 0.9$), further action is required including the estimation of the *AUC* ratio with a consideration of parallel pathways of elimination for the victim drug, which is presented in Section 4.3. Because of the higher perpetrator concentrations experienced in the gut, the cutoff values are different [1]. For example, when $[I_g]$ is calculated using Dose/250 mL, the cutoff for *R* is 11 instead of 1.1.

17.4.2.1 Example Applications of the Basic Model

Example 17.1 Fluconazole, nefazodone, and paroxetine are all reversible inhibitors of CYP2C9. In studies with warfarin as the victim drug, their K_i values have been reported as 5.5, 8.5, and 65 µM, respectively [12]. Based on $C_{\max}$ values for the inhibitors of 5.65, 1.39, and 1.00 µM, respectively, rate their predicted inhibitory effects.

$$R_1 = \frac{Cl_{\text{int}}}{Cl_{\text{int}}^I} = (1 + [I]/Ki)$$

$$\text{Fluconazole: } R_1 = \frac{Cl_{\text{int}}}{Cl_{\text{int}}^I} = (1 + 1.11/3.1) = 2$$

$$\text{Nefazodone: } R_1 = \frac{Cl_{\text{int}}}{Cl_{\text{int}}^I} = (1 + 1.39/8.5) = 1.16$$

$$\text{Paroxetine: } R_1 = \frac{Cl_{\text{int}}}{Cl_{\text{int}}^I} = (1 + 1.00/65) = 1.02$$

TABLE 17.4   Parameter Values and Typical C_{max} ([I]) Concentrations for Three Time-Dependent Inhibitors

Inhibitor	K_I (unbound) (μM)	k_{inact} (min^{-1})	k_{inact} (h^{-1})	k_{inact}/K_I (mL.min^{-1}. μmol^1)	[I] mg/L	[I] μM
Clarithromycin	18.9	0.053	3.18	2.80	1.07	1.43
Diltiazem	1.15	0.027	1.62	23.4	0.037	0.0892
Erythromycin	13.5	0.041	2.46	3.04	0.73	0.995

Thus, fluconazole would be expected to produce the greatest inhibition *in vivo* and paroxetine the least.

Example 17.2   Clarithromycin, diltiazem, and erythromycin are all TDI inhibitors of CYP3A4. Their K_I and k_{inact} values estimated using midazolam as the victim drug (see [3]) are shown in Table 17.4, which also shows typical C_{max} concentrations for each inhibitor.

Using a k_{degrad} value for CYP3A4 of 0.0192 h^{-1} [3] and the inhibitor concentrations shown in the table, determine the value of R_2 for the three inhibitors.

The molecular weights of the clarithromycin, diltiazem, and erythromycin are 748, 415, and 734 Da, respectively. Thus, [I] values are 1.43, 0.0892, and 0.995 μM, respectively.

Clarithromycin R_2

$$R_2 = \frac{k_{degrad} + \dfrac{k_{inact} * [I]}{K_I + [I]}}{k_{degrad}}$$

$$R_2 = \frac{0.0192 + \dfrac{3.18 * 1.43}{18.9 + 1.43}}{0.0192} = 12.6$$

Similar calculations give:

$$\text{Diltiazem } R_2 = 7.07$$
$$\text{Erythromycin } R_2 = 9.80$$

Thus, clarithromycin is predicted to cause the greatest inhibition, followed by erythromycin and then diltiazem.

Recalculate the values using each drug's K_I as the inhibitor concentration. The R_2 values for clarithromycin, diltiazem, and erythromycin are now 83.8, 43.2, and 65.1, respectively. The rank order is now the same as the rank order of the k_{inact}, and it illustrates that clarithromycin has the potential to be the most potent inhibitor when its concentration is high.

Example 17.3   Rifampin and carbamazepine are both inducers of several CYP enzymes. For induction of the metabolism of midazolam, the E_{max} and EC50 of rifampin have been reported as 23.2-fold increase and 0.943 μM, respectively and those of carbamazepine

39.1-fold increase and 14.9 μM, respectively (see [13]). Determine their R_3 values using C_{max} values of rifampin and carbamazepine of 7.9 and 21 μM, respectively.

$$R_3 = \frac{Cl_{int}}{Cl_{int}^{Ind}} = \frac{1}{1 + \dfrac{E_{max} * [I]}{EC50 + [I]}}$$

$$R_3 = \frac{1}{1 + \dfrac{23.2 * 7.9}{0.943 + 7.9}} = 0.046$$

Carbamazepine

$$R_3 = \frac{1}{1 + \dfrac{39.1 * 21}{14.9 + 21}} = 0.042$$

The value of R indicates that the inducers would have similar effects on the induction of the metabolism of midazolam.

17.4.3   Predictive Models Incorporating Parallel Pathways of Elimination (*fm*)

17.4.3.1   AUC and fm

Most drugs are eliminated by multiple pathways of elimination, only one of which is affected by a perpetrator. The impact of a change in activity of a single pathway to the overall *AUC* will depend on the importance of that pathway to the overall clearance and bioavailability of the drug. If the altered pathway constitutes only a minor pathway of elimination of the drug, changes in its activity will be much less important than if it is a major or sole pathway of elimination. The fraction of the dose metabolized by the affected pathway (*fm*) is defined as the fractional contribution of a single enzymatic pathway to the overall *AUC*. Note, *fm* is defined a little differently from *fe*, the fraction of the dose excreted unchanged in the urine (see Chapter 5) because the *AUC* derived from an enzymatic pathway is controlled not only by hepatic clearance but also by hepatic bioavailability.

Assume a drug is eliminated totally by the hepatic route ($Cl = Clh$; $Fg = 1$). Let Clh and Fh be the total clearance and hepatic bioavailability. Let Clh_1 and Fh_1 be clearance and bioavailability of the pathway affected by a perpetrator. The fractional contribution of the affected pathway to the overall *AUC*, (*fm*), is:

$$fm = \frac{Cl_1/Fh_1}{Cl/Fh} \tag{17.15}$$

Using the expression for oral hepatic clearance presented previously [equation (17.12)]

$$fm = \frac{Cl_1/Fh_1}{Cl/Fh} = \frac{Cl_{int1}}{Cl_{int}} \tag{17.16}$$

The *AUC* ratio in the presence and absence of a perpetrator was given in equation (17.14) and is reproduced below:

$$AUCR = \frac{AUC^P}{AUC} = \frac{Cl_{int}}{Cl_{int}^P} \tag{17.17}$$

Partitioning total intrinsic clearance into the affected pathway ($Cl_{int1} = Cl_{int} * fm$ (in the absence of a perpetrator); Cl^P_{int1} (in the presence of a perpetrator)) and unaffected pathway ($Cl_{int} * (1 - fm)$):

$$AUCR = \frac{Cl_{int} * fm + Cl_{int}(1 - fm)}{Cl^P_{int1} + Cl_{int}(1 - fm)} \qquad (17.18)$$

Dividing through by Cl_{int}

$$AUCR = \frac{1}{\dfrac{Cl^P_{int1}}{Cl_{int}} + (1 - fm)} \qquad (17.19)$$

But from (17.16), $Cl_{int} = Cl_{int1}/fm$
Thus,

$$AUCR = \frac{1}{fm * \dfrac{Cl^P_{int1}}{Cl_{int1}} + (1 - fm)} \qquad (17.20)$$

Thus, the change in the *AUC* of a victim drug brought about by an inhibitor or inducer that affects only one of several pathways of metabolism can be predicted based on the ratio of intrinsic clearance in the presence and absence of the perpetrator and the fraction of the victim drug metabolized by the affected enzyme (*fm*). The ratio of the intrinsic clearance in the presence and absence of any of the three types of modifiers is the perpetrator's *R* value. The *R* values for each type of perpetrator [equations (17.2), (17.4), and (17.6)] can be incorporated in turn into equation (17.20) to provide the relevant equations for the three types of perpetrators. Note the simulation models presented in the next sections demonstrate the critical importance of obtaining accurate values for *fm*, especially when *fm* is high (>0.8).

17.4.3.2 Reversible Inhibitors of Hepatic Enzymes

Substituting the expression for R_1 [equation (17.3)] into equation (17.20), the *AUCR* for reversible inhibitors is given by:

$$AUCR = \frac{1}{fm * \left(\dfrac{1}{1 + [I]/Ki}\right) + (1 - fm)} \qquad (17.21)$$

Example and Simulation: http://web.uri.edu/pharmacy/research/rosenbaum/sims

1. *Calculate the estimated AUCR for the inhibition of the hepatic metabolism of mida-zolam (fm = 0.93) by fluconazole (K_i = 3.4 µM [12]). Use an estimated C_{max} of 6.72 mg/L or (1000 * 6.92/306 = 21.96 µM) for fluconazole (MW = 306 Da) after a 400-mg single dose.*

$$AUCR = \frac{1}{0.93 * \left(\dfrac{1}{1 + (21.96/3.4)}\right) + (0.07)} = 5.14$$

2. *Open simulation model 15, DDI 3 Reversible Inhibition: Fluconazole and Midazo-lam, which can be found at http://web.uri.edu/pharmacy/research/rosenbaum/sims/Model15. In addition to the parameters noted above, the following parameters for midazolam are used [14]: fu = 0.016; BP = 0.653; Cl = 4.74 mL/min/kg; fe = 0; Vd = 0.78 L/kg; Fa = 1 and Fg = 1 (in a later model in Section 4.4.2, Fg is also incorporated into the predictive model). A first-order absorption rate constant of 6 h^{-1} was assumed and the default oral dose of midazolam is 10 mg. The simulation model assumes a body weight of 70 Kg.*

3. *Perform a simulation with the inhibitor button switched off. Note the values of Cl, Clh, Fh, and t1/2. Turn on the inhibitor switch and repeat the simulation. Note the value of AUCR, which is determined using a built-in calculator and displayed on the model interface. Also note, fluconazole increases midazolam's Fh 1.4-fold and Cl (plasma) decreases to 26.6% its normal value. Midazolam's Cl_{int} can be calculated as described in Chapter 5 or from $Clb_h/Fh = Cl_{int} * fb$ or $Cl_h/Fh = Cl_{int} * fu$. Thus, in the absence of the inhibitor, Cl_{int} is 1661 L/h and in the presence of the inhibitor, Cl_{int} is 223 L/h.*

4. *Alter the inhibitor concentration ($C_{max}(mg/L)$) from 2.5, 5, 10, 20, 50, 75, and 100 mg/L. Note the value of AUCR for each value of C_{max}. Plot the data and note the hyperbolic shape. Also note that the inhibitory effects appear to be reaching a maximum at higher concentrations.*

5. *The value of fm varies among drugs. Note the values of AUCR when fm changes through 0.2, 0.3, 0.4, 0.5, 0.6, 0.7, 0.8, 0.85, 0.9, 0.95, 0.99, and 1. Plot AUCR as a function of fm. Note how AUCR increases exponentially with increases in fm. At low fm values, AUCR increases gently as fm increases. In contrast, beyond fm values of 0.8, there is a very steep relationship between AUCR and fm. This illustrates the importance of obtaining accurate values of fm when estimating the magnitude of interactions, particularly when a drug's fm approaches 1.*

17.4.3.3 Models for Time-Dependent Inhibitors

Substituting the expression for R_2 [equation (17.4) into equation (17.20)], the *AUCR* for TDI is given by:

$$AUCR = \frac{1}{fm * \dfrac{k_{degrad}}{\left(k_{degrad} + \frac{k_{inact}*[I]}{K_I+[I]}\right)} + (1-fm)} \qquad (17.22)$$

Example and Simulation: http://web.uri.edu/pharmacy/research/rosenbaum/sims

Investigate the potential interaction between paroxetine, a TDI of CYP2D6, and desipramine ($fm_{CYP2D6} = 0.85$). Use the following parameters for paroxetine [15]: unbound $K_I = 0.315\ \mu M$, $k_{inact} = 10.2\ h^{-1}$, and $[I] = 5\ nM$. Use a k_{degrad}, CYP2D6 of 0.0136 h^{-1}.

1. *Calculate the [I]:K_I and the k_{inact}:k_{degrad} ratio. Note the [I]/K_I ratio of 0.016 indicates low potency but note the k_{inact}:k_{degrad} ratio of 750 is indicative of powerful inactivation.*

2. *Calculate the estimated AUCR for the interaction*

$$AUCR = \frac{1}{0.85 * \dfrac{0.0136}{\left(0.0136 + \frac{10.2*0.005}{0.315+0.005}\right)} + (0.15)} = 4.59$$

3. Open simulation model 16, DDI 4 Time Dependent Inhibition-Paroxetine and Desipramine, which can be found at *http://web.uri.edu/pharmacy/research/ rosenbaum/sims/Model16*. The model has been created using the parameters listed above as well as the following parameters for desipramine (see [16]): $fu = 0.18$, $Cl_{int} = 701$ L/h, $fm_{CYP2D6} = 0.85$, and $BP = 0.96$. Additionally, $Fa = 1$, $Fg = 1$, and $Vd = 2065$ L (based on a reported value of Vd_{ss}/F of 2950 L [17] and an assumed bioavailability of 0.7) and $ka = 0.6$ h^{-1}(based on an observed peak at 4–6 h).

4. Perform a run with the inhibitor button turned off. Observe the Cp–time profile and desipramine's Cl, Fh, and t1/2. Turn to inhibitor button on and simulate the effects of paroxetine on desipramine. Check the displayed value of AUCR with the value calculated above. Note the values of Cl, Fh, and the t1/2 and the pharmacokinetic parameters. Observe the predicted plasma concentration–time profiles in the absence and presence of paroxetine. Compare the values of desipramine's C_{max} displayed in the graph. Based on the change in all these parameters, do you predict that paroxetine affects the clearance and/or the bioavailability of desipramine?

5. Clear the graph and adjust the paroxetine concentration. Start at 0.5 nm and successively double it. Note the inhibitor's action reaches a maximum value.

6. Note the values of AUCR when fm changes through 0.2, 0.3, 0.4, 0.5, 0.6, 0.7, 0.8, 0.85, 0.9, 0.95, 0.99, and 1. Plot AUCR as a function of fm. Note how AUCR increases exponentially with increases in fm. As observed for reversible inhibitor, AUCR increases exponentially with fm. When fm > 0.8, a very steep relationship exists between AUCR and fm and AUCR becomes highly sensitive to changes in fm. As was the case for reversible inhibition, this illustrates the importance of obtaining accurate values of fm when estimating the magnitude of interactions, particularly when a drug's fm approaches 1.

7. Reset all devices and clear the graph and perform a simulation. Note the values of the ratios: k_{inact}/K_I, $[I]:K_I$, and the $k_{inact}:k_{degrad}$, which can all be used to assess TDIs. Reduce the values of K_I (inhibitor is getting more potent) and note the values of the AUCR and the ratios. Return K_I to its default value 0.315, and now decrease k_{inact}, that is, make the inhibitor less destructive. Note the values of the AUCR and the ratios.

17.4.3.4 Model for Inducers of the Drug-Metabolizing Enzymes

Substituting the expression for R_3 [equation (17.6)] into equation (17.20), the AUCR for an inducer is given by:

$$AUCR = \cfrac{1}{fm * \left(1 + \cfrac{E_{max} * [I]}{EC50 + [I]}\right) + (1 - fm)}$$

Example: A drug is primarily eliminated by CYP3A4 elimination ($fm = 0.93$). Estimate the AUCR when it is administered in conjunction with rifampin (EC50 = 0.943, E_{max} = 23.2-fold increase and $[I] = 7.9$ μM. [13])

$$AUCR = \cfrac{1}{0.93 * \left(1 + \cfrac{23.2 * 7.9}{0.943 + 7.9}\right) + (1 - 0.93)} = 0.49$$

17.4.4 Models Incorporating Intestinal Extraction

17.4.4.1 Model for Intestinal Extraction

A review of intestinal presystemic metabolism and the models used to predict intestinal extraction has recently been published [18]. Although the human intestine expresses a number of drug-metabolizing enzymes, CYP3A is the most abundant, constituting about 80% of total intestinal CYP enzymes and as a result has been the most extensively studied. Other cytochrome P450 enzymes are present but in much lower concentrations. For example, CYP2C9, the next most abundant, accounts for only about 14% of the total intestinal CYP. UDP-glucuronosyltransferases (UGTs) are also present and are believed to be important for the intestinal extraction and low bioavailability of raloxifene and troglitazone. However, the intestinal UGTs have not been well studied to date.

Intestinal extraction by CYP3A will be the focus of the following discussion. Despite its low expression (1%) compared to the liver, it plays an important role in limiting the bioavailability of several drugs. For example, values of 0.11, 0.07, 0.14, and 0.57 have been reported for the intestinal bioavailability (*Fg*) of buspirone, lovastatin, tacrolimus, and midazolam, respectively. It is believed that the much lower blood flow to the enterocytes compared to the liver (248 versus 1500 mL/min) provides the enterocytes with a greater opportunity to metabolize drugs and results in a more efficient extraction process. Drugs that experience high intestinal extraction can be subject to highly clinically significant DDIs. For example, grapefruit juice, a selective inhibitor of intestinal CYP3A4, increases the *AUC* of buspirone (*Fg* ~ 0.11) an average of about 9.2-fold and that of midazolam (*Fg* = 0.57) only 1.5-fold. Likewise, regular strength grapefruit juice has a much more profound effect on the pharmacokinetics of simvastatin (3.6-fold increase in *AUC* [19]), which undergoes extensive intestinal extraction (*Fg* ~ 0.14) compared to atorvastatin (1.4-fold increase in the *AUC*) [20], which undergoes more modest extraction (*Fg* ~ 0.38).

Predictive DDI models at the intestinal level apply the well-stirred venous equilibrium model (see Chapter 5 and equation 5.53) to develop an expression for the intestinal extraction ratio [21]. Thus:

$$Eg = \frac{Cl_{\text{intg}} * fu}{Q_g + Cl_{\text{intg}} * fu} \tag{17.23}$$

where *Eg* is the extraction ratio for intestinal metabolism, Q_g is the blood flow to the enterocytes, Cl_{intg} is the unbound intestinal intrinsic clearance, and *fu* is the unbound drug fraction.

An expression for *Fg*, which is equal to $1 - Eg$, can be obtained from equation 17.23:

$$Fg = \frac{Q_g}{Q_g + Cl_{\text{intg}} * fu} \tag{17.24}$$

Let Fg^{p} and Cl_{intg}^{P} be the intestinal bioavailability and intrinsic clearance, respectively, in the presence of a perpetrator.

$$\frac{Fg^{P}}{Fg} = \frac{Q_g + Cl_{\text{intg}} * fu}{Q_g + Cl_{\text{intg}}^{P} * fu} \tag{17.25}$$

Rearranging

$$\frac{Fg^P}{Fg} = \frac{1}{\dfrac{Q_g}{Q_g + Cl_{intg} * fu} + \dfrac{Cl_{intg}^P * fu}{Q_g + Cl_{intg} * fu}} \tag{17.26}$$

Multiplying the second term in the denominator by Cl_{intg}

$$\frac{Fg^P}{Fg} = \frac{1}{\dfrac{Q_g}{Q_g + Cl_{intg} * fu} + \dfrac{Cl_{intg} Cl_{intg}^P * fu}{(Q_g + Cl_{intg} * fu) Cl_{intg}}} \tag{17.27}$$

The first expression in the denominator is Fg [equation (17.24)] and the second expression contains the expression for $(1 - Fg)$ [equation (17.23)]; substituting for these:

$$\frac{Fg^P}{Fg} = \frac{1}{Fg + (1 - Fg) * \dfrac{Cl_{intg}^P}{Cl_{intg}}} \tag{17.28}$$

If the perpetrator brings no changes in Fa, Fh, or Cl

$$AUCR = \frac{AUC^P}{AUC} = \frac{Fg^P}{Fg} = \frac{1}{Fg + (1 - Fg) * \dfrac{Cl_{intg}^P}{Cl_{intg}}} \tag{17.29}$$

Thus, in common with modifiers of hepatic metabolism, changes in the AUC brought about by perpetrators that alter the activity of intestinal enzymes can also be predicted by the ratio (R) of intrinsic clearance (intestinal) in the presence and absence of a perpetrator.

The $AUCR$ from reversible inhibitors, TDI, and inducers can be estimated by substituting equations (17.2), (17.5), and (17.6), respectively, for Cl_{intg}^P/Cl_{intg} in equation (17.29).

Predictive AUC Ratio ($AUCR$) for Reversible Inhibitors of Intestinal Metabolism

$$AUCR = \frac{1}{Fg + (1 - Fg) * \dfrac{1}{(1 + [I_g]/Ki)}} \tag{17.30}$$

Predictive $AUCR$ for TDIs of Intestinal Metabolism

$$AUCR = \frac{1}{Fg + (1 - Fg) * \dfrac{k_{degrad}}{\left(k_{degrad} + \dfrac{k_{inact} * [I_g]}{K_I + [I_g]} \right)}} \tag{17.31}$$

It is difficult to obtain estimates for the degradation constant (k_{degrad}) of intestinal CYP3A4, and published values vary widely. A value of 0.0288 h^{-1} is recommended (see [18]).

Predictive *AUCR* for Inducers of Intestinal Metabolism

$$AUCR = \frac{1}{Fg + (1 - Fg) * \left(1 + \dfrac{E_{max} * [I_g]}{EC50 + [I_g]}\right)} \tag{17.32}$$

Most drugs that undergo intestinal extraction also undergo hepatic metabolism. Consequently, the simulation model and example for intestinal extraction presented in Section 4.4.3 also incorporate hepatic metabolism.

17.4.4.2 Combined Hepatic and Intestinal Extraction
The predictive models for hepatic metabolism and intestinal extraction are usually combined because a perpetrator that alters the activity of CYP3A has the potential to alter both hepatic and intestinal metabolism. The combined model for a reversible inhibitor is shown below:

$$AUCR = \frac{AUC^P}{AUC} = \frac{1}{fm * \dfrac{1}{(1 + [I_h]/Ki)} + (1 - fm)} * \frac{1}{Fg + (1 - Fg) * \dfrac{1}{(1 + [I_g]/Ki)}} \tag{17.33}$$

Example: The model presented earlier on fluconazole's reversible inhibition of midazolam will now be extended to also incorporate intestinal metabolism.

Assume that *fm* and *Fg* for midazolam are 0.93(4) and 0.57(11), respectively, and that fluconazole has a $K_i = 3.4$ μM. Use an $[I_h]$ of 7.2 μM and an $[I_g] = 59.3$ μm [11] and calculate the *AUCR* for this potential interaction

$$AUCR = \frac{1}{0.93 * \dfrac{1}{(1 + 7.2/3.4)} + (1 - 0.93)} * \frac{1}{0.57 + (1 - 0.57) * \dfrac{1}{(1 + 59.3/3.4)}} = 4.5$$

Note the value of *AUCR* reported in a clinical study was 3.60 (see [11]).

17.4.4.3 Simulation and the Estimation of Fg Using Grapefruit Juice:
http://web.uri.edu/pharmacy/research/rosenbaum/sims
The combined hepatic and intestinal predictive model will be further studied using simulation model 17, DDI 5 Hepatic and Intestinal Metabolism, which can be found at: http://web.uri.edu/pharmacy/research/rosenbaum/sims/Model17.

The model has been created with default parameters based on the interaction between fluconazole and oral midazolam. In addition to the parameters of fluconazole and midazolam noted above, the following pharmacokinetic parameters were used for midazolam [14]: fu = 0.016; BP = 0.653; Cl = 4.74 mL/min/kg; fe = 0; Vd = 0.78 L/kg; a first-order absorption rate constant of 6 h^{-1} was used.

Based on fu = 0.016 and Q_g = 14.9 L/h, intestinal intrinsic clearance (Cl_{intg}) was estimated

$$Fg = \frac{Q_g}{Q_g + Cl_{intg} * fu}$$

thus, Cl_{intg} = 702 L/h

1. *Perform a simulation to evaluate midazolam's pharmacokinetics in the absence and presence of fluconazole (inhibitor). Compare the value of AUCR displayed in the simulation model to the value calculated above (Section 4.4.3). If you wish to compare this value to the one estimated using the model considering only hepatic metabolism only (Section 6.2), the inhibitor concentration in the latter model will have to be adjusted to match the one used in this simulation.*

2. *Grapefruit juice is a TDI of intestinal but not hepatic CYP3A4. It inhibits intestinal metabolism and extraction but leaves hepatic metabolism unaltered. These characteristics have led to its use in the estimation of Fg. Turn the inhibitor switch off. Perform a run and note the value of oral clearance (Cl/F), which is a parameter that is easily and frequently measured in clinical studies. Note F = Fa * Fh * Fg. If it is assumed Fa = 1 then Cl/F = Cl/(Fh * Fg). Turn on the grapefruit switch and note the value of oral clearance, which assuming complete inhibition of intestinal extraction and Fg = 1 is now Cl/Fh. Use the two values of oral clearance to work backwards to estimate Fg.*

   1. *Control (no grapefruit juice)*

   (a) *Estimate oral clearance of the CYP3A4 pathway*

   $$\left(\frac{Clh}{Fh * Fg}\right)_{CYP3A4} = \frac{Cl}{Fh * Fg} * fm = 50.1 * 0.93 = 46.5 \text{ L/h}$$

   (b) *Estimate blood oral clearance of the CYP3A4 pathway*

   $$\left(\frac{Clb_h}{Fh * Fg}\right)_{CYP3A4} = \left(\frac{Clh}{Fh * Fg}\right)_{CYP3A4} * \frac{1}{BP} = \frac{46.5}{0.653} = 71.21 \text{ L/h}$$

   2. *Test (grapefruit juice)*

   (c) *Estimate oral clearance of the CYP3A4 pathway assuming no change in hepatic CYP34 activity and complete inhibition of intestinal CYP3A4 (Fg = 1)*

   $$\left(\frac{Clh}{Fh}\right)_{CYP3A4} = \frac{Cl}{Fh} * fm = 28.6 * 0.93 = 26.6 \text{ L/h}$$

   (d) *Estimate blood oral clearance of the CYP3A4 pathway*

   $$\left(\frac{Clb_h}{Fh}\right)_{CYP3A4} = \left(\frac{Clh}{Fh}\right)_{CYP3A4} * \frac{1}{BP} = \frac{26.6}{0.653} = 40.73 \text{ L/h}$$

   Calculate Fg
   Assuming Fa = 1, F = Fh * Fg, and that Fg = 1 in the presence of grapefruit juice

   $$\left(\frac{Clb_h}{Fh * Fg}\right)_{CYP3A4} = 71.21 \text{ and } \left(\frac{Clb_h}{Fh}\right)_{CYP3A4} = 40.73 \text{ thus } \frac{39.2}{Fg} = 71.21$$

   Fg = 0.57

3. *Probe the effects of different values of fm, Cl_{intg}, and inhibitor concentrations, which will bring about equal changes to $[I_h]$ and $[I_g]$.*

4. *Compare the profiles obtained with very high inhibitor concentrations to those obtained with grapefruit juice.*

17.4.5 Models Combining Multiple Actions of Perpetrators

Perpetrators of DDIs may have effects on more than one of the hepatic CYP enzymes. Additionally, perpetrators may simultaneously act as reversible inhibitors, TDI, and/or inducers. In such cases, the various predictive models may be combined to accommodate all the actions of a perpetrator [11].

Let

$$A_h = \left(\frac{1}{1 + [I_h]/Ki} \right)$$

$$B_h = \frac{k_{\text{degrad}}}{\left(k_{\text{degrad}} + \frac{k_{\text{inact}} * [I_h]}{K_I + [I_h]} \right)}$$

$$C_h = \left(1 + \frac{E_{\text{max}} * [I_h]}{EC50 + [I_h]} \right)$$

$$A_g = \frac{1}{(1 + [I_g]/Ki)}$$

$$B_g = \frac{k_{\text{degrad}}}{\left(k_{\text{degrad}} + \frac{k_{\text{inact}} * [I_g]}{K_I + [I_g]} \right)}$$

$$C_g = \left(1 + \frac{E_{\text{max}} * [I_g]}{EC50 + [I_g]} \right)$$

For combined effects

$$AUCR = \left(\frac{1}{[A_h * B_h * C_h] * fm + (1 - fm)} \right) * \left(\frac{1}{[A_g * B_g * C_g] * (1 - Fg) + Fg} \right)$$

Example: Erythromycin (MW = 734 DA) is both a reversible inhibitor and TDI of CYP3A. When midazolam was used as a victim drug, the following parameters were reported: $K_i = 9$ µM, $K_I = 13.5$ µM, and $k_{\text{inact}} = 2.46$ h^{-1} (see [3]). After a 500-mg dose of erythromycin, the C_{max} is estimated to be 0.950 µM. Assume the following for erythromycin: $fu = 0.162$, $Fa = 1$, and $ka = 1.8$ h^{-1}.

Use values of the k_{degrad} for CYP3A4 of 0.0192 and 0.0288 h^{-1} for the liver and enterocytes, respectively, and blood flow to the liver and hepatocytes of 88.2 and 14.9 L/h, respectively, and calculate the estimated $AUCR$ for midazolam ($fm = 0.98$ and $Fg = 0.57$). Use the unbound C_{maxu} of 0.154 µM for $[I_h]$ for the TDI model and a value of 1.06 µM for the maximum unbound hepatic inlet concentration for reversible inhibition. For intestinal extraction, use an estimated concentration of 45.7 µM for erythromycin's enterocyte concentration after a 500-mg dose.

$$A_h = \left(\frac{1}{1 + 1.06/9} \right) = 0.89$$

$$B_h = \frac{0.0192}{\left(0.0192 + \frac{2.46 * 0.154}{13.5 + 0.154} \right)} = 0.41$$

$$A_g = \frac{1}{(1 + 45.7/9)} = 0.164$$

$$B_g = \frac{0.0288}{\left(0.0288 + \dfrac{2.46 * 45.7}{13.5 + 45.7}\right)} = 0.0149$$

$$AUCR = \left(\frac{1}{[0.41 * 0.89] * 0.93 + 0.07)}\right) * \left(\frac{1}{[0.0149 * 0.164] * 0.43 + 0.57}\right) = 4.2$$

The *AUCR* observed in a clinical study was 3.8.

17.5   PREDICTIVE MODELS FOR TRANSPORTER-BASED DDIs

Clinically, significant drug transporter-based DDIs are being increasingly recognized. Most commonly, the perpetrator drug alters the absorption, hepatic metabolism, or renal excretion of the victim drug. For example, induction or inhibition of intestinal permeability glycoprotein can decrease and increase digoxin absorption, respectively, exposing a patient to potentially serious subtherapeutic or toxic concentrations of digoxin, respectively. Inhibition of hepatic organic anion transporting polypeptide (OATP) family of transporters by cyclosporine, gemfibrozil, and rifampin can produce large increases in the *AUC* of drugs such as the statins and sartans that depend on OATPs (OATP1B1, OATP1B3, and OATP2B1) for uptake into the liver for their subsequent hepatic elimination. The prototypic organic anion transporter (OAT) inhibitor probenecid decreases the renal clearance of several drugs including methotrexate. Gemfibrozil, which as noted above inhibits OATP, is also an inhibitor of renal OAT. The clinically significant increase in the *AUC* of pravastatin when coadministered with gemfibrozil is thought to be the result of both a reduction in renal clearance via OAT and a reduction in hepatic clearance via OATP. In light of the risks associated with altered transporter activities, the predictive models based on those developed for metabolism are now being applied to transporter-based DDIs.

17.5.1   Kinetics of Drug Transporters

Transporter systems are assumed to follow Michaelis–Menten kinetics:

$$\text{Rate of Transport} = \frac{J_{max} * C}{Km_t + C} \tag{17.34}$$

where J_{max} is the maximum rate of transport, Km_t is the Michaelis–Menten constant for the process, and C is the driving concentration. Assuming that Km_t is much greater than C, the process can be viewed as first order:

$$\text{Rate of Transport} = \frac{J_{max}}{Km_t} * C = Cl_{intact,t} * C \tag{17.35}$$

where J_{max}/Km_t is referred to as transporter intrinsic clearance ($Cl_{intact,t}$).
   The effect of a reversible inhibitor of a transporter is given by:

$$\frac{Cl_{intact,t}}{Cl_{intact,t}^I} = (1 + [I]/Ki) \tag{17.36}$$

where $Cl_{intact,t}{}^I$ is the transporter intrinsic clearance in the presence of the inhibitor, $[I]$ is the inhibitor concentration, and K_i is the inhibitor's dissociation constant, which is determined *in vitro* using recombinant cell lines or hepatocytes. As discussed in Appendix E, the K_i is difficult to estimate and the IC50 is often measured in transporter studies. The relationship between K_i and the IC50 was discussed in Appendix E. Using the IC50 for the inhibitory potency:

$$\frac{Cl_{intact,t}}{Cl_{intact,t}{}^I} = (1 + [I]/IC50) \tag{17.37}$$

The same predictive equations discussed earlier can also be applied to DDIs involving transporters. The recommendations of International Transporter Consortium for evaluating transporter-based DDIs have been published [22]. For example, for inhibitors of hepatic OATPs, initially the ratio of the maximum unbound plasma concentration ($[I]$) and the K_i (or IC50) is determined. If this ratio is greater than or equal to 0.1, the R value should then be calculated based on an inhibitor concentration equal to the maximum unbound concentration in the portal vein ($[I]_{u,hi,max}$) [equation (17.7)] as follows:

$$R = \frac{Cl_{intact,t}}{Cl_{intact,t}{}^I} = (1 + [I]_{u,hi,max}/K_i) \tag{17.38}$$

An R value of greater than 2 for an OATP inhibitor is indicative of a potentially clinically significant interaction and should be followed with a clinical study using a well-known OATP substrate such as atorvastatin, pravastatin, pitavastatin, or rosuvastatin [22].

Example 1 (see [22]). The IC50 for lopinavir's inhibition of OATP is 0.1 μM. After 400 mg doses, its estimated C_{max} is 15–20 μM and its *fu* value is 0.015. Estimate the $[I]/IC50$ ratio based on the unbound drug concentration.

$$\frac{[I]}{IC50} = \frac{0.3}{0.1} = 3$$

This is greater than 0.1. Calculate the R value based on an $[I]_{u,hi,max}$ of 0.491 μM (*fu* = 0.015; dose = 400 mg; ka = 0.03 min^{-1}, Fa = 1; and Q = 1500 mL/min; MW = 629 DA)

$$R = \frac{Cl_{intact,t}}{Cl_{intact,t}{}^I} = \left(1 + \frac{[I]_{u,hi,max}}{IC50}\right) = \left(1 + \frac{0.491}{0.1}\right) = 5.91$$

This R value suggests that lopinavir could bring about clinically significant drug interactions for those drugs whose clearance is highly dependent on OATP.

Example 2, A study on inhibition of the OATP-mediated uptake of a new drug found gemfibrozil's and cyclosporine's K_i for the inhibition to be 7.4 and 0.82 μM, respectively. Calculate R based on the maximum unbound concentration in the portal vein ($[I]_{u,hi,max}$) using the following values:

Gemfibrozil (MW = 250 DA), Dose = 600 mg; C_{maxb} = 138 μM; fu_b = 0.05; ka = 0.025 min^{-1}; and Fa = 1.

Cyclosporine (MW = 1203 DA), Dose = 800 mg; C_{maxb} = 1.37 μM; fu_b = 0.1; ka = 0.1 min^{-1}; and Fa = 0.5.

(a) Gemfibrozil

$$[I]_{u,hi,max} = fu_b * \left(C_{maxb} + \frac{Dose * ka * Fa}{Q_h} \right)$$

$$= 0.05 * \left(138 + \frac{600 * 1000/250 * 0.025 * 1}{1.5} \right) = 8.9 \, \mu M$$

$$R = \left(1 + \frac{[I]}{K_i} \right) = \left(1 + \frac{8.9}{7.4} \right) = 2.19$$

(b) Cyclosporine

$$[I]_{u,hi,max} = fu_b * \left(C_{maxb} + \frac{Dose * ka * Fa}{Q_h} \right)$$

$$= 0.1 * \left(1.37 + \frac{800 * 1000/1203 * 0.1 * 0.5}{1.5} \right) = 2.35 \, \mu M$$

$$R = \left(1 + \frac{[I]}{K_i} \right) = \left(1 + \frac{2.35}{0.82} \right) = 3.87$$

The R values suggest that both gemfibrozil and cyclosporine could have a clinically significant interaction with the victim drug and that cyclosporine effect would be more pronounced.

The extent to which inhibition of a transporter affects the overall clearance of a victim depends on the importance of the transporter to the overall clearance of the drug. For example, the overall effect of the inhibition of a drug's OATP hepatic uptake will depend on extent to which hepatic clearance contributes to the overall clearance and the extent to which the drug's hepatic clearance is dependent on OATP uptake. More refined predictive models consider the fractional contribution of transporter clearance to overall clearance (ft) [23]. This is analogous to the use of the fraction of the dose metabolized along the affected pathway (fm) for metabolism-based interactions. Thus, for reversible inhibition:

$$AUCR = \frac{1}{ft * \left(\frac{1}{1 + [I]/Ki} \right) + (1 - ft)}$$

For example, if the hepatic uptake of a drug by OATP1B1 controls hepatic clearance and if the drug also undergoes renal clearance with an fe value of 0.10, ft could be set to 0.9.

The application of the models to predict transporter-based DDIs is evolving and is an area of active area of research. Compared to the drug-metabolizing enzymes, less is known about the transporters themselves including their abundance in different tissues. Transporter predictive models are also complicated by several additional factors. First, many of the perpetrators of transporter-based interactions lack specificity and frequently alter not only the activity of more than one transporter but also may alter the activity of the drug-metabolizing enzymes. This makes it difficult to isolate an effect on a single transporter. Additionally, the absorption and elimination processes frequently proceed along a number of sequential steps that involve the interplay of several transporter systems and the drug-metabolizing enzymes. For example, although the rate-limiting step in the hepatic elimination of many of the statins is believed to be active hepatic uptake by the OATP1B1 and OATP1B3 transporters, once in the hepatocytes these drugs undergo metabolism by the CYP enzymes and biliary excretion mediated by efflux transporters. Predictive DDI models that isolate only the hepatic uptake may not be able to accurately predict the impact of a perpetrator on the overall elimination. Complex mechanistic models (extended clearance models, see Chapter 18, Figure 18.6) that incorporate transporter systems, biliary excretion and metabolism have been developed to address this problem [24, 25]. Additionally, dynamic PBPK models that simulate drug concentrations in different tissues may be better suited for the development of these complex predictive models. The commercial PBPK software packages such as Simcyp incorporate detailed models for drug absorption and hepatic elimination, which can be more easily adapted to study a potential perpetrator's effect at several levels.

17.6 APPLICATION OF PHYSIOLOGICALLY BASED PHARMACOKINETIC MODELS TO DDI PREDICTION: THE DYNAMIC APPROACH

PBPK modeling, which is introduced in Chapter 18, is becoming an increasingly used tool in drug development and one of its most important and widespread applications is in the prediction of DDIs *in vivo*. Between 2008 and 2011, the FDA received 25 submissions containing PBPK modeling and 60% of these were on their use in predicting DDIs [26]. The approach is based on the same techniques and models used to estimate changes in the activity (Cl_{int}) of enzymes and/or transporters, but differs from the static models discussed above in that the concentrations of the perpetrator and victim drugs are continuously modeled over time after a dose. Also, because the PBPK models incorporate real tissues including the liver and the gut, the concentration of the perpetrator at the site of the interaction (liver, gut, etc.) can be estimated, which should provide more accurate predictive estimates and fewer false positive predictions compared to the more conservative static approaches. PBPK models are also very versatile and can be easily adapted to address more complex scenarios. For example, the PBPK approach was used to evaluate interactions for a victim drug metabolized by both CYP3A and CYP2D6. Once the model had been validated and had been shown to reproduce plasma concentrations–time profiles observed *in vivo*, it was used to simulate the effects of CYP3A inhibitors in individuals who were poor metabolizers of CYP2D6 [26]. This was particularly useful because this is a difficult issue to address in a clinical study. Additionally, as detailed in Chapter 18, increasingly sophisticated PBPK models are being developed, which simultaneously incorporate hepatic and intestinal metabolism as well as transporters at relevant sites in the body, making PBPK ideally suited to assess the impact of perpetrators that act on one or more enzymes and/or transporters. In light of the increasing use of PBPK modeling in predicting DDIs, a review of best practices required for regulatory submissions has recently been published [26]. More details of PBPK models are provided in Chapter 18.

17.7 CONCLUSION

The models presented in this chapter describe how drug parameters primarily determined in vitro can be applied to predict changes in the *in vivo AUC* of a drug that is victim to DDIs. The models are driven by a relatively small number of parameters: the inhibitors' fraction unbound; K_i, for reversible inhibitors: k_{inact}, and K_I for TDI; and E_{max} and **EC50** for inducers. All of these parameters are determined *in vitro* using preparations containing viable human metabolizing enzymes, such as microsomal preparations or human hepatocytes. In addition to the drug-specific parameters noted above, TDI models also require a system-specific parameter, the $k_{dregrad}$ of the affected enzyme. The fraction of the drug metabolized by an affected enzyme (*fm*) is the only parameter needed for the victim drug, unless the victim drug is a 3A4 substrate, in which case *Fg* is also needed. If the maximum unbound concentration in the portal vein is used as the inhibitor concentration, the inhibitor's *Fa* and *ka* are also needed. These models have now been expanded to the prediction of transporter-based DDIs. Their application continues to be associated with some uncertainties and problems. One issue is the need to identify and harmonize the optimum experimental conditions required to obtain accurate and reproducible estimates of the drug parameters *in vitro*. Additionally, the most appropriate choice for the perpetrator concentration in the static models has not been established. Nevertheless, the ability of these models to identify perpetrators and optimize the study of DDIs has made them a valuable tool for increasing the efficiency and reducing the cost of DDI studies in drug development. Studies have demonstrated that, although the models tend to overestimate the magnitude of DDIs, they are associated with a very low false negative error and thus achieve the goal of successfully identifying perpetrators likely to cause problems in clinical practice. Dynamic or PBPK models are being used increasingly in this area. As outlined in Chapter 18, this approach has many advantages. The models are able to simulate the whole time course of the concentrations of the perpetrator and victim drug in any tissue of interest (liver, intestine, and kidney). Furthermore, their built-in highly detailed submodels for drug absorption and hepatic elimination are ideally suited to studying the effects of perpetrators that act on several systems simultaneously.

PROBLEMS

17.1 Paroxetine reversibly inhibits several CYP enzymes. The *in vitro* K_i's for competitive inhibition of CYP1A2, 2C9, and 2C19 have been reported to be 4.2, 65, and 11 μM, respectively [12]. Rank their effect on the activity of the different CYPs based on the *in vitro* K_i.

17.2 Ketoconazole is a reversible inhibitor of several CYP enzymes including CYP 2C9, CYP2C19, and CYP2D6. The K_i's for these enzymes were reported as 2.9, 4.7, and 14 μM, respectively. Rank ketoconazole's potency for these enzymes.

17.3 Fluconazole and ketoconazole are both reversible inhibitors of CYP2C19. When omeprazole was used as a victim drug, their K_i's were reported as 2.9 and 4.7 μM, respectively. Estimate the *AUCR* for their interaction with omeprazole (*fm* = 0.87) using C_{max} values of fluconazole and ketoconazole of 29.4 and 1.87 μM, respectively. Also estimate *AUCR* using the unbound concentration of the inhibitors (*fu* values of fluconazole and ketconazole are 0.89 and 0.01, respectively).

17.4 When warfarin (*fm* = 0.91) was used as a victim drug, the K_i for fluconazole's reversible inhibition of CYP2C9 was found to be 5.5 μM [12]. Calculate the estimated *AUCR* for the interaction between fluconazole and warfarin. Use an inhibitor concentration of 29.4 μM.

17.5 Clarithromycin and erythromycin are both TDIs of CYP3A4. Use k_{inact} and K_I values for clarithromycin of 3.18 h^{-1} and 19 μM, respectively, and k_{inact} and K_I values for erythromycin of 2.46 h^{-1} and 13.5 μM, respectively, and:

(a) Compare their potency by calculating k_{inact}/K_I.

(b) Calculate their R_2 values for the effect on the hepatic enzyme. Use 0.0192 h⁻¹ as the k_{degrad} for hepatic CYP3A4 (see [11]).

(c) Estimate there $AUCR$ values for midazolam ($fm = 0.93$ and $Fg = 0.57$) assuming only hepatic extraction.

(d) Estimate their $AUCR$ values assuming both hepatic and intestinal extraction. Use 0.029 h⁻¹ for k_{degrad} for intestinal CYP3A4 (see [11]). Use the estimated concentration of the perpetrator in the enterocyte during absorption.

$$[I_g] = \frac{Dose * Fa * ka}{Q_{ent}}$$

Assume $Q_{ent} = 14.9$ L/h and Fa and ka values of 1 and 1.8 h⁻¹ for both inhibitors and doses of 500 and 1500 mg, respectively, for clarithromycin (MW = 748) and erythromycin (MW = 734).

17.6 Paroxetine is a TDI of CYP2D6. One study reported its K_I and first-order inactivation rate constant to be 0.315 µM and 0.17 min⁻¹, respectively [15]. The same study reported the first-order degradation constant of CYP2D6 as 0.0136 h⁻¹. Calculate the value of R_2 for paroxetine's action on CYP2D6. Use an unbound inhibitor concentration of 0.0059 µM. Calculate the estimated $AUCR$ for respiridone ($fm = 0.89$).

17.7 In their analysis of the TDI model, Obach *et al.* 2007 [4] reported the following values for zileuton and ticlopidine's TDI of CYP2D6:

Inhibitor	k_{inact} (min⁻¹)	k_{inact} (h⁻¹)	K_I (µM)
Ticlopidine	0.011	0.66	5.2
Zileuton	0.11	6.6	89

(a) Calculate the k_{inact}/K_I ratio and predict which may be the most potent inhibitor.

(b) Using total C_{max} inhibitor concentrations of 3 and 21 µM for ticlopidine and zileuton, respectively, and a k_{degrad} of 0.0178 h⁻¹ for CYP2D6 predict the $AUCR$ for theophylline in the presence and absence of ticlopidine and zileuton. Assume the values of fm_{CYP1A2} and BP for theophylline are 0.8 and 0.85, respectively [27].

REFERENCES

1. U.S. Department of Health and Human Services, Food and Drug Administration, Center for Drug Evaluation and Research (CDER). (2012) *Guidance for Industry, Drug Interaction Studies – Study Design Data Analysis, Implications for Dosing, and Labeling Recommendations.*

2. European Medicine Agency (EMA), Committee for Human Medicinal Products (CHMP). (2012) *Guideline on the Investigation of Drug Interactions.*

3. Fahmi, O. A., Hurst, S., Plowchalk, D., Cook, J., Guo, F., Youdim, K., Dickins, M., Phipps, A., Darekar, A., Hyland, R., and Obach, R. S. (2009) Comparison of different algorithms for predicting clinical drug-drug interactions, based on the use of CYP3A4 in vitro data: predictions of compounds as precipitants of interaction, *Drug Metab Dispos, 37*, 1658–1666.

4. Obach, R. S., Walsky, R. L., and Venkatakrishnan, K. (2007) Mechanism-based inactivation of human cytochrome p450 enzymes and the prediction of drug-drug interactions, *Drug Metab Dispos*, *35*, 246–255.

5. Venkatakrishnan, K., Obach, R. S., and Rostami-Hodjegan, A. (2007) Mechanism-based inactivation of human cytochrome P450 enzymes: strategies for diagnosis and drug-drug interaction risk assessment, *Xenobiotica*, *37*, 1225–1256.

6. Niemi, M., Backman, J. T., Fromm, M. F., Neuvonen, P. J., and Kivisto, K. T. (2003) Pharmacokinetic interactions with rifampicin: clinical relevance, *Clin Pharmacokinet*, *42*, 819–850.

7. Kato, M., Chiba, K., Horikawa, M., and Sugiyama, Y. (2005) The quantitative prediction of in vivo enzyme-induction caused by drug exposure from in vitro information on human hepatocytes, *Drug Metab Pharmacokinet*, *20*, 236–243.

8. Vieira, M. L., Kirby, B., Ragueneau-Majlessi, I., Galetin, A., Chien, J. Y., Einolf, H. J., Fahmi, O. A., Fischer, V., Fretland, A., Grime, K., Hall, S. D., Higgs, R., Plowchalk, D., Riley, R., Seibert, E., Skordos, K., Snoeys, J., Venkatakrishnan, K., Waterhouse, T., Obach, R. S., Berglund, E. G., Zhang, L., Zhao, P., Reynolds, K. S., and Huang, S. M. (2014) Evaluation of various static in vitro-in vivo extrapolation models for risk assessment of the CYP3A inhibition potential of an investigational drug, *Clin Pharmacol Ther*, *95*, 189–198.

9. Kanamitsu, S., Ito, K., and Sugiyama, Y. (2000) Quantitative prediction of in vivo drug-drug interactions from in vitro data based on physiological pharmacokinetics: use of maximum unbound concentration of inhibitor at the inlet to the liver, *Pharm Res*, *17*, 336–343.

10. Prueksaritanont, T., Chu, X., Gibson, C., Cui, D., Yee, K. L., Ballard, J., Cabalu, T., and Hochman, J. (2013) Drug-drug interaction studies: regulatory guidance and an industry perspective, *AAPS J*, *15*, 629–645.

11. Fahmi, O. A., Maurer, T. S., Kish, M., Cardenas, E., Boldt, S., and Nettleton, D. (2008) A combined model for predicting CYP3A4 clinical net drug-drug interaction based on CYP3A4 inhibition, inactivation, and induction determined in vitro, *Drug Metab Dispos*, *36*, 1698–1708.

12. Obach, R. S., Walsky, R. L., Venkatakrishnan, K., Gaman, E. A., Houston, J. B., and Tremaine, L. M. (2006) The utility of in vitro cytochrome P450 inhibition data in the prediction of drug-drug interactions, *J Pharmacol Exp Ther*, *316*, 336–348.

13. Einolf, H. J., Chen, L., Fahmi, O. A., Gibson, C. R., Obach, R. S., Shebley, M., Silva, J., Sinz, M. W., Unadkat, J. D., Zhang, L., and Zhao, P. (2014) Evaluation of various static and dynamic modeling methods to predict clinical CYP3A induction using in vitro CYP3A4 mRNA induction data, *Clin Pharmacol Ther*, *95*, 179–188.

14. Mitsui, T., Nemoto, T., Miyake, T., Nagao, S., Ogawa, K., Kato, M., Ishigai, M., and Yamada, H. (2014) A useful model capable of predicting the clearance of cytochrome 3A4 (CYP3A4) substrates in humans: validity of CYP3A4 transgenic mice lacking their own Cyp3a enzymes, *Drug Metab Dispos*, *42*, 1540–1547.

15. Venkatakrishnan, K., and Obach, R. S. (2005) In vitro-in vivo extrapolation of Cyp2d6 inactivation by paroxetine: prediction of nonstationary pharmacokinetics and drug interaction magnitude, *Drug Metab Dispos*, *33*, 845–852.

16. Brown, H. S., Griffin, M., and Houston, J. B. (2007) Evaluation of cryopreserved human hepatocytes as an alternative in vitro system to microsomes for the prediction of metabolic clearance, *Drug Metab Dispos*, *35*, 293–301.

17. Gueorguieva, I., Jackson, K., Wrighton, S. A., Sinha, V. P., and Chien, J. Y. (2010) Desipramine, substrate for CYP2D6 activity: population pharmacokinetic model and design elements of drug-drug interaction trials, *Br J Clin Pharmacol*, *70*, 523–536.

18. Galetin, A., Gertz, M., and Houston, J. B. (2010) Contribution of intestinal cytochrome p450-mediated metabolism to drug-drug inhibition and induction interactions, *Drug Metab Pharmacokinet*, *25*, 28–47.

19. Lilja, J. J., Neuvonen, M., and Neuvonen, P. J. (2004) Effects of regular consumption of grapefruit juice on the pharmacokinetics of simvastatin, *Br J Clin Pharmacol*, *58*, 56–60.

20. Fukazawa, I., Uchida, N., Uchida, E., and Yasuhara, H. (2004) Effects of grapefruit juice on pharmacokinetics of atorvastatin and pravastatin in Japanese, *Br J Clin Pharmacol*, *57*, 448–455.

21. Mizuma, T., Tsuji, A., and Hayashi, M. (2004) Does the well-stirred model assess the intestinal first-pass effect well?, *J Pharm Pharmacol*, *56*, 1597–1599.

22. Giacomini, K. M., Huang, S. M., Tweedie, D. J., Benet, L. Z., Brouwer, K. L., Chu, X., Dahlin, A., Evers, R., Fischer, V., Hillgren, K. M., Hoffmaster, K. A., Ishikawa, T., Keppler, D., Kim, R. B., Lee, C. A., Niemi, M., Polli, J. W., Sugiyama, Y., Swaan, P. W., Ware, J. A., Wright, S. H., Yee, S. W., Zamek-Gliszczynski, M. J., and Zhang, L. (2010) Membrane transporters in drug development, *Nat Rev Drug Discov*, *9*, 215–236.

23. Barton, H. A., Lai, Y., Goosen, T. C., Jones, H. M., El-Kattan, A. F., Gosset, J. R., Lin, J., and Varma, M. V. (2013) Model-based approaches to predict drug-drug interactions associated with hepatic uptake transporters: preclinical, clinical and beyond, *Expert Opin Drug Metab Toxicol*, *9*, 459–472.

24. Li, R., Barton, H. A., and Varma, M. V. (2014) Prediction of pharmacokinetics and drug-drug interactions when hepatic transporters are involved, *Clin Pharmacokinet*, *53*, 659–678.

25. Varma, M. V., Pang, K. S., Isoherranen, N., and Zhao, P. (2015) Dealing with the complex drug-drug interactions: towards mechanistic models, *Biopharm Drug Dispos*, *36*, 71–92.

26. Zhao, P., Rowland, M., and Huang, S. M. (2012) Best practice in the use of physiologically based pharmacokinetic modeling and simulation to address clinical pharmacology regulatory questions, *Clin Pharmacol Ther*, *92*, 17–20.

27. Ebden, P., Banks, J., Peel, T., Buss, D. C., Routledge, P. A., and Spragg, B. P. (1986) The disposition of theophylline in blood in chronic obstructive lung disease, *Ther Drug Monit*, *8*, 424–426.

18

INTRODUCTION TO PHYSIOLOGICALLY BASED PHARMACOKINETIC MODELING

Sara E. Rosenbaum

Objectives

The material in this chapter will enable the reader to:

1. Understand how basic PBPK models are built
2. Recognize the drug- and system-specific parameters needed for the models
3. Differentiate the characteristics of PBPK and compartment models
4. Observe the drug concentrations simulated by PBPK models

Basic Pharmacokinetics and Pharmacodynamics: An Integrated Textbook and Computer Simulations,
Second Edition. Edited by Sara E. Rosenbaum.
© 2017 John Wiley & Sons, Inc. Published 2017 by John Wiley & Sons, Inc.

5. Recognize how drug-specific parameters can be estimated

6. Appreciate how PBPK models can be adapted to incorporate detailed processes in ADME

7. Have a general understanding of some of the applications of PBPK models

18.1 INTRODUCTION

Physiological-based pharmacokinetic (PBPK) modeling is an alternative approach to the modeling and simulation of drug concentration data. Conceptually, this approach is in some ways simpler and more logical than the compartmental approach because it eliminates imaginary compartments and instead uses real tissues. Consequently, the PBPK models are parameterized by real physiological parameters of tissue blood flow and volume instead of rate constants and exponents, which can be difficult to conceptualize and relate to real physiological parameters. This makes it easier to interpret PBPK models and to extrapolate them to other situations where the physiological parameters may be altered. PBPK models were introduced to pharmacokinetic modeling in the 1960s, but at that time two of the properties of the models and the modeling process inhibited their wide endorsement. First, because the models include many tissues, they generate a large number of equations that need powerful computer hardware and software to handle. Second, the large number of human and/or laboratory animal physiological parameters (blood flow and tissue volumes) needed to create the models were not generally available at that time.

Today, the landscape is very different. The computing power is no longer an issue. There are a wide range of purpose built and other software packages that can be used to apply PBPK modeling. In addition, the physiological parameters required by the models are now widely available (see [1]). The approach also received an extremely important boost with the development of methods to predict the drug-specific model parameters that the models also need, from a drug's physiochemical characteristics and data obtained from *in vitro* studies. As a result, PBPK models can be applied to drugs even before they are administered to humans or laboratory animals, and they have become a powerful tool for the pharmaceutical industry to use to increase the efficiency of the development process. All these developments have led to a renewed interest in PBPK modeling and the approach has been widely endorsed by academic scientist, the pharmaceutical industry, and drug regulatory bodies. A recent review of published PBPK studies [2] found a steady increase in publications over the last 15 years from nine articles in 2004 up to 94 in 2014. Several excellent reviews on the development and application of these models have recently appeared in the literature [3–6]. Interestingly, the models used to predict the drug-specific parameters of drugs in the absence of *in vivo* data were originally developed in the field of environmental toxicology, where PBPK models have been used extensively to predict human toxicity from environmental chemicals, which cannot be tested directly in humans. Today, PBPK modeling is being applied throughout the whole drug development process. Models based purely on a drug's physiochemical properties and *in vitro* data can be used to help identify molecules with optimum absorption and elimination characteristics. As drugs move along the development process and *in vivo* data become available in animals, the model parameters can be adjusted to better represent observed plasma concentration–time profiles. The models can be used to assist in the establishment of the initial doses used in humans, and then further adjusted in the light of data obtained in humans.

Models developed for a drug in healthy volunteers can be adapted by modifying relevant physiological or elimination parameters to predict drug behavior in different populations including children, the elderly, pregnant women, different ethnic groups, and individuals with renal or hepatic impairment. Virtual populations can be created to probe drug behavior in special populations, such as individuals deficient in CYP2D6, to determine if these populations are susceptible to an altered spectrum of toxicity or adverse events. A further stimulus to the application of PBPK has been the availability of purpose built, user friendly commercial software that can integrate the modeling with extensive libraries of physiological data and algorithms for the prediction of drug-specific parameters. These include ADMEWORKS DDI Simulator®, GastroPlus®, PK-sim®, and SimCYP®.

18.2 COMPONENTS OF PBPK MODELS

The PBPK models are made up of three core parts or components:

1. Physiological parameters. These are primarily the values of blood flow and volume for the different tissues that comprise the model.
2. Drug parameters. The drug parameters needed for the simplest of the models are the steady-state tissue to plasma partition coefficient, protein-binding data, and the intrinsic clearances for the different elimination pathways.
3. Model structure. The structure of the model includes the number and arrangement of the tissues, which tends to be fairly consistent from one model to another. The models mimic the anatomical arrangement in the body in which the tissues are linked by the systemic circulation (Figure 18.1). Arterial blood splits off from the systemic circulation to perfuse the tissues and deliver the drug. The venous blood leaving the tissue is then returned to the systemic circulation. A typical model may consist of around 7–15 tissues.

18.3 EQUATIONS FOR PBPK MODELS

As discussed in Chapter 4, the distribution of a drug to a tissue is a two-step process: The delivery of the drug to the tissue, which is a function of the tissue blood flow; and the uptake of the drug by the tissue, which is controlled by the ability of the drug to diffuse across the capillary and cell membranes within the tissue. The overall rate of distribution is controlled by the slower of these two steps. Given that most drugs are small nonpolar molecules that can easily pass the capillary and cell membranes, distribution is usually blood flow or perfusion limited. As a result, the basic PBPK models assume blood flow limited or perfusion-controlled distribution. The characteristics of the perfusion-limited distribution model are discussed in more detail below.

After the administration of a drug, the drug is delivered to the tissue in the arterial blood. The tissue is viewed as a well-stirred single compartment and diffusion is assumed to occur instantaneously driven by the concentration gradient created by the unbound form of the drug in the blood and in the tissue (Figure 18.2). As the blood emerges from the tissue, it is assumed that drug in the venous blood is in equilibrium with that in the tissue, and that the unbound concentrations are equal. When distribution is complete and a pseudo-equilibrium

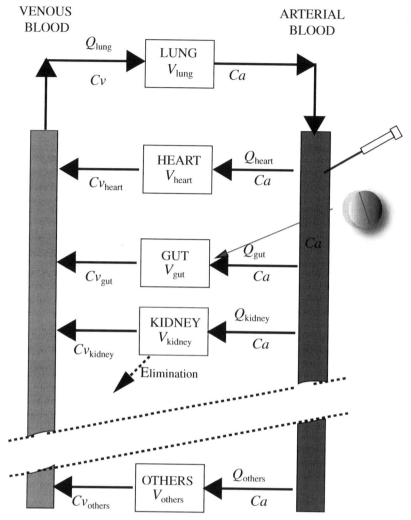

FIGURE 18.1   An abbreviated PBPK model. The tissues of the model are linked by the systemic circulation. Arterial blood delivers drug to the tissues and the venous blood leaving the tissue is then returned to the systemic circulation. The concentration in arterial blood is Ca and that in the venous blood leaving a tissue Cv_t. Drug elimination may occur as the blood flows through the kidney (shown) and liver. The physiological parameters used in the model are tissue blood flow (Q_t) and tissue volume (V_t). This model shows only the lungs, heart, and the kidney. A typical model may consist of around 7–15 tissues. The model shows intravenous drug input directly into the venous blood and oral administration where absorption occurs into the gut. *(For a color version of this figure, see the color plate section.)*

is achieved between the tissue and the blood, and the ratio of the tissue concentration (Ct) to the blood concentration is constant. Recall from Chapter 4, the ratio of the tissue to plasma (Cp) concentrations is the drug's tissue partition coefficient (Kp_t):

$$\frac{Ct}{Cp} = Kp_t \tag{18.1}$$

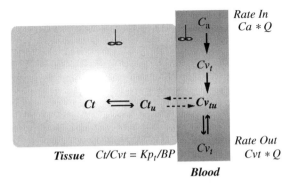

FIGURE 18.2 Perfusion-controlled distribution. The tissue is viewed as a well-stirred single compartment. Drug is delivered to the tissue in arterial blood: Q is the blood flow to the tissue and Ca is the drug concentration in arterial blood. The rate of drug delivery is $Q*Ca$. Drug may bind to proteins and macromolecules in the blood and tissue. The unbound fraction in blood, plasma, and the tissue are fu_b, fu, and fu_t, respectively. The unbound drug concentration in the tissue (Ct_u), venous blood (Cv_{ut}), and plasma (Cp_u) are all equal. The ratio of the total drug concentration in the tissue (Ct) and the concentration in venous blood (Cv_t) can be expressed in terms of the tissue:plasma partition coefficient (Kp_t) and the drugs blood:plasma concentration ratio (BP). The rate the drug leaves the tissue is $Q*Cv_t$. *(For a color version of this figure, see the color plate section.)*

Because drug is delivered to the tissues in the whole blood not just plasma, the partition coefficient needs be expressed in terms of the ratio of the tissue concentrations to blood concentration (Cb):

$$\frac{Ct}{Cb} \tag{18.2}$$

Recall (Chapter 5), the relationship between the blood and plasma concentrations is expressed using the blood:plasma ratio (BP):

$$BP = \frac{Cb}{Cp} \quad \text{and} \quad Cb = Cp * BP \tag{18.3}$$

Substituting for Cb as given in equation (18.3) above into equation (18.2)

$$\frac{Ct}{Cb} = \frac{Ct}{Cp * BP}$$

But, $Kp_t = Ct/Cp$

$$\frac{Ct}{Cb} = \frac{Kp_t}{BP} \tag{18.4}$$

and

$$Cb = \frac{Ct * BP}{Kp_t} \tag{18.5}$$

The time it takes for distribution to go to completion will depend on the rate of delivery of the drug to the tissue and on the final amount of drug in the tissue when distribution is complete. The former is a function of the tissue blood flow. The latter is a function of the drug's tissue partition coefficient and the volume of the tissue (the larger the partition coefficient and the larger the size of the tissue, the greater the amount of drug in the tissue when distribution is complete). A drug's partition coefficient will vary from one tissue to another depending on the drug's physiochemical characteristics, its solubility in various spaces within the cells of different tissues, and the extent to which it binds to macromolecules (proteins and lipoproteins) in different tissues. Once distribution is complete in all tissues, the unbound drug concentration is assumed to be equal throughout the body.

During the distribution process, the rate of distribution to a tissue can be expressed as the difference between the rate a drug enters and leaves a tissue (Figure 18.1). Thus:

Rate of change of the amount of drug in the tissue over time, $\dfrac{dAt}{dt}$:

$$\frac{dAt}{dt} = \text{Rate In} - \text{Rate Out}$$

$$\frac{dAt}{dt} = Qt * Ca - Qt * Cvt \tag{18.6}$$

where Qt is the tissue blood flow (volume of blood per unit time), Ca is the concentration of the drug in arterial blood (amount per unit volume), and Cvt is the drug concentration in the venous blood emerging from the tissue. Cvt will vary among tissues depending on how much drug is taken up as the blood passes through a particular tissue. As discussed above, it is assumed that the drug in the venous blood emerging from a tissue (Cvt) is in equilibrium with the drug concentration in the tissue (Ct). The relationship between the drug concentration in the venous blood [Cb in equation (18.5)] and the tissue concentration is given in equation (18.5). Thus:

$$Cvt = \frac{Ct * BP}{Kp_t} \tag{18.7}$$

Substituting for Cvt into equation (18.6)

$$\frac{dAt}{dt} = Qt * Ca - Qt * \frac{Ct * BP}{Kp_t} \tag{18.8}$$

or:

$$\frac{Vt * dCt}{dt} = Qt * Ca - Qt * \frac{Ct * BP}{Kp_t} \tag{18.9}$$

where Vt and Ct are the tissue volume and drug concentration, respectively. Equation (18.9) is then repeated for each noneliminating tissue in the model.

Organs of Elimination: The organs of elimination (liver and kidney) need an additional component to their equations to reflect any loss of drug due to elimination. Drug elimination is modeled using a drug's intrinsic clearance driven by the unbound tissue concentration. Thus, the PKPB equation for an organ of elimination is:

$$\frac{Vt * dCt}{dt} = Qt * Ca - \frac{Qt * Ct * BP}{Kp_t} - Cl_{\text{int}} * Ct_u \tag{18.10}$$

where Ct_u is the unbound tissue concentration of the drug, and Cl_{int} is the overall intrinsic clearance for all pathways of elimination in the tissue. As discussed previously, the unbound

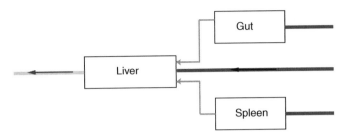

FIGURE 18.3   Unique blood flow pattern to the liver.

concentrations throughout the tissue blood and plasma are all assumed to be equal. Thus, Ct_u is equal to the unbound concentration in the venous plasma (Cp_{ut}) leaving the tissue. But as shown in (18.1) $Cp = Ct/Kp_t$ and $Cp_{ut} = Cp * fu$:

$$Ct_u = Cp * fu = \frac{Ct}{Kp_t} * fu \tag{18.11}$$

where *fu* is the unbound fraction in the plasma. Substituting for Ct_u into equation (18.10)

$$\frac{Vt * dCt}{dt} = Qt * Ca - \frac{Q * Ct * BP}{Kp_t} - Cl_{int} * \frac{Ct}{Kp_t} * fu \tag{18.12}$$

Liver, Spleen, and Gut Blood Flow: Venous blood flow from the spleen and gut passes through the liver before returning to the circulation (Figure 18.3). The equations for the gut and spleen are the same as for other noneliminating tissues, but they are structured into the model to reflect this unique arrangement. The equations for drug input into the liver must reflect blood from all sources, and the blood flow from the liver will be the sum of all blood flows entering the liver. Assuming no elimination in the liver, the equation for the rate of change of the amount of drug in the liver is:

$$\frac{VtdC_{liver}}{dt} = \text{Amount received from (hepatic artery + gut + spleen)} - \text{Amount leaving}$$

Or

$$\frac{VtdC_{liver}}{dt} = Q_{h,ha} * Ca + Q_{gut} * \left(\frac{BP * C_{gut}}{Kp_{gut}} \right) + Q_{spleen} * \left(\frac{BP * C_{spleen}}{Kp_{spleen}} \right)$$
$$- Q_h * \left(\frac{BP * C_{liver}}{Kp_{liver}} \right)$$

where Q_h is the total blood flow to and from the liver [sum of blood flow from the hepatic artery ($Q_{h,\,ha}$), the spleen (Q_{spleen}), and gut (Q_{gut})].

18.4 BUILDING A PBPK MODEL

An interactive model will now be built for a drug based on physiological parameters provided in the paper of Jones and Rowland-Yeo [4]. The model will be used to simulate drug concentrations after either an intravenous or an oral dose. The parameters have been calculated assuming 70-kg body weight, a tissue density of 1, and a total body volume of

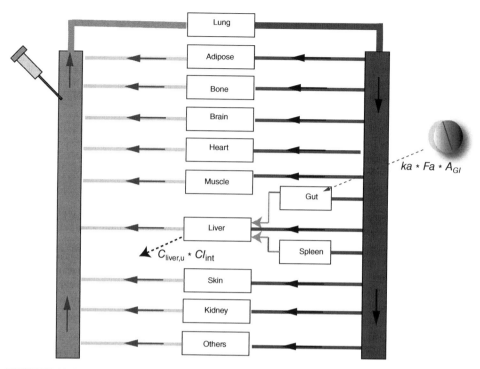

FIGURE 18.4 A full PBPK model. This model consists of 11 specific tissues and the remaining tissues grouped as "Others." In this model, elimination is modeled from the liver with a rate equal to the product of the unbound drug concentration and the drug's intrinsic metabolic clearance (Cl_{int}). It is assumed that there is no renal elimination. Oral absorption is modeled as a first-order process controlled by the absorption rate constant (ka), the fraction of the dose absorbed into the GI membrane (Fa), and the amount of drug in the GI tract (A_{GI}). (*For a color version of this figure, see the color plate section.*)

70 L. The model includes the following tissues and organs: lungs, adipose tissue, bone, brain, heart, muscle, skin, liver, kidney, gut, and spleen, and the remaining tissues will be grouped as "Others" (Figure 18.4). The physiological parameters needed in the model are shown in Table 18.1

For an oral dose, all tissue and blood concentrations are set to zero at time zero. For an intravenous dose, tissue and arterial blood concentrations are set to zero, and it is assumed that the drug will distribute throughout the venous blood instantaneously. At the time of the injection, the concentration of drug in the venous blood (Cv) is:

$$Cv = \frac{Av}{Vv} = \frac{Dose}{Vv} \tag{18.13}$$

where A_v and V_v are the amount of drug in the venous blood and the volume of the venous blood, respectively. Using the value of V_v from Table 18.1:

$$Cv = \frac{Dose \text{ mcg}}{3.6 \text{ L}} \text{mcg/L} \tag{18.14}$$

TABLE 18.1   Physiological Parameters Used in the PBPK Model

Tissue/Organ	Blood Flow (L/h)	Volume (L)
Lung	390	0.53
Adipose tissue	19.5	14.9
Bone	19.5	6.0
Brain	46.8	1.4
Heart	15.6	0.33
Muscle	66.3	28
Skin	19.5	2.6
Liver	20.2 (artery)	1.47
Kidney	74.1	0.31
Gut	57.1	1.2
Spleen	6.72	0.18
Others[a]	44.7	7.68
Arterial blood	N/A	1.8
Venous blood	N/A	3.6
Plasma		3.0

Source: Data from Reference [4].

[a]The volume of the other tissues was calculated by summing the volumes of the tissue specifically included in the model and subtracting their total volume from 70 L. The total cardiac output is 390 L/h and the sum of the blood flow to the tissues specifically included in the model is 345.3 L. Thus, blood flow to the tissues grouped as "Others" is 390 − 345.3 = 44.7 L/h.

The venous blood takes the drug to the lungs, which receives the full cardiac output. The arterial blood leaving the lungs then branches out to each of the tissues to deliver the drug.

For simplicity, the blood-plasma ratio of the drug has been set to 1, as have all the plasma-tissue partition coefficients and the fraction unbound in the plasma. The drug is assumed to be eliminated completely in the liver with an intrinsic clearance of 40 L/h.

The drug concentration in arterial blood, Ca, is given by:

$$Ca = \frac{Aa}{Va} \tag{18.15}$$

where Aa is the amount in the arterial blood, and Va is the volume of arterial blood (1.8 L see Table 18.1). At time zero after an intravenous injection, $Aa = 0$.

Tissue Equations

1. Lungs

   The equation for the lungs is a little different because the venous blood enters the lungs and arterial blood leaves the lungs:

   $$\frac{V_{lungs}dC_{lungs}}{dt} = Q_{lungs} * Cv - Q_{lungs} * \frac{BP * C_{lungs}}{Kp_{lungs}}$$

   Substituting values from Table 18.1 and assuming that $BP = 1$ and $Kp = 1$:

   $$\frac{0.532dC_{lungs}}{dt} = 390 * Cv - 390 * C_{lungs}$$

   The expression for Cv is given in equation (18.13)

2. Other Noneliminating Tissues

The same equation is used for the other tissues not involved in drug elimination. As an example, the equation for the heart will be presented.

$$\frac{VtdC_{\text{heart}}}{dt} = Q_{\text{heart}} * Ca - Q_{\text{heart}} * \frac{BP * C_{\text{heart}}}{Kp_{\text{heart}}}$$

Substituting values from Table 18.1:

$$\frac{1.2dC_{\text{heart}}}{dt} = 15.6 * Ca - 15.6 * C_{\text{heart}}$$

The expression for Ca is given in equation (18.15).

These equations are repeated for all the tissues in the model.

3. Eliminating Tissues

The equation for an eliminating tissue has an additional expression for the rate of elimination that occurs within the tissue. In this example, the drug will be assumed to be eliminated completely in the liver with an intrinsic clearance of 40 L/h. The equation for the rate of change of the amount of drug in the liver over time will be:

$$\frac{VtdC_{\text{liver}}}{dt} = Q_{h,ha} * Ca + Q_{\text{gut}} * \frac{BP * C_{\text{gut}}}{Kp_{\text{gut}}} + Q_{\text{spleen}} * \frac{BP * C_{\text{spleen}}}{Kp_{\text{spleen}}}$$
$$- Q_h * \frac{BP * C_{\text{liver}}}{Kp_{\text{liver}}} - Cl_{\text{int}} * C_{\text{liver,u}} \qquad (18.16)$$

where Cl_{int} is the intrinsic metabolic clearance, and $C_{\text{liver,u}}$ is the unbound drug concentration in the liver. But as presented in equation (18.11)

$$Ct_u = \frac{Ct}{Kp_t} * fu$$

$$\frac{VtdC_{\text{liver}}}{dt} = Q_{h,ha} * Ca + Q_{\text{gut}} * \frac{BP * C_{\text{gut}}}{Kp_{\text{gut}}} + Q_{\text{spleen}} * \frac{BP * C_{\text{spleen}}}{Kp_{\text{spleen}}}$$
$$- Q_h * \frac{BP * C_{\text{liver}}}{Kp_{\text{liver}}} - \frac{Cl_{\text{int}} * Ct * fu}{Kp_{\text{liver}}}$$

Substituting the values from Table 18.1, $Q_h = 20.2 + 57.1 + 6.72 = 84.02$ L/h and assuming fu, BP, and all Kps equal 1 and an unbound intrinsic clearance of 40 L/h

$$\frac{VtdC_{\text{liver}}}{dt} = 20.2 * Ca + 57.1 * C_{\text{gut}} + 6.72 * C_{\text{spleen}} - 84.02 * C_{\text{liver}} - 40 * \frac{C_{\text{liver}}}{Kp_{\text{liver}}} * fu$$

4. Drug Administration

The model will simulate drug concentrations after either an oral or intravenous dose. For the oral dose, it is assumed that the drug is absorbed into the gut by a first-order process, with an absorption rate constant of 0.6 h^{-1}.

$$\text{Rate of Absorption} = Fa * Fg * ka * A_{GI}$$

where *Fa* is the fraction of the dose entering the apical side of the gut membrane, *Fg* is the fraction of the drug in the enterocyte-escaping metabolism, *ka* is the first-order absorption constant, and A_{GI} is the amount of drug in the gastrointestinal tract.

It is assumed that $Fa = 1$, $Fg = 1$ and at time zero, $A_{GI} = Dose$

Initial conditions for the model

For an oral dose (10,000 μg), at time zero:

All tissue concentrations $= 0$

$Ca = 0$

$Cv = 0$

For the intravenous dose (1000 μg)

All tissue concentrations $= 0$

$Ca = 0$

$Cv = Dose/Vv$

As presented in equation (18.14), $Cv = 1000/3.6 = 278$ μg/L.

18.5 SIMULATIONS: http://web.uri.edu/pharmacy/research/rosenbaum/sims

The model (model 18, Example PBPK Model) can be found at http://web.uri.edu/pharmacy/ research/rosenbaum/sims/Model18.

Simulations

(a) Click the "Build the Model" button to see how the model is constructed.

(b) Concentrations will be simulated over an 10-h period. When a simulation is performed, the model enables tissue concentrations in any of the tissues included in the model to be simulated. Perform a run with the default route of administration (oral) and a dose of 10 mg. For simplicity, only the tissue concentrations of the venous blood, heart, muscle, and adipose tissue are shown. Note that distribution proceeds

TABLE 18.2 Tissue Perfusion Values for the Tissues Included in the Model

Tissue/Organ	Tissue Perfusion Blood Flow/Vol Tissue (L/h/L)
Lung	733
Kidney	241
Gut	47.7
Heart	47.4
Spleen	36.9
Brain	33.4
Liver	13.7
Skin	7.5
Others	5.8
Bone	3.3
Muscle	2.4
Adipose	1.3

faster in tissues with the higher perfusions (Table 18.2). The graph shows the very rapid distribution to the heart (perfusion: 15.6 L/h/0.329 L = 47.4 L/h/L), where the tissue concentrations almost immediately essentially superimpose over those of the venous blood. In contrast, distributions to the muscle (perfusion: 66.3 L/h/28 L = 2.37 L/h/L) and the adipose tissue (perfusion: 19.5 L/h/14.9 L = 1.3 L/h/L) proceed more slowly.

(c) *Go to the IV Administration page. Perform a simulation with the default IV dose of 1 mg. Note the drug concentrations over the first hour after administration are displayed. Again, only drug concentrations in the venous blood, heart, muscle, and adipose tissue are shown. Note that because distribution proceeds so rapidly in the heart, concentrations in the heart rise very quickly and achieve very high concentrations. In contrast, the concentrations in the muscle, where distribution proceeds more slowly, rise more slowly and never achieve the high concentrations seen in the heart. Nevertheless, distribution is complete in these tissues after 0.25 h, after which the concentrations fall in parallel with those of venous blood.*

(d) *Observe the effect of Kp on a tissue profile. Go to the Alter Kp page. Tissue concentrations will be simulated after oral absorption. The graph shows concentrations in the venous blood and adipose tissue over time. Adjust the adipose tissue Kp from 1 to 5 to 10. Note the tissue concentrations and the time to reach equilibrium increase as Kp increases.*

(e) *Observe the effect of altering tissue perfusion. Perform a run. Note how easily the model can be adapted to changing liver blood flows. Note normal total liver blood flow is 83 L/h. Alter hepatic blood flow first to 40 and then to 160 L/h. Note the change in the time course of venous drug concentrations. Similar changes can be made to the blood flows of any or all of the tissues in PBPK models to match known changes in the physiological parameters in different populations.*

This model can be adapted to other drugs by changing the drug-specific parameters of fu, the tissue Kp_t values, BP, Cl_{int}, Fa, and ka. It can also be altered to other special populations by altering the physiological parameters of blood flow and tissue volume.

18.6 ESTIMATION OF HUMAN DRUG-SPECIFIC PARAMETERS

A powerful and valuable application of PBPK modeling is its ability to simulate plasma and tissue concentrations of a drug in humans even before the drug is administered to an animal (laboratory animal or human). Various methods can be used to estimate the drug-specific parameters. Some of the parameters, such as Kp_t, can be estimated using the physiochemical properties of a drug (log[P], pKa, etc). Others, such as intrinsic metabolic clearance and a drug's binding characteristics, can be estimated by extrapolating or scaling drug parameters estimated in *in vitro* systems. Other biological parameters, such as renal clearance, can be estimated by extrapolating values determined in laboratory animals. This method of model building is known as the "bottom-up" approach to modeling and simulation. In contrast, the traditional compartmental models use a "top-down" approach because plasma concentration data (top) obtained in humans are needed to begin the modeling process. The data are used to select the most appropriate model (e.g., one, two, or three compartments), which is then used to model the data and estimate the drug's pharmacokinetic parameters (bottom). PBPK models built using the bottom-up approach contain a large number of parameters, some of which may be associated with some uncertainty. As a result, once *in vivo* data become available, the parameters of a PBPK model that are associated with the greatest uncertainty can be altered or optimized to try to better replicate the observed plasma concentration–time profiles. This process of optimizing the parameters of a PBPK model using clinical data is referred to as the "middle out" approach. The bottom-up approach is a valuable feature of PBPK modeling, and the following sections present the methods used to estimate the drug-specific parameters.

18.6.1 Tissue Plasma Partition Coefficient

The plasma-tissue partition coefficient (Kp_t) is the ratio of a drug's concentration (total) in a tissue to that in the plasma at steady state. Historically, Kp_t values were measured by administering drugs to laboratory animals, sacrificing them, and then assaying the drug concentration in the plasma and each of the tissues of interest. This is an expensive, timing-consuming process that results in the sacrifice of a large number of laboratory animals. Mechanistic methods have been developed that allow a drug's partition coefficient for different tissues to be calculated based on the physiological and biochemical composition of a tissue, a drug's physiochemical properties, and the drug's binding characteristics measured *in vitro*. The total concentration of the drug in a tissue is made up of free drug, drug that partitions into lipids and phospholipids, and drug that binds to proteins and lipoproteins. Differences in the compositions of the plasma and the tissues result in differences in the total concentration between these two spaces and result in Kp_t values that do not equal to 1. Further, each tissue has its own unique make-up of lipids, phospholipids, proteins, and lipoproteins, resulting in Kp_t values that vary from one tissue to another. Models have been developed to predict a drug's Kp_t in specific tissues based on the composition of the tissue (neutral lipids, neutral and charged phospholipids, and proteins and lipoproteins), the drug's lipophilicity (LogP), and the drug's *in vitro* binding characteristics (*fu*). Assuming that a drug distributes into a tissue by passive diffusion, it has been traditionally assumed that at steady state, the free drug concentration in the plasma and blood is equal to the free concentration in the tissues. The initial approaches used to predict Kp_t have been further refined to accommodate the behavior of charged drugs, where a slight difference in pH between the plasma (7.4) and the tissue intracellular water (7.0) can result in different degrees of ionization of a drug in the plasma and tissues and, in turn differences in the unbound concentrations in these two spaces. A recent evaluation of some commonly used tissue composition formula found that the models of Rogers *et al.* [7,8] were the most accurate and that in 77% of cases were able to estimate Kp_t values within threefold of experimentally determined values [9]. The specific formula used to estimate a drug's Kp_t values is chosen according to whether a drug is basic, acidic, or a zwitterion. The formula requires only a drug's *fu* value, pKa, and partition coefficient (n-octanol:water, except of adipose tissue which uses the vegetable oil:water coefficient). The tissue-specific parameters required by the formula are given in the literature [7–9].

18.6.2 Volume of Distribution

A drug's steady-state volume of distribution (*Vd*ss) can be estimated using a classic pharmacokinetic equation based on a drugs tissue:plasma partition coefficient in the different tissues:

$$Vdss = \sum (Vt * Kp_t) + Vp$$

Incorporating the drug found in the erythrocytes

$$Vdss = \sum (Vt * Kp_t) + (Ve * EP) + Vp$$

where Ve is the volume of the erythrocytes, and EP is the erythrocyte:plasma ratio, which is a function of a drugs' distribution between the plasma and blood and the hematocrit value:

$$EP = \frac{BP - (1 - Ht)}{Ht}$$

For the drug used in the simulation model above, assuming $Ve = 2.43$ L, a hematocrit of 0.45, and a $BP = 1$:

$$Vdss = 34.719 + 2.43 + 2.968 = 40.1 \text{ L}$$

18.6.3 Clearance

Intrinsic hepatic clearance can be estimated from *in vitro* studies using preparations of active human enzymes, such as hepatocytes, microsomes, or recombinant enzymes. The enzymes involved in the metabolism of a drug are first identified and the intrinsic clearance for each pathway is estimated *in vitro*. The *in vivo* intrinsic clearance is estimated by scaling from the *in vitro* system to the whole organ *in vivo*. Usually, the unbound clearance in the *in vitro* system ($Cl_{\text{intin vitro}}$) is determined in units of volume per unit time per mg of microsomal protein. This has to be scaled to a value in a human.

For example,

Let $Cl_{\text{intin vitro}} = 10 \, \mu\text{L/min/mg}$ microsomal protein.

Assuming a normal value of 45 mg microsomal protein per gram of liver:

$Cl_{\text{int}} = 10 * 45 = 450 \, \mu\text{L/min/g}$ of liver

Assuming a normal liver weighs 1.47 kg or 1470 g:

$Cl_{\text{int}} = 450 * 1470 \, \mu\text{L/min} = 661{,}500 \, \mu\text{L/min} = 39.7 \text{ L/h}$

Human renal clearance is a function of three processes that occur in the nephron: glomerular filtration of the unbound drug in the plasma, tubular secretion, and passive tubular reabsorption (see Chapter 5). As a result, it cannot be measured *in vitro* and is primarily estimated using allometry to scale values determined in laboratory animals to humans. Allometry assumes that the only difference in renal clearance between different species is size of the species. A typical allometric formula for renal clearance across different species is:

$$Clr = a * BW^b$$

where a and b are the coefficient and exponent, respectively, that relate renal clearance (Clr) to body weight (BW) among different species. Typically, the exponent for clearance among species is around 0.75. The formula predicts that clearance will increase as body weight increases but less than proportionally. Consequently, when clearance is expressed

TABLE 18.3 **Values of Human and Rat Unbound Renal clearances (Clr_u).**
Note the rat:human ratio is approximately equal to the ratio of the GFR in
these species

Drug	Rat Clr_u (mL/min/kg)	Human Clr_u (mL/min/kg)	Rat:Human Ratio (GRF ratio = 4.8)
Cefoperazone	4.7	1.2	3.5
Cimetidine	35	7.0	5.0
Enalapril	18	3.1	5.8
Lisinopril	11	1.7	6.5

Source: Data from Reference [10].

per unit body weight, the formula predicts that clearance will decrease as the weight of the whole animal increases. The disadvantage of this approach is that values of renal clearance are needed in several species in order to estimate the coefficient and exponent. An alternative estimation approach that uses only rat renal clearance [10] assumes that the unbound renal clearance between two species is a function of the ratio of their glomerular filtration rates. Thus, if the unbound renal clearance is known in the rat, it can be estimated in humans based on the fact that the glomerular filtration rate in the rat (per unit body weight) is about 4.8 times that of humans [10]. Thus:

$$Clr_{u,\text{human}}(\text{mL/min/kg}) = \frac{Clr_{u,\text{rat}}\ (\text{mL/min/kg})}{4.8}$$

Table 18.3 shows the unbound renal clearance of several drugs in rats (GFR = 1.8 mL/min/kg) and humans (8.7 mL/min/kg). It demonstrates that the rat:human ratio of the values is approximately equal to 4.8, the ratio of rat:human GFR.

18.7 MORE DETAILED PBPK MODELS

The PBPK model developed previously is an example of a basic model. Distribution to all tissues was assumed to be perfusion controlled and driven by the passive diffusion of the drug across membranes. Oral absorption was modeled as a first-order process across the intestinal membrane. This basic model is widely used and many examples of its application can be found in the literature. However, the need to more accurately replicate drug concentrations observed *in vivo* as well as the desire to expand the application of the models has resulted in the development of models that incorporate an increasing amount of detail about the processes of absorption, distribution, metabolism, and excretion (ADME).

18.7.1 Permeability-Limited Distribution

Most drugs are small lipophilic molecules that can easily diffuse across membranes in the body. As a result, their distribution is controlled by tissue perfusion. Large polar molecules, on the other hand, may experience difficulty passing biological membranes. Typically, as discussed in Chapter 4, these molecules do not experience difficulty passing across the capillary membranes, which are very loose and permeable to most drugs. However, the membranes of the cells of the tissues may present a barrier to them, and distribution may become limited by the drug's ability to diffuse across the cell membrane. Models have

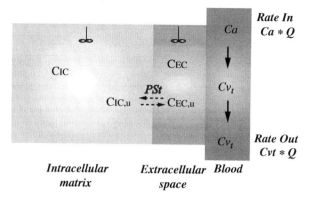

FIGURE 18.5 Permeability-limited distribution. The tissue is compartmentalized into two units, the extracellular compartment (tissue blood and extracellular space) and the intracellular tissue compartment. Drug is delivered by arterial blood, concentration Ca (blood flow Q). Distribution between the blood and the extracellular fluid is perfusion controlled. It occurs rapidly and the drug concentrations in the venous blood (Cv_t) and the extracellular space (C_{EC}) are equal. The movement of unbound drug back and forth across the cell membrane is controlled by the drug's permeability surface area product (PS_t) and the concentration gradient of the unbound drug in the extracellular ($C_{EC,u}$) and intracellular ($C_{IC,u}$) spaces. *(For a color version of this figure, see the color plate section.)*

been developed for diffusion or permeability-limited distribution, which compartmentalize the tissue into two units, the extracellular compartment (tissue blood and extracellular space) and the intracellular tissue compartment (Figure 18.5) [11–13].

It is assumed that the drug can easily pass through the capillary membrane and that a rapid equilibrium is achieved between the tissue blood and the extracellular space. As a result, the drug concentration in the extracellular space (C_{EC}) is equal to concentration in the venous blood (Cv_t) (fraction unbound is fu_b). Diffusion across the cell membrane into the intracellular space is controlled by the drug's permeability and the surface area of the membrane. Permeability and the surface area are combined into a single parameter, the permeability-surface area product (PS_t), which is also referred to as the passive diffusion clearance. The permeability-limited model produces two equations per tissue: one for the intracellular tissue compartment (IC) and one for the extracellular space (EC). The equations associated with the tissue displayed in Figure 18.5 are shown below:

$$\frac{dA_{EC}}{dt} = \text{Uptake From Blood} + \text{Passive Diffusion In} - \text{Passive Diffusion Out}$$

$$= Q_T * Ca - Q_T * C_{EC} + C_{IC} * fu_{IC} * PS_t - C_{EC} * fub * PS_t$$

$$\frac{dA_{IC}}{dt} = (\text{Passive Diffusion In} - \text{Passive Diffusion Out})$$

$$= C_{EC} * fu_b * PS_t - C_{IC} * fu_{IC} * PS_t \qquad (18.17)$$

where C_{EC} is the concentration in extracellular space (equal to the concentration in the venous blood leaving the liver), PS_t is the permeability surface area product, C_{IC} is the concentration in the intracellular space, fu_{IC} is the fraction unbound in the intracellular compartment and fu_b is the unbound fraction in the blood. Recall from Chapter 5:

$$fu_b = \frac{fu}{BP}$$

The expression for fu_{IC} can be obtained as follows. Assuming the unbound concentration is equal throughout the tissue:

$$C_{IC,u} = Cp_u$$

$$C_{IC} * fu_{IC} = Cp * fu \tag{18.18}$$

Rearranging,

$$\frac{C_{IC}}{Cp} = \frac{fu}{fu_{IC}} \quad \text{thus} \quad Kp = \frac{fu}{fu_{IC}} \tag{18.19}$$

Rearranging

$$fu_{IC} = \frac{fu}{Kp} \tag{18.20}$$

More detail about the equations used for permeability-controlled distribution can be found in the references cited above. A PBPK permeability controlled simulation model, Model 32, PBPK Permeability Controlled Model With Transporters, can be found at http://web.uri.edu/pharmacy/research/rosenbaum/sims/Model32.

18.7.2 Drug Transporters

Drug transporters are involved in the absorption distribution and elimination of many drugs. Consequently, in order to accurately replicate drug concentrations observed *in vivo*, it may be necessary to include them in the PBPK models of some drugs. The kinetics of drug transporters are assumed to follow Michaelis–Menten kinetics, and as discussed in Chapter 5, assuming the drug's Km is much greater than the drug concentrations, the transport of drugs will follow first-order kinetics:

$$\text{Rate of Transport} = \frac{J_{\max_t}}{Km_t} * C = Cl_{\text{intact},t} * C$$

where $J\max_t$ and Km_t are the maximum rate of transport and the Michaelis–Menten constant for the transporter, respectively. C is the drug concentration driving the transport, and $Cl_{\text{intact},t}$ is the intrinsic clearance for the transport process, which is equal to the transporter's $J\max_t/Km_t$.

Drug transporters are most likely to play an important role for the tissue uptake of those drugs that experience difficulty penetrating cell membranes. Consequently, when included in PBPK models, they are most commonly incorporated with a permeability-controlled distribution model for the tissue. For some drugs such as rosuvastatin and pravastatin, transporter-mediated hepatic uptake is so critical to their elimination that models that include only intrinsic metabolic clearance under predict their hepatic clearance *in vivo*. An example of a model for hepatic elimination that includes transporter-mediated uptake and efflux and metabolism (extended clearance model) is shown in Figure 18.6.

In this example of hepatic elimination, the drug's elimination incorporates an uptake transporter on the basolateral membrane and an efflux transporter on the canalicular side of the hepatocyte membrane. Each transporter has its corresponding intrinsic clearance

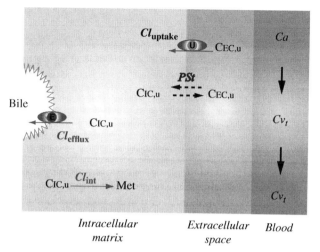

FIGURE 18.6 Liver model incorporating the action of transporters. Transporters are usually added to permeability-limited distribution models. In this model for hepatic elimination, the drug's elimination incorporates an uptake transporter on the basolateral membrane and an efflux transporter on the canalicular side of the hepatocyte membrane. Drug may pass into the hepatocyte by passive diffusion (permeability surface area product, PS_t) and/or through the action of the uptake transporter (intrinsic clearance, Cl_{uptake}). Once inside the cell, the drug may diffuse passively back into the blood; undergo metabolism (intrinsic clearance, Cl_{int}); and/or be subject to efflux into the bile (intrinsic clearance, Cl_{efflux}). See Figure 18.5 for the definition of other symbols. *(For a color version of this figure, see the color plate section.)*

(Cl_{uptake} and Cl_{efflux}, respectively). The transporter clearance for a drug can be estimated *in vitro* using immortalized cell lines expressing the transporter, isolated cells, or sandwich-cultured hepatocytes for hepatic transporters [14]. The values determined *in vitro* are then scaled up to the whole human. At this time, the scaling process for transporters has been found to be challenging because of the deficiency of information on the relative abundance of transporters *in vivo* systems. Empirically determined scaling factors are often needed to adequately replicate observed human concentrations. In the model shown in Figure 18.6, drug may pass into the hepatocyte by passive diffusion (permeability surface area product, PS_t) and/or through the action of the uptake transporter (intrinsic clearance, Cl_{uptake}). Once inside the cell, the drug may diffuse passively back into the blood; undergo metabolism (intrinsic clearance, Cl_{int}); and/or be subject to efflux into the bile (intrinsic clearance, Cl_{efflux}).

The equations associated with the model for hepatic elimination shown in Figure 18.6 would take the following form:

$$\frac{1}{V_{EC}} * \frac{dC_{EC}}{dt} = (\text{Inputs-Outputs})$$

$$= (\text{uptake from blood}) + (\text{passive diffusion in}) - (\text{passive diffusion out})$$
$$- (\text{transporter uptake into cell})$$
$$= (Q_{ha} * Ca + Q_{pv} * Cv_{pv} - Q_{hv} * C_{EC}) + (C_{IC} * fu_{IC} * PS_L)$$
$$- (C_{EC} * fub * PS_L) - (C_{EC} * fub * Cl_{uptake}) \tag{18.21}$$

and

$$\frac{1}{V_{IC}} * \frac{dC_{IC}}{dt} = \text{(Inputs-Outputs)}$$

$$= \text{(passive diffusion in)} + \text{(transporter uptake)} - \text{(passive diffusion out)}$$

$$- \text{(efflux into bile)} - \text{(metabolism)}$$

$$= (C_{EC} * fub * PS_L) + (C_{EC} * fub * Cl_{uptake}) - (C_{IC} * fu_{IC} * PS_L)$$

$$- (C_{IC} * fu_{IC} * Cl_{efflux}) - (C_{IC} * fu_{IC} * Cl_{int}) \qquad (18.22)$$

where V_{IC} and V_{EC} are the volumes of the intracellular and extracellular space, respectively (e.g., 1.14 and 0.439 L, respectively [15]); Cl_{uptake}, Cl_{efflux}, and Cl_{int} are the intrinsic clearances for the uptake transporter, the efflux transporter, and metabolism; Ca, C_{pv}, and C_{EC} and C_{IC} are the drug concentrations in the hepatic artery, hepatic portal vein, extracellular, and intracellular space, respectively; and Q_{ha}, Q_{pv}, and Q_{hv} are blood flows of the hepatic artery, portal vein, and hepatic vein, respectively. See the previous permeability-controlled model and equation (18.17) for the other definitions.

The above model is based on the well-stirred venous equilibrium model for hepatic clearance. To better replicate drug concentrations observed *in vivo*, an alternative model for the liver has been developed in which the extracellular and intracellular spaces of the liver are divided into five sequential compartments to represent flow or transit of drug through the liver [16, 17] (Figure 18.7). This approach has been used to incorporate the active and passive hepatic uptake, hepatic metabolism, and biliary efflux of several drugs including pravastatin, cerivastatin, valsartan, and repaglinide [17]. The parameters for each of these processes were initially scaled from values obtained from the sandwich-cultured human hepatocyte system, and then subsequently empirically scaled to replicate observed plasma concentration time profiles of these drugs.

A PBPK permeability controlled simulation model, Model 32, PBPK Permeability Controlled Model With Transporters, can be found at http://web.uri.edu/pharmacy/research/rosenbaum/sims/Model32.

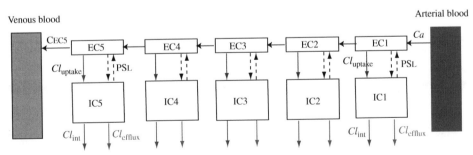

FIGURE 18.7 Transit through the liver modeled using five compartments. The model is essentially the same as the previous model (Figure 18.6) but in this case, the extracellular and intracellular spaces of the liver are divided into five units. EC represents the extracellular space and IC the intracellular space. Black dashed lines indicate passive diffusion (liver permeability surface area product (PS_L)); blue lines indicate transporter-mediated uptake (clearance, Cl_{uptake}); purple lines indicate hepatic metabolism (intrinsic clearance, Cl_{int}); and red lines indicate transporter-mediated efflux into the bile (clearance, Cl_{efflux}). *(For a color version of this figure, see the color plate section.)*

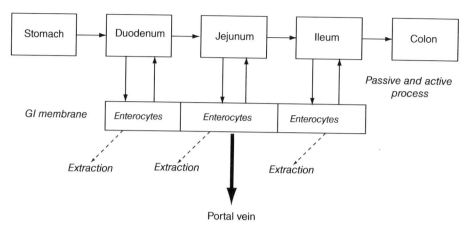

FIGURE 18.8 Mechanistic model for gastrointestinal drug absorption.

18.7.3 Models for Oral Absorption

Drug absorption across the gastrointestinal membrane and bioavailability are critical in determining the feasibility of the oral route and the pharmacokinetics of drugs that are given orally. As a result, much research has been directed toward developing models that incorporate as many as possible of the processes and factors involved in drug absorption. Mechanistic absorption models have been developed for absorption that include dissolution, drug-degradation in the gastrointestinal fluid, intestinal permeability, transporter systems, and intestinal extraction. These models compartmentalize the gastrointestinal tract into several sections from the stomach to the colon to replicate the different sections of the gastrointestinal tract through which a dosage form and a drug transits (see [3]). For example, Figure 18.8 shows a model that uses five compartments. Each compartment is assigned the unique characteristics, such as the pH, permeability, blood flow, and CYP3A4 abundance corresponding to the area the compartment represents. Drug dissolution in gastrointestinal fluid can be incorporated into models by separating the dissolved and undissolved form of the drug. For CYP3A4 substrates that undergo intestinal extraction in the enterocytes, the intestinal membrane is incorporated as a tissue of elimination using the drug's intrinsic clearance (Figure 18.8). When relevant, drug transporter systems for common intestinal transporters, such as permeability glycoprotein and organic anion transporting polypeptide (OATP), can also be incorporated.

The additional drug-specific properties required for these models include the drug's permeability in different areas of the intestine, molecular weight, pKa, particle size, and aqueous solubility or solubility in simulated gastrointestinal fluid, which contains bile salts and other substances that can aid the dissolution of poorly soluble drugs. These drug properties can be estimated in silico and *in vitro* and, once validated the models can be used to predict the rate of absorption, *Fa* and *Fg*. The absorption models are very useful in selecting drug candidates in early drug development, and later in development for optimizing oral drug formulations, predicting food effects, and designing sustained release preparations. The absorption submodels are incorporated into many of the commercially available PBPK software packages such as GASTRO-Plus® and SimCYP®, which makes the application of these models quite straightforward.

18.7.4   Reduced Models

The sheer number of tissues included into a full physiological model creates complexity. The models have a large number of equations, require a large number of tissue and drug parameters, and can require a significant amount of computing time. Furthermore, the value of some of the model parameters may be associated with some uncertainty, which can add bias to the model output and predications. In some applications, it may not be necessary nor desired to simulate drug concentrations in all the tissues of a full physiological model. For example, models used to predict the magnitude of a drug–drug interaction (DDI) between a potential perpetrator and victim drugs may want to simulate the liver concentrations of these drugs but not those in other tissues. In order to simplify the models and to reduce the number of parameters, equations, and computing time, reduced models may be developed for use in these applications. Reduced, hybrid, or semiphysiological models can be created by separating the tissue of interest, for example, the liver from other tissues which are then lumped or grouped together into one or more compartments, which can take the form of traditional compartments [18, 19].

18.8   APPLICATION OF PBPK MODELS

PBPK models are being used extensively in the pharmaceutical industry from early drug discovery throughout the development process. They are being used to optimize lead molecule identification and decrease the risk of developing a drug that will subsequently found to have unsatisfactory pharmacokinetic properties. PBPK modeling is also being used to increase the efficiency and reduce the cost of development by aiding in the selection of the most critical clinical studies and helping to optimize the design of the studies. It also has the further benefit of reducing the number of preclinical studies and the number of laboratory animals needed to support drug development.

The ability to estimate drug-specific parameters in silico and *in vitro* enables models to be built well before a drug is administered to humans. Even though such early models may possess uncertainties and may not ultimately accurately predict human behavior, they can be useful in eliminating drug candidates with poor pharmacokinetic properties, such as low bioavailability or rapid elimination. As drugs continue through the development process, the availability of *in vivo* data in animals provides the opportunity to validate the models and refine them to more accurately simulate observed concentrations. This process is referred to as "learn, confirm and refine" [4]. The refinement process continues as more animal and human *in vivo* data become available. If there is confidence in the ability of the models to predict human concentrations, they can then be used to determine initial doses in humans, where they have the advantage of being able to predict concentrations in tissues where the drug may act, and thus in theory possess the ability to more accurately calculate optimum doses. Once a model has been validated for a normal population, the models can be applied to special populations known to have altered physiological parameters and/or altered drug clearance. Thus, PBPK models can be used to evaluate a drug's pharmacokinetic properties and optimal doses in children, the elderly, pregnant women, different ethnic groups, and people with renal and/or hepatic impairment. A process that can significantly reduce the number of clinical studies is needed in these groups.

An important application of PBPK modeling is the prediction of DDIs. A recent analysis of PBPK studies published in the literature between 2004 and 2014 found that the majority

(28%) addressed the prediction of DDIs [2]. In contrast to the "static" models discussed in detail in Chapter 17 that use a single measure of a perpetrators concentration to predict DDI risk, PBPK models are able to predict the whole time course of a perpetrator's concentration in the target tissue, which should result in more accurate predictions. Additionally, the more mechanistic models that incorporate intestinal extraction, and transporters at various sites involved in ADME, are ideally suited to study more complex DDIs such as perpetrators that act on multiple enzymes and/or transporters [20]. Commercially available PBPK custom software packages such as SimCYP® offer the additional advantage of having the capability to generate virtual populations in which to study DDI risk. Their large data base of patient demographics and correlated physiological parameters can be used to construct virtual populations made up of individuals with a variety of demographic characteristics, including genetic polymorphism in enzymes (e.g., CYP2D6 and CYP2C9) and transporters (e.g., OAPT). Thus, in addition to identifying the risks and responses in a typical individual, they offer the opportunity to identify any unusual adverse effects (toxicity and subtherapeutic drug concentrations) that may be experienced by special populations that are usually poorly represented in traditional clinical studies.

REFERENCES

1. Brown, R. P., Delp, M. D., Lindstedt, S. L., Rhomberg, L. R., and Beliles, R. P. (1997) Physiological parameter values for physiologically based pharmacokinetic models, *Toxicol Ind Health*, *13*, 407–484.

2. Sager, J. E., Yu, J., Ragueneau-Majlessi, I., and Isoherranen, N. (2015) Physiologically based pharmacokinetic (PBPK) modeling and simulation approaches: a systematic review of published models, applications, and model verification, *Drug Metab Dispos*, *43*, 1823–1837.

3. Rowland, M., Peck, C., and Tucker, G. (2011) Physiologically-based pharmacokinetics in drug development and regulatory science, *Annu Rev Pharmacol Toxicol*, *51*, 45–73.

4. Jones, H., and Rowland-Yeo, K. (2013) Basic concepts in physiologically based pharmacokinetic modeling in drug discovery and development, *CPT Pharmacometrics Syst Pharmacol*, *2*, e63.

5. Jones, H. M., Chen, Y., Gibson, C., Heimbach, T., Parrott, N., Peters, S. A., Snoeys, J., Upreti, V. V., Zheng, M., and Hall, S. D. (2015) Physiologically based pharmacokinetic modeling in drug discovery and development: a pharmaceutical industry perspective, *Clin Pharmacol Ther*, *97*, 247–262.

6. Espie, P., Tytgat, D., Sargentini-Maier, M. L., Poggesi, I., and Watelet, J. B. (2009) Physiologically based pharmacokinetics (PBPK), *Drug Metab Rev*, *41*, 391–407.

7. Rodgers, T., Leahy, D., and Rowland, M. (2005) Physiologically based pharmacokinetic modeling 1: predicting the tissue distribution of moderate-to-strong bases, *J Pharm Sci*, *94*, 1259–1276.

8. Rodgers, T., and Rowland, M. (2006) Physiologically based pharmacokinetic modelling 2: predicting the tissue distribution of acids, very weak bases, neutrals and zwitterions, *J Pharm Sci*, *95*, 1238–1257.

9. Graham, H., Walker, M., Jones, O., Yates, J., Galetin, A., and Aarons, L. (2012) Comparison of in-vivo and in-silico methods used for prediction of tissue: plasma partition coefficients in rat, *J Pharm Pharmacol*, *64*, 383–396.

10. Lin, J. H. (1998) Applications and limitations of interspecies scaling and in vitro extrapolation in pharmacokinetics, *Drug Metab Dispos*, *26*, 1202–1212.

11. Gertz, M., Houston, J. B., and Galetin, A. (2011) Physiologically based pharmacokinetic modeling of intestinal first-pass metabolism of CYP3A substrates with high intestinal extraction, *Drug Metab Dispos*, *39*, 1633–1642.

12. Thompson, M. D., and Beard, D. A. (2011) Development of appropriate equations for physiologically based pharmacokinetic modeling of permeability-limited and flow-limited transport, *J Pharmacokinet Pharmacodyn*, *38*, 405–421.

13. Li, R., Barton, H. A., Yates, P. D., Ghosh, A., Wolford, A. C., Riccardi, K. A., and Maurer, T. S. (2014) A "middle-out" approach to human pharmacokinetic predictions for OATP substrates using physiologically-based pharmacokinetic modeling, *J Pharmacokinet Pharmacodyn*, *41*, 197–209.

14. Zamek-Gliszczynski, M. J., Lee, C. A., Poirier, A., Bentz, J., Chu, X., Ellens, H., Ishikawa, T., Jamei, M., Kalvass, J. C., Nagar, S., Pang, K. S., Korzekwa, K., Swaan, P. W., Taub, M. E., Zhao, P., and Galetin, A. (2013) ITC recommendations for transporter kinetic parameter estimation and translational modeling of transport-mediated PK and DDIs in humans, *Clin Pharmacol Ther*, *94*, 64–79.

15. Yoshida, K., Maeda, K., and Sugiyama, Y. (2013) Hepatic and intestinal drug transporters: prediction of pharmacokinetic effects caused by drug-drug interactions and genetic polymorphisms, *Annu Rev Pharmacol Toxicol*, *53*, 581–612.

16. Watanabe, T., Kusuhara, H., Maeda, K., Shitara, Y., and Sugiyama, Y. (2009) Physiologically based pharmacokinetic modeling to predict transporter-mediated clearance and distribution of pravastatin in humans, *J Pharmacol Exp Ther*, *328*, 652–662.

17. Jones, H. M., Barton, H. A., Lai, Y., Bi, Y. A., Kimoto, E., Kempshall, S., Tate, S. C., El-Kattan, A., Houston, J. B., Galetin, A., and Fenner, K. S. (2012) Mechanistic pharmacokinetic modeling for the prediction of transporter-mediated disposition in humans from sandwich culture human hepatocyte data, *Drug Metab Dispos*, *40*, 1007–1017.

18. Quinney, S. K., Zhang, X., Lucksiri, A., Gorski, J. C., Li, L., and Hall, S. D. (2010) Physiologically based pharmacokinetic model of mechanism-based inhibition of CYP3A by clarithromycin, *Drug Metab Dispos*, *38*, 241–248.

19. Gertz, M., Tsamandouras, N., Sall, C., Houston, J. B., and Galetin, A. (2014) Reduced physiologically-based pharmacokinetic model of repaglinide: impact of OATP1B1 and CYP2C8 genotype and source of in vitro data on the prediction of drug-drug interaction risk, *Pharm Res*, *31*, 2367–2382.

20. Varma, M. V., Pang, K. S., Isoherranen, N., and Zhao, P. (2015) Dealing with the complex drug-drug interactions: towards mechanistic models. *Biopharm Drug Dispos*, *36*, 71–92.

19

INTRODUCTION TO PHARMACODYNAMIC MODELS AND INTEGRATED PHARMACOKINETIC–PHARMACODYNAMIC MODELS

Drs. Diane Mould and Paul Hutson

Objectives

The material in this chapter will enable the reader to:

1. Understand classic receptor theory of drug action
2. Understand the basis and application of the sigmoidal E_{max} or I_{max} and related models
3. Understand the time course of drug response based on the sigmoidal E_{max} model

Basic Pharmacokinetics and Pharmacodynamics: An Integrated Textbook and Computer Simulations,
Second Edition. Edited by Sara E. Rosenbaum.
© 2017 John Wiley & Sons, Inc. Published 2017 by John Wiley & Sons, Inc.

19.1 INTRODUCTION

Mathematical models are important tools for the study of drug actions *in vivo*. To be complete, such models should include a pharmacodynamic component for the concentration–response relationship and a pharmacokinetic component for the dose–plasma concentration relationship. In theory, such integrated pharmacokinetic–pharmacodynamic (PK–PD) models could predict responses at any time, after any dose, administered by any route. These models would be of enormous value for estimating doses and dosing intervals to achieve specific desired responses. They could also be used to gain insight into the behavior of a drug in situations not yet studied.

For example, if an appropriate PK–PD model is identified and the model parameters determined after a single dose of a drug, simulations can be performed to predict steady-state responses and optimum dosing regimens to achieve desired responses. Integrated PK–PD models are being applied increasingly to optimize the design of clinical trials, increase the efficiency of these studies, and decrease the cost of drug development [1, 2]. Integrated PK–PD models are also being used increasingly in translational research in which parameters identified *in vitro* and small animals are used to predict drug response in humans [2, 3]. These studies are proving to be valuable during drug discovery to help identify the specific molecules most likely to progress successfully throughout the development process and succeed in humans. Recently, an integrated PK–PD model has been developed specifically for clinical practice to estimate optimum doses of several anticancer drugs in individual patients [4].

As discussed in Chapter 1, the development of mathematical models for concentration–response relationships in humans has been hampered by several factors. Among these are the inability to measure the drug concentration at the site of action, the difficulty in measuring the response to a drug, and the complex and varied nature of the chain of events between receptor activation and the emergence of response. The processes associated with the pharmacodynamic phase of drug response are much more varied and complex in nature than those involved in the pharmacokinetic phase. A drug's pharmacokinetics are driven primarily by passive diffusion and the common pathways of renal excretion and hepatic metabolism, which are usually simple first-order processes. By contrast, the interaction of a drug with its receptors can lead to a vast array of disparate effects. The intended drug response may occur almost immediately or may take several days or even weeks to become apparent. The response may initiate homeostatic processes or tolerance that can further complicate the model needed to describe the effect of the drug. Thus, in comparison to pharmacokinetics, the design of models of drug response is much more challenging, and a greater diversity of models is required to accommodate different types of processes. Often the goal of drug treatment occurs over a prolonged period, or the prevention of a discrete, event. Responses to such drugs in human beings can usually not be measured to guide titration of dose. This problem has been overcome to a large extent by the identification of biomarkers or surrogates of drug response. A *biomarker* may be defined as a concrete biological characteristic that can be measured objectively as a parallel indicator of a drug response [5]. Ideally, biomarkers used for the development of pharmacodynamic models should possess the following qualities:

- Valid for the response being assessed.
- Measured objectively rather than relying on subjective evaluations of a patient or health care provider.

- Continuous rather than an all-or-none response.
- Sensitive for the response; that is, changes in the response should lead consistently to changes in the biomarkers.
- Specific for the response. Ideally, changes in the biomarker should be associated with the drug response, not with other events.
- Reproducible from one occasion to another and from one clinical center to another.
- Occurs in the same concentration range as the therapeutic response.
- Repeatable in the same patient at later times to enable the response to be evaluated over an extended period. Evaluations that are invasive or those that may involve learning would not meet this criterion.

Examples of biomarkers include measurement of the amplitude of certain frequency bands on an electroencephalograph to evaluate the effects of centrally acting drugs, and the measurement of relevant endogenous compounds such as proteins in biological fluids. For example, reductions in amyloid β peptide levels in the cerebrospinal fluid and increased concentrations of tau protein have been used as biomarkers in Alzheimer's disease.

In this chapter, we discuss the receptor theory of direct drug action, classic pharmacodynamic models, and the parameters that are used to evaluate a drug's pharmacodynamic characteristics. We also discuss the development and application of the pharmacodynamic models most commonly used to model drug response *in vivo*. These direct action models of drug effect presume that the effect of the drug is directly related to the drug concentration and its affinity for binding to the corresponding receptor.

In the following chapter, more complex PD models will be presented that accommodate drug effects that are not directly linked to the time and concentration of drug exposure.

19.2 CLASSIC PHARMACODYNAMIC MODELS BASED ON RECEPTOR THEORY

The classic receptor theory of drug action is an important starting point for understanding drug action *in vivo* and the development of pharmacodynamic models in humans. The classic receptor-based models have been developed primarily through a study of drug action in the more controlled and isolated *in vitro* environment, where response and the drug concentration at the site of action can easily be measured. Additionally, the action of a drug *in vitro* can be studied in isolation without the interference of homeostatic and other competing processes.

As discussed in Chapter 1, most drugs exert their effects by interacting with their receptors in a reversible manner. The interaction of an agonist with its receptor leads to a conformational change in the receptor that results in a signal or stimulus. The stimulus then initiates other actions that ultimately result in a biological response (Figure 19.1). The events between generation of the stimulus and the final response constitute what is called the *response chain*. This can be a simple direct process such as the opening or closing of an ion channel, or it may involve a long transduction process that includes a cascade of several events and the action of second messengers. The overall intensity of drug response is a function of two types of properties: drug-specific and tissue- or system-specific properties. The *drug-specific properties* are the ability of the drug to interact with the receptors (affinity) and the ability of the drug to produce a stimulus per unit receptor (intrinsic efficacy).

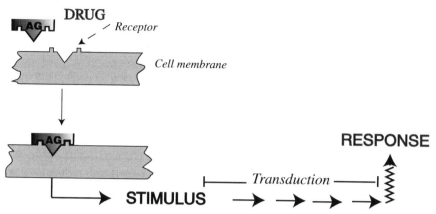

FIGURE 19.1   Diagrammatic representation of the drug–receptor interaction. The drug interacts with the receptor to produce a conformational change in the receptor. This results in a stimulus. The stimulus initiates the events that culminate in the biological response.

The *tissue-specific properties* are the number or density of the receptors and the process that converts the initial signal into a response and the maximal response possible. Ideally, a pharmacodynamic model should separate these two types of properties.

The first mathematical model for the relationship between agonist drug response and concentration was developed in 1937 by Clark. Over the years, this model was modified—by Ariens (in 1954), Stephenson (in 1956), and Furchgott (in 1966) (see [6])—but key elements of the original model remain. Based on their work, two models that have relevance to drug evaluation in humans are presented. The first is the simpler model of Ariens, the *intrinsic activity model*, which incorporates the term *intrinsic activity*. The second model, the *efficacy model*, a more sophisticated extension of the first model, incorporates a parameter for a drug's efficacy to accommodate the concept of spare receptors. Both models are based on the assumption that drug action is a function of a drug's quality of binding to its receptors. Thus, the characteristics of receptor binding are fundamental to both models.

19.2.1 Receptor Binding

The response to a drug is assumed to be a function of the number of receptors occupied. Receptor occupancy is another example of a capacity-limited process that is described by the *law of mass action*:

$$C + R \underset{k_{\text{off}}}{\overset{k_{\text{on}}}{\rightleftharpoons}} RC \tag{19.1}$$

where C is the molar concentration of drug, R is the molar concentration of unoccupied receptors, RC is the molar concentration of the drug's receptor complex, k_{on} is the rate constant for the forward process, and k_{off} is the rate constant for the backward process.

Once equilibrium is established, the rates of the forward and backward processes become equal:

$$(R_T - RC) \cdot C \cdot k_{\text{on}} = RC \cdot k_{\text{off}} \tag{19.2}$$

where R_T is the total molar concentration of receptors. After rearrangement, we have

$$RC = \frac{R_T \cdot C}{K_d + C} \tag{19.3}$$

or

$$\frac{RC}{R_T} = \frac{C}{K_d + C} \tag{19.4}$$

where K_d is the drug's dissociation constant (k_{off}/k_{on}) and is a reciprocal measure of the drug's affinity for the receptors. As affinity increases, K_d decreases and there is greater binding at a given drug concentration. Note that because k_{on} is a second-order rate constant, the units of K_d are those of concentration, and it follows that K_d is the concentration at which drug has bound to half of the total receptors.

Because the system has only a finite number of receptors, the concentration of occupied receptors (RC) in equation (19.3) is limited by the total concentration (or capacity) of receptors in a system (R_T). As a result, the relationship between occupancy and drug concentration has the hyperbolic shape typical of *capacity-limited* processes (Figure 19.2). At low concentrations ($K_d \gg C$), there is a large excess of free receptors, and the concentration of the complex can increase in direct proportion to increases in concentration. As the concentration approaches and exceeds K_d, the ratio of bound to total receptors no longer increases in proportion to the drug concentration. Eventually, all the receptors are occupied, the concentration of the drug–receptor complex achieves its maximum value and increases in drug concentration have no further effect on the concentration of the complex.

19.2.2 Concentration-Response Models

Response to a drug is assumed to be a function of the number or fraction of the total receptors that are occupied. The relationship between response and drug concentration is usually either hyperbolic (Figure 19.3) or sigmoidal in nature; that is, high drug concentrations

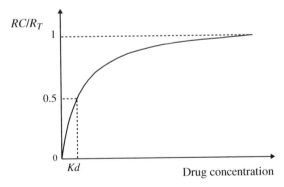

FIGURE 19.2 Relationship between fraction of receptors occupied and drug concentration. The fraction of the receptors occupied (RC/R_T) is shown as a function of the drug concentration (C). Binding of a drug to its receptors is an example of a capacity-limited process. At high drug concentrations, binding is limited by the number or capacity of the receptors. RC is the concentration of the drug–receptor complex, and R_T is the total concentration of receptors. When $\frac{RC}{R_T} = 0.5$, $C = K_d$, the dissociation constant.

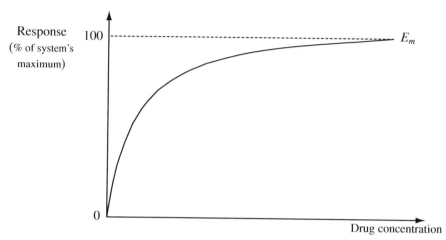

FIGURE 19.3   Relationship between the response and drug concentration. The response increases with drug concentration, but the increase gets proportionally less as the drug concentration increases (law of diminishing returns). Eventually, at higher drug concentrations, a maximum response is achieved. In this figure, the drug is able to achieve the system's maximum response (E_m).

produce a maximum response, and once this has been achieved, further increases in concentration produce no additional increases in response. The two models presented below differ in their assumptions regarding the origin of the capacity-limited nature of the response–concentration relationship.

During the course of this discussion, several pharmacodynamic parameters will be introduced:

1. E_m, the maximum response of a system. If the effect of a drug is to decrease a response, the maximal inhibition is represented instead as I_m.

2. E_{max}, the maximum response of a drug; for a full agonist, $E_{max} = E_m$. If the effect of a drug is to decrease a response, the maximal response of the drug is represented instead as I_{max}.

3. EC_{50}, the drug concentration that produces half the drug's maximum response. If the effect of a drug is to decrease a response, the drug concentration that produces half the drug's maximum response is represented instead as IC_{50}.

4. K_d, the drug concentration that results in 50% receptor occupancy.

5. α, the intrinsic activity or fraction of the system's maximum response that an agonist can illicit.

6. n, the slope factor in the sigmoid E_{max} model, modifies the slope and shape of the curve (Figure 19.9). When $n = 1$, the sigmoid E_{max} model collapses to the basic E_{max} model.

19.2.2.1 Intrinsic Activity Model

The simplest pharmacodynamic model, the *intrinsic activity model*, assumes that the capacity-limited nature of the response–concentration relationship is a direct consequence of the capacity-limited nature of receptor occupancy. In this model, developed by Ariens, response is assumed to be directly proportional to receptor occupancy. Specifically, the fraction of maximum response (E/E_m) is assumed to be proportional to the fraction of the total receptors occupied (RC/R_T), and the constant of proportionality is the intrinsic activity:

$$\frac{E}{E_m} = \alpha \cdot \frac{RC}{R_T} \tag{19.5}$$

where E is the response, E_m is the system's maximum possible response, and α is an efficacy term that Ariens called *intrinsic activity*. Equations (19.4) and (19.5) can be combined to

$$E = \frac{\alpha \cdot E_m \cdot C}{K_d + C} \tag{19.6}$$

Note the similarity of the equation to the Michaelis–Menten equation describing the mixed order elimination of drugs by enzymes and transporters (15.6). Here, $\alpha \bullet E_m$ is the maximal effect possible for a drug (E_{max}), analogous to the maximum rate of elimination of the drug, V_{max}.

The maximum response that a specific drug can achieve (E_{max}) may be equal to or less than the maximum response that the system can produce (E_m) (Figure 19.4). Intrinsic activity is the constant of proportionality between the system's maximum response and the drug's maximum response. Full agonists will have an intrinsic activity of 1; a partial agonist will have an intrinsic activity greater than 0 and less than 1. For example, a drug that can produce only 60% of the system's maximum effect ($E_{max} = 0.6 E_m$) will have an α value of 0.6 (Figure 19.4). An antagonist will have an intrinsic activity of zero. According to this model, the same degree of receptor occupancy for a series of full agonists ($\alpha = 1$) will result in the same response.

19.2.2.2 Efficacy Model
A more complex *efficacy model* may be required to explain drug effect when the simple intrinsic, direct model cannot account for the observation that some drugs are able to

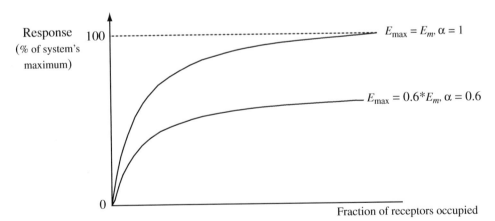

FIGURE 19.4 Response–concentration relationship based on the intrinsic activity model. The fractional response is directly proportional to the fraction of the total receptors occupied. The constant of proportionality is intrinsic activity (α). Drugs that have intrinsic activities of 1 (full agonist) and 0.6 (partial agonist) have maximum responses (E_{max}) of 100% and 60% of the system's maximum response (E_m), respectively.

produce a maximum response at less than maximum receptor occupancy. To accommodate this observation:

1. The concept of *spare receptors*, receptors that are not occupied when some drugs produce a maximal response, was introduced.

2. The model separated the two stages of drug response (Figure 19.1). First, the drug interacts with its receptors to produce a conformational change in the receptor and generate a stimulus. Second, the tissue translates the stimulus into a biological response, a process that may involve signal transduction and second messengers.

3. It is assumed that the intensity of the stimulus that results from a given level of receptor occupancy is not the same among drugs. Drugs that possess high efficacy are able to produce a larger stimulus per occupied receptor than drugs with lower efficacy. Further, drugs with high efficacy are able to produce the system's maximum response at less than full receptor occupancy. Drugs with lower efficacy may need to occupy all the receptors to produce a full response, while others are unable to produce the system's maximum response (partial agonists) even when all the receptors are occupied.

4. It is assumed that submaximal response despite high drug concentrations relationship can arise from weak agonists or partial agonists, or by an unknown process farther down the response chain. Such downstream processes are often associated with tolerance to a drug, and may be modeled using the precursor depletion concept described later in this chapter.

The value of the drug stimulus depends on two factors: the fraction of the receptors occupied (drug concentration and affinity) and the *efficacy* (e), the efficiency with which the drug translates its binding to the receptors into the stimulus. The value of the stimulus can be expressed as:

$$S = e \cdot \frac{RC}{R_T} \tag{19.7}$$

where S is the value of the stimulus, and e is the efficacy of the drug.

Solving for e, it can be seen (19.8) that this efficacy term for a given drug is a constant that relates the magnitude of the stimulus to the fraction of receptors that are occupied.

$$e = \frac{S}{\left(\frac{RC}{R_T} \right)} \tag{19.8}$$

A drug's *efficacy* (the efficiency with which the receptor binding is converted into the initial stimulus) is a function not only of the drug efficacy but also of the number of receptors. The efficacy of a drug can be expressed per unit receptor. This is known as the *intrinsic efficacy* (ε):

$$\varepsilon = \frac{e}{R_T} \tag{19.9}$$

Substituting into equation (19.8), the intrinsic efficacy of a drug can also be described as the unit of stimulus per occupied receptor:

$$\varepsilon = \frac{S}{RC} \tag{19.10}$$

Because the stimulus does not represent the fraction of maximal response (E/E_m), it can achieve values greater than 1 (E/E_m cannot be greater than 1). As a result, unlike intrinsic activity, efficacy can achieve a value greater than 1. In contrast to the simple intrinsic activity model in which full agonists have an intrinsic activity of 1, the value of efficacy can vary among full agonists, which allows the model to distinguish the different efficacies of full agonists.

The system then converts the stimulus into a biological response. This may be a fast, simple process in equilibrium with plasma drug concentrations, or may involve a cascade of several steps and may require a significant amount of time as described in the next chapter. The magnitude of response is a function of the value of the initial stimulus and may be expressed as:

$$\frac{E}{E_m} = f(S) \tag{19.11}$$

To accommodate the capacity-limited characteristics of the relationship between response and drug concentration (as discussed above, E/E_m has a maximum value of 1), the right-hand side of the equation must resolve to a value between zero (the stimulus produces no response) and 1 (the stimulus produces the maximum response), so a hyperbolic function [$E/E_m = S/(1 + S)$] is frequently used for the relationship between the value of the stimulus and the magnitude of the biological effect. To obtain this hyperbolic function, we combine equations (19.7) and (19.11) to yield

$$\frac{E}{E_m} = f\left(\frac{e \cdot RC}{R_T}\right) \tag{19.12}$$

and substituting for RC/R_T from equation (19.4) gives us

$$\frac{E}{E_m} = f\left(\frac{e \cdot C}{K_d + C}\right) \tag{19.13}$$

Equation (19.13) can incorporate equation (19.9) to yield

$$\frac{E}{E_m} = f\left(\frac{\varepsilon \cdot R_T \cdot C}{K_d + C}\right) \tag{19.14}$$

From a mechanistic basis, it can be seen (19.14) that the effect produced by a given drug concentration is dependent on:

1. The magnitude of stimulus expected from the fraction of bound/total receptors (e).
2. The affinity of the drug for the receptor, which is expressed using the dissociation constant (K_d), which is a reciprocal measure of affinity. It is equal to the drug concentration when 50% of the receptors are occupied. Low values of K_d are associated with high affinity, and vice versa.
3. The tissue property (f) that translates the initial stimulus into the biological response.

The parameters of this model thus separate the drug-specific parameters of intrinsic efficacy (ε) and affinity (K_d) from tissue-specific properties of the total concentration of receptors (R_T) and the tissue property that converts the stimulus into the biological response (f) discussed in the next section. It can also be seen that the constant α of the intrinsic activity

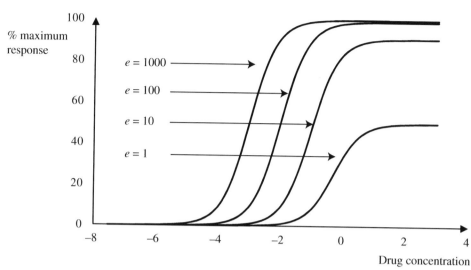

FIGURE 19.5 Semilogarithmic plots of response against drug concentration for a series of agonists with different efficacies (e). The affinity of all four drugs is the same. In the figure, the drugs that have efficacies of 1 and 10 are partial agonists because they cannot produce the maximum response produced by other drugs (full agonists).

model is analogous to the term e (also equal to $\varepsilon \cdot R_T$) of the efficacy model. It is reassuring that the more complex efficacy (19.13) model has the same form of the more fundamental intrinsic activity model (19.6). The notable difference is that the intrinsic activity α has values from 0 to 1, whereas the efficacy e can have any positive value, including zero. The ratio of $E/E_{\max}$ cannot exceed 1, so the right side of (19.14) is similarly constrained. The result is that systems with drug efficacy e > 2 can reach maximal effect E_m even when the concentration is not greater than K_d, which for a drug with efficacy e = 1 would yield only 50% of maximal effect. Higher efficacy will often allow less frequent dosing, as the effect of such drugs will persist long into the elimination of the drug.

Figure 19.5 shows the typical concentration–response profile associated with the efficacy model. In the figure, drugs with efficacies of 1 and 10 are partial agonists because they cannot produce the maximum response produced by other drugs (the full agonists). Note that at low concentrations, drugs with higher efficacies produce larger responses at equivalent concentrations (i.e., they are more potent). At very high concentrations, there is no difference among full agonists in the magnitude of the response which cannot exceed 100%, but partial agonists produce lower maximum responses. Note that although the two curves on the left both represent responses to full agonists, they are not superimposed because the agonists producing them differ in efficacy.

Figure 19.6 shows how the value of a drug's affinity influences the response–concentration relationship for a series of full agonists with the same efficacy. As affinity increases (K_d decreases), response at a given concentration increases. Figures 19.5 and 19.6 demonstrate that a drug's potency is a function of both its affinity and efficacy. A summary of some of the pharmacodynamic terms introduced in this section is provided below.

1. *Affinity*. The affinity of a drug is a measure of the strength with which the drug binds to the receptor and is the reciprocal of the dissociation constant (i.e., $1/K_d$). K_d is equal to the drug concentration when half the receptors are occupied. Drugs that have

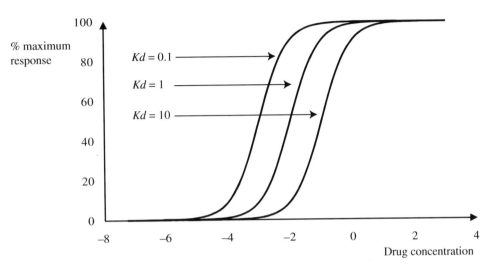

FIGURE 19.6   Semilogarithmic plot of response against drug concentration for a series of agonists with different values of affinity. The efficacy of all three drugs is the same. A drug's K_d value is a reciprocal form of affinity; as K_d increases, affinity decreases.

high affinities (K_d small) require a lower concentration to occupy half the receptors compared to drugs with relatively low affinities.

2. *Efficacy and intrinsic efficacy. Efficacy* is an expression of the efficiency with which a drug converts its interaction with the receptors of a system into a stimulus. Full agonists have large values of efficacy that may vary among drugs. Partial agonists will have low efficacies, and antagonists will have zero efficacy. *Intrinsic efficacy* is a measure of a drug's efficacy per unit receptor. As such, in contrast to efficacy, it is dependent only on the drug and is a pure measure of the drug's ability to produce a stimulus from its interaction with a receptor. Affinity and intrinsic efficacy constitute the drug-specific parameters that control the response–concentration relationship. Their individual roles in the response chain are shown in Figure 19.7.

3. *Intrinsic activity.* Intrinsic activity is the fraction of the full system response that a drug can produce. A full agonist that can produce the maximal system response has an intrinsic activity of 1, a partial agonist has an intrinsic activity between 0 and 1, and an antagonist has an intrinsic activity of 0. In contrast to pure efficacy, intrinsic activity does not make any distinction among full agonists—they all have intrinsic activities of 1.

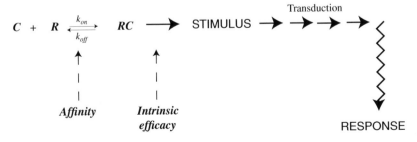

FIGURE 19.7   Affinity and intrinsic efficacy in the drug response chain.

4. *Potency*. Potency reflects the concentration of a drug that is required to produce a given effect. Most commonly, it is expressed as the EC_{50}, the drug concentration that produces half the drug's maximum response. A drug with high potency will produce a given effect at a lower concentration than will one with low potency. Potency, a function of tissue and drug factors, is controlled by the drug factors of affinity and intrinsic efficacy. Affinity controls the number of receptors occupied at a certain drug concentration, and intrinsic efficacy determines the magnitude of the effect that results from the occupancy. Potency is also controlled by two tissue-specific factors: the number of receptors present in a system and how the receptor stimulus is converted into a response. Within a biological system, the relative potency of two drugs is dependent on affinity and intrinsic efficacy. Note that in the efficacy model, if a drug has high efficacy, its EC_{50} will be much less than the K_d value.

19.3 DIRECT EFFECT PHARMACODYNAMIC MODELS

As discussed previously, the evaluation of drug response in humans is complicated by several factors. These include the difficulty in measuring drug concentrations at the site of action, the identification of the events that constitute the response chain, the potential involvement of homeostatic mechanisms, and the difficulty associated with measuring drug response. Recognizing the capacity-limited nature of the response–concentration relationship *in vivo*, Wagner [7] proposed using an empirical, capacity-limited model, to describe the relationship between response and concentration. This equation, developed initially by Hill to describe the binding of oxygen to hemoglobin [8], expresses the binding of a ligand to a macromolecule and is known as the E_{max} or *sigmoidal E_{max} model*.

19.3.1 E_{max} and Sigmoidal E_{max} Models

The sigmoidal E_{max} model and the simpler E_{max} model are among the most frequently used pharmacodynamic models. The E_{max} *model* is summarized as:

$$E = \frac{E_{max} * C}{EC_{50} + C} \tag{19.15}$$

and the sigmoidal E_{max} model is similar to

$$E = \frac{E_{max} * C^n}{EC_{50}^n + C^n} \tag{19.16}$$

where E is the drug effect or response, E_{max} is the maximum effect of the drug, C is the drug concentration, and EC_{50} is the concentration that produces 50% maximum response. The slope factor n in the sigmoid E_{max} model modifies the slope and shape of the curve and is added to improve the fit of the model. When $n = 1$, the sigmoid E_{max} model collapses to the basic E_{max} model. The value of n has been suggested to be the number of drug molecules binding to the receptor, analogous to the binding of oxygen to hemoglobin in the Hill hemoglobin dissociation equation that inspired the sigmoid E_{max} model. However, the value of n is often a noninteger, and should be considered an empirically derived value that serves to improve the ability of the resulting pharmacodynamic model to fit observed data.

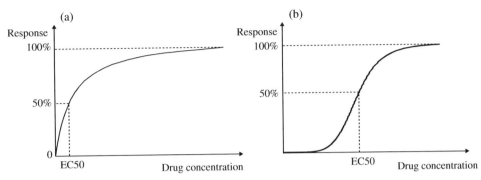

FIGURE 19.8   Relationship between response and drug concentration at the site of action for the E_{max} model (a) and the sigmoidal E_{max} model (b). The EC_{50} is the concentration that produces half the drug's maximum response.

The entire sigmoidal E_{max} model is empirical and makes no assumptions about mechanistic factors that are responsible for the capacity-limited or saturation characteristics of the response–concentration relationship. However, the E_{max} model bears a close resemblance to the simple intrinsic activity model, which assumed that response was directly proportional to receptor occupancy, did not incorporate the concept of spare receptors, and combined the processes of stimulus generation and transduction. The similarities of the empiric E_{max} models are clear from a comparison of equation (19.13) to the equation for the simple intrinsic activity model that was derived using mechanistic concepts of drug–receptor interactions (19.7).

In considering the relationship between response and concentration, it is helpful to recall the very similar Michaelis–Menten model for the rate of an enzymatic reaction (see 5.4.6). The hyperbolic relationship between the drug effect and concentration is shown in Figure 19.8a. At low concentrations, the system is well below saturation, and the effect increases almost linearly with concentration. As the concentration increases further, some saturation of the system is observed and the effect can no longer increase proportionately with concentration. Eventually, when the system is fully saturated, the maximum effect is observed. In common with Michaelis–Menten kinetics, it is the relationship between the concentration and the EC_{50} (K_m in the Michaelis–Menten equation) that determines the nature of the response–concentration relationship. When drug concentrations are much lower than EC_{50} (the response is less than 20% maximum), a linear relationship is observed between the response and the concentration. As the concentration increases, the increase in response with concentration becomes nonlinear, and eventually, at high concentrations, the response approaches maximum. At this point, increases in concentrations produce little increase in effect. Additionally, after the administration of a dose that approaches maximum effect, the dissipation of the response will be slow because there is little change in response with concentration at high drug concentrations.

A summary of the parameters of the model follows.

1. EC_{50}, the concentration of a drug that produces 50% of its maximum response. It is a measure of a drug's potency. It is dependent on a drug's affinity and its intrinsic efficacy. It will also depend on how the biological system relays the stimulus that results from activation of the receptor to generate the response.

2. E_{max}, an efficacy parameter, is dependent not only on a drug's efficacy but also on the biological system. Specifically, it will be dependent on the number of receptors

and how the stimulus resulting from receptor activation is relayed to generate the response. If the E_{max} of a series of drugs were measured in the same system, the values could be compared to provide values of their relative intrinsic activity and thus distinguish between full and partial agonists.

3. n is a factor that expresses the slope of the response–concentration relationship.

Baseline Effects and Drug-Induced Decreases in Response The basic equation for the sigmoidal E_{max} model (19.16) predicts that the response to an agonist will be zero when the drug concentration is zero and that the response will increase with concentration. In many cases, a nonzero baseline effect (E_0) is present (e.g., heart rate). The sigmoidal E_{max} model can easily be adapted to account for both of these situations:

$$E = E_0 + \frac{E_{max} * C^n}{EC_{50}^n + C^n} \tag{19.17}$$

where E_0 is the baseline state of the system. Equation (19.17) is often modified to solve for the change in effect from baseline caused by the effect of the drug:

$$E - E_0 = \frac{E_{max} * C^n}{EC_{50}^n + C^n} \tag{19.18}$$

19.3.2 Inhibitory *I*max and Sigmoidal *I*max Models

The effect of a drug commonly will serve to decrease an effect, such as inhibition of enzyme activity. In such cases, it is typical to modify the E_{max} or sigmoidal E_{max} models by corresponding substitution with I_{max} and IC_{50} in either equation [(19.15) and (19.16)]. The use of I_{max} serves to clarify the direction of the drug action.

$$E = \frac{I_{max} * C}{IC_{50} + C} \tag{19.19}$$

When a baseline activity or effect is present, equation (19.19) can be modified to reflect the new activity arising from drug-induced loss of function

$$E = E_0 - \frac{I_{max} * C^n}{IC_{50}^n + C^n} \tag{19.20}$$

which can also be represented as a change from the baseline.

$$E_0 - E = \frac{I_{max} * C^n}{IC_{50}^n + C^n} \tag{19.21}$$

The decrease in heart rate with β-adrenergic antagonists such as propranolol is an example of a case in which the use of an inhibitory I_{max} model can be used [9].

19.3.3 Linear Adaptations of the E_{max} and *I*max Model

Prior to the availability of computer software to perform nonlinear regression analysis, linear forms of the E_{max} model were useful. These models may still be of value in situations

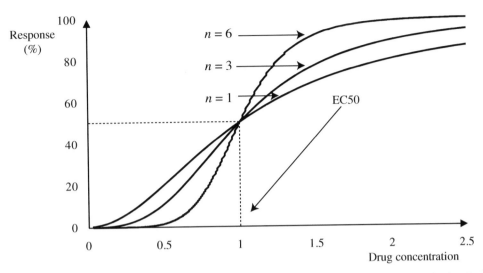

FIGURE 19.9 Effect of the slope factor n on the response–concentration relationship in the sigmoidal E_{max} model. It can be seen that as n increases, the slope of the response–concentration curve gets steeper.

where it may not be possible to approach the maximum effect of a drug, possibly because of toxicity. Without such data at the maximal effect, a simpler model often must be utilized. Two linearized versions of the E_{max} model exist: the linear model and the logarithmic model.

Linear Model Note in equation (19.15) that when $C \ll EC_{50}$, the denominator resolves to EC_{50}, which leads to the *linear model*, where there is a linear relationship between effect and concentration:

$$E = \frac{E_{max} \cdot C}{EC_{50}} \qquad (19.22)$$

or

$$E = a \cdot C \qquad (19.23)$$

where a is a proportionality constant equal to E_{max}/EC_{50}. This can be seen at low concentrations in Figure 19.10. The linear model holds in the range 0–20% maximum response. Similar approximations can be made when $C \ll IC_{50}$. The disadvantage of this model is that it predicts that the response will continue to increase indefinitely in a proportional manner as concentration increases. It does not reflect clinically observed responses at higher concentrations.

Logarithmic Model In the logarithmic model, response is expressed as a function of the logarithm of concentration. There is no mechanistic reason for this; it simply allows a greater range of concentrations to be plotted. However, in the response range 20–80%, a linear relationship exists between response and the logarithm of concentration (Figure 19.11).

$$E = a + b \cdot \log C \qquad (19.24)$$

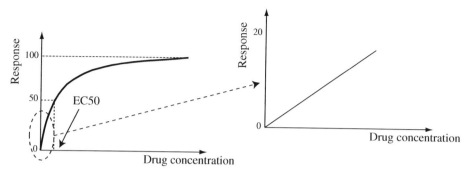

FIGURE 19.10   Linear model at concentrations producing less than 20% maximum response.

The logarithmic model suffers from several disadvantages. In common with the simple linear model, it predicts that the effect or extent of inhibition will rise indefinitely with increases in concentration. The logarithmic model cannot predict effects when the concentration is zero, and if the maximum response is not known, it is difficult to identify the lower (20%) and upper (80%) bounds of the model. Further, the logarithmic model is impaired by the inability to model a maximum effect as concentrations are increased. Because of these limitations, the E_{max}, sigmoidal E_{max}, or the corresponding I_{max} models are used when possible.

19.4   INTEGRATED PK–PD MODELS: INTRAVENOUS BOLUS INJECTION IN THE ONE-COMPARTMENT MODEL AND THE SIGMOIDAL E_{MAX} MODEL

To create a complete model of drug response, a pharmacokinetic model that describes the plasma concentration at any time after the administration of a dose of a drug must be linked to a pharmacodynamic model that describes the response produced by any given concentration at the site of action (Figure 19.12). A drug's pharmacokinetic parameters, such as

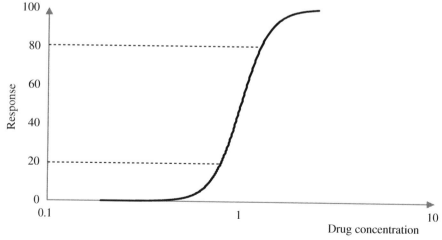

FIGURE 19.11   Log-linear model. A linear relationship between response and the logarithm of drug concentration exists in the region of 20–80% maximum response.

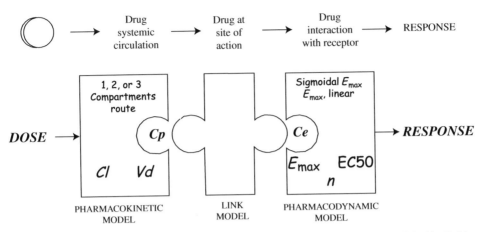

FIGURE 19.12 Modeling the complete dose–response relationship can be accomplished by linking a pharmacokinetic model to a pharmacodynamic model.

clearance and volume of distribution, determine the plasma concentration at any time after the dose. The pharmacodynamic parameters, such as E_{max} and EC_{50}, determine the response to any concentration at the site of action. When they are linked, the response at any time after a dose can be estimated. The simplest approach to linking the two models is to assume that the concentration at the site of action is always in equilibrium with the plasma concentration (Figure 19.13). As a result, the plasma concentration (Cp) can be used as the concentration that drives response:

$$E = \frac{E_{max} \cdot Cp}{EC_{50} + Cp}$$
(19.25)

Figure 19.14 shows the plasma concentration and response simulated when a model for an intravenous bolus injection is linked to an E_{max} model. Note that the units of time in Figure 19.14 are elimination half-lives and the units of concentration are EC_{50} equivalents. It can be seen that the initial plasma concentration falls by 50% in one unit of time, and falls an additional 50% over each subsequent unit of time. In contrast, the initial fall in response is much less steep. In one elimination half-life (one unit of time), the initial response falls by

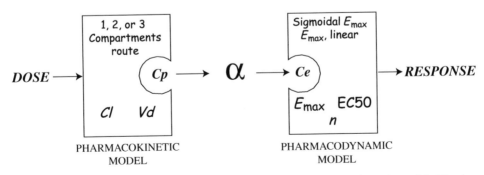

FIGURE 19.13 Direct link between the pharmacokinetic and pharmacodynamic models. The drug concentration at the site of action is assumed to be in equilibrium with the plasma at all times. This allows response in the pharmacodynamic model to be driven by the plasma concentration.

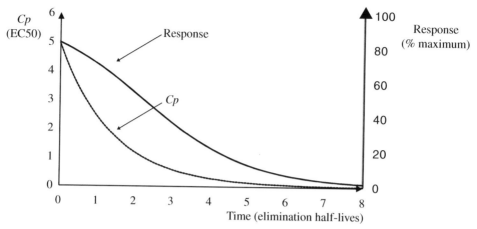

FIGURE 19.14   Graph illustrating the plasma concentration after an intravenous bolus dose E_{max} linked to an E_{max} pharmacokinetic model. Note that time has units of the drug's elimination half-life, and the units of concentration are multiples of the drug's EC_{50}.

only about 10%. The differing slopes of the fall in response and concentration are illustrated further in Figure 19.15, which shows plasma concentration and response over time after a low dose (10 units) (Figure 19.15a) and a high dose (1000 units) (Figure 19.15b). It can be seen that the initial plasma concentration from the high dose is 100 concentration units, or 100 times greater than the drug's EC_{50}. Under these conditions, a maximum response of 100% is obtained. The system is saturated and there is excess drug available to produce maximum response. As a result, even as drug is eliminated from the body, sufficient drug is still available to sustain the maximum response. When the drug concentration is much greater than the drug's EC_{50} (or when the response is around maximal response), the fall in response is much less steep than the fall in the plasma concentration, and response lingers. Under these conditions, it takes several elimination half-lives for the initial response to fall by 50% (Figure 19.15b). In contrast, a small dose that achieves an initial concentration

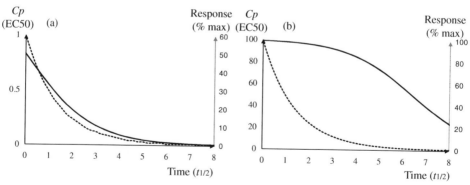

FIGURE 19.15   Graph of plasma concentration and corresponding E_{max} response model plotted against time after a small (a) and a large (b) dose. Note that time has units of the drug's elimination half-life, and the units of concentration are multiples of the drug's EC_{50}. After a small dose (a), the plasma concentrations (dashed line) approximate or are less than the drug's EC_{50}, and response (solid line) falls almost in parallel with plasma concentration. After larger doses (b) yielding plasma concentrations (dashed line) much larger than the EC_{50}, the fall in response (solid line) is much slower than the fall in the plasma concentration.

around EC_{50} produces around 50% maximal response, and the fall in response approximately parallels the fall in plasma concentration (Figure 19.15a). This phenomenon has several implications, among which is its impact on dosing regimen design. Drugs that are administered in doses that achieve plasma concentrations much larger than their EC_{50} values and which, as a result, produce responses approaching maximal can be administered using dosing frequencies much longer than their half-lives. For example, atenolol has a half-life of about 6 h but can be administered daily because it is used in doses that produce close to maximum response [10].

19.4.1 Simulation Exercise: http://web.uri.edu/pharmacy/research/rosenbaum/sims

Open model 19, Drug Response, Sigmoidal E_{max} Model, which can be found at http://web.uri.edu/pharmacy/research/rosenbaum/sims/Model19.

The model consists of a one-compartment model with intravenous input linked to a sigmoidal E_{max} model. The model is set up so that time is in units of elimination half-lives and concentration is in units of EC_{50}. The parameters have the following default values: $Vd = 10$ L, $Cl = 6.93$ L/$t_{1/2}$, $E_{max} = 100$, and $EC_{50} = 1$ EC_{50}; dose units are $EC_{50} \cdot L$.

1. *Explore the model and note the model summary.*
2. *Go to the "Cp and Response" page. Give a dose and observe that when $Cp = EC_{50}$, response is 50% maximum. Note that the fall in response does not parallel the fall in Cp. It takes one unit of time (one elimination $t_{1/2}$) for the initial Cp to fall by 50%. In the same period, response falls by only about 10%. Note that at 6 units of time, the response is about 20%, and it takes about one unit of time (one elimination half-life) for it to fall by 50%.*
3. *Go to the "Effect of Cp:EC_{50} Ratio" page. Give a dose of 10 units. Note that Cp takes one unit of time to fall by 50%, and during this time the response also falls by about 50%. When Cp is small compared to the EC_{50} ($Cp \ll EC_{50}$), the fall in response parallels the fall in Cp. Give a dose of 1000 units. Note that the initial Cp is 100 times greater than the EC_{50} and the initial response is maximal. In addition, during the first elimination half-life, Cp falls by 50% but response does not change. Under these circumstances, it takes about six elimination half-lives for the response to fall by 50%. When $Cp \gg EC_{50}$, the response is maximal or close to maximal. The system is saturated and there is an excess amount of drug at the site of action. Even after drug has been eliminated, there is still enough drug to elicit a large response. Under these circumstances, the fall in response is much slower than the fall in Cp. Drugs that are administered in doses that produce a close to maximal effect ($Cp \gg EC_{50}$) do not have to be administered every half-life to avoid wide changes in response. The dosing interval can be much greater than the half-life.*
4. *Observe the maximum response (R_{max}) from doses of 10, 100, and 1000 units. Note that R_{max} is not proportional to dose. The response concentration relationship is nonlinear.*
5. *Go to the "Effect of n" page. Without clearing the graph between doses, give doses using n values of 0.5, 1, 2, and 5. Note that as n increases, the steepness of the concentration–response curve increases. When n is large, small increases in the concentration can lead to large increases in response. Note that changes in n do not alter the EC_{50}.*

19.5 PHARMACODYNAMIC DRUG–DRUG INTERACTIONS

The concurrent use of more than one medication raises the potential of some form of drug–drug interaction (DDI). As discussed in Chapter 17, DDIs most commonly have a pharmacokinetic basis in which the perpetrator drug brings about changes in the activity of a protein, notably an enzyme or a transporter involved in the absorption, distribution, and/or elimination of the victim drug. This can result in changes in the concentration versus time profile of the victim drug (see Chapters 5 and 17) and an increase or decrease drug exposure, which can impact safety or efficacy.

Pharmacodynamic DDIs are also possible, and may exist concurrently with pharmacokinetic DDIs. For example, consider two drugs that both act as agonists at the same receptor and have similar affinity for the receptor, but have different intrinsic efficacies (ε). If both drugs are concurrently present at equal concentrations, the agonist with the lower ε will appear to antagonize the more potent agonist, since fewer receptors are occupied by the drug with the higher intrinsic efficacy [11].

Using an $E_{\max}$ model, this pharmacodynamic interaction can be modeled by the additive effect of the two drugs:

$$E = \frac{E_{\max A} \cdot C_A}{\mathrm{EC}_{50A} \left(1 + \frac{C_B}{\mathrm{EC}_{50B}}\right) + C_A} + \frac{E_{\max B} \cdot C_B}{\mathrm{EC}_{50B} \left(1 + \frac{C_A}{\mathrm{EC}_{50A}}\right) + C_B} \tag{19.26}$$

Here the subscripts A and B identify the two drugs and their corresponding EC50 and $E_{\max}$ values. This relationship is a general one for drugs that bind to the same receptor. When one drug has no activity when bound to the receptor, it is considered a pure antagonist. If Drug B is considered a pure antagonist when bound to the same receptor as Drug A, (19.26) collapses to

$$E = \frac{E_{\max A} \cdot C_A}{\mathrm{EC}_{50A} \left(1 + \frac{C_B}{\mathrm{EC}_{50B}}\right) + C_A} \tag{19.27}$$

It can be seen that if the pure antagonist Drug B is present at a concentration equal to EC_{50B}, it will double the EC_{50A}, the concentration of Drug A required to elicit 50% of $E_{\max}$. If a pure antagonist with a low EC50 is administered, the amount of agonist required to elicit the required response will increase dramatically. This is a desirable characteristic of reversal drugs such as naloxone for opioid toxicity that quickly raise the EC50 of the intoxicating drug above the concentrations that led to the toxicity.

19.5.1 Simulation Exercise:
http://web.uri.edu/pharmacy/research/rosenbaum/sims

Open model 20, Pharmacodynamic DDI, which can be found at http://web.uri.edu/ pharmacy/research/rosenbaum/sims/Model20.

The model consists of a one-compartment model with intravenous input for two drugs A and B acting at the same receptor. The model is set up so that time is in units of elimination half-lives and concentration is mg/L. Drug A is administered as an IV infusion with a loading dose such that steady state is achieved immediately. Drug B is given as in IV bolus. The default pharmacokinetic and pharmacodynamic parameters of drugs A and B are the *same and are as follows: $Vd = 10$ L, $Cl = 7$ $L/t_{1/2}$, $E_{maxA} = 100\%$, $E_{maxB} = 100\%$, $EC_{50A} = 10$ mg/L, $EC_{50B} = 10$ mg/L; dose units are mg.*

1. *Go to the "Simulation Page". Give an infusion of Drug A at 70 $mg/t_{1/2}$ (this will give a steady state Cp_A of 10 mg/L—the value of the EC50) but no Drug B and observe that, as expected, response is 50% of maximum.*

2. *Set the infusion of A to zero and give a dose of Drug B of 400 mg. This will give an initial Cp_B of 40 mg/L and will decay to 10 mg/L (EC50) after at 2 $t_{1/2}$, the unit of time. Observe when $t = 2$ $t_{1/2}$, $Cp_B = EC50$ and response is 50% of maximum.*

3. *Set the infusion of Drug A back to 70 $mg/t_{1/2}$, and maintain the dose of B at 400 mg. Note that the initial effect of adding the agonist Drug B is to increase the overall response, even though the contribution from Drug A is initially decreased by competition for the receptor. As Drug B is eliminated, its effect decreases, and that of Drug A increases back to its baseline. Now decrease the value of E_{maxB} from 100 to 25. Note how the overall effect of adding Drug B is to decrease the effect, since it is acting as an antagonist due to its lesser intrinsic efficacy relative to Drug A.*

4. *Clear the graphs and reset to the default EC50 values (10), and set E_{maxB} to 0 to establish it as a pure antagonist to Drug A, and increase the infusion rate of Drug A to 700 to simulate an inadvertent drug overdose. Note how the addition of the antagonist Drug B decreases the overall effect. Now decrease the EC50B from 10 to 1 to presume a higher affinity of the antagonist for the receptor. Note how the effect on Drug A is more dramatic, but how this decrease is temporary as the concentration of Drug B decreases after its bolus. In the clinic, it must be remembered that boluses of naloxone administered to reverse opioid toxicity will only have a temporary effect. In patients receiving extended release opioid formulations, patches, or methadone with its long elimination half-life, repeated doses or infusions of naloxone will be required to reverse opioid toxicity until the opioid concentrations decrease.*

PROBLEMS

19.1 The dosing regimen for nosolatol ($Cl = 12.6$ L/h, $Vd = 210$ L/70 kg, and $S = 1$) was calculated in Chapter 12 using pharmacokinetic principles. A dosing regimen of 200 mg every 12 h was selected based on a target average steady-state plasma concentration of 1.2 mg/L, a $t_{1/2}$ value of about 12 h, and the desire to have the plasma concentrations fall no more than about 50% in a dosing interval and stay between 750 and 1900 mg/L.

The pharmacodynamics of nosolatol have recently been studied. The response (reduction in exercise heart rate) and the plasma concentration were measured after several doses and the data fit to a one-compartment pharmacokinetic model linked to an E_{max} model. The values of nosolatol's pharmacokinetic parameters agreed well with previous estimates, and the estimated pharmacodynamic parameters of nosolatol were ($\pm$S.D.) $E_{max} = 30 \pm 3.2$ beats per minute (bpm) and $EC_{50} = 75 \pm 15$ μg/L. Ideally, the drug's effect should always be in the range of 28–22 bpm response (reduction in exercise heart rate). Assume that the drug is administered as a multiple IV bolus injections and that there is no hysteresis or delay in its effect. Use equation (19.20) to identify the desired peak and trough concentrations. Determine a dosing regimen to achieve the desired response profile.

REFERENCES

1. Peck, C. C., Barr, W. H., Benet, L. Z., Collins, J., Desjardins, R. E., Furst, D. E., Harter, J. G., Levy, G., Ludden, T., Rodman, J. H., Sanathanan, L., Schentag, J. J., Shah, V. P., Sheiner, L. B., Skelly, J. P., Stanski, D. R., Temple, R. J., Viswanathan, C. T., Weissinger, J., and Yacobi, A. (1994) Opportunities for integration of pharmacokinetics, pharmacodynamics, and toxicokinetics in rational drug development, *J Clin Pharmacol*, *34*, 111–119.

2. Danhof, M., de Jongh, J., De Lange, E. C., Della Pasqua, O., Ploeger, B. A., and Voskuyl, R. A. (2007) Mechanism-based pharmacokinetic–pharmacodynamic modeling: biophase distribution, receptor theory, and dynamical systems analysis, *Annu Rev Pharmacol Toxicol*, *47*, 357–400.

3. Mager, D. E., Woo, S., and Jusko, W. J. (2009) Scaling pharmacodynamics from *in vitro* and preclinical animal studies to humans, *Drug Metab Pharmacokinet*, *24*, 16–24.

4. Wallin, J. E., Friberg, L. E., and Karlsson, M. O. (2009) A tool for neutrophil guided dose adaptation in chemotherapy, *Comput Methods Programs Biomed*, *93*, 283–291.

5. Wagner, J. A. (2009) Biomarkers: principles, policies, and practice, *Clin Pharmacol Ther*, *86*, 3–7.

6. Clarke, W. P., and Bond, R. A. (1998) The elusive nature of intrinsic efficacy, *Trends Pharmacol Sci*, *19*, 270–276.

7. Wagner, J. G. (1968) Kinetics of pharmacologic response: I. Proposed relationships between response and drug concentration in the intact animal and man, *J Theor Biol*, *20*, 173–201.

8. Hill, A. (1910) The possible effects of the aggregation of the molecules of haemoglobin on its dissociation curves, *J Physiol*, *40*, IV–VII.

9. Lalonde, R. L., Straka, R. J., Pieper, J. A., Bottorff, M. B., and Mirvis, D. M. (1987) Propranolol pharmacodynamic modeling using unbound and total concentrations in healthy volunteers. *J Pharmacokinet Biopharm*, *15*, 569–582.

10. Tozer, T. N., and Rowland, M. R. (2006) *Introduction to Pharmacokinetics and Pharmacodynamics*, Lippincott Williams & Wilkins, Baltimore.

11. Ariens, E. J., and Simonis, A. M. (1964) A molecular basis for drug action: the interaction of one or more drugs with different receptors, *J Pharm Pharmacol*, *16*, 289–312.

20

SEMIMECHANISTIC PHARMACOKINETIC–PHARMACODYNAMIC MODELS

Drs. Diane Mould and Paul Hutson

Objectives

The material in this chapter will enable the reader to:

1. Understand the limitations of the simple sigmoidal E_{max} model to characterize a drug's pharmacodynamic properties and to summarize the time course of drug response

2. Appreciate the value of several examples of semimechanistic pharmacodynamic models

3. Identify the structure and characteristics of the semimechanistic pharmacodynamic models for indirect effects, transduction and transit compartments, tolerance, irreversible drug effects, and disease progression

20.1 INTRODUCTION

The sigmoidal E_{max} model is used extensively in clinical pharmacology and has proven to be valuable in modeling response data from a wide variety of drugs, including both agonists and antagonists. Models developed for individual drugs have provided a better understanding of the dose–response or exposure relationship, assisted in the determination of dose requirements, and helped identify situations where pharmacodynamics and dose requirements may be altered and thus dose adjustments are necessary. However, the model is essentially empirical and, as such, suffers from several disadvantages.

The sigmoidal E_{max} model can be used to link the steady-state response to exposure or can be used when the drug effect is directly related to drug concentration (such as with some

1. Simple PK-PD models

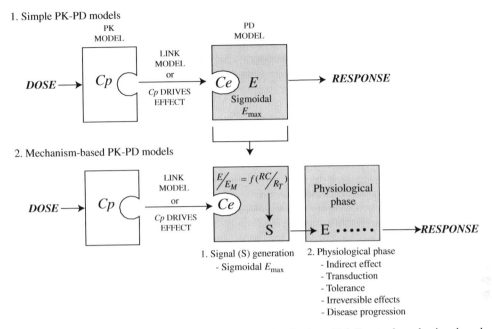

FIGURE 20.1 Diagrammatic representation of the simple sigmoidal E_{max} and mechanism-based pharmacodynamic models. S is the initial stimulus resulting from the drug receptor interaction, and E is the direct biological response.

antihypertensive agents). When used to link a steady-state response to exposure, however, the sigmoid E_{max} model effectively condenses the observed response into a single capacity-limited process driven by drug concentration or exposure. In this setting, consideration is not given to any of the events along the response chain (Figure 20.1). Although the assumptions are different, it can be considered to be equivalent to the intrinsic activity model (19.2.2.1). The sigmoid E_{max} model does not accommodate time delays between receptor activation and the emergence of the response. An effect compartment can be added to explain short delays, usually attributed to drug distribution, and is sometimes imposed empirically for disease progression models to account for the delay seen between initiating treatment and seeing a measurable response. However, in some situations, the mechanism of action of the drug may suggest that the delay in response has a pharmacodynamic, and not a pharmacokinetic basis. For example, the peak effect in response to a single dose of warfarin occurs at a time when most of a dose has already been eliminated from the body. This delay cannot be explained by a delay in the drug reaching its site of action, but rather that warfarin acts by inhibiting vitamin K epoxide reductase, an enzyme that recycles oxidized vitamin K1 to its reduced form following the carboxylation of several blood coagulation proteins, mainly prothrombin and factor VII. Thus, the mechanism of action of warfarin is not a direct effect on blood coagulation. Additionally, the sigmoidal E_{max} model cannot support the possibility of exposure-dependent changes in the concentration–response relationship, such as the development of tolerance.

Finally, the sigmoidal E_{max} model does not separate drug-specific (efficacy and affinity) and tissue-specific (receptor density) parameters. The drug-specific pharmacodynamic parameters have been found to be remarkably consistent among different species and from *in vitro* studies [1]. Thus, if a pharmacokinetic–pharmacodynamic (PK–PD) model for drug response *in vivo* separated the drug- and tissue-specific parameters, it would be possible to estimate drug response in humans based on parameters found in laboratory animals or *in vitro*. This translational research could have a major impact on drug development. It could allow drug candidates with the greatest chance of success to be identified early during development and could help to optimize the design of clinical trials, which could decrease both the cost and time of drug development. The sigmoidal E_{max} parameters are usually dependent on both the drug and the system in which they were determined. As a result, this model has limited applications in translational research.

The shortcomings of the sigmoidal E_{max} model have been addressed through the development of a range of semimechanistic pharmacodynamic models that incorporate additional steps in the chain of events between receptor activation and the emergence of the response [1–3] or allow for a delay between exposure and response. A description of some of these models is presented below.

20.2 HYSTERESIS AND THE EFFECT COMPARTMENT

Measured drug concentration from the blood, plasma, or serum is generally used to drive response in pharmacodynamic models because it is the concentration that can be measured easily. If a simple direct effect E_{max} model is applied, this approach is justified as long as the drug concentration at the site of action is in equilibrium with the plasma. However, when these two concentrations are not in equilibrium, strange response–concentration profiles can be observed. These unusual effects must be understood and addressed before pharmacodynamic modeling can be conducted.

Frequently, in clinical pharmacodynamic studies, a plot of drug response versus plasma concentration appears as a counterclockwise circular path such as the profile shown in Figure 20.2. For comparison, the figure also shows the relationship that would be expected based on the E_{max} model. This phenomenon is called *hysteresis*, a word derived from a Greek word meaning to be behind or to be late. It occurs when there is a time lag between the rise and fall of plasma concentration and the rise and fall in response.

Hysteresis can have several different causes, including indirect drug effects and a long transduction process. But a simple and common cause is a slow distribution of a drug to its site of action. The phenomenon may be understood by recognizing, first, that it is the drug at the site of action, not that in the plasma, which drives the response. Second, it is important to appreciate that distribution of the drug from the plasma to the site of action may be slow and that the peak concentration at the site may occur later than that in the plasma. Figure 20.2b shows the drug concentration–time profile for the plasma and the drug's site of action when distribution is slow. The overall curve has been split into three phases. It can be seen that the peak plasma concentration (solid line) occurs earlier than the peak at the site of action. In the initial period after drug administration (phase 1), there is a slow distribution of the drug to the site: The concentration at the site of action increases and the response increases. During this phase, the plasma concentration is also increasing. Eventually, the plasma reaches its peak concentration, and in phase 2 the plasma concentration falls. During this phase, the concentration at the site continues to increase, and as a result so does the response. Thus, it is in this area (plasma concentration falling and response increasing) that the plot of response against the plasma concentration begins to move in a counterclockwise pattern. This pattern continues until the concentration at the site of action begins to fall (Figure 20.2, area 3). In phase 3, the concentration at the site, the concentration in the plasma, and the effect all decrease. Note that hysteresis would be eliminated if the response

(a)

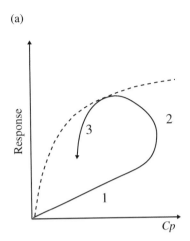

(b)

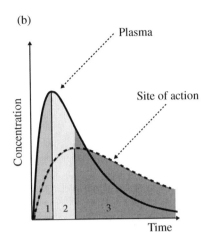

FIGURE 20.2 Hysteresis due to a distributional delay. Panel (a) shows response plotted as a function of plasma concentration (solid line). Also shown is the expected response–plasma concentration relationship (dashed line). Panel (b) shows the drug concentrations in the plasma (solid line) and at the site of action (dashed line) as a function of time after a dose. As a result of slow distribution, the peak concentration at the site of action occurs later than the peak plasma concentration. It is important to appreciate that the response is driven by the drug concentration at the site of action, not that in the plasma. Note in area 1 of part (b) that the plasma concentration and the concentration at the site of action both increase. Because of the latter, the effect increases. In area 2, the concentration at the site continues to increase; thus, the effect increases, but the plasma concentration is decreasing. It is at this point that the curve of response against Cp begins to move in a counterclockwise direction [panel (a)]. Eventually, the concentration at the site of action decreases. As a result, response decreases (area 3).

was plotted as a function of the drug concentration at the site of action rather than in the plasma. Hysteresis is discussed further and illustrated in simulation model 21 (see Simulation Model, Section 20.2.1).

The distributional delay to the site of action can be accommodated using a hypothetical "effect compartment" to link the pharmacokinetic and pharmacodynamic models [4] (Figure 20.3). The effect compartment represents the site of action or biophase, and it is attached to the central compartment of multicompartment models (Figure 20.4). Drug distribution to and redistribution from the compartment are modeled as first-order processes. The rate of change of the drug concentration in the effect compartment may be expressed as:

$$\frac{dCe}{dt} = Cp \cdot k_{1e} - Ce \cdot k_{e0} \tag{20.1}$$

where Ce is the concentration of drug in the effect compartment or the concentration at the site of action, Cp is the plasma concentration, and k_{1e} and k_{e0} are the first-order rate constants for distribution into and out of the effect compartment, respectively.

The amount of drug that distributes to the site of action is assumed to be very small. As a result, drug redistributing from the effect compartment is not returned to the system but is assumed to be lost (Figure 20.4). This simplifies the pharmacokinetics of the drug.

The prominence of hysteresis and the amount of delay in the response is determined by the time it takes for the effect site to equilibrate with the plasma. Just as a drug's elimination rate constant or elimination half-life controls the time to reach steady state during

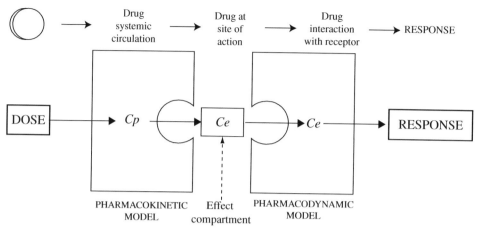

FIGURE 20.3 An effect compartment is used to link the pharmacokinetic and pharmacodynamic models when there is a delay in drug reaching the site of action.

an infusion or any other type of chronic drug administration, k_{e0} controls the time it takes the effect compartment to equilibrate with the plasma. Thus, minimal hysteresis is associated with large k_{e0} values, and significant hysteresis is associated with small k_{e0} values. Since redistribution or loss of drug from the site is a first-order process, the k_{e0} half-life $(0.693/k_{e0})$ can be used to estimate the time it takes for drug distribution to be complete $(3–5t_{1/2,ke_0})$. Once distribution to the site is complete, the ratio of the concentration of drug in the plasma and the site of action will be fairly constant and the concentrations will generally parallel each other. At this time, a normal relationship between response and the plasma concentration will be observed. Thus, hysteresis is not observed when plasma concentrations and concentrations at the site of action are at steady state but is only observed in nonsteady-state conditions, such as the period after initial drug administration.

The value of the k_{e0} can be estimated from the hysteresis curve and the time course of drug response. It is not possible to estimate k_{1e}, and as a result it is not possible to estimate drug concentrations at the site of action. The value of k_{1e} is usually assumed to be equal to

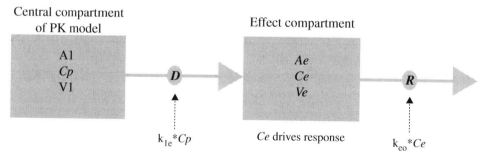

FIGURE 20.4 The effect compartment is linked to the central compartment of the pharmacokinetic model. The distribution (D) and redistribution (R) of the drug to and from the effect compartment are first-order processes with rate constants of k_{1e} and k_{e0}, respectively. The amount of drug that distributes to the effect compartment is assumed to be so small that rather than returning it to the system, it can be assumed to be lost from the system. A, C, and V represent the amount, concentration, and volume, respectively, and 1 and e signify the central and effect compartments, respectively.

k_{e0}, and as a result, after distribution has gone to completion, Ce will be equal to Cp. As a result, when the effect compartment is linked to an E_{max} model, the value of the EC_{50} will be expressed in terms of the plasma concentration. Examples of drugs whose effects have been modeled using the effect compartment include d-tubocurarine (muscle paralysis), digoxin (left ventricular ejection time shortening), disopyramide (QT prolongation), and fentanyl (respiratory depression) [5].

20.2.1 Simulation Exercise:
http://web.uri.edu/pharmacy/research/rosenbaum/sims

Open model 21, Effect Compartment, which can be found at http://web.uri.edu/pharmacy/research/rosenbaum/sims/Model21.

The model is a one-compartment model with first-order absorption linked through an effect compartment to an E_{max} model. The default model parameters are Vd = 20 L, Cl = 4 L/h (this results in k and $t_{1/2}$ of 0.2 h^{-1} and 3.5 h, respectively), F = 1, k_a = 1 h^{-1}, E_{max} = 100, EC_{50} = 1 mg/L, k_{e0} = 0.5 h^{-1}, and dose = 20 mg.

1. *Explore the model and review the model summary.*

2. *Review the video.*

3. *Go to the "Effect of k_{eo}" page. The graph on the left shows the values of Cp and Ce after each simulation. The graph on the right shows the response after each simulation. The graph on the right will not be cleared after a simulation, so the response from different simulation runs can be compared. Give doses using values of k_{e0} of 0.5, 1, 2, and 4 h^{-1}. Note that as k_{e0} increases, the time lag between the rise and fall of Cp and that of Ce decreases. Note that the delay in response also decreases. It can also be seen that changes in the value of k_{e0} influence the duration of action. If the response must be greater than 20% to be therapeutic, the onset of action would increase and the duration of action would decrease as k_{e0} increased. Comparing k_{e0} values of 0.5 and 4 h^{-1}, the onset of action would decrease from around 1.5 to 0.5 h, and the duration of action would decrease from around 8.8 to 7.6 h, respectively.*

4. *Go to the "Effect of Dose" page. Give doses of 20, 50, 100, and 200 mg and observe how R_{max} (the maximum response) and T_{max} (the time of maximum response) are influenced by dose. Note that the relationship between response and dose is not linear. Increases in dose result in less than proportional increases in response. Eventually, when a peak plasma concentration produces the maximum response (E_{max}), further increases in dose will not produce larger responses. Note that T_{max} is the same for each dose. This is an important feature of hysteresis produced by distributional delays that distinguishes it from other causes of hysteresis and delays in response.*

20.3 PHYSIOLOGICAL TURNOVER MODELS
AND THEIR CHARACTERISTICS

The direct action of a drug can be modeled using the sigmoidal E_{max} model, any of its derived models (E_{max} and linear models), or the operational model of agonism. Mechanism-based PK–PD models address the events that occur along the response chain subsequent to the receptor activation and the generation of the initial stimulus (Figure 20.1). For example, models have been developed to address long transduction processes, the

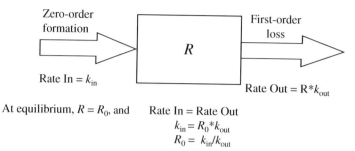

$$k_{in} = R_0 \cdot k_{out}$$
$$R_0 = k_{in}/k_{out}$$

FIGURE 20.5   Turnover model for the formation and loss of a biological factor or response variable (R). Its formation is assumed to be a zero-order process (k_{in}), and loss is assumed to be first order with a rate constant of k_{out}.

development of tolerance, indirect drug effects, irreversible drug effects, and the impact of drugs on an underlying disease that changes over time (disease progression models). A variety of different models have been developed to address these issues, and many incorporate a physiological turnover model for the synthesis and degradation of a biological quantity or factor (Figure 20.5). These turnover models were first introduced into pharmacodynamics as the so-called "indirect effect models" [7–11] and have subsequently been incorporated or reparameterized into other models in diverse and creative ways. In pharmacodynamic models, the biological response (R) that is being produced in the turnover model is an entity that is usually involved in mediating either the disease mechanism or impacts on clinical response. As a result, R is often referred to as the response variable. In models, R has been a variety of different things, including the amount or concentration of an endogenous compound, an enzyme, white blood cells, red blood cells, platelets, and gastric acid secretion. The formation of the biological quantity R is assumed to be a zero-order process with a rate constant often referred to as k_{in}. Loss or degradation of R is assumed to be a first-order process with a rate constant referred to as k_{out}.

The physiological system for the production and degradation of the biological factor is shown in Figure 19.15. The assumptions and characteristics of the system are as follows:

- It is assumed that the precursor for the biological factor is not depleted. As a result, it is assumed to be formed by a constant continuous (zero order) process: rate = k_{in}.
- The response R is assumed to be degraded or removed by a first-order process, the rate of which is dependent on the value of R and a first-order rate constant k_{out}.
- The rate of change of R with time is given by

$$\frac{dR}{dt} = k_{in} - k_{out} \cdot R \tag{20.2}$$

where R is a biological response, k_{in} is a zero-order rate constant for the formation of R, and k_{out} is a first-order rate constant for the loss of R.

- Under normal circumstances, the system is stationary and at equilibrium. The biological factor (R) will be constant and has a baseline level of R_0. At baseline, the rate of production is equal to the rate of degradation multiplied by the baseline response

$$k_{in} = R_0 \cdot k_{out} \tag{20.3}$$

Rearranging yields

$$R_0 = \frac{k_{in}}{k_{out}} \tag{20.4}$$

20.3.1 Points of Drug Action

External factors such as drugs, concomitant medications or treatments, and/or disease can interfere with the physiological system through actions on k_{in} and/or k_{out}, or by effecting R. These actions would destroy the equilibrium and produce changes in R. An inhibition of k_{in}, a stimulation of k_{out}, or direct destruction of the biological factor would all result in a decrease in its value. In contrast, stimulation of k_{in} or inhibition of k_{out} would increase the value of the biological factor.

20.3.2 System Recovery After Change in Baseline Value

Assuming that the action of the external influence is transient, once the influence is removed, the system would return to equilibrium and its previous baseline level. Figure 20.6

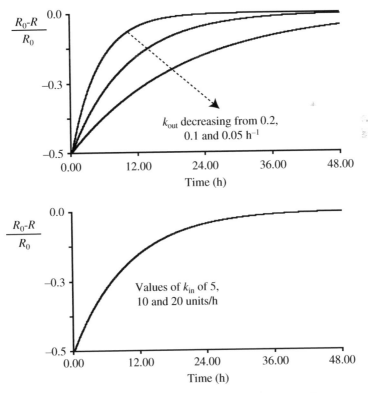

FIGURE 20.6   Influence of the values of the rate constants on the time it takes a system to restore equilibrium when the baseline is reduced by 50%. Values of k_{out} of 0.05, 0.1, and 0.2 h^{-1} were used, and k_{in} was set to 10 units/h. Values of k_{in} of 5, 10, and 20 units/h were used, and k_{out} was fixed at 0.1 h^{-1}. Response is fractional change from baseline.

shows how the values of k_{in} and k_{out} influence the return to baseline after an external influence reduced the response variable to 50% of its normal baseline value. It can be seen that the time for the system to restore equilibrium is dependent on k_{out} and independent of k_{in}. Since the loss of the biological response is a first-order process, it takes about four degradation (k_{out}) half-lives for equilibrium to be restored (Appendix B). The system is analogous to the kinetics of an intravenous infusion, where the time to steady state is dependent on a drug's elimination half-life and independent of the infusion rate and the value of the steady-state plasma concentration. In common with the infusion model, the time it takes for the system to restore equilibrium is also independent of the magnitude of the initial change. Thus, if the baseline is disrupted by 20%, 50%, or 70%, it will still take four degradation (k_{out}) half-lives for equilibrium to be restored.

In summary:

- The time it takes the system to restore the usual baseline level is dependent on the value of k_{out}. As a first-order process, it will take 3–5 k_{out} half-lives for the system to return to baseline.
- The time it takes the system to restore the usual baseline level is independent of the value of k_{in}.
- The time it takes the system to restore the usual baseline level is independent of the magnitude of the change from baseline.

20.4 INDIRECT EFFECT MODELS

20.4.1 Introduction

The product of a physiological system such as the one discussed above may be a natural ligand (R) that is directly responsible for a physiological response. For example, R could be gastric acid production, a substance that clots blood, or a low-density lipoprotein. A drug could exert its action by affecting the concentration of R. It could reduce R either by inhibiting its formation or by stimulating its degradation. Alternatively, it could increase R by either stimulating its production or inhibiting its degradation. Such drugs are said to *act indirectly*. Warfarin is an example of a drug that acts indirectly. Warfarin is used therapeutically to inhibit the clotting of blood, but it does not have any direct effect on this process. Instead, it inhibits the synthesis of clotting factors that play an integral part in the clotting of blood, and it is the concentration of these clotting factors (response variables) that is directly related to the action of warfarin.

Pharmacodynamic models for drugs that act indirectly need to incorporate, in addition to the model for the drug's direct action (e.g., E_{max} model), the physiological turnover system described above. The four potential ways that drugs can interfere with the physiological turnover models [inhibition or stimulation of either k_{in} or k_{out} (Figure 20.7)] give rise to four basic indirect models that are consistently numbered Models I–IV [7]:

- Inhibition of k_{in}:   Model I
- Inhibition of k_{out}:   Model II
- Stimulation of k_{in}:   Model III
- Stimulation of k_{out}:   Model IV

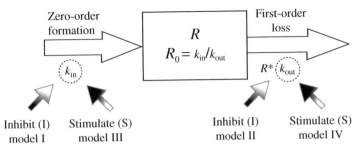

FIGURE 20.7   Four indirect effect models. Drugs could inhibit k_{in} or k_{out} (models I and II, respectively) or stimulate k_{in} or k_{out} (models III and IV, respectively).

The direct action of a drug on the physiological system is usually modeled using the E_{max} or sigmoidal E_{max} model. To differentiate the four models, the "effect" is categorized as either stimulation (S) or inhibition (I), and it is measured as the fractional change in the rate constant affected. Thus, the stimulatory (S) or inhibitory (I) effect of 0.3 would mean a 30% increase or a 30% decrease, respectively, in the rate constant affected. The equations for the direct effect of the drug are

$$I = \frac{I_{max} \cdot Cp}{IC_{50} + Cp} \tag{20.5}$$

$$S = \frac{S_{max} \cdot Cp}{SC_{50} + Cp} \tag{20.6}$$

where I and S represent the fractional change in the rate constant, I_{max} is the maximal possible fraction inhibition that a drug can produce [(I_{max} can vary between zero (no inhibition) and 1 (complete inhibition)], IC_{50} is the drug concentration that produces 50% of I_{max}, S_{max} is the maximal fraction stimulation that a drug can produce (S_{max} can be any number greater than zero), and SC_{50} is the drug concentration that produces 50% of S_{max}. Cp is the plasma concentration, which is assumed to drive the direct effect.

The action of the drug on k_{in} or k_{out} is then incorporated into the differential equation for the physiological model [equation (20.2)]. For example, for model I, the inhibition of k_{in}, the inhibitory action of the drug, would be incorporated as follows:

$$\frac{dR}{dt} = k_{in}(1 - I) - k_{out} \cdot R \tag{20.7}$$

Substituting I from equation (20.5) into equation (20.7), we have

$$\frac{dR}{dt} = k_{in} \left(1 - \frac{I_{max} \cdot Cp}{IC_{50} + Cp} \right) - k_{out} \cdot R \tag{20.8}$$

The equations for all four indirect effect models are shown in Figure 20.8. It is not possible to solve the differential equations to obtain explicit solutions. As a result, simulations are extremely useful in understanding the characteristics of indirect effect models.

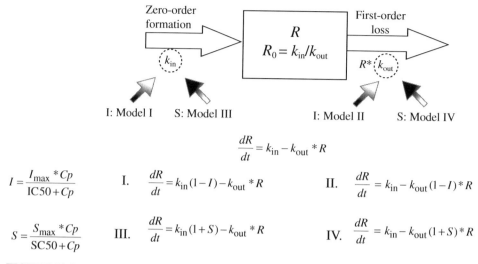

$$\frac{dR}{dt} = k_{in} - k_{out} * R$$

$$I = \frac{I_{max} * Cp}{IC50 + Cp}$$

I. $\quad \frac{dR}{dt} = k_{in}(1 - I) - k_{out} * R$

II. $\quad \frac{dR}{dt} = k_{in} - k_{out}(1 - I) * R$

$$S = \frac{S_{max} * Cp}{SC50 + Cp}$$

III. $\quad \frac{dR}{dt} = k_{in}(1 + S) - k_{out} * R$

IV. $\quad \frac{dR}{dt} = k_{in} - k_{out}(1 + S) * R$

FIGURE 20.8 Equations for the four indirect models. The rate of change of the response variable (R) with time is equal to the rate in minus the rate out. The direct effect of the drug to either inhibit (I) or stimulate (S) k_{in} or k_{out} is modeled using the E_{max} model. The direct effect is expressed in terms of the fraction decrease (inhibition) or increase (stimulation) in the rate constant affected.

20.4.2 Characteristics of Indirect Effect Drug Responses

Indirect effect models have been used extensively to model the response of a variety of drugs, including the action of warfarin on the synthesis of clotting factors; the inhibitory action of H_2-blockers on acid secretion; the inhibition of water reabsorption by furosemide, bronchodilation produced by β_2-agonists; and the action of terbutaline in reducing potassium concentrations [11].

In two of the four models, the drug reduces the response variable (inhibition of k_{in} and stimulation of k_{out}), while in the other two models the drug increases the response variable above its baseline (stimulation of k_{in} and inhibition of k_{out}). Figure 20.9 shows the typical response profiles from the four indirect effect models at three dose levels. The data were simulated by connecting a one-compartment model with intravenous bolus input to each of the four indirect effect models. Two special characteristics of these models are clearly visible in Figure 20.9. First, the response is delayed relative to the plasma concentration (with an intravenous injection, the peak plasma concentration occurs at time zero). Second, although, as expected, the maximum response (R_m) increases with dose, unusually, the time of the maximum response (T_{R_M}) also increases with dose.

The four models share many characteristics and some have their own unique features. A detailed discussion of the properties of the models, the selection of an appropriate model for a specific drug effect, and the estimation of model parameters are beyond the scope of this discussion but can be found in the literature [8–10]. The discussion below will provide a general description of the models, with particular emphasis on how the model parameters affect the time course of drug response (the onset, magnitude, and duration) and how this affects the design of dosing regimens. The discussion is presented using model I, the inhibition of k_{in}, as the example. Interactive simulation models of all four indirect models are provided to allow readers to evaluate the characteristics of all the indirect effect models.

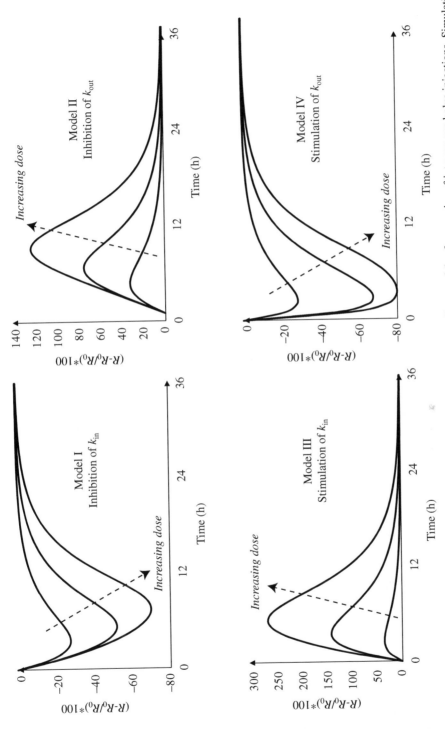

FIGURE 20.9 Response (percent change from baseline) profiles of the four indirect effect models after a series of intravenous bolus injections. Simulations were performed using doses of 10, 100, and 1000 mg in each of the four models. The models had the following parameters: $Vd = 20$ L, $k = 0.7$ h^{-1}, $k_{in} = 10$ units/h, $k_{out} = 0.2$ h^{-1} (models I and II), I_{max} (models I and II) = 1, S_{max} (models III and IV) = 5, IC$_{50}$ (models I and II) = 0.1 mg/L, and SC$_{50}$ (models III and IV) = 1 mg/L.

20.4.3   Characteristics of Indirect Effect Models Illustrated Using Model I

In the indirect effect model I, the drug inhibits the zero-order rate constant (k_{in}) for the production of the response variable. This model has been applied to the action of warfarin, which is used widely to increase the clotting time of blood in patients who are susceptible to blood clots and at risk for strokes. Warfarin exerts its action by inhibiting the synthesis of clotting factors that are involved in the clotting process. Indirect effect model I results in a decrease in the value of the response variable according to the equation

$$\frac{dR}{dt} = k_{in} \left(1 - \frac{I_{max} \cdot Cp}{IC_{50} + Cp} \right) - k_{out} \cdot R \tag{20.9}$$

If high concentrations of the drug are able to inhibit k_{in} completely, $I_{max} = 1$ and the parameter can be removed from the numerator. Initially, when no drug is present, the response is at its equilibrium baseline value (k_{in}/k_{out}) (see Figure 19.15). After an intravenous dose, assuming no distributional delays, the drug will immediately inhibit k_{in}, and the synthesis of the response variable will fall. Translation of the drug action into a decrease in the response variable itself will depend on the time it takes for the existing response variable to be removed, which will depend on the value of k_{out}.

The characteristics of the model will be demonstrated using simulations. A one-compartment model with intravenous bolus input was combined with the indirect effect model. The simulations were carried out using the following default parameter values: dose = 100 mg, $k = 0.7$ h^{-1}, $Vd = 20$ L, $IC_{50} = 0.1$ mg/L, $I_{max} = 1$, $k_{in} = 10$ units/h, and $k_{out} = 0.2$ h^{-1}. Note that for these simulations, $k > k_{out}$; the loss of the response variable is rate limiting (the drug's elimination half-life is shorter than the half-life for the turnover of the response variable). The model used to simulate these figures may be found at http://web.uri.edu/pharmacy/research/rosenbaum/sims/Model22.

20.4.3.1   Time Course of Response
Note that for clarity, the elimination half-life of the drug has been set to 1 h. The time course of the response can be observed in Figure 20.10; the plasma concentration (dashed line) is

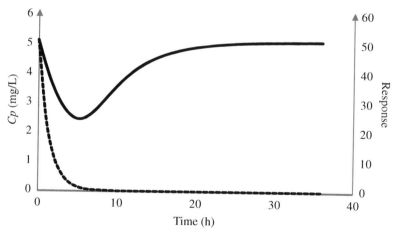

FIGURE 20.10   Plasma concentration (dashed line) and response (solid line) after an intravenous bolus injection (100 mg). Simulations were carried out using parameter values for model I given in the legend of Figure 20.5.

at its peak at time zero, but the maximum response does not occur until about 5 h (five elimination half-lives). At this time, the drug has been almost completely removed from the body. For drugs with indirect action, the time course of the drug action extends beyond the drug's presence in the body. In this example, it takes about 16 h (16 drug elimination half-lives) for the baseline to return to about 90% of its original value. Recall from Section 20.3.2 that once the external force is removed, it takes about four k_{out} half-lives for the system to be restored to equilibrium. In this example, the $t_{1/2}$ of k_{out} is 3.5 h.

20.4.3.2 Effect of Dose

It was shown previously (Figure 20.9) that as the value of the dose increases, the response increases. Note, however, that the dose–response relationship is nonlinear. In model I, a dose of 10 produces a maximum response (R_m) of about a 25% change from baseline, a dose of 100 produces an R_m of about a 50% change from baseline, and a dose of 1000 mg produces an R_m of about a 70% change from baseline. Also note that the time for the maximum response (T_{R_M}) increases with dose. This is a characteristic of these models and can be used to distinguish delays in response caused by indirect effects from delays caused by a slow distribution of the drug to its site of action. Recall that in the effect compartment model, the time for the maximum response remains constant with dose (see Section 20.2). The time of the maximum effect in the indirect models increases with dose because larger doses produce greater saturation of the system (e.g., receptors) and, as a result, the duration of the direct action of the drug is longer, as was seen with direct effect models in Chapter 19. Because k_{in} is inhibited for a longer period at higher doses, the peak or maximum response occurs later. Thus, the duration of action increases with dose.

20.4.3.3 Maximum Response and Maximum Achievable Response of a Drug

At the peak response (R_m), the rate of production of the response variable equals the rate of removal, and the rate of change of R with time is momentarily zero:

$$\frac{dR}{dt} = 0 \tag{20.10}$$

Substituting into (20.19) and rearranging gives us

$$R_m = \frac{k_{in}}{k_{out}} \left(1 - \frac{I_{max} \cdot Cp}{IC_{50} + Cp} \right) \tag{20.11}$$

Substituting for k_{in}/k_{out} according to equation (20.4) yields

$$R_m = R_0 \left(1 - \frac{I_{max} \cdot Cp}{IC_{50} + Cp} \right) \tag{20.12}$$

As the dose increases, the drug's effect (I) approaches I_{max} and R_m approaches the maximum effect the drug can achieve (R_{max}), since $Cp \gg IC_{50}$, $IC_{50} + Cp \approx Cp$ and:

$$R_{max} = R_0(1 - I_{max}) \tag{20.13}$$

If a drug has the maximum possible value of I_{max} (1), R_{max} tends to zero and the response expressed as the percentage change from baseline tends to 100%. Thus, the maximum response possible in model I is zero.

20.4.3.4 Influence of Physiological System Parameters

When the physiological turnover system was studied in isolation earlier in the chapter, it was shown that the time for complete recovery of the system after its equilibrium has been disturbed, is dependent on k_{out}, and independent of k_{in}. The independence of recovery on k_{in} for the indirect effect model is shown in Figure 20.11a, which shows the time course of the therapeutic response (expressed as a percentage change from baseline) at three values of k_{in}. The influence of k_{out} on the system is shown in Figure 20.11b. Note that k_{out} controls both the onset of action and the recovery of the system. The larger the value of k_{out}, the faster the onset, the shorter and the faster the recovery. This has important implications for dosing regimen design. Small values of k_{out} will result in a long duration of action and will enable the drug to be administered less frequently. When the k_{out} is 0.05 h^{-1} (k_{out} $t_{1/2} = 14$ h), the action of the drug persists for over 36 h. Thus, this drug could easily be administered daily, even though it has an elimination half-life of 1 h.

Figure 20.11c shows the influence of k_{out} in a system where $k_{out} > k$ (elimination is rate controlling). Note that the time scale of this plot has been expanded to 72 h. Under these circumstances ($k < k_{out}$), k_{out} has little influence on the duration of action. Elimination is a rate-limiting process and it controls the duration of action. The dosing interval of the drug would then be based on the pharmacokinetic, not the pharmacodynamic characteristics of the drug.

The initial values of k_{in} and k_{out} determine the baseline value of the biological variable. As a result, when the initial value of either parameter is altered, the baseline and the absolute change in R will be affected (Figure 20.12). It can be seen that smaller values of k_{in} are associated with lower baseline values of R. The response curve is shifted downward and the maximum response is greater, but recall from Figure 20.12a that the relative change in R is the same for all values of k_{in}. It can be seen that as the initial value of k_{out} increases, the baseline decreases and the response curve is shifted downward. A given dose produces a larger maximum response, which occurs earlier (recall from Figure 20.12b that larger initial values of k_{out} also produce larger relative responses). The smaller the value of k_{out}, the longer it takes to return to baseline.

20.4.3.5 Influence of Pharmacokinetics: Elimination Rate Constant

The elimination rate constant is a measure of the rate of drug elimination. It can be seen (Figure 20.11d) that slower elimination (smaller values of the elimination rate constant) results in increased maximum responses, an increase in T_{R_M}, and a more prolonged duration of action of the drug. Slower elimination results in a more prolonged inhibition of k_{in}, which will result in a more profound, longer lasting therapeutic effect. The value of k does not affect the onset of response (the initial slope).

20.4.3.6 Pharmacodynamic Parameters of the Drug: Effect of IC_{50} and I_{max}

Variability in IC_{50} is essentially the same as variability in the dose. A decrease in the value of IC_{50} (the potency of the drug increases) is equivalent to an increase in the dose. Thus, when IC_{50} decreases, the response and the time for maximum response increase (Figure 20.13a). In contrast, as the I_{max} value increases, the response increases but the time for maximum response remains the same (Figure 20.13b). Note that variability in I_{max} produces proportional changes in R_m.

20.4.3.7 Time to Steady State During an Intravenous Infusion

The time to steady-state response during a constant, continuous intravenous infusion is shown in Figure 20.14. Figure 20.14a shows the response over time for model I and, for

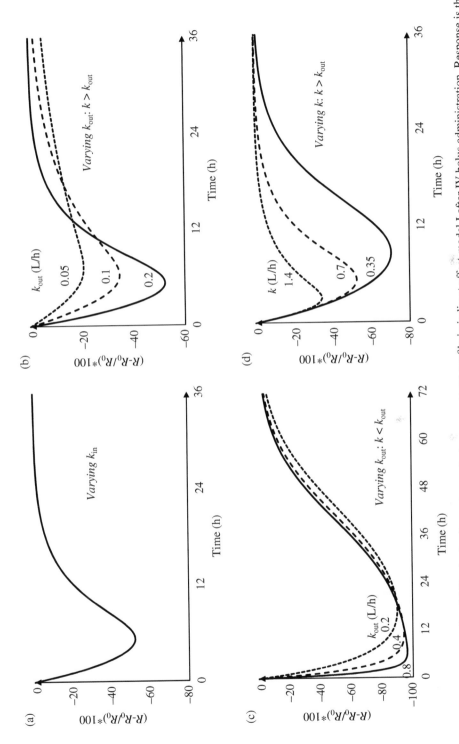

FIGURE 20.11 Effect of variability in the three rate constants on a response profile in indirect effect model I after IV bolus administration. Response is the percent change from baseline. In part (a), k_{in} was varied (5, 10, and 20 units/h); in part (b), k_{out} was varied (0.05, 0.1, and 0.3 h^{-1}), with k at its default value (0.7 h^{-1}); in part (c), k_{out} was varied (0.2, 0.4, and 0.8 h^{-1}) with k set to 0.1 h^{-1}; and in part (d), k was varied (0.35, 0.7, and 1.4 h^{-1}). The dose was set to 100 mg. Unless otherwise stated, all other parameters were set to the default values given in the legend of Figure 20.10.

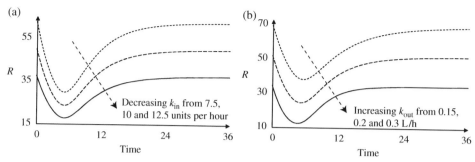

FIGURE 20.12 Effect of changes in k_{in} and k_{out} on the absolute value of the response variable (R). The values of the rate constants that were varied are given in the figure. All other parameter values were set to their default values given in the legend of Figure 20.10.

comparison, Figure 20.14b shows the response for model IV (stimulation of k_{out}), which also produces a reduction in the response variable below baseline. Note that for model I (Figure 20.14a), the time to steady-state response is about the same for the various infusion rates, and it is approximately 24 h. In contrast, the time to steady-state response in model IV decreases as the infusion rate increases (Figure 20.14b). This is because the value of k_{out} controls the time to steady-state response. In model I, k_{out} does not vary with dose; it is constant (0.2 h^{-1}, k_{out} $t_{1/2} = 3.5$ h), and by about seven k_{out} half-lives (24.5 h), the response is at steady state. In contrast, k_{out} is the subject of the drug's action in model IV. Larger infusion rates will produce larger stimulations of k_{out}, and as a result (k_{out} $t_{1/2}$ decreases), it will take less time to reach steady state. If these data are available, the time to steady-state response from different infusion rates can be used to distinguish models I and IV. Simulations using the other indirect effect models will demonstrate that the time to steady state is constant for model III (stimulation of k_{in}) but varies with the infusion rate for model II. Specifically, for model II (inhibition of k_{out}), as the infusion rate increases, a greater inhibition of k_{out} is observed and the time to steady-state response increases.

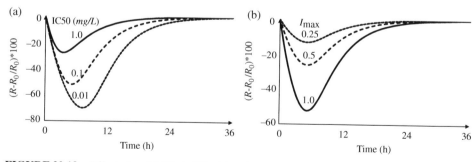

FIGURE 20.13 Effect of variability in IC$_{50}$ (a) and I_{max} (b) on the response profile of indirect effect model I after IV bolus administration. Response (percent change from baseline) was simulated using values of IC$_{50}$ of 0.01, 0.1, and 1 mg/L (a) and values of I_{max} of 0.25, 0.5, and 1 (b). A dose of 100 mg was used, and unless otherwise stated, all other parameters were set to the default values given in the legend of Figure 20.10.

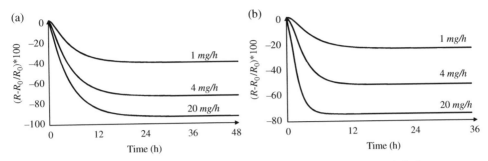

FIGURE 20.14   Effect of the infusion rate on the time to steady-state response in indirect response models I (a) and IV (b). Parameter values for the models are those given in the legend of Figure 20.10.

The characteristics of the three other models can be investigated by computer simulations. The default parameter values of the simulation models are shown in Table 20.1, and the individual models can be found at the following sites:

- Indirect Effect Model I (Model 22): http://web.uri.edu/pharmacy/research/rosenbaum/sims/Model22.
- Indirect Effect Model II (Model 23): http://web.uri.edu/pharmacy/research/rosenbaum/sims/Model23.
- Indirect Effect Model III (Model 24): http://web.uri.edu/pharmacy/research/rosenbaum/sims/Model24.
- Indirect Effect Model IV (Model 25): http://web.uri.edu/pharmacy/research/rosenbaum/sims/Model25.

A summary of the characteristics of the four models is shown in Table 20.2, which also shows the limiting value of the maximum achievable response (R_{max}) in the four models. These values were identified using the same approach for model I as presented in equations (20.10)–(20.13).

20.4.3.8 Distinguishing Between Competing Indirect Effect Models

During model development, it is important to determine the most appropriate structural pharmacodynamic model to describe data. However, the four basic indirect effect pharmacodynamic models have some overlap in the response–time profiles. For example,

TABLE 20.1   Default Parameters Used in the Simulation Models for the Four Indirect Effect Models

Parameter	Model I	Model II	Model III	Model IV
Dose (mg)	100	500	500	500
k (h^{-1})	0.7	0.7	0.7	0.7
Vd (L)	20	20	20	20
k_{in} (units/h)	10	10	10	10
k_{out} (h^{-1})	0.2	0.2	0.2	0.2
I_{max} or S_{max}	1	1	5	5
IC$_{50}$ or SC$_{50}$ (mg/L)	0.1	0.1	1	1

TABLE 20.2 **Summary of the Characteristics of the Four Indirect Response Models**

	Model I: Inhibition: k_{in}	Model II Inhibition: k_{out}	Model III Stimulation: k_{in}	Model IV Stimulation: k_{out}
As dose ↑:	Response ↑ T_{R_M} ↑	Response ↑ T_{R_M} ↑	Response ↑ T_{R_M} ↑	Response ↑ T_{R_M} ↑
As k_{in} ↑	R_0 ↑ Relative R ↔	R_0 ↑ Relative R ↔	R_0 ↑ Relative R ↔	R_0 ↑ Relative R ↔
As k_{out} ↑	R_0 ↓ Relative R ↑ Time of onset ↓ Duration ↓	R_0 ↓ Relative R ↑ Time of onset ↓ Duration ↓	R_0 ↓ Response ↑ Time of onset ↓ Duration ↓	R_0 ↓ Response ↑ Time of onset ↓ Duration ↓
As k ↑	Response ↓ T_{R_M} ↓ Duration ↓	Response ↓ T_{R_M} ↓ Duration ↓	Response ↓ T_{R_M} ↓ Duration ↓	Response ↓ T_{R_M} ↓ Duration ↓
As IC_{50}/SC_{50} ↑	Response ↓ T_{R_M} ↓	Response ↓ T_{R_M} ↓	Response ↓ T_{R_M} ↓	Response ↓ T_{R_M} ↓
As I_{max}/S_{max} ↑	Response ↑ T_{R_M} ↔	Response ↑ T_{R_M} ↑	Response ↑ T_{R_M} ↔	Response ↑ T_{R_M} ↓
Time to steady state	↔ Dose	↑ Dose	↔ Dose	↓ Dose
R_{max}	$= R_0 \cdot (1 - I_{max})$; tends to zero	$= R_0/(1 - I_{max})$; tends to ∞	$= R_0 \cdot (1 + S_{max})$	$= R_0/(1 + S_{max})$

Models 1 and 4 produce very similar profiles, which can make determination of the appropriate structural model difficult. As was seen previously, the time to steady-state response on infusion can serve as one diagnostic but data from such long-term infusions can be difficult to obtain. However, varying the administered dose can produce distinguishing differences in the response profiles that will allow the selection of a reasonable model. Figure 20.15 shows that when the dose is varied over a 10-fold range, Model 1 produces a maximal response at varying times for each dose, whereas Model 4 has the same time to maximal response regardless of the dose administered. Having data from several doses therefore can be a key component in model identification.

Similarly, varying the input rate can also produce distinguishing differences although somewhat less concrete. Figure 20.16 shows the profile differences when input rate is varied. While these examples are based on IV infusions, administering orally using daily, twice daily, and three times daily or using an immediate release versus a sustained release will also help to provide distinguishing information. It should be noted that for any study aimed at determining the pharmacodynamics of a new therapeutic agent, obtaining data during the phase where drug effect is wearing off is important.

Finally, if data with varying dose or input rate are not available, selecting a structural model that is consistent with the known or expected mechanism of action of a drug or is consistent with other drugs in the same class is a good alternative.

20.5 OTHER INDIRECT EFFECT MODELS

Effect compartment models are generally used for very short lag between exposure and measured response (seconds to hours). Simple indirect effect models allow for longer lags

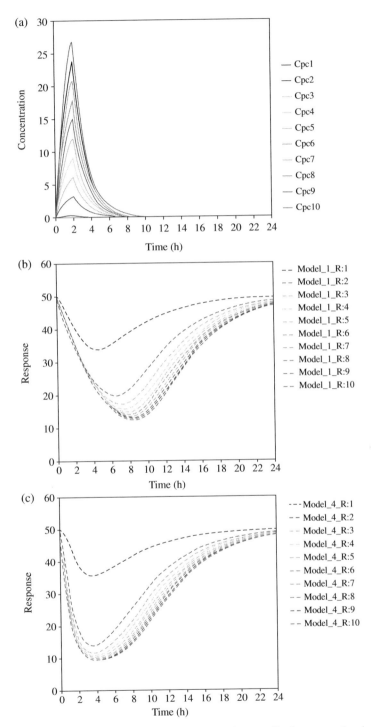

FIGURE 20.15   Effect of changing dose on response–time profile for competing indirect effect models. The pharmacokinetic profile (a) Model 1 (b) and Model 4 (c). Parameter values for the models are those given in the legend of Table 20.1. (*For a color version of this figure, see the color plate section.*)

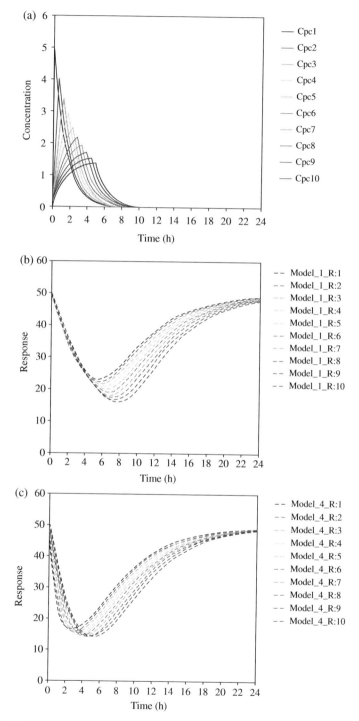

FIGURE 20.16 Effect of changing input rate on response–time profile for competing indirect effect models. The pharmacokinetic profile (a) Model 1 (b) and Model 4 (c). Parameter values for the models are those given in the legend of Table 20.1. (*For a color version of this figure, see the color plate section.*)

(hours to days). Although the basic indirect effect models are useful to describe many pharmacodynamic responses, there are occasions when the response is separated from drug exposure over a long period. When the gap between exposure and response is prolonged, the indirect effect models can be modified by including additional compartments into a chain. The precursor pool model for tolerance described in a later section is just such a modification. However, this model can also be used to describe longer delays without tolerance. Models with more than one additional compartment are commonly referred to as "transit" models.

20.5.1 Transit Compartment Models

Transduction refers to the process and steps involved in the conversion of drug–receptor interaction into a measured biological response. During transduction, the stimulus that is generated from the drug–receptor interaction is relayed along a sequence of cascading events that may involve G-protein activation, second messengers, ion-channel activation, and/or gene transcription. If the process is slow, it may become rate limiting and there may be a significant time lag between the changes in response and changes in the plasma concentrations of the drug. The delayed response–time profile that occurs as a result of transduction can be captured using a series of transit compartments to relay or transfer the initial stimulus [12]. Generally, it is not possible to determine either the number of transduction steps or the duration of each step. Thus, the number of transit compartments and the time for the response to move between compartments are modeled empirically to fit the response data. A model with three transit compartments is shown in Figure 20.17.

Generation of the initial stimulus or biosignal (E) that results from interaction of a drug with its receptors can be modeled using any of the models presented previously, such as the E_{max} model (Figure 20.17). If it is assumed that there is rapid distribution of the drug to its site of action, plasma concentrations can be used as the driving force in the equation.

The stimulus is then transmitted throughout the transit compartments. These models are usually parameterized for the mean transit time (MTT) for the entire process and for the number of compartments (n). The individual intercompartmental transit times (τ) for the various compartments are usually fixed to the same value, MTT/($n + 1$). A transit time is equivalent to the reciprocal of a first-order rate constant, and the transfer of the effect

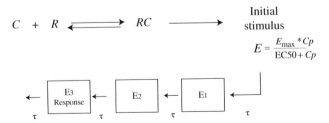

FIGURE 20.17 Transit compartment model with three transit compartments. In this model, the magnitude of the initial signal (E) is estimated from the E_{max} model. The signal is then transferred throughout a series of transit compartments, each of which has an intercompartmental transit time of τ.

between compartments can be modeled using first-order kinetics. Generally, the following equation can be used for the effect (E) in each compartment:

$$\frac{dE_n}{dt} = \frac{1}{\tau} \cdot E_{n-1} - \frac{1}{\tau} \cdot E_n = \frac{1}{\tau} \cdot (E_{n-1} - E_n) \tag{20.14}$$

The equations for each compartment are:

$$\frac{dE_1}{dt} = \frac{1}{\tau} \cdot \left(\frac{E_{max} \cdot Cp}{EC_{50} + Cp} - E_1 \right) \tag{20.15}$$

$$\frac{dE_2}{dt} = \frac{1}{\tau} \cdot (E_1 - E_2) \tag{20.16}$$

$$\frac{dE_3}{dt} = \frac{1}{\tau} \cdot (E_2 - E_3) \tag{20.17}$$

where E_n is the effect in the nth transit compartment, and $\tau = MTT/(n + 1)$ is the intercompartmental transit time. A power function can be added to the value of the effect in any compartment to amplify or dampen the effect during transduction [12].

Response data simulated using four transit compartment models are shown in Figure 20.18. It can be seen that as the response is transferred from one compartment to the next, the response is delayed, and it is dampened. As it moves through successive compartments, the peak of the signal is lower and the overall profile becomes wider and more symmetrical.

Figure 20.19 shows how the number of compartments influences the profile. The data were simulated by fixing the total MTT (6 h) and using between one and four transit compartments. The number of compartments has the clearest impact on the time of the final response. Even though the total MTT is the same in the various simulations (a–d), as the number of compartments increases the delay in the final response increases. Also, as the initial stimulus is divided into an increasing number of compartments, the profiles in equivalent compartments (e.g., compartment 2 of two compared to compartment 2 of four) become

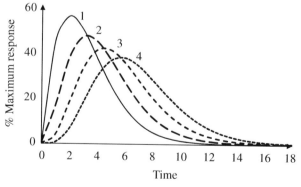

FIGURE 20.18   Value of the signal as it is transferred through four transit compartments. The data were simulated using an IV bolus injection (dose = 100 mg, Vd = 20 L, and $k = 0.7$ h^{-1}) with a direct link to an E_{max} model (EC_{50} = 1 mg/L and E_{max} = 100). The initial signal was then transferred throughout four transit compartments with a total transit time of 6 h and an intercompartmental transit time of 6/5 = 1.2 h.

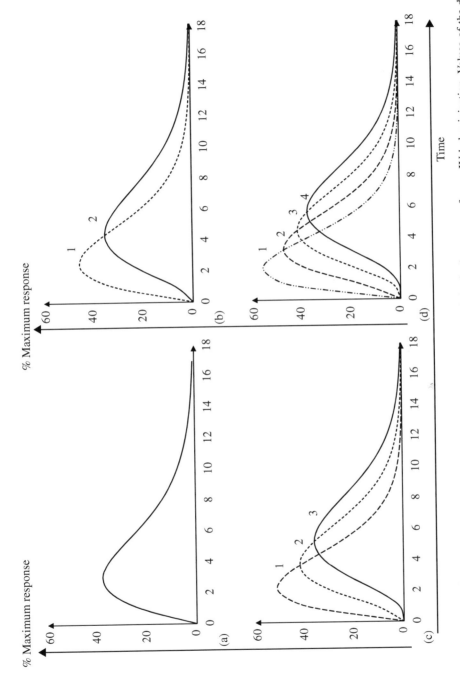

FIGURE 20.19 Effect of the number of transit compartments on the shape of the final response after an IV bolus injection. Values of the dose, pharmacokinetic, and pharmacodynamic are the same as those in the legend of Figure 20.12. The total mean transit time was maintained constant at 6 h, and response was generated using one (a), two (b), three (c), and four (d) transit compartments, with intercompartmental transit times of 3, 2, 1.5, and 1.2 h, respectively. The solid line represents the final response.

sharper, larger, and the peak occurs sooner. As a result, when a large number of compartments are used, the final response can be larger than that obtained in a model with fewer compartments. For example, in Figure 20.19, the peak response in the four-compartment model is 37%, whereas that in the two-compartment model is 35%. The model for the hematological toxicity of anticancer drugs that is presented in Section 20.5.2 is an example of a transit compartment model.

20.5.1.1   Simulation Exercise:
http://web.uri.edu/pharmacy/research/rosenbaum/sims
Open model 26, Transit Compartment Model of Drug Response, which can be found at http://web.uri.edu/pharmacy/research/rosenbaum/sims/Model26.

The model consists of a pharmacokinetic model of a one-compartment model ($Vd = 20\,L$ and $k = 0.7\,h^{-1}$) with intravenous bolus input. The generation of the stimulus is modeled using an E_{max} model ($E_{max} = 100$ and $EC_{50} = 1\,mg/L$) linked to Cp. The stimulus is transferred through a series of transit compartments. For each model, the intercompartmental transit time and the transit time for the dissipation of the final response are all the same and equal to the total MTT/(n + 1), where n is the number of transit compartments. The default value of n and the total MTT are 4 and 6 h, respectively.

1. *Explore the model and note its structure.*
2. *Go to the "Response Profiles" page. Choose a dose and note the time profiles of the plasma concentration, the initial stimulus, and the response in the different transit compartments.*
     Observe:
     - *Cp falls monoexponentially from its maximum value at time zero.*
     - *There is no delay in the generation of the initial stimulus; its maximum value corresponds to the maximum value of the plasma concentration at time zero. The stimulus decreases as plasma concentrations decay.*
     - *Transit compartments produce a delay in response. The response in each compartment starts at zero and gradually increases to reach a peak and then decreases.*
     - *The time of the peak response increases with each successive compartment. Note that the peak of the final response in compartment 4 occurs at around 6 h, by which time all the drug will have been eliminated ($t_{1/2} = 1\,h$).*
     - *The compartments have a dampening effect on the response. This dampening effect increases as the response moves through the compartments. Thus, the maximum response decreases and the profile widens and becomes more symmetrical in each successive compartment.*
3. *Go to the "Effect of Dose" page. Perform simulations with the default model with four compartments and a total MTT of 6 h. Choose doses of 10, 100, and 1000 mg. Note that the maximum response is not proportional to dose. The time of the maximum response increases with dose.*
4. *Go to the "Number of Compartments (No. Comp.) and MTT" page. Observe in turn how:*
     - *The total MTT affects the profile when the number of compartments is maintained constant.*
     - *The number of compartments affects the profile when the total MTT is held constant.*
     - *Probe different ways to obtain a peak response at 4 h.*

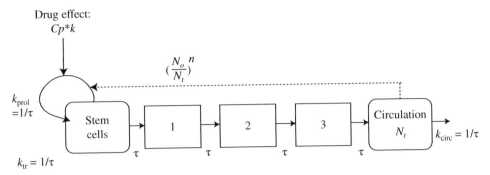

FIGURE 20.20 Pharmacodynamic component of the integrated PK–PD model for the neutropenia brought about by anticancer drugs. The neutrophils are assumed to be produced in the stem cells. Their prolonged maturation prior to release in the circulation is modeled using three transit compartments, each of which has the same intercompartmental transit time (τ). The proliferation rate of the neutrophils is dependent on the proliferation rate constant (k_{prol}), the number of precursor cells and a feedback mechanism that is dependent on the baseline neutrophil count (N_0), and the number circulating at any time (N_t). Feedback is equal to $(N_0/N_t)^n$, where n is a power function. Drug toxicity is modeled as an action on k_{prol}, where k_{tr} and k_{circ} are first-order rate constants for progression between compartments and the loss of neutrophils, respectively.

20.5.2 Model for Hematological Toxicity of Anticancer Drugs

Doses and the duration of therapy for many anticancer drugs, including docetaxel, paclitaxel, etoposide, and topotecan, are limited by drug-induced neutropenia. This is a serious toxicity that can put patients at risk for serious life-threatening infections. An integrated PK–PD model has been developed for the time course of this effect [13] (Figure 20.20). The model contains some unique elements as well as components of the models discussed previously. The model is outlined below.

1. A unique part of the model is the formation of neutrophils from the stem cell pool in the bone marrow. Their formation is assumed to be a first-order process driven by the number of precursor cells and a first-order rate constant (k_{prol}). A feedback process is incorporated into the rate of proliferation of the neutrophils based on the baseline neutrophils count (N_0) and the number of neutrophils circulating at any time (N_t):

$$\text{feedback} = \left[\frac{N_0}{N_t}\right]^n \tag{20.18}$$

where n is a power factor. The feedback process becomes operative whenever the circulating neutrophil count deviates from the normal circulating baseline value.

Overall, the rate of proliferation of the neutrophils is given by

$$\text{rate of proliferation} = \text{number in pool} \cdot k_{prol} \cdot \text{feedback} \tag{20.19}$$

2. Once new cell proliferation begins, it takes about 90–135 h for the cells to develop fully and to be released into the circulation [13]. This extended development process is modeled using the transit compartment transduction model. A series of three

transit compartments are incorporated between the stem cells and the circulation (Figure 20.20). The intercompartmental transit time between each compartment is set to the same value. For example, if the total time for cell development (total MTT) is 135 h, the transit time between compartments is $135/4 = 33.75$ h, which is equivalent to a first-order rate constant of $0.0296\ \mathrm{h^{-1}}$.

3. The target of the drug action is assumed to be the first-order rate constant for neutrophil proliferation (k_{prol}). Thus, this component of the model is similar to that of an indirect response model (model I, inhibition of k_{in}), and similarly, the effect of the drug is assessed in terms of the fractional inhibition of k_{prol}:

$$k_{prol} = k_{prol_0}(1 - I) \qquad (20.20)$$

where k_{prol} is the first-order rate constant for proliferation, k_{prol0} is the rate constant in the absence of the drug, and I is the inhibitory effect of the drug.

4. The inhibitory action of the drug on k_{prol} is modeled as a linear function of the plasma concentration and is expressed as:

$$I = Cp \cdot \mathrm{KF} \qquad (20.21)$$

where I is the effect (fractional inhibition of k_{prol}) and KF is the kill factor, which has units of reciprocal concentration and is often called the slope. It is the constant of proportionality that determines the potency of the drug in inhibiting proliferation.

Owing to the difficulty assessing the rate constants for proliferation (k_{prol}) and the loss of neutrophils from the circulation (k_{circ}), as well as to keep the number of model parameters to a minimum, these rate constants are both set equal to the rate constant for progression between the transit compartments (Figure 20.19).

Pharmacodynamic models of hematological toxicity have been developed for several anticancer drugs, including docetaxel, paclitaxel, etoposide [13], and topotecan [14]. The system-specific parameters (MTT and the power factor n for the feedback control of circulating neutrophils) of the models were found to be consistent among the various drugs [13]. A typical model-predicted profile of the plasma concentration and neutrophil count after a cycle of five daily doses of a myelotoxic drug is shown in Figure 20.21. These plots were generated for a fictitious myelotoxic drug, mirotecan, using parameter values similar

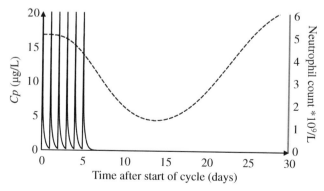

FIGURE 20.21 Typical plasma concentration (solid line) and neutrophil count (dashed line) after five daily infusions of an anticancer drug that causes neutropenia. The data were simulated using parameters of the fictitious drug mirotecan. The parameter values are given in the text.

TABLE 20.3   Neutropenia Classification System

Grade of neutropenia	1	2	3	4
Neutrophil count (10^9/L)	2.0−1.5	1.5−1.0	1.0−0.5	<0.5

to those reported in the literature. The parameters used for the simulation are provided in Section 7.2.1. For comparison, the published values of topotecan are also provided. From Figure 20.21, it can be seen that the nadir neutrophil count occurs about 12 days after the start of therapy, at which time drug from all five doses has been eliminated. Notice that by 21 days, the time when the next cycle of doses is typically administered, the neutrophil count has recovered. In fact, it can be seen that at around 22–24 days, the neutrophil count overshoots its original baseline value. This phenomenon occurs as a result of the feedback mechanism, which stimulates proliferation when the circulating neutrophil count is low.

The application of these models in cancer chemotherapy offers the potential of providing a way to optimize doses for individual patients. From a therapeutic perspective, doses of these drugs should be as large as possible to maximize their effects on cancer cells, but their hematological toxicity limits the dose. The importance of the dose in determining patient outcome has been illustrated in studies, which indicate that patients who experience midlevel neutropenia (grades 2–3) (Table 20.3) have a higher survival rate than do those who experience milder (grade 1) or more severe neutropenia (grade 4) [15]. Doses are generally based on body surface area or weight and do not address the possibility that a patient's pharmacokinetic or pharmacodynamic parameters may be significantly different from average. Some patients may require lower-than-average doses, due, for example, to slow elimination (pharmacokinetic), a high kill factor (pharmacodynamic), or a low baseline neutrophil count. This group of patients will be at risk for developing severe neutropenia. Usually, these patients are identified as a result of routine monitoring of the neutrophils, which is usually performed during treatment. If patients are found to have severe neutropenia, a standard protocol is used to reduce their dose and/or to delay the next drug cycle.

The pharmacokinetic and/or pharmacodynamic properties in other patients may result in higher than normal dose requirements, and since there are no measurable indicators of this situation, it may go unnoticed and can result in patients being chronically under dosed. The group of scientists who first developed these models has now developed software to estimate optimum doses of etoposide in individual patients [15, 16]. The software uses the model for hematological toxicity in conjunction with a patient's pretreatment baseline neutrophil count and a measured neutrophil count during therapy.

20.5.2.1 Simulation Exercise
A simulation model (Hematological Toxicity of Anticancer Drugs, Model 27) based on the published models [13] and parameters has been created for a fictitious drug (mirotecan) and may be found at the link http://web.uri.edu/pharmacy/research/rosenbaum/sims/Model27.

Mirotecan is assumed to follow two-compartmental pharmacokinetics with the following parameters: Cl = 15 L/h, Cld = 18 L/h, V_1 = 26 L, and V_2 = 45 L. The parameters of the pharmacodynamic model are baseline neutrophil count = 5 × 10^9/L, total MTT = 135 h, kill factor = 0.25 L/μg, and power function for feedback loop (n) = 0.18. For comparison, the published pharmacokinetic and pharmacodynamic parameters for topotecan are Cl = 25 L/h (normal renal function), Cld = 49.9 L/h, V_1 = 39.9 L/70 kg, and V_2 = 44.5 L. The baseline neutrophil count = 4.89 × 10^9/L, total MTT = 116 h, kill factor = 0.183 L/μg, *and power function for feedback loop (n) = 0.130 [14]. The dosing schedule for mirotecan is five daily doses of 1.0 mg administered intravenously as short infusions over a 30-min period. Explore the pharmacokinetic and pharmacodynamic models.*

1. *Go to the "Plasma Concentration and Cell Profile" page. Give the doses and observe the time course of plasma concentrations and neutrophil count. Note that the nadir of the neutrophil level occurs at around 12 days. The typical patient will experience a nadir of about 1.3×10^9 neutrophils/L, which is a grade 2 neutropenia.*

2. *Go to the "PK and PD Variability" page. Observe the effects of pharmacokinetic and pharmacodynamic variability on response.*

   (a) *Select parameter values that would represent the worst-case scenario of a patient who would be most resistant to the effects of the drug. Observe the nadir of the neutrophil count and recovery time in this patient.*

   (b) *Select parameter values that would represent the worst-case scenario of a patient who would be most sensitive to the effects of the drug. Observe the nadir of the neutrophil count and recovery time in this patient.*

20.5.3 Alternate Parameterizations of Transit Models

While the parameterization of the transit model for neutrophil counts works well, some cell types exhibit different growth and lifespan properties. For example, the red blood cell has been shown to have a much longer lifespan than white cells [17], and although the lifespan is considerably shorter in patients with end stage renal disease [18] the traditional transit model parameterization does not work well for evaluation of the effects of red cell transfusions, iron supplementation, or the administration of epoetin on hemoglobin or red cell counts. The initial proposal for dealing with a physiologic lifespan involved the use of delayed differential equations [19] in which the pharmacodynamic system is represented twice, once at a previous time point and once at the current time point. However, such systems are difficult to work with and are computationally far more intensive than the more simplistic transit models. However, the performance of the delayed differential functions has been shown to be reasonably consistent with transit models [20] and when the transit compartments are summed together the transit and delayed differential equations are virtually identical. Thus, the transit model can be reparameterized to sum the contents of each of the transit compartments to produce a response curve that is more reflective of a longer lived response [21]. Figure 20.22 depicts response time curves following the administration of an inhibitory function using the standard transit model parameterization where the response is taken from the last transit compartment and compares it to the result of summing the contents of the theoretical transit compartments. Note that with the latter summed model, a more "squared" response profile with more rapid response to drug stimulus becomes apparent.

20.6 MODELS OF TOLERANCE

20.6.1 Introduction to Pharmacologic Tolerance

Tolerance may be defined as a process that results in a reduction in the response to a specific drug concentration following repeated drug exposure. This definition of tolerance excludes pharmacokinetics tolerance, which can, for example, arise with a drug that induces its own

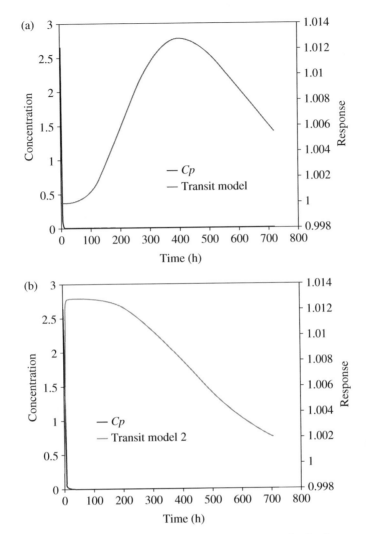

FIGURE 20.22   Response time profiles with the traditional parameterization for a transit model (a) and when the transit compartments are summed (b). If five transit compartments ($E_1,..,E_5$) are assumed, each containing its own erythrocyte (RBC) count arising from the effect of a drug decreasing the rate of RBC into E_1 that is passed into subsequent transit compartments, the response in the transit model in panel (a) is measured only at the final compartment, E_5. Panel (b) shows the effect of a summed transit model in which the response is taken as the sum of the response (e.g., RBCs) in each of the theoretical transit compartments.

metabolism. Only pharmacodynamic-based tolerance is addressed in this section. A model for the time course (onset and duration) and the magnitude of tolerance would be useful to use to probe potential modifications of dosing regimens to minimize its impact as well as to estimate the type of dose adjustments that may be necessary to overcome its effect.

Owing to the complex underlying biological processes associated with the development of tolerance, most approaches to modeling tolerance use empirical models that attempt to explain the observations. Some very simple models for receptor downregulation and desensitization have been created using decay and growth functions. Thus, receptor downregulation has been modeled by adding a decay function (e^{-kt}) to the E_{max} parameter of the sigmoidal E_{max} model. Desensitization has been modeled by adding a growth function to the drug's EC_{50}.

Pharmacodynamic-based tolerance can develop through several mechanisms, one of which is the production of a compensatory or counter-regulatory response called *homeostatic tolerance*. Tolerance can occur by depletion or restriction of the availability of a precursor or agonist pool. Tolerance can also occur due to changes in the chain of events between receptor activation and the production of a response. These include desensitization of the receptors, downregulation of the receptors, and the depletion of endogenous compounds, such as second messengers, which play an important role in mediating the response.

20.6.2 Counter-Regulatory Force Tolerance Model

A common approach that has been used to model tolerance is to assume that the drug or its response stimulates the production of a *counter-regulatory compound* or *force*. The latter can be modeled to either produce the opposite effect of the drug or to act as an antagonist or a partial agonist to the drug. This approach has been used to model tolerance from nicotine, nitroglycerin, caffeine, and morphine [22–24]. The specific details of the models used for different drugs vary somewhat, but the model used for the development of the tolerance for nicotine represents a clear example. Tolerance of the chronotropic effect of nicotine was assumed to be the result of the formation of a hypothetical nicotine antagonist [22]. This antagonist or tolerance mediator is assumed to be formed from the drug in the central compartment, but since it is only hypothetical, its production does not deplete or in any way influence the amount of drug in the central compartment. The rate of production of the mediator is assumed to be first order, driven by the plasma concentration of the drug (Figure 20.23). The mediator is assumed to be lost by a first-order process:

$$\frac{dCm}{dt} = Cp \cdot k_{1m} - Cm \cdot k_{m0} \tag{20.22}$$

where Cm is the concentration of mediator or counter-regulatory compound, k_{1m} is a first-order rate constant for the formation of the mediator, and k_{m0} is the first-order rate constant for its destruction.

Often, k_{1m} and k_{m0} are set equal to each other, and as a result, at steady state, the concentration of the hypothetical mediator is the same as the plasma concentration of the drug. This model is very similar to the effect compartment model presented in Chapter 16. In common with the effect compartment model, the rate constant for the loss of the mediator controls the onset and dissipation of tolerance. Thus, it will take 3–5 $t_{1/2,km0}$ for tolerance to reach its maximum value at a given drug concentration, and it will take the same time to dissipate once the drug has been withdrawn.

Any of the pharmacodynamic models discussed previously, such as the sigmoidal E_{max} model, can be used for the direct action of the drug. The plasma concentration could be used as the driving force for the response, or an effect compartment could be incorporated. The model for tolerance to the chronotropic action of nicotine did not incorporate an effect compartment and used a linear pharmacodynamic model on the assumption that the nicotine concentration is always much less than the EC_{50}:

$$E = E_0 + S \cdot Cp \tag{20.23}$$

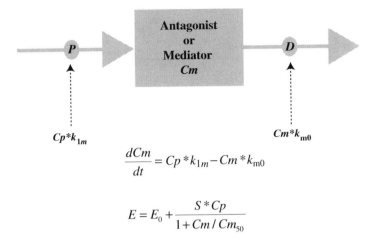

$$\frac{dCm}{dt} = Cp * k_{1m} - Cm * k_{m0}$$

$$E = E_0 + \frac{S * Cp}{1 + Cm / Cm_{50}}$$

FIGURE 20.23   Pharmacodynamic model for tolerance. Tolerance is assumed to be produced by the action of a hypothetical metabolite of the parent drug. The metabolite is assumed to be produced and removed by first-order processes driven by the concentration of the parent drug (Cp) and the hypothetical metabolite (Cm), respectively. The rate constants for formation (k_{1m}) and loss (k_{m0}) are usually set equal to each other. The effect of the drug is modeled as the change from baseline (E_0) using linear model with a slope of S. The metabolite is assumed to act as an antagonist, and Cm_{50} is the steady-state concentration of the metabolite that produces 50% maximum tolerance. This is the model used for the development of tolerance to nicotine. From [22].

where E is the heart rate, E_0 is the resting heart rate, Cp is the plasma concentration of nicotine, and S is the slope factor.

The pharmacodynamic model is then modified to account for the action of the modifier (Figure 20.23). In the nicotine example, the modifier was modeled as a noncompetitive antagonist. Thus, the overall effect of the drug was expressed as:

$$E = E_0 + \frac{S \cdot Cp}{1 + Cm/Cm_{50}} \tag{20.24}$$

where E is the net effect, Cm is the concentration of the counter-regulatory mediator, and Cm_{50} is the steady-state concentration of the mediator that produces 50% maximum tolerance.

The pharmacokinetic parameters are estimated from the plasma concentration data. The pharmacodynamic parameters S, k_{m0}, Cm_{50}, and E_0 are estimated from the time course of response. Figure 20.24 shows the plasma concentration and response (heart rate) simulated from the model parameters reported for nicotine [22]. Data were simulated after two short infusions of 5 mg of nicotine over 30 min. It can be seen in Figure 20.24a that as a result of accumulation, the nicotine concentration after the second dose is higher than that after the first. In contrast, and as a result of tolerance, the response after the second dose is lower than that after the first. When response is plotted as a function of nicotine concentration, a circular or clockwise relationship between response and concentration is observed. This phenomenon is known as *proteresis*, which means "comes earlier." In Figure 20.24b, it can be seen that proteresis becomes apparent on the downward fall in the plasma concentration, when the response at a given concentration is less than it was during the initial upward movement in the concentration. Thus, while a counterclockwise hysteresis is indicative of

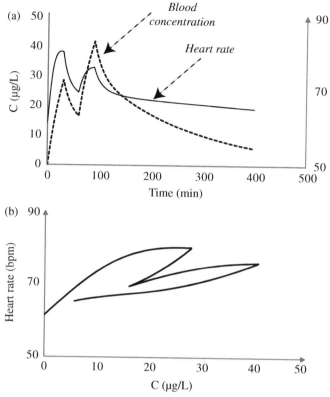

FIGURE 20.24   Tolerance to nicotine. The nicotine blood concentration (µg/L) (dotted line) and response (heart rate) (solid line) against time are shown after two successive infusions of nicotine (a). Figure 20.24(b) shows response (heart rate) plotted against nicotine blood concentration after the two infusions. Based on data from [22].

a lag between concentration and response, clockwise proteresis is indicative of tolerance occurring.

The same approach can be used to describe the development of tolerance using a competitive antagonist model [6] where there are two effect compartments, one for the agonist and a second for the antagonist:

$$E = E0 - \frac{\left(\frac{CE}{EC50}\right)^{\gamma E} + T\max\left(\frac{CT}{TC50}\right)^{\gamma T}}{1 + \left(\frac{CE}{EC50}\right)^{\gamma E} + \left(\frac{CT}{TC50}\right)^{\gamma T}} \tag{20.25}$$

where CE is the concentration of the parent drug in the effect compartment, EC50 is the concentration at half-maximal response, and γE is the Hill coefficient reflecting the steepness of the concentration effect relationship. CT is the concentration of a hypothetical tolerance drug in an additional compartment, TC50 is the concentration at half-maximal tolerance, and γT is the Hill coefficient for the concentration/tolerance relationship. This approach has been used to describe acute tolerance to opiates [25] and benzodiazepines [26]. A similar model was used for the development of tolerance to nitroglycerin, where in this case the hypothetical mediator was assumed to produce an action (Ec, vasoconstrictor) in opposition to that of the drug (Ed, vasodilatory) [24]. The net effect of nitroglycerin was the sum of the vasodilatory and vasoconstrictor effects (*Ed + Ec*). A comparison of the different approaches to tolerance has been reviewed [27]. The operational model of agonism has also proved to be useful for studying tolerance. For example, it has been used to study the mechanism behind the development of tolerance to the μ-opioid agonists [28] and to investigate the relationship between efficacy and tolerance [29].

20.6.2.1 *Simulation Exercise*

Open model 28, Drug Tolerance: Hypothetical Antagonist Model, which can be found at http://web.uri.edu/pharmacy/research/rosenbaum/sims/Model28.

   The model is based on the published model of tolerance to the cardio-accelerating effects of nicotine [22]. The pharmacokinetic model consists of a two-compartment pharmacokinetic model with parameters k_{10}, k_{12}, and k_{21} of 0.0112, 0.03, and 0.0325 min^{-1}, respectively, and Vc = 114 L. Note that these parameters give an elimination half-life of nicotine of about 150 min. The pharmacodynamic model consists of a linear effect model [equation (20.23)] with tolerance produced by a hypothetical noncompetitive antagonist [equations (20.22) and (20.24)]. The pharmacodynamic parameters are as follows: $k_{1m} = k_{m0} = 0.020$ min^{-1}, S = 1.31 bpm per μg/L, Cm_{50} = 7.72 μg/L, and E_0 = 61.2 bpm. Drug administration is modeled as two short (30 min) intravenous infusions of 5 mg.

1. *Explore the model and review the "Model Summary" page.*
2. *Simulate plasma concentration and the response. Note that although the plasma concentration increases with the second dose, the effect decreases.*
3. *Try to increase the value of the second dose to achieve the same response as that obtained after the first dose.*
4. *Go to the "k_{m0} and Cm_{50}" page. Probe the influence of k_{m0}. Note that as the value of k_{m0} increases, tolerance occurs more quickly and is more prominent (the effect of nicotine is less). Tolerance also wears off faster so the fall in response is more gentle because the effects of nicotine are greater.*
5. *Conduct simulation changing the value of Cm_{50}. This is the concentration of the "antagonist" that produces a 50% effect. Since it is nicotine that drives the tolerance and since the concentration of nicotine at steady state is the same as that of the antagonist, Cm_{50} can be considered the steady-state nicotine concentration that produces 50% tolerance. As Cm_{50} decreases, tolerance becomes more prominent at a given drug concentration; the nicotine-induced increase in the heart rate is smaller.*
6. *Go to the "Change τ" page, which allows the time between the multiple doses to be altered. Note that as the dosing interval is increased, the tolerance effect on the next dose becomes less. The loss of tolerance is controlled by k_{m0}, which is about 1.2 h^{-1}, and has a half-life of 0.58 h. Thus, tolerance should dissipate in about 7×0.58 h = 4 h. The elimination half-life of nicotine (about 2 h) also controls the duration of tolerance. Reduce the elimination half-life by increasing the value of k_{10}. Note that when k_{10} is increased to large values (rapid elimination), tolerance dissipates about 4 h after a dose.*

20.6.3 Precursor Pool Model of Tolerance

Tolerance would occur if a drug's action is dependent on an endogenous compound (precursor) that is depleted during the response to the drug. The full action of the drug would

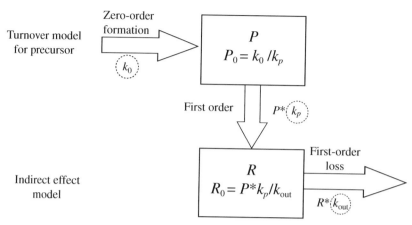

FIGURE 20.25 Precursor pool depletion model. The response variable (R) is produced by a first-order process (rate constant k_p) from a precursor (P) that gets depleted. The loss of the response variable is a first-order process with a rate constant k_{out}. The precursor is formed by a zero-order process (k_0). The drug stimulates the formation of the response variable by increasing k_p. Based on data from Reference [22].

only be restored once the amount of the endogenous compound returned to its normal resting value. The precursor pool indirect response model (Section 20.4) has been applied to model this phenomenon [30].

In previous discussions of the basic indirect model, it was assumed that the precursor pool for the production of the response variable was large and could never be depleted. Thus, the production of the response variable was modeled as a constant (zero order) process. In the precursor pool depletion model for tolerance, this assumption is not made. The response variable (R) is assumed to be produced from its precursor (P) by a first-order process with a rate constant (k_p) (Figure 20.25). The loss of the response variable is modeled in the usual way as a first-order process with a rate constant k_{out}.

$$\frac{dR}{dt} = k_p P - k_{out}R \tag{20.26}$$

The drug is assumed to increase the amount of the response variable by stimulating its rate constant for production (k_p). The direct action (E) is the fractional stimulation of (k_p).

$$\frac{dR}{dt} = k_p(1 + E)P - k_{out}R \tag{20.27}$$

The direct effect of the drug can be modeled using the E_{max} or sigmoidal E_{max} model:

$$E = \frac{E_{max} * Cp}{EC_{50} + Cp} \tag{20.28}$$

The usual turnover model is used for the precursor pool (Figure 20.25). The precursor is usually assumed to be produced by a zero-order process and lost by a first-order process through its conversion to the response variable:

$$\frac{dP}{dt} = k_0 - P * k_p \tag{20.29}$$

where $P \cdot k_p$ is the rate of the appearance of the drug response, R.

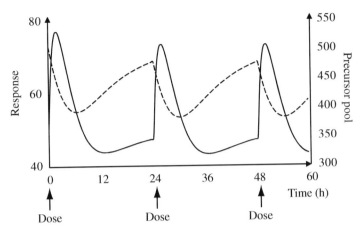

FIGURE 20.26 Precursor model predicted plot of response (solid line) and precursor pool status (dashed line) against time. The simulation was conducted with multiple IV bolus injections (100 mg every 24 h) and the following parameters: $Vd = 20$ L, $k = 0.4$ h^{-1}, $k_0 = 50$ units/h, $k_p = 0.1$ h^{-1}, $k_{out} = 1$ h^{-1}, EC$_{50} = 1$ mg/L, and $E_{max} = 1$.

Drug Effect on P   In the absence of the drug, the precursor pool is in equilibrium and $P_0 = k_0/k_p$. When the drug stimulates k_p to increase the response variable, P decreases (Figure 20.26). Once the drug's action stops, the return of P to equilibrium value (P_0) is determined by the value of (k_p). If a second dose of the drug is administered before the precursor pool is restored, the second dose will not be able to produce the same magnitude of effect as the first dose.

Drug Effect on R   In the absence of the drug, R is at its baseline value ($R_0 = k_p * P_0/k_{out}$). The drug stimulates k_p and increases the response R. When the drug action ceases, R decreases toward R_0 (Figure 20.26). However, because of the time it takes P to return back to P_0, R can achieve a value that is less than R_0 (Figure 20.26). This is known as rebound. If P has not been able to return to its baseline value by the time a second dose is given, the effect from this second dose will be less than that after the first. Similar behavior is seen when the effect of drug is to inhibit the conversion of precursor to elicit the response R. Inhibition of k_p will decrease R, and after removal of the drug there can be rebound with transient response higher than was present at baseline.

20.6.3.1 Simulation Exercise
Open model 29, Tolerance: Precursor Pool Depletion Model, which can be found at http://web.uri.edu/pharmacy/research/rosenbaum/sims/Model29.
  The model has the following parameter values: $k = 0.4$ h^{-1}, $Vd = 20$ L, $k_p = 0.1$ h^{-1}, $k_0 = 50$ units per h, $P_0 = k_0/k_p = 500$ units, $k_{out} = 1$ h^{-1}, $R_0 = k_p * P_0/k_{out} = 50/L = 50$ units, $EC_{50} = 1$ unit/L, $E_{max} = 1$, dose = 100 mg, and dosing interval = 24 h.

  1. *Explore the model. Perform a simulation on the "Response Profile" page. The drug stimulates the production of the response variable (R) (response), which depletes the precursor pool (P). As the drug effect dissipates, R decreases toward its baseline value, but it overshoots the original value. This is known as rebound and occurs*

because P is still depleted. Note that even by the time a second dose is given, P is not yet fully restored to its baseline value (500 units). As a result, the response to the second dose is less than that to the first.

2. *Go to the "Dosing Regimen" page. Note that as the dose increases, the rebound effect and tolerance are more prominent. Restore the default setting and probe the influence of the dosing interval. Note that tolerance and rebound become more prominent with smaller dosing intervals. When the dosing interval is increased to 48 h, P is able to return to its original baseline value and tolerance is not observed, but the rebound effect is still present.*

20.7 IRREVERSIBLE DRUG EFFECTS

Some drugs bind covalently to their receptors. As a result, the target is destroyed and its function returns only when it has been replaced by newly synthesized product. The target may be a protein, DNA, an enzyme, or a cell at any stage of development. The proton pump inhibitors are examples of drugs that act irreversibly. They bind to and destroy the H^+,K^+-ATPase pumps in the parietal cells of the gastric mucosa, and normal proton secretion is restored only when the pumps are replaced by newly synthesized functioning pumps (i.e., the usual turnover time of the system). For proton pumps, the turnover time is over 24 h, and as a result, proton pump inhibitors can be administered daily, even though most of them have very short elimination half-lives. For example, the duration of action of omeprazole ($t_{1/2} <$ 1 h) is sufficiently long to allow it to be administered daily. Aspirin is another example of a drug that acts irreversibly. Aspirin reacts covalently with prostaglandin cyclooxygenase, an enzyme that is responsible for the formation of thromboxane B_2, which in turn promotes platelet aggregation when platelets become fractured. Aspirin destroys the activity of the enzyme, and as a result it can no longer synthesize thromboxane B_2. Aspirin's action persists until new platelets are synthesized with functional cyclooxygenase that can resume the synthesis of thromboxane. Once again, although aspirin has a very short elimination half-life (around 15 min), the drug can be given daily because of prolonged inhibition of cyclooxygenase.

Cancer chemotherapy also provides examples of irreversibly acting drugs, including the alkylating agents, such as cyclophosphamide and chlorambucil, which bind covalently to DNA, and drugs such as etoposide and topotecan, which destroy developing white blood cells in the bone marrow. Additionally, some inhibitors of drug metabolism act by binding irreversibly to, and destroying the activity of, enzymes. Again, the action of the inhibitor can last long after it has been eliminated from the body, and will persist until the damaged enzyme is turned over and replaced with new, functioning enzyme.

20.7.1 Application of the Turnover Model to Irreversible Drug Action

The physiological turnover model presented in Section 20.3 has been used to model the irreversible effects of several drugs, including proton pump inhibitors. In this application, the target of the drug is the biological factor, or response variable, itself (Figure 20.27). As usual, the response variable is assumed to be synthesized by a zero-order process, with a rate constant equal to k_{in} and degraded by a first-order process with a rate constant k_{out}. The

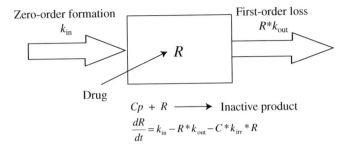

FIGURE 20.27   Model for an irreversible pharmacological effect. The model consists of a physiological turnover model with zero-order formation (k_{in}) and first-order loss (rate constant k_{out}) of the response variable (R). The irreversible interaction of the drug with the response variable is driven by the drug concentration (C) and expressed using the second-order rate constant k_{irr}.

irreversible drug effect is modeled by incorporating drug concentration-dependent destruction of the response variable, R, according to the equation

$$C + R \xrightarrow{\quad k_{irr} \quad} \text{product} \qquad\qquad (20.30)$$

where C is the drug concentration, R is the response variable and target of the drug action, and k_{irr} is a second-order rate constant for the concentration-dependent effect of the drug on the factor.

Based on the model shown in Figure 20.27, an expression can be written for the action of the drug on the response variable:

$$\frac{dR}{dt} = k_{in} - R \cdot k_{out} - C \cdot k_{irr} \cdot R \qquad\qquad (20.31)$$

This model has been used to model the action of proton pump inhibitor pantoprazole using the rate of acid output as the response variable [31]. Thus, R is the rate of acid secretion, k_{in} is a zero-order rate constant for the rate of acid production, k_{out} is a first-order rate constant for the natural endogenous degradation of the rate of acid secretion, and C is the plasma concentration of the drug. A simulation model has been built for the fictitious drug disolvprazole based on the published model for pantoprazole.

20.7.1.1 Simulation Exercise
The model developed for pantoprazole [31] was used as the basis of an integrated PK–PD model for the fictitious drug disolvprazole. The characteristics of this model will be demonstrated through simulation. The model Proton Pump Inhibitors-Model for Irreversible Effects (Model 30), may be found at the link http://web.uri.edu/pharmacy/research/rosenbaum/sims/Model30.

The pharmacokinetic model consists of a one-compartment model with first-order absorption with the parameters presented previously for disolvprazole: Cl = 12 L/h, Vd = 35 L, F = 0.5, and $k_a = 3\,h^{-1}$. The elimination half-life is 2 h. The pharmacodynamic model consists of a physiological turnover model that incorporates drug concentration–dependent irreversible destruction of the response variable (acid production). The pharmacodynamic *parameters are based on those of pantoprazole, but were modified slightly when appropriate to match the characteristics of disolvprazole discussed previously. They are as follows: $k_{in} = 0.8$ mmol/h/h and $k_{out} = 0.03$ h^{-1} $k_{irr} = 1$ L/mg/h. These compare to the following pharmacodynamic parameters of pantoprazole: $k_{in} = 0.416$ mmol/h/h, $k_{out} = 0.031$ h^{-1} $k_{irr} = 0.751$ L/mg/h [31].*

1. *Review the model.*
2. *Notice the time course of the plasma concentration and the response. Note that:*
   (a) *The maximum response is delayed with respect to the plasma concentration.*
   (b) *The effect of the drug persists long after the drug is eliminated.*
3. *Go to the "Dose and τ" page. For doses of 25, 50, 100, and 200 mg, observe that:*
   (a) *Response increases with dose but not in a proportional manner.*
   (b) *As the dose increases, the peak effect occurs earlier.*
4. *Increase τ to observe how long the effect from a single dose persists. Note that even though the drug's elimination half-life is 2 h, the effect of a single dose lasts over 3 days.*

This simulation model is required to answer Problem 20.4.

20.8 DISEASE PROGRESSION MODELS

Many diseases that are treated with drugs are not static, but worsen or improve over time. Chronic progressive diseases such as Parkinson's disease, Alzheimer's disease, and osteoporosis deteriorate over time. Other conditions such as postoperative pain or recovery from an injury are self-limiting and gradually resolve even without drug treatment. In many cases, drugs used to treat these conditions have no effect on healthy, disease-free individuals. Thus, models for the response of these diseases to drugs must incorporate a model for the underlying disease, and this model must address the continuously changing status of the disease. These models, called *disease progression models,* must consider the pharmacokinetics of the drug, its mechanism of action, and the natural history of the symptoms or disease being treated.

20.8.1 Drug Pharmacokinetics

An understanding of the pharmacokinetics of the active drug is fundamental to effective modeling of disease progression. In the examples below, drug input will be modeled using a constant continuous intravenous infusion.

20.8.2 Pharmacodynamics

As previously presented in this chapter and preceding chapters, drug action that results from drug–receptor interaction can be generated using a pharmacokinetic model linked to any of the previously discussed pharmacodynamic models, such as the sigmoidal E_{max} model or linear model. If necessary, an effect compartment or transit compartments can be added to accommodate delays in the response of the disease to the drug. In this discussion, the simple E_{max} model without delays will be used to model the direct effect of the drug.

20.8.3 Disease Activity Models

A *disease activity model* represents how a disease changes over time in the absence of drug therapy. The disease status may be evaluated by measuring a symptom of the disease, an outcome of the disease (e.g., blood pressure and bone density), or a biomarker. Three models of disease progression are presented: the linear model, the exponential decay or zero asymptotic model, and the exponential model with nonzero maximum disease status. These models have been used successfully to model a variety of conditions, such as Parkinson's disease, Alzheimer's disease, muscular dystrophy, and the treatment of HIV disease [32–35]. Disease (or symptom) activity may be cyclical, such as when linked to menstrual periods or relapsing/remitting multiple sclerosis. It is important to recognize that models of disease progression are often empirically derived, and their mathematical construct is not necessarily mechanistically founded.

Drugs can broadly interact with diseases in three ways:

1. Drugs can relieve the symptoms without altering the underlying progression of a disease. This is called *symptomatic action*. When a symptomatic drug is withdrawn, the disease is at the same place that it would have been at without the treatment.
2. Drugs can halt or slow the progression of a disease. This is known as a *protective action*. In this case, the improvement in disease status remains even when the drug is withdrawn.
3. Drugs can cure the disease. Most commonly associated with antibiotics or chemotherapy, these models often include components of competing pathogen or tumor growth against first-order cell kill.

20.8.4 Disease Progression Models

A *disease progression model* incorporates all three factors listed above: what is the concentration of the active drug expected to be in the action compartment; what is the effect of the drug concentration expected to be on the disease; and what is the disease activity expected to be in the absence of effective drug concentrations?

20.8.4.1 Linear Disease Progression Model

The *linear model* is frequently used to model the progression and treatment of chronic progressive diseases. It simply assumes that the disease deteriorates at a constant rate and can carry on doing so indefinitely. The disease status (S_t) at a given time is given by

$$S_t = S_0 + \alpha \cdot t \tag{20.32}$$

where S_t is the status of the disease at time t, S_0 is the status of the disease at time zero, and α is the slope representing the rate at which the status of the disease changes over time.

Depending on how disease status is measured, it may increase or decrease during the natural progression of a disease. For example, the loss of bone density due to osteoporosis decreases as the disease progresses, and if renal function is assessed using serum creatinine, the disease status will increase over time. Thus, α may be positive or negative. For this discussion, a positive slope will be used. Because many chronic conditions deteriorate very slowly, the period over which the diseases and their treatment are studied can be extremely long and may span several years.

Symptomatic Drugs   The action of symptomatic drugs, which reduce the disease status without altering the underlying progression, is modeled by incorporating an additive term, E_t, to represent the action of the drug at time t. Thus, the linear disease progression model will be modified as follows:

$$S_t = S_0 + \alpha \cdot t - E_t \tag{20.33}$$

where E_t is the effect of the drug.

The effect of a symptomatic drug in a linear model is shown in Figure 20.28, which shows that as the symptomatic action is characterized by an immediate change in the disease status, the curve is shifted downward but the slope is unchanged. In practice,

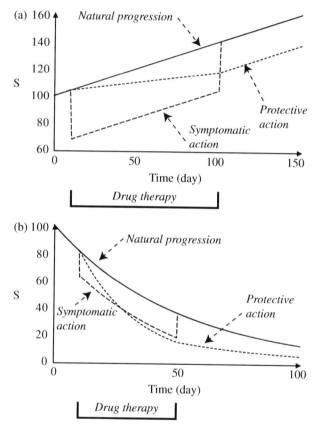

FIGURE 20.28   Linear (a) and exponential (b) disease progression models. Disease status (S) is shown as a function of time. Data were simulated using an IV infusion of 100 mg/h in a one-compartment model ($Vd = 20$ L and $Cl = 4$ L/h). The linear progression model has an initial disease status of 100 units and a slope of 0.4 unit/day. The symptomatic and protective effects were modeled using the E_{max} model with an EC_{50} of 10 mg/L and E_{max} values of 50 units and 0.35 day^{-1}, respectively. The infusion ran from day 10 to day 100. The exponential model has an initial disease status of 100 units and a k_{prog} of 0.02 day^{-1}. The EC_{50} of the drug was 10 mg/L, and E_{max} values of 25 units and 0.03 day^{-1} were used for the symptomatic and protective effects, respectively. The infusion ran from day 10 to day 50.

frequently, there is a lag time before the effects of the drug become apparent and a more gradual onset of action is observed. This can be accommodated in a model by incorporating a link model, such as a series of transit compartments. As soon as the drug is withdrawn, the status reverts back to the value that it would have had without drug therapy. This feature distinguishes the symptomatic effect from the protective effect (see below). However, in practice, a symptomatic drug effect may wear off more slowly than is shown in Figure 20.28, and the difference between the symptomatic and protective effects becomes less noticeable.

Protective Drugs   Protective drugs slow the progression of a disease. Their action is modeled by an effect on the progression slope:

$$S_t = S_0 + (\alpha - E_t) \cdot t \qquad (20.34)$$

Thus, the drug effectively reduces the slope (Figure 20.28). It can be seen that the effect of protective drugs is more gradual than those of symptomatic drugs. When the drug is withdrawn, the slope will return to its original value, but the patient is left with a lower (better) disease status than that of a patient who had no treatment.

20.8.4.2 *Exponential Decay or Zero Asymptotic Model*

Diseases that are only transient in nature and resolve themselves over time can be viewed as conditions that eventually decay to zero. These diseases are modeled by adding a decay function to the disease status:

$$S_t = S_0 \cdot e^{-k_{\text{prog}} \cdot t} \qquad (20.35)$$

where k_{prog} is a first-order rate constant for disease progression. In this model, S decays to a minimum (zero), and as a result this model is called an *asymptotic model*.

Symptomatic Drugs   Once again, the action of symptomatic drugs is modeled using an additive term:

$$S_t = S_0 \cdot e^{-k_{\text{prog}} \cdot t} - E_t \qquad (20.36)$$

The effect of a symptomatic drug in an exponential model is shown in Figure 20.29. In the zero asymptotic model, the action of the drug is in the same direction as the disease progression. In common with the linear model, the symptomatic action is rapid, the curve is shifted downward, the slope is unchanged, and when the drug is withdrawn, the status reverts back to the value that it would have had without drug therapy. Once again, a more gradual onset of action can be accommodated using a link model.

Protective Drugs   In the exponential model, the action of protective drugs is incorporated into k_{prog}. In the treatment of a self-resolving condition, the drug increases the value of k_{prog} to expedite the decay to zero. The action of protective drugs is modeled as follows:

$$S_t = S_0 \cdot e^{-(k_{\text{prog}} + E_t) \cdot t} \qquad (20.37)$$

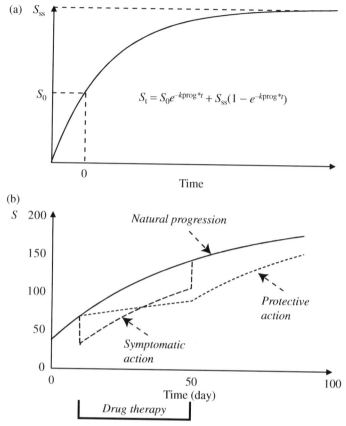

FIGURE 20.29   Maximum asymptotic disease progression model. Disease status (S) is shown over time. Time is measured from the first measured disease status value (S_0) (a). S_{ss} represents the maximum terminal value for the disease status, and k_{prog} is the rate constant for disease progression. Part (b) shows the profile for symptomatic and protective drug effects on k_{prog}. The data were simulated using an intravenous infusion of 100 mg/h in a one-compartment model ($Vd = 20$ L and $Cl = 4$ L/h). The infusion ran from day 10 to day 20. The progression model had k_{prog} and S_{ss} of 0.02 day^{-1} and 200 units, respectively. The symptomatic and protective effects were modeled using the E_{max} model with an EC$_{50}$ of 10 mg/L and E_{max} values of 50 units and 0.5, respectively.

It can be seen in Figure 20.29 that as was the case for the linear model, the protective effect has a more gradual onset of action, and once again when the treatment is withdrawn, the slope reverts to its original value but the patient is in a better place because of the treatment. These types of conditions that resolve naturally often are much shorter in duration than chronic progressive conditions. This leads to several important points. First, because of their faster onset of action, drugs that act symptomatically may be superior to disease-modifying drugs. Also, because these conditions resolve naturally, it is not as important that the natural progression of the disease be affected. Second, when evaluating the action of drugs, it is important to assess their effect early in the treatment process. If their effect is assessed too late, the disease may have almost resolved itself, and the drug may appear to be no different from a placebo.

20.8.4.3 *Exponential Model with a Nonzero Maximum Disease Status*

Some degenerative diseases deteriorate to a final concluding maximal state. These diseases can be modeled using a model for exponential growth (Figure 20.29a). The equation for this profile is

$$S_t = S_{ss} \cdot (1 - e^{-k_{prog} \cdot t}) \tag{20.38}$$

where k_{prog} is the first-order rate constant for disease progression, S_{ss} is the terminal status of the disease, and t is the time since the beginning of the disease.

The equation is modified because the time when the disease started is usually unknown and progression is assessed relative to when it is first measured (baseline) (Figure 20.29a). Thus, the equation for progression takes the form

$$S_t = S_0 \cdot e^{-k_{prog} \cdot t} + S_{ss} \cdot (1 - e^{-k_{prog} \cdot t}) \tag{20.39}$$

where S_0 is the measured baseline, and t is the time from the baseline measurement.

Symptomatic drug treatment is modeled by an additive term:

$$S_t = S_0 \cdot e^{-k_{prog} \cdot t} + S_{ss} \cdot (1 - e^{-k_{prog} \cdot t}) - E_t \tag{20.40}$$

Protective action can be modeled through an effect on k_{prog}:

$$S_t = S_0 \cdot e^{-(k_{prog} - E_t) \cdot t} + S_{ss} \cdot (1 - e^{-(k_{prog} - E_t) \cdot t}) \tag{20.41}$$

Figure 20.29b shows the typical profile of symptomatic and protective effects from this model.

Alternatively, the protective effect can be modeled through an effect on the terminal state of the disease:

$$S_t = S_0 \cdot e^{-k_{prog} \cdot t} + (S_{ss} - E_t) \cdot (1 - e^{-k_{prog} \cdot t})c \tag{20.42}$$

These models have been further adapted to incorporate placebo effects, which can be very important for some drugs, such as antidepressants. Other models have combined both symptomatic and protective effects. An alternative approach to modeling the effects of drugs on disease progression has been proposed based on the physiological turnover system [36] discussed at the beginning of this chapter. In this application, the biological quantity or response variable is the disease status (S_t). Under normal conditions of health, the disease status, which is a disease symptom or a biomarker used to assess the disease, is constant, as are k_{in} and k_{out} ($S = k_{in}/k_{out}$). Disease is assumed to disrupt homeostasis by decreasing either k_{in} or k_{out}. In effect, these disease progression models are essentially models I and II of the indirect effect models with ongoing modification of k_{in} and k_{out}. This approach was used to model the action of several hypoglycemic drugs in the treatment of type 2 diabetes [37].

20.8.4.4 *Weibull Function Models*

Weibull functions belong to the class of semiempirical models to describe disease progression. Pennypacker *et al.* [38] first proposed using the Weibull function to describe the progression of plant diseases. Although commonly employed in models of plant disease, Weibull functions have not been used widely to describe the time course of human disease. Freeman *et al.* [39] used this function to describe the progression from hepatitis C to cirrhosis. Similarly, Foucher *et al.* [40] implemented the Weibull function with a Markov chain to describe the progression of HIV through various states as life without disease, appearance of symptoms, disease progression, and eventual death. Owing to the inherent flexibility of Weibull functions, they can be used to describe a wide variety of diseases not easily described using more traditional functions.

The function was evaluated for numerical stability by Thal *et al.* [41]. The authors reported that the Weibull function was generally robust and allowed for a variety of inflection points that made this function suitable for describing a variety of disease progression scenarios such as those with relapsing/remitting behavior. The authors, however, also pointed out that if the parameters exhibited high correlation, simplification of the Weibull function could provide more reasonable confidence intervals for the parameters.

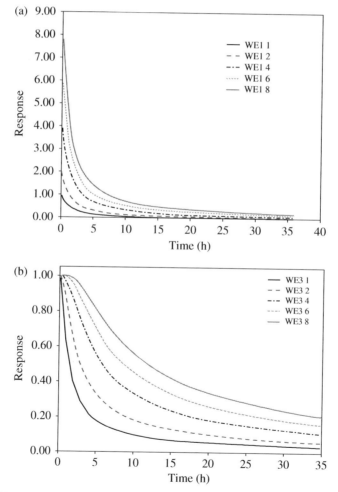

FIGURE 20.30 A simplified Weibull function where WEI1 is modified (a) and WEI3 is modified (b).

In order to maintain numerical plausibility, a modified Weibull function with three parameters may be implemented. This function can take on several characteristics depending on the value of the shape function parameter WE3. When all parameters are constrained to be positive and the parameter WE3 is at or below 1, the function mimics an exponential model, which describes a rapid fall off from a baseline value to a new lower plateau in the time course of response. However, as WE3 increases to values greater than 1, the function approximates a Weibull model, which allows for a delay in the onset of change before the function falls to a plateau. The rate of change of the score between baseline and plateau is controlled by the parameter WE2, and WE1 describes the maximum decrease from the baseline value. $S_i(t)$ is the Weibull function value at a given time "t."

$$S_i(t) = WE1 \cdot (1 - e^{-(WE2/t)^{WE3}})   \tag{20.43}$$

Depending on the Weibull parameter values, the function can either be used to describe a decay over time as shown in Figure 20.30 or it can be used to describe an increase in disease score over time to a new higher plateau. The effects of modifying WEI1 and WEI3 show the overall flexibility of this function.

PROBLEMS

20.1 The pharmacokinetics and pharmacodynamics of a new antihistamine are being evaluated in human volunteers. The response is assessed by measuring the inhibition of a wheal generated in response to a subcutaneous injection of histamine in the forearm. Volunteers received a 10-mg oral dose of the drug. Plasma concentration and response were measured at various times after the dose, and the data are provided in Table P20.1A.

TABLE P20.1A   Plasma Concentrations and Inhibition of the Wheal at Various Times After Administration of an Antihistamine

Time (h)	Cp (µg/L)	Response (% inhibition)
0	0	0.0
0.4	1.69	5.1
1	3.05	23.1
2	3.76	44.0
2.4	3.78	48.7
3	3.69	53.5
3.8	3.45	57.1
4	3.39	57.6
5	3.04	59.1
5.4	2.9	59.2
6	2.7	59.0
7	2.39	58.1
8	2.11	56.5
10	1.65	52.2
12	1.29	46.9
16	0.78	35.8
18	0.61	30.4

The data are to be used to assess the concentration–response relationship and identify a multiple dosing schedule.

(a) Plot the response as a function of Cp. If, for example, a response of 60% inhibition is desired, is it possible to identify therapeutic plasma concentrations?

(b) Previous studies have shown that the drug has a bioavailability of 0.5. The worksheet used for the analysis of oral data can be used to perform pharmacokinetic analysis on the data. It will be found that the drug has the following pharmacokinetic parameters: $Cl = 123$ L/h, $Vd = 1000$ L, and $k_a = 1$ h^{-1}.

Nonlinear regression analysis was used to model the data to the E_{max} model with an effect compartment. The following parameter values were obtained: $E_{max} = 100\%$, $EC_{50} = 2$ µg/L, and $k_{e0} = 0.4$ h^{-1}. As a result, the concentration of drug at the site of action could be estimated in units of plasma concentration. These data are shown in Table P20.1B. Plot the data and comment on the concentration–effect relationship.

Develop a multiple intravenous dosing regimen that will provide a steady-state peak effect of about 80% and a trough effect of about 40% inhibition of the wheal. Assume that at steady state, the effect compartment is in equilibrium with the plasma.

TABLE P20.1B   Concentrations at the Site of Action and Inhibition of the Wheal at Various Times After Administration of an Antihistamine

Time (h)	Ce (Cp equivalents) µg/L	Response (% inhibition)
0	0	0.0
0.4	0.11	5.1
1	0.6	23.1
2	1.57	44.0
2.4	1.9	48.7
3	2.3	53.5
3.8	2.66	57.1
4	2.72	57.6
5	2.89	59.1
5.4	2.9	59.2
6	2.88	59.0
7	2.77	58.1
8	2.6	56.5
10	2.18	52.2
12	1.77	46.9
16	1.11	35.8
18	0.87	30.4

20.2   The pharmacokinetics and pharmacodynamics of a new antihistamine are being evaluated in human volunteers. The response is assessed by measuring the inhibition of a wheal generated in response to a subcutaneous injection of histamine in the forearm. Volunteers received a 10-mg oral dose of the drug. Plasma concentration and response were measured at various times after the dose, and the data are provided in Table P20.2A.

TABLE P20.2A   Plasma Concentration and Response Data After an Oral Dose of an Antihistamine

Time (h)	Cp (µg/L)	Response (% inhibition)
0	0	0.0
0.4	1.69	5.1
1	3.05	23.1
2	3.76	44.0
2.4	3.78	48.7
3	3.69	53.5
3.8	3.45	57.1
4	3.39	57.6
5	3.04	59.1
5.4	2.9	59.2
6	2.7	59.0
7	2.39	58.1
8	2.11	56.5
10	1.65	52.2
12	1.29	46.9
16	0.78	35.8
18	0.61	30.4

The data are to be used to assess the concentration–response relationship and identify a multiple dosing schedule.

(a) Plot the response as a function of Cp. If, for example, a response of 60% inhibition is desired, is it possible to identify therapeutic plasma concentrations?

TABLE P20.2B   Drug Concentrations at the Site of Action and Response Data After an Oral Dose of an Antihistamine

Time (h)	Ce (Cp equivalents) µg/L	Response (% inhibition)
0	0	0.0
0.4	0.11	5.1
1	0.6	23.1
2	1.57	44.0
2.4	1.9	48.7
3	2.3	53.5
3.8	2.66	57.1
4	2.72	57.6
5	2.89	59.1
5.4	2.9	59.2
6	2.88	59.0
7	2.77	58.1
8	2.6	56.5
10	2.18	52.2
12	1.77	46.9
16	1.11	35.8
18	0.87	30.4

(b) Previous studies have shown that the drug has a bioavailability of 0.5. The work-sheet used for the analysis of oral data can be used to perform pharmacokinetic analysis on the data. It will be found that the drug has the following pharmacokinetic parameters: $Cl = 123$ L/h, $Vd = 1000$ L, and $k_a = 1$ h^{-1}.

Nonlinear regression analysis was used to model the data to the E_{max} model with an effect compartment. The following parameter values were obtained: $E_{max} = 100\%$, EC$_{50} = 2$ μg/L, and $k_{e0} = 0.4$ h^{-1}. As a result, the concentration of drug at the site of action could be estimated in units of plasma concentration. These data are shown in Table P20.2B. Plot the data and comment on the concentration–effect relationship.

Develop a multiple intravenous dosing regimen that will provide a steady-state peak effect of about 80% and a trough effect of about 40% inhibition of the wheal. Assume that at steady state, the effect compartment is in equilibrium with the plasma.

20.3 An intravenous dosing regimen of 25 mg of lipoamide every 8 h was developed in Section 20.7.2.1. The regimen was designed on pharmacokinetic principles, based on the belief that peaks and troughs of around 90 and 25 μg/L, respectively, are desirable. Based on lipoamide's reported bioavailability of 0.21, the equivalent oral dose would be about 120 mg. Prior to starting a clinical trial with lipoamide, a more thorough understanding of the dose–response relationship is desired so that optimum dosing regimens can be used in the trial. A small integrated PK/PD study was conducted in which response of lipoamide was measured by observing the reduction in body temperature. The data from a single patient are shown in Table P20.3.

TABLE P20.3   Plasma Concentration and Response After a Single Oral Dose (120 mg) of Lipoamide

Time (h)	Cp (μg/L)	Reduction in Temp °F
0	0.0	0
0.5	49.9	1.15
1	53.2	2.25
1.5	50.2	2.9
2	46.7	3.27
2.5	43.3	3.46
3	40.2	3.55
4	34.7	3.56
6	25.8	3.32
8	19.2	2.98
12	10.6	2.25
14	7.9	1.9

(a) Plot concentration and response against time. Plot response against concentration. Comment on these profiles.

Is it possible to determine the optimum concentration to produce a particular response? Suggest models that could be applied to the response data?

(b) Several mechanism-based models were evaluated to see if they would fit the data. The best fit of the data was obtained with indirect effect model I (inhibition of k_{in}), which has been used previously to model antipyretic activity [42]. Fever is assumed to be the result of the action of a response variable. Lipoamide's antipyretic activity is assumed to be the result of its inhibition of the synthesis of this substance.

The model used to fit the lipoamide data may be found at http://web.uri.edu/pharmacy/research/rosenbaum/sims/Model31.

Use the model to probe optimum dosing regimens for this drug. Ideally, a sustained antipyretic action is desired that will maintain the temperature at or below 100°F during the dosing interval. If possible, a dosing interval of either 12 or 24 h would be preferred to 8 h. More recent studies indicate that the incidence of side effects is minimal if the plasma concentration is below 300 μg/L. Can the dosing regimen based on pharmacokinetics (120 mg q 8 h) be improved upon?

20.4 A model to examine the action of a fictitious proton pump inhibitor, disolvprazole, is provided at the link http://web.uri.edu/pharmacy/research/rosenbaum/sims/Model30.

Open the model and go to the "Problem" page. Flip the switch to observe the effects of single doses. Observe the effects of changing the rate constants individually while maintaining all the others at their default value. Use the following values for each of the rate constants when they are altered individually:

k_{in}: 0.4, 0.8, and 1.6 mmol/h/h (Note that every time the graphs are cleared, the single-dose switch will have to be turned on again.)

k_{out}: 0.015, 0.03, and 0.06 h^{-1}

k_{irr}: 15, 30, and 60 L/mg/h

k: 0.17, 0.34, and 0.68 h^{-1}

Answer the following questions:

(a) When all the parameters have their default values, what is the maximum effect? What is the duration of action of the drug? How does it compare to the drug's elimination half-life?

(b) Summarize how each individual parameter affects the intensity and duration of the effect.

(c) How would you predict that inhibitors of the metabolism of the proton pump inhibitors would affect their therapeutic effect?

20.5 A drug is under development for the treatment of an autoimmune disease that appears to be mediated by a newly identified protein that has been called μ-in. Studies in animals show that the drug reduces the concentrations of the protein and that the symptoms of the disease (response), which is assessed using a biomarker, improve. Trials are being conducted in humans. Three separate oral doses of the drug (100, 50, and 25 mg) were administered to several patients with the autoimmune disease, and plasma concentrations of the drug and the fall in the level of the biomarker were measured at different times. The data from one subject are given in Table P20.5.

(a) Plot response against concentration for one of the doses. Comment on the profile and suggest possible explanations and ways in which it could be addressed in the modeling process.

TABLE P20.5   Plasma Drug Concentration (Cp) and Change in Concentration of a Biomarker (R) at Three-Dose Levels

	Dose					
	100 mg		50 mg		25 mg	
Time (h)	Cp (mg/L)	ΔR	Cp (mg/L)	ΔR	Cp (mg/L)	ΔR
0	0.000	0.0	0.000	0.0	0.000	0.0
3	2.919	−23.9	1.460	−22.8	0.730	−20.9
6	2.049	−42.7	1.024	−40.9	0.512	−37.9
10	0.979	−59.4	0.490	−56.3	0.245	−51.0
14	0.442	−68.3	0.221	−62.9	0.111	−54.5
15	0.362	−69.5	0.181	−63.2	0.090	−54.1
16	0.296	−70.1	0.148	−63.1	0.074	−53.3
17	0.242	−70.4	0.121	−62.6	0.060	−52.0
18	0.197	−70.2	0.099	−61.6	0.049	−50.4
24	0.059	−61.3	0.029	−49.2	0.015	−37.1
40	0.002	−20.0	0.001	−14.1	0.001	−9.6

(b) Plot response against time for the three doses on the same chart. Based on the profile, do you think that an effect compartment model or an indirect effect model would be more appropriate for these data?

(c) The drug's pharmacokinetic parameters are $k = 0.02\,\text{h}^{-1}$ and $V_d = 20\,\text{L}$. Based on pharmacokinetics alone, how frequently do you think the drug should be dosed? Revise your estimate of the dosing frequency based on the response–time profiles. How do you explain the difference between the two estimates?

20.6 A double-blind clinical trial was conducted on a new corticosteroid for the treatment of muscular dystrophy. Trial participants were split randomly into two groups. The test group took a 40-mg daily dose of the drug under study. The control group took placebo daily. Response was assessed from tests of muscle strength. After 8 months, the trial had to be discontinued due to the concern of toxicity. The average data for the test (drug) and placebo group are given in Table P20.6. Additionally, data are provided on the natural progression of the disease in the absence of intervention. Plot the data and comment on the effects of placebo and the drug relative to the natural progression. Do you think the drug has a protective or a symptomatic effect?

TABLE P20.6   Response (Change in Average Muscle Strength) at Various Times

Time (months)	Natural Progression	New Drug	Placebo
0	10.0	10.0	10.0
1	9.2	11.6	9.8
2	8.4	11.5	9.0
3	7.6	10.7	7.8
4	6.8	9.9	6.8
5	6.0	9.1	6.0
6	5.2	6.0	5.2
7	4.4	4.4	4.4

20.7 A totally new class of drug was evaluated for the treatment of Alzheimer's disease. The clinical status of each patient was evaluated using a dementia score based on the Alzheimer's Disease Assessment Scale, which tests memory, language, orientation, reason, praxis, and concentration. The total score could vary from 0 (no impairment) to 100 (maximum impairment). Response was evaluated as the mean change from baseline. The patients were enrolled in the trial and monitored over a 10-week period. At 10 weeks, half of the participants in the trial took an existing medication for Alzheimer's disease, and the remainder received the new treatment. The drugs were discontinued after 100 weeks. The average data for the test (drug) and control (existing medication) are given in Table P20.7. Additionally, data are provided on the natural progression of the disease in the absence of any interventions. Plot the data and comment on the effect of the new drug.

TABLE P20.7   Progression of Alzheimer's Disease in the Absence of Treatment, in the Presence of a New Drug, and in the Presence of Existing Therapy

Time (weeks)	Natural Progression	New Drug	Existing Therapy
0	1.0	1.0	1.0
2	1.8	1.8	1.8
6	3.4	3.4	3.4
10	5.0	5.0	5.0
15	7.0	6.9	−2.2
20	9.0	8.1	−14.5
24	10.6	8.8	−18.0
28	12.2	9.4	−18.3
32	13.8	9.9	−19.2
36	15.4	10.4	−15.8
42	19.8	11.2	−13.4
48	20.2	11.9	−11.1
56	23.4	12.9	−7.8
64	26.6	14.0	−4.7
72	29.8	15.0	−1.5
80	33.0	16.0	1.8
88	36.2	19.0	5.0
96	39.4	18.0	8.2
100	41.0	18.5	9.8
102	41.8	18.8	11.3
104	42.6	19.1	16.8
106	43.4	19.5	24.3
108	44.2	20.0	31.4
112	45.8	21.3	41.0
120	49.0	24.3	48.6

REFERENCES

1. Danhof, M., De Jongh, J., De Lange, E. C., Della Pasqua, O., Ploeger, B. A., and Voskuyl, R. A. (2007) Mechanism-based pharmacokinetic-pharmacodynamic modeling: biophase distribution,

receptor theory, and dynamical systems analysis, *Annu Rev Pharmacol Toxicol*, *47*, 357–400.

2. Mager, D. E., Wyska, E., and Jusko, W. J. (2003) Diversity of mechanism-based pharmacodynamic models, *Drug Metab Dispos*, *31*, 510–518.

3. Mager, D. E., Woo, S., and Jusko, W. J. (2009) Scaling pharmacodynamics from in vitro and preclinical animal studies to humans, *Drug Metab Pharmacokinet*, *24*, 16–24.

4. Sheiner, L. B., Stanski, D. R., Vozeh, S., Miller, R. D., and Ham, J. (1979) Simultaneous modeling of pharmacokinetics and pharmacodynamics: application to d-tubocurarine, *Clin Pharmacol Ther*, *25*, 358–371.

5. Lalonde, R. L. (1992) Pharmacodynamics, in *Applied Pharmacokinetics*, 2nd ed. (Evans, W. E., Schentag, J. J., and Jusko, W. J., Eds.), Applied Therapeutics, Vancouver, WA.

6. Holford, N. H., and Sheiner, L. B. (1982) Kinetics of pharmacologic response, *Pharmacol Ther*, *16*, 143–166.

7. Dayneka, N. L., Garg, V., and Jusko, W. J. (1993) Comparison of four basic models of indirect pharmacodynamic responses, *J Pharmacokinet Biopharm*, *21*, 457–478.

8. Sharma, A., and Jusko, W. J. (1996) Characterization of four basic models of indirect pharmacodynamic responses, *J Pharmacokinet Biopharm*, *24*, 611–635.

9. Sharma, A., and Jusko, W. J. (1998) Characteristics of indirect pharmacodynamic models and applications to clinical drug responses, *Br J Clin Pharmacol*, *45*, 229–239.

10. Krzyzanski, W., and Jusko, W. J. (1998) Mathematical formalism and characteristics of four basic models of indirect pharmacodynamic responses for drug infusions, *J Pharmacokinet Biopharm*, *26*, 385–408.

11. Jusko, W. J., and Ko, H. C. (1994) Physiologic indirect response models characterize diverse types of pharmacodynamic effects, *Clin Pharmacol Ther*, *56*, 406–419.

12. Mager, D. E., and Jusko, W. J. (2001) Pharmacodynamic modeling of time-dependent transduction systems, *Clin Pharmacol Ther*, *70*, 210–216.

13. Friberg, L. E., Henningsson, A., Maas, H., Nguyen, L., and Karlsson, M. O. (2002) Model of chemotherapy-induced myelosuppression with parameter consistency across drugs, *J Clin Oncol*, *20*, 4713–4721.

14. Leger, F., Loos, W. J., Bugat, R., Mathijssen, R. H., Goffinet, M., Verweij, J., Sparreboom, A., and Chatelut, E. (2004) Mechanism-based models for topotecan-induced neutropenia, *Clin Pharmacol Ther*, *76*, 567–578.

15. Wallin, J. E., Friberg, L. E., and Karlsson, M. O. (2009) Model-based neutrophil-guided dose adaptation in chemotherapy: evaluation of predicted outcome with different types and amounts of information, *Basic Clin Pharmacol Toxicol*, *106*, 234–242.

16. Wallin, J. E., Friberg, L. E., and Karlsson, M. O. (2009) A tool for neutrophil guided dose adaptation in chemotherapy, *Comput Methods Programs Biomed*, *93*, 283–291.

17. Ricketts, C., Jacobs, A., and Cavill, I. (1975) Ferrokinetics and erythropoiesis in man: the measurement of effective erythropoiesis, ineffective erythropoiesis and red cell lifespan using 59Fe, *Br J Haematol*, *31*, 1, 65–75.

18. Ly, J., Marticorena, R., and Donnelly, S. (2004) Red blood cell survival in chronic renal failure, *Am J Kidney Dis*, *44*, 4, 715–719.

19. Krzyzanski, W., and Ruixo, J. J. P. (2012) Lifespan based indirect response models, *J Pharmacokinet Pharmacodyn*, *39*, 1, 109–123.

20. Budha, N. R., Kovar, A., and Meibohm, B. (2011) Comparative performance of cell life span and cell transit models for describing erythropoietic, *Drug Effects AAPS J*, *13*, 4, 650–661.

21. Wu, L., Mould, D. R., Perez Ruixo, J. J., and Doshi, S. (2015) Assessment of hemoglobin responsiveness to epoetin alfa in patients on hemodialysis using a population pharmacokinetic pharmacodynamic model, *J Clin Pharmacol*, *55*, 10, 1157–1166.

22. Porchet, H. C., Benowitz, N. L., and Sheiner, L. B. (1988) Pharmacodynamic model of tolerance: application to nicotine, *J Pharmacol Exp Ther*, *244*, 231–236.

23. Shi, J., Benowitz, N. L., Denaro, C. P., and Sheiner, L. B. (1993) Pharmacokinetic–pharmacodynamic modeling of caffeine: tolerance to pressor effects, *Clin Pharmacol Ther*, *53*, 6–14.

24. Bauer, J. A., and Fung, H. L. (1994) Pharmacodynamic models of nitroglycerin-induced hemodynamic tolerance in experimental heart failure, *Pharm Res*, *11*, 816–823.

25. Gårdmark, M. L., Ekblom, M., Bouw, R., and Hammarlund-Udenaes, M. (1993) Quantification of effect delay and acute tolerance development to morphine in the rat, *J Pharmacol Exp Ther*, *267*, 3, 1061–1067.

26. Ihmsen, H., Albrecht, S., Hering, W., Schüttler, J., and Schwilden, H. (2004) Modeling acute tolerance to the EEG effect of two benzodiazepines, *Br J Clin Pharmacol*, *57*, 2, 153–161.

27. Gardmark, M., Brynne, L., Hammarlund-Udenaes, M., and Karlsson, M. O. (1999) Interchangeability and predictive performance of empirical tolerance models, *Clin Pharmacokinet*, *36*, 145–167.

28. Cox, E. H., Kuipers, J. A., and Danhof, M. (1998) Pharmacokinetic-pharmacodynamic modeling of the EEG effect of alfentanil in rats: assessment of rapid functional adaptation, *Br J Pharmacol*, *124*, 1534–1540.

29. Madia, P. A., Dighe, S. V., Sirohi, S., Walker, E. A., and Yoburn, B. C. (2009) Dosing protocol and analgesic efficacy determine opioid tolerance in the mouse, *Psychopharmacol (Berl)*, *207*, 413–422.

30. Sharma, A., Ebling, W. F., and Jusko, W. J. (1998) Precursor-dependent indirect pharmacodynamic response model for tolerance and rebound phenomena, *J Pharm Sci*, *87*, 1577–1584.

31. Ferron, G. M., McKeand, W., and Mayer, P. R. (2001) Pharmacodynamic modeling of pantoprazole's irreversible effect on gastric acid secretion in humans and rats, *J Clin Pharmacol*, *41*, 149–156.

32. Chan, P. L., and Holford, N. H. (2001) Drug treatment effects on disease progression, *Annu Rev Pharmacol Toxicol*, *41*, 625–659.

33. Holford, N. H., Chan, P. L., Nutt, J. G., Kieburtz, K., and Shoulson, I. (2006) Disease progression and pharmacodynamics in Parkinson disease: evidence for functional protection with levodopa and other treatments, *J Pharmacokinet Pharmacodyn*, *33*, 281–311.

34. Griggs, R. C., Moxley, R. T., 3rd, Mendell, J. R., Fenichel, G. M., Brooke, M. H., Pestronk, A., and Miller, J. P. (1991) Prednisone in Duchenne dystrophy: a randomized, controlled trial defining the time course and dose response. Clinical investigation of Duchenne dystrophy group, *Arch Neurol*, *48*, 383–388.

35. Mould, D. R. (2007) Developing models of disease progression, in *Pharmacometrics: the Science of Quantitative Pharmacology*, (Ette, E. I., and Williams, P. J., Eds.), pp. 547–581, Wiley, Hoboken, NJ.

36. Post, T. M., Freijer, J. I., DeJongh, J., and Danhof, M. (2005) Disease system analysis: basic disease progression models in degenerative disease, *Pharm Res*, *22*, 1038–1049.

37. De Winter, W., DeJongh, J., Post, T., Ploeger, B., Urquhart, R., Moules, I., Eckland, D., and Danhof, M. (2006) A mechanism-based disease progression model for comparison of long-term effects of pioglitazone, metformin and gliclazide on disease processes underlying type 2 diabetes mellitus, *J Pharmacokinet Pharmacodyn*, *33*, 313–343.

38. Pennypacker, S. P., Knoble, H. D., Antle, C. E., and Madden, V. (1980) A flexible model for studying plant disease progression, *Phytopathology*, *70*, 232–235.

39. Freeman, A. J., Law, M. G., Kaldor, J. M., and Dore, G. J. (2003) Predicting progression to cirrhosis in chronic hepatitis C virus infection, *J Viral Hepatol*, *10*, 285–293.

40. Foucher, Y., Mathieu, E., Saint-Pierre, P., Durand, J. F., and Daures, J. P. (2005) A semi-Markov model based on generalized Weibull distribution with an illustration for HIV disease, *Biom J*, *47*, 825–833.

41. Thal, W. M., Campbell, C. L., and Madden, L. V. (1984) Sensitivity of Weibull model parameter estimates to variation in simulated disease progression data, *Phytopathology*, *74*, 1425–1430.

42. Garg, V., and Jusko, W. J. (1994) Pharmacodynamic modeling of nonsteroidal anti-inflammatory drugs: antipyretic effect of ibuprofen, *Clin Pharmacol Ther*, *55*, 87–88.

APPENDIX A

REVIEW OF EXPONENTS AND LOGARITHMS

Sara E. Rosenbaum

A.1   EXPONENTS

When a number is expressed in exponential notation, it takes the following form:

$$\text{number} = \text{base}^{\text{exponent}}$$

The following are examples of exponential expressions using different bases:

$$2^3, 6^3, 10^6, 15^8, e^3, 20^2$$

Basic Pharmacokinetics and Pharmacodynamics: An Integrated Textbook and Computer Simulations,
Second Edition. Edited by Sara E. Rosenbaum.
© 2017 John Wiley & Sons, Inc. Published 2017 by John Wiley & Sons, Inc.

Exponents to the base 10 and base e are the most common, and the base 10 form is used most frequently in everyday life. Examples include

$$10^6 = 1,000,000$$
$$10^3 = 1000$$
$$10^1 = 10$$
$$10^0 = 1$$
$$10^{-1} = 0.1$$

The base e form is used most frequently in the mathematical sciences, including pharmacokinetics. This exponent form is introduced into a formula when calculus is used to integrate equations.

$$e = 2.718$$

Examples of exponents to the base e:

$$e^2 = 7.389$$
$$e^1 = 2.718$$
$$e^{0.639} = 2$$
$$e^0 = 1 \quad \textit{important to know}$$
$$e^{-1} = 0.368 \,(1/e \text{ or } 1/2.718)$$
$$e^{-\infty} = 0 \quad \textit{important to know}$$

In pharmacokinetics, it is necessary to know how to use a calculator to solve exponent expressions such as $e^{6.8}$, $e^{-0.43}$, and $e^{-0.3 \times 2}$. (*answers*: 897.8, 0.651, and 0.549).

A.2 LOGARITHMS: LOG AND LN

The *logarithm* of a number is the power or exponent when that number is converted into exponential form. The power or exponent will clearly depend on the base. If the base 10 is used, the logarithm is known as the *log*. Examples are provided in Table A.1.

When the base e is used, the logarithm is known as the *natural logarithm* or *ln*. Examples are provided in Table A.2.

TABLE A.1   Examples of Base 10 Logarithms (Logs)

Number	Exponential Form	Log
1000,000	10^6	6
100	10^2	2
40	$10^{1.6}$	1.6
2	$10^{0.301}$	0.301
10	10^1	1
1	10^0	0
0.1	10^{-1}	−1

TABLE A.2   Examples of Natural Logarithms (Lns)

Number	Exponential Form	Ln
7.389	e^2	2
2	$e^{0.693}$	0.693
2.718	e^1	1
1	e^0	0
0.368	e^{-1}	-1

When the base 10 logarithm scale is used for expressions containing e, it may be necessary to convert a log to an ln. This is done using the factor 2.303:

$$\ln X = \log X \times 2.303$$

Thus, if $\log 5 = 0.6989$, then

$$\ln 5 = 0.6989 \times 2.303 = 1.609$$

If $\log 2 = 0.3010$, then

$$\ln 2 = 0.3010 \times 2.303 = 0.693$$

Generally, there is no longer any reason to use the base 10 logarithms in pharmacokinetics. They were used in the past because it was the most convenient scale to use on semilogarithmic graph paper to plot pharmacokinetic data. Now, data can be plotted easily using spreadsheets on computers, where the natural logarithm scale can be used as easily as the base 10 scale.

A.3   PERFORMING CALCULATIONS IN THE LOGARITHMIC DOMAIN

A.3.1   Multiplication

To multiply two numbers, they can be converted to logarithm form and added. Consider $10^2 \times 10^3$:

$$\begin{array}{cc} \textit{Nonlog domain} & \textit{Log domain} \\ 100 \times 1000 = 100,000 & 2 + 3 = 5 \end{array}$$

Thus,

$$10^2 \times 10^3 = 10^{2+3} = 10^5$$

$B \cdot C \cdot D$:

$$\ln(B \cdot C \cdot D) = \ln B + \ln C + \ln D$$

3×5:

$$\ln(3 \times 5) = \ln 3 + \ln 5 = 1.10 + 1.61 = 2.71 \quad {}^*\text{anti-ln}(2.71) = 15$$

*The conversion from the logarithm domain back to the nonlogarithm domain is referred to as taking an antilogarithm.

$B \cdot e^3$:

$$\ln(B \times e^3) = \ln B + \ln e^3 = \ln B + 3$$

A.3.2 Division

To divide two numbers, they can be converted to the logarithm domain and subtracted.
B/A:

$$\ln(B/A) = \ln B - \ln A$$

3/5:

$$\ln(3/5) = \ln 3 - \ln 5 = 1.10 - 1.61 = -0.51 \quad \text{anti-ln}(-0.51) = 0.6$$

A.3.3 Reciprocals

The reciprocal of a number is the negative ln of the number.

$$\ln(1/A) = -\ln(A)$$
$$\ln(B/A) = -\ln(A/B)$$
$$Proof: -\ln(A/B) = -(\ln A - \ln B) = \ln B - \ln A = \ln(B/A)$$
$$\ln(1/10) = -\ln 10 = -2.303 \quad \text{anti-ln}(-2.303) = 0.1$$

A.3.4 Exponents

To determine the solution of an exponential expression, in the logarithmic domain, exponents are multiplied.
A^b:

$$\ln A^b = b \cdot \ln A$$

8^2:

$$\ln 8^2 = 2 \cdot \ln 8 = 2 \times 2.08 = 4.16 \quad \text{anti-ln}(4.16) = 64$$

A.4 CALCULATIONS USING EXPONENTIAL EXPRESSIONS AND LOGARITHMS

Example A.1   Solve for x in the following expressions: (a) $e^x = 3$, (b) $e^x = 23$, (c) $e^x = 106$, and (d) $e^x = 563$.

Solution

(a) $e^x = 3$
$\quad x = \ln 3 = 1.10$
(b) 3.14

(c) 4.66

(d) 6.33

Example A.2 Solve for x in the following expressions: (a) $\ln x = 4.3$, (b) $\ln x = -1.4$, and (c) $\ln x = -0.3$.

Solution

(a) $\ln x = 4.3$

$x = e^{4.3}$

$x = 73.7$

(b) 0.247

(c) 0.741

Example A.3 Evaluate $e^{-1.3}$.

Solution

$$e^{-1.3} = 0.273$$

Example A.4 Find the value of k in the following expression: $e^{-1.3k} = 2$.

Solution Take the logarithms

$$k \cdot \ln e^{-1.3} = \ln 2$$
$$k \cdot (-1.3) = 0.693$$
$$-1.3\,k = 0.693$$
$$k = -\frac{0.693}{1.3} = -0.533$$

Example A.5 A common expression in pharmacokinetics is $Cp = Cp_0 \cdot e^{-kt}$. Evaluate Cp when $Cp_0 = 35$, $k = 1.5$, and $t = 2$.

Solution

$$Cp = 35e^{-1.5 \times 2} = 35e^{-3} = 35 \times 0.0498 = 1.74$$

Example A.6 Given that $Y = Y_0 \cdot e^{-k}$, convert the equation to the ln domain.

Solution

$$\ln Y = \ln Y_0 - kt \qquad\qquad (A.1)$$

Expression (A.1) is the equation for a straight line ($y = a - bx$) with a slope of $-k$ and an intercept of $\ln Y_0$ (Figure A.1).

Example A.7 Given that $Y = Y_0 \cdot e^{-kt}$, calculate k given that $Y_1 = 66.3$ mg, $t_1 = 2$ h, $Y_2 = 29.2$ mg, and $t_2 = 6$ h.

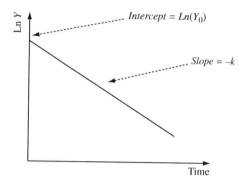

FIGURE A.1   Plot of ln Y against time.

Solution $k = -$ slope of the plot of ln Y against time:

$$\text{slope} = \frac{\ln \ Y_1 - \ln Y_2}{t_1 - t_2} \quad \text{or} \quad \frac{\ln(Y_1/Y_2)}{t_1 - t_2}$$

$$= \frac{\ln(29.2/66.3)}{6 - 2}$$

$$= -0.205$$

$$k = -\text{slope} = 0.205 \ \text{h}^{-1}$$

Example A.8   Given that $Y = Y_0 \cdot e^{-kt}$, calculate the intercept, Y_0.

Solution   Use either data pairs to substitute in the basic equation (A.1):

$$\ln(66.3) = \ln Y_0 - 0.205 \times 2 \quad \text{or} \quad \ln(29.2) = \ln Y_0 - 0.205 \times 6$$

$$4.19 = \ln Y_0 - 0.41 \quad \text{or} \quad 3.37 = \ln Y_0 - 1.23$$

$$\ln Y_0 = 4.19 + 0.41 = 4.6 \qquad \ln Y_0 = 3.37 + 1.23 = 4.6$$

$$Y_0 = 100 \qquad\qquad Y_0 = 100$$

A.5   DECAY FUNCTION: e^{-kt}

This is an extremely important expression in pharmacokinetics and is utilized in almost all pharmacokinetic equations. It is important to understand this expression and *not* be intimidated by it. It is actually very simple, and a little time spent considering and understanding this function will demystify all pharmacokinetic equations and help prevent calculation errors.

$$e^{-kt} \ \text{is a} \ decay \ function$$

where k is a constant, and t is the time, which starts at zero and increases to ∞.

$$\text{At } t = 0 : \quad e^{-kt} = 1$$

$$\text{At } t = \infty : \quad e^{-kt} = 0$$

That is, *as time increases, e^{-kt} decays from 1 to zero*. The rate constant k controls the speed with which e^{-kt} decays: The larger the value of k, the more rapidly the expression decays toward zero.

A.6 GROWTH FUNCTION: $1 - e^{-kt}$

The growth function is also frequently encountered in pharmacokinetics and runs counter to the decay function (e^{-kt}):

$$1 - e^{-kt} \text{ is a } growth \text{ } function$$

where k is a constant, and t is the time, which starts at zero and increases to ∞.

$$\text{At } t = 0: \quad (1 - e^{-kt}) = 0$$
$$\text{At } t = \infty: \quad (1 - e^{-kt}) = 1$$

That is, *as time increases, $1 - e^{-kt}$ grows from zero to 1*. The rate constant k controls the speed with which the expression grows toward 1. The larger the value of k, the more rapidly the expression grows toward 1.

A.7 DECAY FUNCTION IN PHARMACOKINETICS

$$Cp = A \cdot e^{-kt}$$

This is *the* most important *mathematical* equation in pharmacokinetics. In basic pharmacokinetics, it appears in the following forms:

$$\text{A} \cdot Cp = A \cdot e^{-kt}.$$
$$\text{B} \cdot Cp = A \cdot e^{-k_1 t} + B \cdot e^{-k_2 t}, \quad \text{where } k_1 > k_2.$$
$$\text{C} \cdot Cp = A \cdot (1 - e^{-kt}).$$
$$\text{D} \cdot Cp = A \cdot (e^{-k_1 t} - e^{-k_2 t}), \quad \text{where } k_2 > k_1.$$

These equations represent the fundamental form of the pharmacokinetic equations associated with an intravenous bolus injection in a one-compartment model (A); an intravenous bolus injection in a two-compartment model (B); constant continuous drug input in a one-compartment model (C); and first-order drug absorption in a one-compartment model (D).

If the expressions e^{-kt} and $1 - e^{-kt}$ are understood, equations A to D all become very simple.

Example A.9 Evaluate equations A through D above for Cp at time zero and infinity.

Solution

$$\text{A} \cdot t = 0, Cp = A; t = \infty, Cp = 0$$
$$\text{B} \cdot t = 0, Cp = A + B; t = \infty, Cp = 0$$
$$\text{C} \cdot t = 0, Cp = 0; t = \infty, Cp = A$$
$$\text{D} \cdot t = 0, Cp = 0; t = \infty, Cp = 0$$

Example A.10   In equations B and D, which exponent term gets to zero first?

Solution   The one with the larger value of k: Equation B. k_1; Equation D. k_2.

Example A.11   Write out the shortened forms of equations B and D when the first exponent term has reached zero.

Solution

$$B \quad Cp = B \cdot e^{-k_2 t};$$
$$D \quad Cp = A \cdot e^{-k_1 t}.$$

Both are simple expressions of monoexponential decay.

PROBLEMS

A.1   The following equation, $Cp = 100e^{-0.347 \times t}$, represents the monoexponential decay of the plasma concentration after an intravenous dose of a drug, where the plasma concentration (Cp) is mg/L, t is time (h), and 0.347 h^{-1} is the first-order elimination rate constant. Evaluate for Cp when

  (a) $t = 0$ h
  (b) $t = 2$ h
  (c) $t = 6$ h
  (d) $t = 8$ h
  (e) $t = 10$ h
  (f) $t = 14$ h
  (g) $t = 20$ h

    What are the ranges of Cp from time zero to infinity?

A.2   The equation $Cp = 100e^{-1.386 \times t}$ represents the monoexponential decay of the plasma concentration after an intravenous dose of a drug, where the plasma concentration (Cp) is mg/L, t is time (h), and 1.386 h^{-1} is the first-order elimination rate constant. Evaluate for Cp when:

  (a) $t = 0$ h
  (b) $t = 0.5$ h
  (c) $t = 1.5$ h
  (d) $t = 2$ h
  (e) $t = 2.5$ h
  (f) $t = 3.5$ h
  (g) $t = 5$ h

    What are the ranges of Cp from zero to infinity? How do these answers compare to the answers in Problem A.1, and what accounts for the difference?

A.3   The equation $Cp = 100(1 - e^{-0.347 \times t})$ represents the growth in the plasma concentration when a drug is administered at a constant continuous rate (e.g., during an intravenous infusion), where the plasma concentration (Cp) is mg/L, t is time (h), and 0.347 h^{-1} is the first-order elimination rate constant. Evaluate for Cp when:

  (a) $t = 0$ h
  (b) $t = 2$ h

    (c) $t = 6$ h

    (d) $t = 8$ h

    (e) $t = 10$ h

    (f) $t = 14$ h

    (g) $t = 20$ h

    What are the ranges of Cp from zero to infinity?

A.4 The equation $Cp = 100 \, (1 - e^{-1.386 \times t})$ represents the growth in the plasma concentration when a drug is administered at a constant continuous rate (e.g., during an intravenous infusion), where the plasma concentration (Cp) is mg/L, t is time (h), and $1.386 \, \text{h}^{-1}$ is the first-order elimination rate constant. Evaluate for Cp when:

    (a) $t = 0$ h

    (b) $t = 0.5$ h

    (c) $t = 1.5$ h

    (d) $t = 2$ h

    (e) $t = 2.5$ h

    (f) $t = 3.5$ h

    (g) $t = 5$ h

    What are the ranges of Cp from zero to infinity? How do these answers compare to the answers in Problem A.3, and what accounts for the difference?

A.5 Given that $Cp = 23e^{-0.3t}$:

    (a) Convert the equation for the logarithm domain.

    (b) Draw a plot of the shape you would expect from a plot of $\ln Cp$ versus t.

A.6 Calculate the slope given that $[\ln 2 - \ln(0.5)]/(1 - 15) = \text{slope}$.

A.7 $C = C_0 \cdot e^{-kt}$, where C is a variable that changes with time, C_0 is C at time $= 0$, k is a constant, and t is time. Given that $C = 22$ mg/L at $t = 2$ h and $C = 5$ mg/L at $t = 10$ h:

    (a) Determine k.

    (b) Determine C_0.

APPENDIX B

RATES OF PROCESSES

Sara E. Rosenbaum

B.1 INTRODUCTION

Pharmacokinetics is the study of the manner in which drug concentrations in the body change over time after the administration of a dose. The plasma concentration (Cp) of the drug is usually the focus in pharmacokinetic studies because it is fairly easy to obtain samples of plasma and analyze them to determine the drug concentration. A goal in pharmacokinetics is to develop fairly simple equations to describe how the plasma concentration changes with time. Clearly, the plasma concentration (dependent variable) at any time will depend on the:

- Dose administered (a constant in a specific situation)
- Time the sample was taken (this is the independent variable)

Basic Pharmacokinetics and Pharmacodynamics: An Integrated Textbook and Computer Simulations,
Second Edition. Edited by Sara E. Rosenbaum.
© 2017 John Wiley & Sons, Inc. Published 2017 by John Wiley & Sons, Inc.

Thus, the pharmacokinetic equation will express the dependent variable as a function of dose and time and generally can be written as:

$$Cp = \text{dose (function) time}$$

These equations will have to include expressions for how the underlying processes of drug absorption, distribution, and elimination (metabolism and excretion) (ADME) influence the plasma concentration–time relationship. As discussed in this book, almost all processes in pharmacokinetics are either first or zero order. Thus, pharmacokinetic equations must incorporate mathematical expressions for the rates of zero- or first-order processes in ADME when appropriate. The equations and characteristics of zero- and first-order processes are presented in this appendix.

B.2   ORDER OF A RATE PROCESS

The rate of many chemical and physical processes, such as chemical reactions, radioactive decay, and the draining of liquid from a tank, is proportional to the concentration or amount of one or more of the participants or dependent variables. In pharmacokinetics, which involves primarily simple zero- and first-order processes, the order of the process can be considered to be the number of participants involved in this relationship.

B.3   ZERO-ORDER PROCESSES

The rate of a zero-order process is *constant* and *independent* of the dependent variable (none of the reactants control the rate). Examples of zero-order processes include filling a car with gas, removing water from a boat or basement using a pump, and the administration of a drug by an intravenous infusion.

Consider a tank being filled with water by an electric pump:

$$\text{rate of filling} = k_0(\text{L/h}) \tag{B.1}$$

where k_0 represents the rate of filling. It is a constant controlled by the pump setting. The volume of water (Y) is the dependent variable. As time increases, the filling process proceeds, the volume of water in the tank changes (increases), but the rate of filling does not change.

B.3.1   Equation for Zero-Order Filling

- Let the volume of water in the tank be Y.
- Let the initial volume be Y_0 (e.g., 5 mL).
- Let the rate of filling be k_0 (e.g., 10 mL/min).

What volume of water (Y) is in the vessel after 15 min of filling?

Fifteen minutes of filling at a rate of 10 mL/min will add $15 \times 10 = 150$ mL of water. The tank already contained 5 mL, so the total volume now is $150 + 5 = 155$ mL of water.

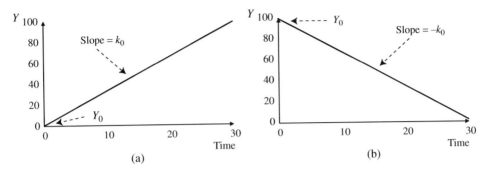

FIGURE B.1   Plot of volume (Y) against time for zero-order fill (a) and zero-order emptying (b) processes.

More generally, for a zero-order process,

$$Y = Y_0 + k_0 \cdot t \qquad (B.2)$$

Thus, a plot of Y as a function of time will yield a straight line with a slope equal to the rate of filling, k_0 and an intercept equal to the initial volume, Y_0 (Figure B.1a). In the graph Y_0 is shown as zero.

B.3.2   Equation for Zero-Order Emptying

Similarly, it can be shown that for zero-order emptying:

$$Y = Y_0 - k_0 \cdot t \qquad (B.3)$$

Equation (B.3) is also the equation of a straight line. In this case, the slope of the line (the rate) is negative (Figure B.1b).

Example B.1   A tank containing 100 L of a liquid is being emptied by a pump which is set at 5 L/h. How many liters would remain after 10 h?

Solution

$$Y = Y_0 - k_0 \cdot t$$
$$= 100 - 5 \times 10 = 50 \text{ L}$$

Thus, after 10 h, 50 L of liquid would remain.

B.3.3   Time for Zero-Order Emptying to Go to 50% Completion

At 50% completion of a zero-order emptying process, the amount (volume) is half the original amount: $Y = Y_0/2$. Substituting in equation (B.3) yields

$$\frac{Y_0}{2} = Y_0 - k_0 \cdot t$$
$$\frac{Y_0}{2} = k_0 \cdot t \qquad (B.4)$$
$$t = \frac{Y_0}{k_0 \cdot 2}$$

Thus, the time for a zero-order process to go to 50% completion is dependent on the zero-order rate constant k_0 and the initial amount of the dependent variable. The larger the initial quantity, the longer it takes for it to fall by 50%.

B.4 FIRST-ORDER PROCESSES

There are many examples of first-order processes in both nature and medicine. These include radioactive decay, natural degradation of substances, drug absorption from the gastrointestinal tract, and the elimination of drugs from the body. The growth of money in a savings account is type of a first-order process. A first-order process is characterized by a rate that is proportional to the quantity either growing or shrinking under its influence (the dependent variable).

For example, consider a tank full of water being drained through a hole in the bottom. The emptying process is driven by the volume of water in the tank (more specifically, the height of the water). The volume or height of the water is also the quantity being affected by the process—it is the dependent variable. As the process continues, the volume and the height decrease, so the rate of draining also decreases. The rate of a first-order process changes in direct proportion to changes in the dependent variable. Mathematically,

$$\text{rate of draining} \propto Y (\text{volume of water})$$

$$-\frac{dY}{dt} \propto Y$$

$$-\frac{dY}{dt} = k \cdot Y \tag{B.5}$$

where k is a constant of proportionality or **first order rate constant,** with the units t^{-1}. The rate of this process is dependent on the amount of a single dependent variable (Y) and as a result, it is a first-order process.

B.4.1 Equation for a First-Order Process

The expression for the rate of emptying is given by equation (B.5). To get an expression for the dependent variable Y, it is necessary to integrate this equation. Rearranging and integrating the equation yield

$$\frac{dY}{Y} = -k \cdot dt \tag{B.6}$$

$$\int_0^\infty \frac{dY}{Y} = -k \int_0^\infty dt \tag{B.7}$$

$$\ln Y = -kt + c \tag{B.8}$$

when $t = 0$, $Y = Y_0$; thus,

$$\ln Y = \ln Y_0 - kt$$
$$Y = Y_0 \cdot e^{-kt} \tag{B.9}$$

Thus, Y decays monoexponentially from Y_0 at time $= 0$ to zero at $t = \infty$. The relationship between the dependent variable (Y) and time is shown in Figure B.2.

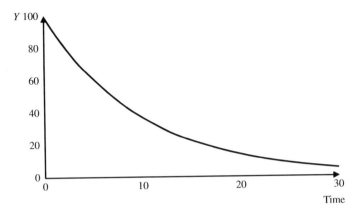

FIGURE B.2 Plot of volume (Y) against time for a first-order emptying process.

Example B.2 Assume that a tank with an initial volume of 100 mL is being emptied by a first-order process with a rate constant of 0.1 h^{-1}. Determine the volume at 2, 3.5, 7, and 10 h.

Solution

Let $Y_0 = 100$ mL and $k = 0.1$ h^{-1}.
Starting conditions: At $t = 0$, $Y = Y_0 = 100$.
Finishing conditions: At $t = \infty$, $Y = 0$.
When $t = 2$ h, $Y = 100^{-0.1 \times 2}$ and $Y = 81.9$ mL.
When $t = 3.5$ h, $Y = 70.5$ mL.
When $t = 7$ h, $Y = 50$ mL.
When $t = 10$ h, $Y = 36.8$ mL.

B.4.2 Time for 50% Completion: the Half-Life

The half-life ($t_{1/2}$) of a first order process is defined as the time it takes for the process to go to 50% completion: When $t = t_{1/2}$, $Y = Y_0/2$. Substituting into equation (B.15) yields

$$\frac{Y_0}{2} = Y_0 \cdot e^{-kt_{1/2}} \tag{B.10}$$

$$\frac{1}{2} = e^{-kt_{1/2}} \tag{B.11}$$

Taking the reciprocal of each side gives us

$$2 = e^{kt_{1/2}} \tag{B.12}$$

and taking natural logarithms gives us

$$\ln 2 = kt_{1/2} \tag{B.13}$$

TABLE B.1   Comparison of Key Characteristics of Zero- and First-Order Processes

	Zero-Order Decay Process	First-Order Decay Process
Equation	$Y = Y_0 - kt$	$Y = Y_0 \cdot e^{-kt}$
Rate: dY/dt	k_0	$Y \cdot k$
Shape of relationship between Y and time	Straight line	Exponential curve
Time for original quantity to fall by 50%	$Y_0/(2 \cdot k_0)$	$0.693/k^a$
Time for process to go to completion	Y_0/k_0	$3–5\ t_{1/2}{}^a$

^{a}Covered in the next section.

Rearranging, we have

$$t_{1/2} = \frac{0.693}{k} \tag{B.14}$$

Note: The time it takes a first-order process to go to 50% completion is independent of the initial value of the dependent variable.

The $t_{1/2}$ is a reciprocal form of k. Thus, large values of k are associated with small values of $t_{1/2}$, and vice versa. They are constants for a process, and both reflect the rate at which the process proceeds. Note that in the previous example, the half-life of the process is 7 h (0.693/0.1), and after 7 h the initial volume had fallen by half.

B.5   COMPARISON OF ZERO- AND FIRST-ORDER PROCESSES

Table B.1 compares key characteristics for zero- and first-order processes.

B.6   DETAILED EXAMPLE OF FIRST-ORDER DECAY IN PHARMACOKINETICS

B.6.1   Equations and Semilogarithmic Plots

There are many examples of first-order processes in pharmacokinetics, including drug absorption, distribution, and elimination. This example concentrates on first-order elimination. Consider the situation where a dose of a drug is injected as an intravenous bolus. Thus, the entire dose is injected at once. In this example, it is assumed that the only process that affects the amount of drug in the body is elimination, a first-order process. At time zero, the entire dose is put into the body. Thereafter, the amount of drug in the body (Ab) is solely under the influence of first-order elimination.

When the amount in the body is large at time zero, the rate of elimination is relatively high. But as the amount decreases due to elimination, the rate of the process will also decrease. As a result, the relationship between the amount in the body and time is not linear (Figure B.3a).

The amount of drug in the body decays according to the equation for first-order decay:

$$Ab = Ab_0 \cdot e^{-kt} \quad \text{or} \quad Ab = \text{dose} \cdot e^{-kt} \tag{B.15}$$

where Ab_0 is the initial amount of drug in the body, which is equal to the dose, and k is first-order rate constant for elimination.

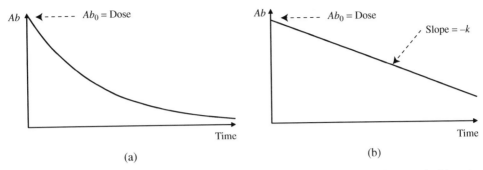

FIGURE B.3 Plot of amount of drug in the body (*Ab*) against time on a linear scale (a) and a semilogarithmic scale (b).

Semilogarithmic Plot of Dependent Variable (Ab) Versus Time. Taking the natural logarithms of equation (B.15), we have

$$\ln Ab = \ln(Ab_0) - kt \quad \text{or} \quad \ln Ab = \ln(\text{dose}) - kt \tag{B.16}$$

These are the equations of a straight line. Thus, a plot of $\ln(Ab)$ against time yields a straight line of slope $(-k)$, and at the intercept, $Ab = Ab_0$ or dose (Figure B.3b). The slope may be calculated as follows:

$$\text{slope} = \frac{\ln(Ab_1/Ab_2)}{t_1 - t_2} \tag{B.17}$$

The elimination rate constant can be determined:

$$k = -\text{slope} = \frac{\ln(Ab_1/Ab_2)}{t_2 - t_1} \tag{B.18}$$

B.6.2 Half-Life

As shown previously,

$$t_{1/2} = \frac{0.693}{k}$$

The $t_{1/2}$ is a reciprocal form of k. They are constants for a particular drug, and both reflect the rate at which a drug is eliminated from the body. Obviously, if k is high (i.e., $t_{1/2}$ is short), elimination (decay) will proceed rapidly. If k is low (i.e., $t_{1/2}$ is long), the drug will be eliminated slowly (slow decay). Because the half-life has much more conceptual meaning than the rate constant, it is more commonly used clinically when discussing a drug's pharmacokinetics.

B.6.3 Fraction or Percent Completion of a First-Order Process Using First-Order Elimination as an Example

It is often important in pharmacokinetics to get an approximate idea of how long it takes for first-order processes such as drug absorption, drug distribution, or drug elimination to go to completion. For example, it may be important to get an idea of how long it will take to eliminate a drug from the body after a dose.

How long does it take a first-order process to go to completion? The answer is: ∞. Although the answer is accurate, it is of little practical value. An alternative approach to the problem is to determine the time for a first-order process to almost go to completion (e.g., 90% completion). Recall that

$$Ab = Ab_0 \cdot e^{-kt} \qquad (B.19)$$

where Ab is the amount of drug in the body at time t, and Ab_0 is the amount at time zero before decay starts.

The decay function (e^{-kt}), which starts at 1 and decays to 0, represents the fraction of the original quantity remaining at any time. The fraction of completion is the ratio of the amount decayed to the original amount:

$$\text{fraction completion} = \frac{Ab_0 - Ab}{Ab_0} = 1 - \frac{Ab}{Ab_0} = 1 - \frac{Ab_0 \cdot e^{-kt}}{Ab_0} = 1 - e^{-kt} \quad (B.20)$$

If $e^{-kt} = 0.7$, 70% of the original quantity remains $(Ab = 0.7Ab_0)$; and $1 - e^{-kt} = 0.3$, 30% has decayed or been eliminated. The process is 30% complete.

The number of half-lives for a first-order process to go to any fraction of completion can be calculated using equation (B.20). For example, the number of half-lives to go to 90% completion may be calculated as follows. At 90% completion, $1 - e^{-kt} = 0.90$:

$$0.9 = 1 - e^{-kt}$$

But $k = 0.693/t_{1/2}$:

$$0.9 = 1 - e^{-0.693/t_{1/2}t}$$
$$\ln(0.1) = -\frac{0.693}{t_{1/2}} \cdot t$$
$$t = 3.32t_{1/2} \qquad (B.21)$$

Thus, it takes $3.32t_{1/2}$ for a first-order process to be 90% complete.

Table B.2 shows the number of half-lives needed to get to various fractions of completion. These values hold for any first-order process. Depending on a given situation, it

TABLE B.2   Number of Half-Lives for a First-Order Process to Go to Certain Fractions of Completion

Percent Completion	$1 - e^{-kt}$	Time, $t_{1/2}$
10	0.1	$\sim \frac{1}{6}$[a]
20	0.2	$\sim \frac{1}{3}$[a]
50	0.5	1
90	0.90	3.3
95	0.95	4.3
99	0.99	6.6

[a]Approximate values.

is usually considered to take anywhere from 3 to 7 half-lives for a first-order process to go to completion. From a practical standpoint, on average, it can be assumed to take four half-lives for completion.

B.7 EXAMPLES OF THE APPLICATION OF FIRST-ORDER KINETICS TO PHARMACOKINETICS

To answer the following questions, assume that all processes in drug absorption, distribution, metabolism, and excretion are first-order processes.

Example B.3   Antacids impair the absorption of many drugs. How long after the administration of Neoral (cyclosporine) should a patient wait before taking an antacid? The first-order absorption rate constant for cyclosporine in the Neoral formulation is around $1.35\,h^{-1}$.

Solution
The half-life for absorption is $0.693/1.35 = 0.51\,h$. It will take about $4 \times 0.5 = 2\,h$ to absorb cyclosporine. Thus, the patient should wait at least 2 h after a dose of Neoral before taking an antacid.

Example B.4   A physician wishes to give warfarin to a patient who has just stopped taking amiodarone, which has an elimination half-life of around 25 days. Amiodarone is known to inhibit the metabolism of warfarin. How long could the interaction between amiodarone and warfarin last?

Solution
Amiodarone is an inhibitor of several drug-metabolizing enzymes, including one of the enzymes that metabolizes warfarin. The interaction can last until amiodarone is eliminated, which will take about 4 months (four elimination $t_{1/2}$'s).

Example B.5   A child accidentally takes his grandmother's digoxin. At the emergency room, a blood sample reveals a serum concentration of 6 μg/L. The serum concentration should be at least < 2, and ideally, < 1.2 μg/L to avoid toxicity. How long will it take for blood levels to become safe? Assume that the plasma concentration is influenced only by first-order elimination and that digoxin's elimination $t_{1/2}$ is 2 days.

Solution
The blood level will fall by 50% each elimination half-life. Thus, it will take two half-lives, or 4 days, to get to 1.5 μg/L and three half-lives, or 6 days, to get to 0.75 μg/L. The exact time to get to 1.2 μg/L can be estimated using the equation for first-order decay [equation (B.9)], the serum concentration is the dependent variable, and the rate constant is $0.693/t_{1/2} = 0.693/2 = 0.347\,day^{-1}$. This provides an answer of 4.6 days.

Example B.6   The distribution of a drug from the plasma to the tissues is usually a first-order process. The disappearance of the drug from the plasma due to tissue uptake can be described by the equation

$$Cp = A \cdot e^{-\alpha t}$$

where Cp is the plasma concentration, A is a constant, α is a first-order rate constant for distribution, and t is the time.

If gentamicin and digoxin have first-order distribution rate constants of about $0.14\ \text{min}^{-1}$ and $0.52\ \text{h}^{-1}$, respectively. Approximately how long will it take for distribution to go to about 95% completion for each drug?

Solution

It will take $4t_{1/2,\alpha}$ to get to 95% completion. For gentamicin, this will be 4(0.693/0.14), or 19.8 min, and for digoxin it will take 4(0.693/0.52), or 5.4 h.

APPENDIX C

CREATION OF EXCEL WORKSHEETS FOR PHARMACOKINETIC ANALYSIS

SARA E. ROSENBAUM

Conventions

Worksheet Instructions Quantities that actually have to be entered in the cells of the worksheets are presented within quotation marks and are italicized.

Worksheet Layout Data that must be entered into the worksheet are colored red and model parameters are colored green. Other colors are used to distinguish the products of different calculations performed on the given data.

C.1   MEASUREMENT OF AUC AND CLEARANCE

The measurement of the area under the plasma concentration–time curve (AUC) is often an important part of a pharmacokinetic analysis. It is used to assess drug exposure and to calculate clearance (*Cl*). Recall that

$$Cl = \frac{F \cdot D}{\text{AUC}_0^\infty}$$

Basic Pharmacokinetics and Pharmacodynamics: An Integrated Textbook and Computer Simulations,
Second Edition. Edited by Sara E. Rosenbaum.
© 2017 John Wiley & Sons, Inc. Published 2017 by John Wiley & Sons, Inc.

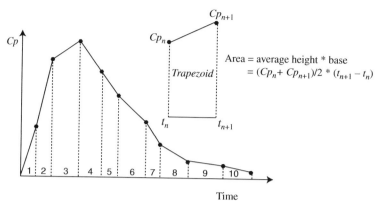

FIGURE C.1   Typical plasma concentration–time profile after oral administration; the curve is segmented into trapezoids using the data points.

where F is the fraction of the dose (D) absorbed. The AUC is most commonly measured using the trapezoidal rule. Descriptions of the trapezoidal rule, the measurement of the AUC, and the estimation of clearance are given below.

C.1.1 Trapezoidal Rule

When a dose of a drug is administered, plasma concentrations can be determined at various times and then plotted against time. Figure C.1 shows the typical profile observed after oral administration.

1. The first step in using the trapezoidal rule to estimate the AUC is to use the measured data points to split the curve into a series of segments, each of which (except the first, which is a triangle) is a trapezoid (a four-sided shape with two parallel sides). In Figure C.1, the 10 measured data points produce 10 segments.

2. The area of each segment must now be determined. The area of a trapezoid (Figure C.1) is given by

$$\text{area of a trapezoid} = \text{average height} \cdot \text{base} \tag{C.1}$$

   Note that this is also the formula for the area of a triangle (the first segment). Thus, the area of each trapezoid produced from the plasma concentration–time data can be calculated as follows:

$$\text{area} = \frac{Cp_n + Cp_{n+1}}{2} \cdot (t_{n+1} - t_n) \tag{C.2}$$

3. The areas of each of the 10 segments are combined to obtain the AUC from zero to the last time point.

4. The AUC from the last time point to infinity must now be calculated. At the time of the last time point, it is assumed that the fall in the plasma concentration is influenced only by first-order elimination (no ongoing absorption or distribution is assumed to occur by this time). Under these conditions, the AUC from the last time point (Cp_{last}) to infinity is given by

$$\text{AUC}_{Cp\text{last}\rightarrow\infty} = \frac{Cp_{\text{last}}}{k}$$

where k is the overall first-order elimination rate constant. When Cp is affected only by first-order elimination, k is the negative slope for the fall in ln Cp with time.

5. All the individual areas are then summed to obtain $AUC_{0 \to \infty}$.

6. The drug's clearance may be determined from the AUC if the bioavailability factor (F) is known:

$$Cl = \frac{F \cdot D}{AUC_0^\infty}$$

If F is not known, the parameter Cl/F, which is known as oral clearance, is determined:

$$\frac{Cl}{F} = \frac{D}{AUC_0^\infty}$$

C.1.2 Excel Spreadsheet to Determine $AUC_{0 \to \infty}$ and Clearance

The empty shell of a worksheet to determine the AUC and clearance is shown in Figure C.2. This will be used as a guide to set up an operational worksheet to determine the AUC and clearance. Open an empty worksheet in Excel and copy the column headings and layout shown in Figure C.2. Save the worksheet as "Worksheet for AUC and Cl" or by a similar appropriate name.

The worksheet will be set up using the plasma concentration–time data in Table C.1. These data were obtained after the oral administration of a 100-mg dose of a drug.

1. Enter the time and Cp data in the upper Given Data section of the worksheet only.

2. Enter the drug dose (100 mg).

3. Plot the data to visualize it and ensure that there are no outliers. Highlight the data (not the column headings), click on the Insert tab on the tool bar, choose Scatter, and then select the Scatter with Straight Lines and Markers. Click on the Layout tab and enter a chart heading and label each axis.

4. All the calculations and data manipulation procedures will be done in the lower section of the worksheet. The given data must be placed in the time and concentration columns in this lower section. Do *not* copy and paste the data into these columns. Instead, the given data cells in the upper section will be referenced. In this way, when new data are entered in the Given Data section, the lower section will automatically update with the new data. The cells containing the data are referenced as follows: In the lower section, go the first cell in the time column and enter "=" (without the quotation marks), then click on the first time cell in the given data column in the upper area. Then hit Enter. Copy this formula throughout the time column. To do this, go back to the first cell containing the reference and point to the lower right-hand corner of the cell. When a cross appears, hold down the mouse and drag it through the rest of the columns. Repeat the entire procedure for the concentration data.

5. Enter the dose in the lower section of the worksheet by referencing the cell containing its value in the upper area.

6. The values for ln Cp for the last three data points will be entered using the Excel Ln function. Thus, in the first of these three ln Cp cells, enter "=Ln(" (without the quotation marks) and then click on the corresponding value of Cp and close the parentheses. Copy this formula throughout the two additional ln Cp cells.

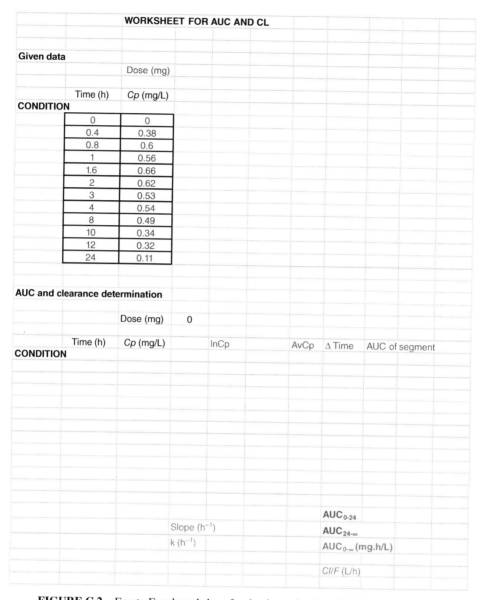

FIGURE C.2   Empty Excel worksheet for the determination of AUC and clearance.

TABLE C.1   Plasma Concentration Time Data After a 100-mg Oral Dose

Time (h)	Cp (mg/L)	Time (h)	Cp (mg/L)
0	0	3	0.530
0.4	0.380	4	0.540
0.8	0.600	8	0.490
1	0.560	10	0.340
1.6	0.660	12	0.320
2	0.620	24	0.110

7. The slope of the ln Cp versus time plot must be determined to calculate k. Enter the cell where for the value of the slope is to appear. The slope is determined using the slope function in Excel. This is one of the function keys that are accessed from the Autosum ($\sum$) symbol on Excel's tool bar. Click on the arrow next to the Autosum key and locate the slope function. It will probably be found in Other Functions, in the Statistical category. Once the slope function has been found, it is necessary to enter the range of y values (ln Cp) and x values (time) that are to be used for the calculation. To do this, click on the known_y's box in the pop-up window and then click throughout the relevant ln Cp cells in the worksheet. Do the same for the known_x's. Make sure that you go in the same direction when you highlight the y's and x's. Hit Enter.

8. Go to the cell where the value of k (equal to the negative slope) is to appear and enter "= -" and then click on the cell containing the value of the slope.

9. The AUC of each trapezoidal segment will be calculated in stages:

   (a) *Average Cp.* The formula $(Cp_n + Cp_{n+1})/2$ must be entered in the cells of the average Cp column. In the top cell enter "=(", then reference the cell containing Cp_n, enter "+" and click on the cell containing Cp_{n+1}, and enter ")/2." Copy the formula throughout the column to the cell corresponding to the next-to-last Cp (there is no another Cp with which to average the last Cp).

   (b) *Time difference.* The formula to calculate delta t, $t_{n+1} - t_n$, now has to be entered in the top cell of the delta t column. Enter "=(", then click on the cell containing t_{n+1}, then enter "−" and click on the cell containing t_n. Close the parenthesis. Copy the formula down through the next-too last cell in the column.

   (c) *Area of each segment.* The formula to calculate the area of each segment, $(Cp_n + Cp_{n+1})/2 * (t_{n+1} - t_n)$, must now be entered in the top cell of this column. Enter "=", then reference on the average Cp value, then enter "*" and reference the corresponding delta t value. Copy the formula throughout the column.

   (d) *AUC from zero to last data point.* Add up all the individual areas (AUC from 0 to Cp_{last}) using the AutoSum function on the tool bar.

   (e) *AUC from last data point to infinity.* The formula Cp_{last}/k to calculate the area from the last Cp value to infinity must be entered the cell where this value is to appear. Enter "=", reference the cell containing the value of the last Cp, then enter "/", reference the value of k, and hit Enter.

   (f) *AUC from zero to infinity.* Use the AutoSum function to calculate $AUC_{0 \to \infty}$.

   (g) *Calculate Cl/F.* (Note: Cl cannot be determined because F is unknown.) Click on the cell where the value of Cl/F is to appear, enter "=", reference the cell containing the dose, then enter "/", reference the value of $AUC_{0 \to \infty}$, and then hit Enter.

Save the completed worksheet as "Worksheet for AUC and Cl." The completed worksheet is shown in Figure C.3.

Note: When this worksheet is used for other data, remember to:

- Reenter the appropriate dose.
- Make sure that all the units are consistent throughout the worksheet and that they are all labeled correctly. For example, if the units of Cp are μg/L, make sure that the dose is entered in μg.

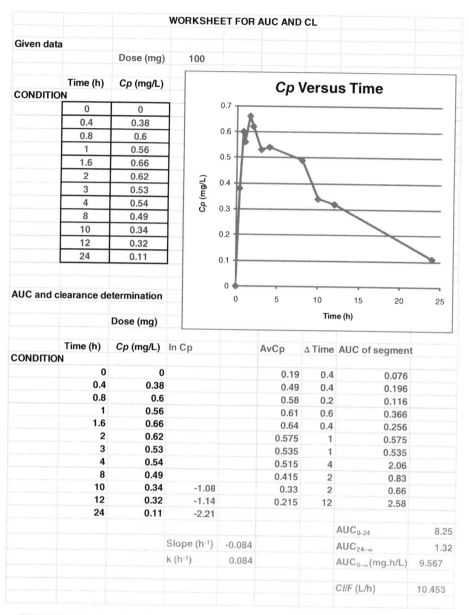

FIGURE C.3   Completed Excel worksheet for the determination of AUC and clearance.

C.2   ANALYSIS OF DATA FROM AN INTRAVENOUS BOLUS INJECTION IN A ONE-COMPARTMENT MODEL

This worksheet will be created by adapting the previous worksheet for the determination of AUC and clearance.

1. Open the completed worksheet for the determination of the AUC and clearance.
2. Change the title of the worksheet to "Worksheet for the Analysis of Data from an IV Bolus Injection in a One-Compartment Model."

TABLE C.2   Plasma Concentrations at Various Times After the IV Administration of a Drug (50 mg)

Time (h)	Cp (mg/L)	Time (h)	Cp (mg/L)
0.1	2.45	3	1.37
0.2	2.40	5	0.92
0.5	2.26	7	0.62
1	2.05	10	0.34
1.5	1.85	12	0.23
2	1.68	15	0.12

3. Save the worksheet as "PK Analysis: One-Compartment Model IV."

4. Delete the diagram and/or the chart or graph.

5. Enter the data obtained after the IV administration of 50-mg dose of a drug from Table C.2 into the upper area of the worksheet. Make sure that the dose is *updated.*

6. The data in the lower calculation area should update automatically.

7. In the upper Given Data area, plot the data on a linear and a semilogarithmic scale to make sure that it appears that the one-compartment model holds for this data set, and that there are no odd data points that are very different from the others.

8. Select the two columns of data (not the headings).

9. Go to Insert; in the Chart area, choose Scatter, Smooth lines, and markers.

10. This first chart will be the linear plot of *Cp* versus time. From the Layout tab, add a title to the graph and label each axis.

11. Copy and paste this graph to create a duplicate alongside it. On the copy, reformat the *y*-axis to the logarithmic scale: right click on the *y*-axis, select Format the Axis, and choose Logarithmic Scale. At this point, it may be appropriate to change the point where the horizontal axis crosses. Modify the graph title and label for the *y*-axis.

12. Rename the lower calculation area "Parameter Determination."

13. Continue the list of model parameters below the cell labeled "*k* (1/h)." Thus, add the following names:

    (a) $t_{1/2}$(h)

    (b) Intercept (I) (note that this will be the ln scale)

    (c) Cp_0 (mg/L) (note that this is the anti-ln of the intercept)

    (d) *Vd* (L)

    (e) *Cl* (*k* * *Vd*) (L/h) (note that this clearance will be determined from *k* and *Vd*)

    (f) *Cl* (Cp_0/*k*) (L/h) (note that this clearance will be determined from AUC calculated from Cp_0 and *k*)

    (g) *Cl* (trapezoidal) (L/h) (note that this clearance will be determined from AUC measured using the trapezoidal rule) Note that in this problem, the area from time zero to the first data point (0–1) must be added (see * in Figure C.4).

14. Extend the calculation of the ln *Cp* values from the third-to-last data point all the way up to the top of the column. Hold the mouse over the bottom right corner of a filled ln *Cp* cell, and drag it up the column.

15. Go to the cell that contains the calculation of the slope. Extend the data points used to calculate the slope to include all the data points.

16. Enter the formula for the listed parameters in the cells adjacent to the label (**_bold italic_** type below indicates that the cell containing the value of that quantity should be referenced):

    (a) $t_{1/2}$(h): Enter "= 0.693/**_k_**" (but not the quotation marks).

    (b) Intercept (I). Note that this is from the ln Cp versus time plot. It will be in the ln scale. Find the intercept function from the list accessed from AutoSum on the upper tool bar. It will be found in the statistical functions. Enter the range of y (lnCp) and x values to be used for its calculation (all of them).

    (c) Cp_0 (mg/L): Enter "= **_EXP(I)_**."

    (d) Vd (L): Enter "= **_Dose/Cp_**$_0$."

    (e) Cl ($k * Vd$): Enter "= **_k_** * **_Vd_**."

    (f) Cl (Cp_0 /k) (L/h)): Enter "**_Dose/(Cp_**$_0$ /**_k_**)."

    (g) Cl (trapezoidal): Enter : $Dose/AUC_0^\infty$.

Note: When this worksheet is used for other data, it is very important to *check the units.* Make sure that all the units are consistent throughout the worksheet and that they are all labeled correctly. For example, if the units of Cp are μg/L, make sure that the dose is entered in μg.

The completed worksheet is shown in Figure C.4.

C.3 ANALYSIS OF DATA FROM AN INTRAVENOUS BOLUS INJECTION IN A TWO-COMPARTMENT MODEL

1. *Set up empty worksheet.* Figure C.5 shows the empty worksheet for the determination of the parameters of the two-compartment model. Use this layout and cell labels to create your own worksheet.

2. *Enter data.* Enter the data from Table E8.1 (page 176), obtained after a 100-mg dose, in the top Given Data section. Plot the data on a semilogarithmic scale to ensure that visually the data appear to fit a two-compartment model.

3. *Reference data in lower calculation area.* Reference the given time and concentration data in the lower Calculation Area of the worksheet. Use these data in the lower area for all future calculations. *Create time and* ln *Cp columns.* Reference the given data to set up time and ln Cp columns.

4. *Determine B and* β. Determine B and β from the last three data points, which are described by the equation $Cp' = B * e^{-\beta t}$, where $Cp' = Cp$ for the last three data points. Use the built-in function to determine the slope and intercept for the ln Cp' versus time relationship for the last three data points. Determine β and B.

5. *Determine A and* α:

    (a) *Calculate Cp′ at early times.* Consider the equation $Cp' = B * e^{-\beta t}$; at later times, $Cp = Cp$, but at earlier times, when distribution is occurring, $Cp' < Cp$. The values of Cp' at these earlier times must be calculated. Use B and β and the equation $Cp' = B * e^{-\beta t}$ to determine the values of Cp' that correspond to the times of the given data (Cp). When doing this, it is important to use the absolute address of the value of B and β since they must remain constant when the formula for Cp' is copied throughout the column. In the example worksheet, B and β are in cells E41 and E39, respectively. The absolute address of a cell is given by including a

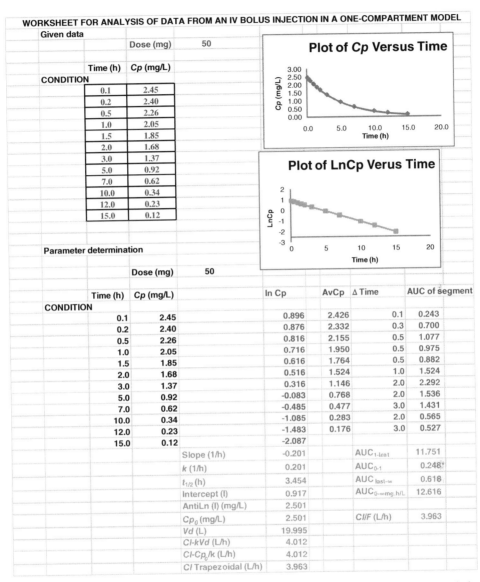

WORKSHEET FOR ANALYSIS OF DATA FROM AN IV BOLUS INJECTION IN A ONE-COMPARTMENT MODEL

FIGURE C.4   Completed Excel worksheet for pharmacokinetic analysis of an intravenous bolus injection in a one-compartment model. *AUC from 0 to the 1st data point at $t = 0.1$ h.

$ sign before the column letter and row number. Thus, the absolute addresses of B and β are \$E\$41 and \$E\$39, respectively. Enter the formula to calculate Cp' in the first Cp' cell: "=\$E\$41 * EXP(-\$E\$39 * G24)." Copy the formula throughout the rest of the Cp' column (time will change for each cell, but B and β will remain constant).

(b) *Calculate $Cp - Cp'$ to isolate the line described by A and α: $Cp - Cp' = A * e^{-\alpha t}$.*
     Calculate $Cp - Cp'$ for those values of Cp' that are less than Cp. Enter the values of $\ln(Cp - Cp')$. Use the built-in functions to determine the slope and intercept of the $\ln(Cp - Cp')$–time relationship. Determine A and α.

Worksheet for the Analysis of Data for an IV Injection in a Two-Compartment Model

GIVEN DATA

Dose (mg)	100

Time(h)	Cp (mg/L)
0.1	7.95
0.2	6.38
0.4	4.25
0.7	2.57
1	1.79
1.5	1.27
2	1.07
3	0.89
4	0.76
6	0.56
8	0.42
12	0.23

Calculation area

GIVEN DATA

		LN SCALE		$Cp'=Bexp^*(-\beta^*t)$		Isolating DistributionExponent					
Time(h)	Cp (mg/L)	Time	LnCp	Time	Cp'	Time	Cp-Cp'	LnCp-Cp'	Time	LnCp'	LnCp-Cp'
0.1	7.95										
0.2	6.38										
0.4	4.25										
0.7	2.57										
1	1.79										
1.5	1.27										
2	1.07										
3	0.89										
4	0.76										
6	0.56										
8	0.42										
12	0.23										
		DOSE(mg)	100								

	βSlope		αSlope		Parameters
	βh^{-1}		$\alpha\ h^{-1}$		T1/2
	LnB		LnA		k21 h-1
	B mg/L		A mg/L		k10 h-1
					k12 h-1
					$AUC_{mg.h/L}$
					Cl L/h
					V1 L
					Vβ L
					Vd_{ss} L
					Cld L/h

FIGURE C.5   Empty Excel worksheet for determination of the parameters of the two-compartment model after an intravenous bolus injection.

6. *Plot lines corresponding to the two exponential functions.* On the farthermost right area, create adjacent columns of time, ln Cp' and $\ln(Cp - Cp')$. Plot a scatter plot of ln Cp' and $\ln(Cp - Cp')$ against time.

7. *Determine the micro rate constants and the pharmacokinetic parameters.* Enter the formula for each parameter (see Sections 8.7.2 and 8.7.3). Reference any parameter from the worksheet that is needed for the calculation.

The complete worksheet is shown in Figure C.6.

C.4   ANALYSIS OF ORAL DATA IN A ONE-COMPARTMENT MODEL

1. *Set up empty worksheet.* Figure C.7 shows the empty worksheet for the determination of the parameters from data obtained after oral administration in a one-compartment model (see Table E9.1A, page 209). Use this layout and cell labels to create your own worksheet.

2. *Enter data.* Enter the data in the top Given Data section. Plot the data on the regular linear and semilogarithmic scales to ensure that visually the data appear to fit a one-compartment model and make sure that there are no outliers.

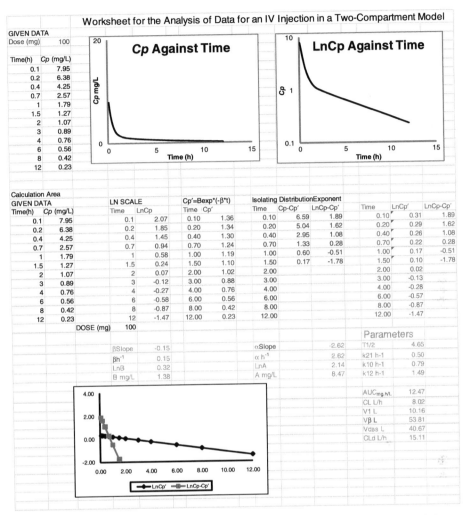

FIGURE C.6 Completed Excel worksheet for determination of the parameters of the two-compartment model after an intravenous bolus injection.

3. *Reference data in lower calculation area.* Reference the given time and concentration data in the lower Calculation Area of the worksheet. Use these data in the lower area for all future calculations.

4. *Create time and ln Cp columns.* Reference the given data to set up adjacent time and ln Cp columns.

5. *Determine I and k.* Determine the intercept (I) and slope (k) of the line created from the last three data points of ln Cp against time. These points are described by the equation $Cp' = I * e^{-kt}$, where $Cp' = Cp$ for the last three data points. Use the built-in slope and intercept function to determine ln I and the slope from the ln Cp' versus time relationship. Determine I [$I = \exp(\ln I)$], and $k = (-\text{slope})$.

6. *Determine k_a and I from the absorption line:*
   (a) *Calculate Cp' at early times.* Consider the equation $Cp' = I * e^{-kt}$; at later times $Cp' = Cp$, but at earlier times, when absorption is underway, $Cp' > Cp$. The values of Cp' at these earlier times must be calculated. Use I and k and the equation $Cp' = I * e^{-kt}$ to determine the values of Cp' that correspond to the times of the

Worksheet for the Analysis of Oral Data in a One-Compartment Model

GIVEN DATA
Dose (mg)   100

Time(h)	Cp (mg/L)
0	0
0.6	2.74
0.8	3.13
1	3.37
1.4	3.55
1.8	3.5
2	3.43
2.6	3.12
3	2.89
4	2.33
7	1.17
12	0.37

Calculation Area
GIVEN DATA

Time(h)	Cp (mg/L)	LN SCALE Time	LnCp	$Cp'=I\,(e^{k*t})$ Time	Cp'	Isolating Absorption Exponent Time	Cp'-Cp	LnCp'-Cp	Time	LnCp'	LnCp'-Cp

DOSE(mg)

Parameters

ElinSlope		AbspSlope	T1/2 h
kh⁻¹		ka h⁻¹	Vd/F L
LnI		LnI	AUC
I mg/L		I mg/L	Cl/F L/h$_{AUC}$
			Cl/F L/h$_{(k*Vd)}$

FIGURE C.7   Empty Excel worksheet for determination of the parameters of the one-compartment model with first-order absorption.

given data (Cp). When doing this, it is important to use the absolute address of the value of I and k since they must remain constant when the formula for Cp' is copied throughout the column. In the example, worksheets I and k are in cells E41 and E39, respectively. The absolute address of a cell is given by including a $ sign before the column letter and row number. Thus, the absolute addresses of I and k are \$E\$41 and \$E\$39, respectively. Enter the formula to calculate Cp' in the first Cp' cell: "=\$E\$41*EXP(-\$E\$39*G24)" Copy the formula throughout the rest of the Cp' column (time will change for each cell, but I and k will remain constant).

(b) *Calculate $Cp' - Cp$ and isolate the line described by k_a: $Cp' - Cp = I * e^{-kat}$.* Calculate $Cp' - Cp$ for those values of Cp' that are greater than Cp. Enter the values of $\ln(Cp' - Cp)$. Use the built-in functions to determine the slope and intercept of the $\ln(Cp' - Cp)$–time relationship. Determine I and k_a.

7. *Plot the lines corresponding to the two exponential functions.* On the farthermost right area, create adjacent columns of time, $\ln Cp'$ and $\ln(Cp' - Cp)$. Plot a scatter plot of $\ln Cp'$ and $\ln(Cp' - Cp)$ against time.

8. *Determine half-life, clearance, and volume of distribution.* Enter the formula for each parameter. $Vd/F = dose * k_a / I * (k_a - k)$ and $Cl/F = dose/AUC$, where $AUC = I * (1/k - 1/k_a)$. Reference any parameter from the worksheet that is needed for the calculation.

The complete worksheet is shown in Figure C.8.

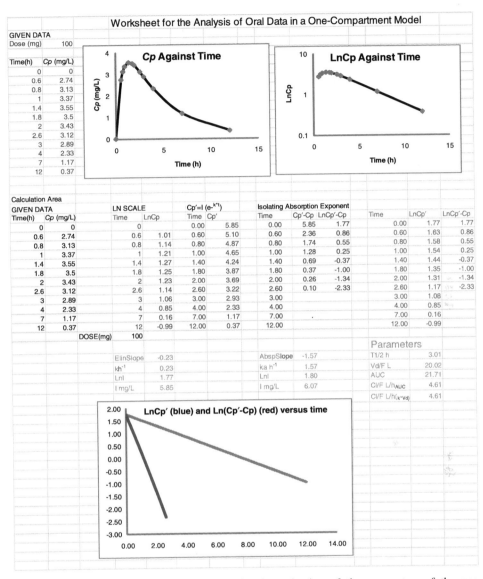

FIGURE C.8   Completed Excel worksheet for determination of the parameters of the one-compartment model with first-order absorption.

C.5   NONCOMPARTMENTAL ANALYSIS OF ORAL DATA

This worksheet will be created to enable AUC, Cl/F, $t_{1/2}$, C_{max}, and T_{max} to be estimated after the administration of a dose by any route. In this example, data obtained after oral administration will be analyzed. The worksheet will be set up to analyze data presented in Chapter 10 from a hypothetical drug–drug interaction study to evaluate if fluconazole alters the pharmacokinetics of fictitious drug lipoamide. The data obtained after a 120-mg oral dose of lipoamide in the absence (control) and in the presence (test) of fluconazole as described in Example 10.3 (Section 10.5, Chapter 10) are provided in Table C.3.

TABLE C.3   Plasma Concentrations of Lipoamide at Various Times After Oral Administration in the Absence and Presence of Fluconazole (Inhibitor)

Time (h)	Cp (μg/L) Control	Cp (μg/L) Inhibitor	Time (h)	Cp (μg/L) Control	Cp (μg/L) Inhibitor
0.0	0.0	0.0	1.2	52.0	160.9
0.2	38.1	117.8	2.0	46.3	143.2
0.4	50.6	156.7	4.0	34.4	106.4
0.6	54.1	167.4	10.0	14.1	43.6
0.8	54.3	168.0	15.0	6.7	20.7
1.0	53.3	165.0	24.0	1.8	5.4

The new worksheet will be created from the worksheet for the determination of the AUC and clearance.

1. Open the completed worksheet for the determination of AUC and Cl. Delete any graphs. Save it as "Worksheet for NCA After Oral Administration."
2. Change the name of the lower calculation area of the worksheet from "AUC and Clearance Determination" to "Parameter Determination Using NCA."
3. Enter (or copy and paste) the control and test data in the upper Given Data area to exactly replace the existing data in the first two columns. There will be one more Cp column in the new worksheet. Insert a scatter chart to view the data. Add a title and label the axis.
4. Enter the value of the dose (make sure that the units are labeled correctly and that they are *uniform throughout* the worksheet).
5. Note that the control data should automatically have been placed in the lower calculation area.
6. In the lower calculation area, change the label k in the cell underneath slope to λ.
7. Underneath the cell labeled Cl/F, add the other parameters to be estimated: $t_{1/2}$, C_{max}, and T_{max}. An entry for Vd/F may be added if desired.
8. Enter the formula to identify C_{max} for the range of concentrations for the control data: from the Excel function keys, select Max and enter the range of Cp values–C28:C39. Enter the following formula to identify T_{max} corresponding to the C_{max} in the range of cells C28 through C39: =OFFSET(B27,MATCH(MAX(C28:C39), C28:C39, 0), 0). Enter the formula for the other new parameters: $t_{1/2} = 0.693/\lambda$ and $Vd/F = Cl/ (F * \lambda)$. (Note this will be V_{β} if the drug follows two-compartment characteristics.)
9. Copy and paste the entire lower calculation area and make a duplicate to the right. Do not worry that the data change to "0" and that #NUM appears in some cells. In the "Phase" row, label the left calculation area "Control" and the right area "Test."
10. Enter the test dose by referencing the dose in the upper area of the worksheet.
11. Enter the test data by referencing the given test data in the upper area of the worksheet. Create a results summary as shown by referencing all the parameters. Enter these parameters into Table C.4.

TABLE C.4   Pharmacokinetic Parameters of Lipoamide in the Absence (Control) and Presence of Fluconazole (Test)

Parameter	Control (Placebo)	Test (Fluconazole)
Cl/F (L/h)		
$t_{1/2}$ (h)		
C_{max} (µg/L)		
T_{max} (h)		

The completed worksheet is shown in Figure C.9.

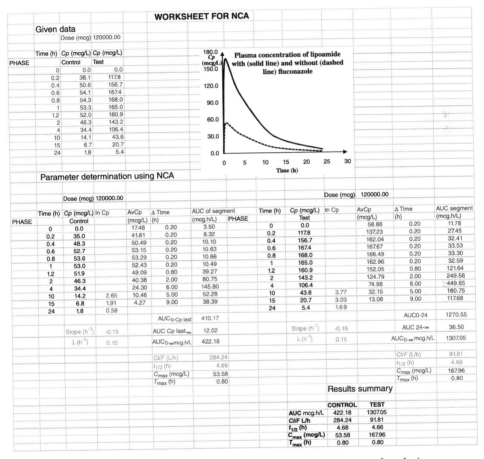

FIGURE C.9   Completed Excel worksheet for noncompartmental analysis.

APPENDIX D

DERIVATION OF EQUATIONS FOR MULTIPLE INTRAVENOUS BOLUS INJECTIONS

Sara E. Rosenbaum

D.1 Assumptions
D.2 Basic Equation for Plasma Concentration After Multiple Intravenous Bolus Injections
D.3 Steady-State Equations

D.1 ASSUMPTIONS

1. All doses are the same.
2. The dosing interval (τ) remains constant.
3. Pharmacokinetic parameters remain constant over entire course of therapy.

For simplicity, F and S are not included as potential modifiers of a dose during the initial derivation of the formula.

D.2 BASIC EQUATION FOR PLASMA CONCENTRATION AFTER MULTIPLE INTRAVENOUS BOLUS INJECTIONS

It is assumed that after a dose, the total amount of drug in the body is equal to the dose plus any drug remaining from previous dose(s). This is known as the *principle of superposition* and is illustrated in Figure D.1.

The maximum and minimum amounts of drug in the body ($Ab_{\max,n}$ and $Ab_{\min,n}$, respectively) after sequential doses will now be calculated, dose by dose. The maximum amount

Basic Pharmacokinetics and Pharmacodynamics: An Integrated Textbook and Computer Simulations,
Second Edition. Edited by Sara E. Rosenbaum.
© 2017 John Wiley & Sons, Inc. Published 2017 by John Wiley & Sons, Inc.

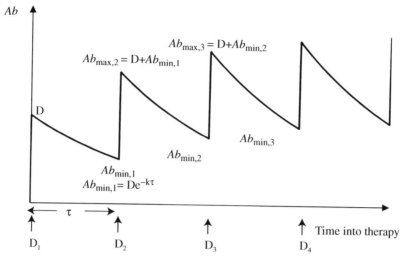

FIGURE D.1 Principle of superposition. The amount of drug in the body after a dose is equal to the dose (D) plus the amount remaining from a previous dose or doses.

of drug in the body after the first dose is the dose (D). During the first dosing interval, this amount decays monoexponentially and at the end of the dosing interval;

$$Ab_{\min,1} = Ab_{\max,1} \cdot e^{-k\tau} = D \cdot e^{-k\tau} \tag{D.1}$$

The second dose is given and the maximum amount in the body is equal to the dose plus what remains from the first dose:

$$Ab_{\max,2} = D + D \cdot e^{-k\tau} = D \cdot (1 + e^{-k\tau}) \tag{D.2}$$

During the second dosing interval, the amount of drug in the body decays monoexponentially and the minimum amount in the body after the second dose is

$$Ab_{\min,2} = Ab_{\max,2} \cdot e^{-k\tau} = D \cdot (1 + e^{-k\tau}) \cdot e^{-k\tau} = D \cdot (e^{-k\tau} + e^{-2k\tau}) \tag{D.3}$$

The results of the calculations are summarized in Table D.1, which also shows the results of the calculations continued through the third dose. A pattern can be observed, and it is possible to use this to predict $Ab_{\max,5}$:

$$Ab_{\max,5} = D \cdot (1 + e^{-k\tau} + e^{-2k\tau} + e^{-3k\tau} + e^{-4k\tau}) \tag{D.4}$$

TABLE D.1   Maximum ($Ab_{\max}$) and Minimum ($Ab_{\min}$) Amounts of Drug in the Body After Sequential Doses

Dose	$Ab_{\max}$	$Ab_{\min}$
1	D	$D \cdot e^{-k\tau}$
2	$D + D \cdot e^{-k\tau}$	$D (1 + e^{-k\tau}) \cdot e^{-k\tau}$
	$D \cdot (1 + e^{-k\tau})$	$D \cdot (e^{-kt} + e^{-2kt})$
3	$D + D \cdot (e^{-k\tau} + e^{-2k\tau})$	$D \cdot (1 + e^{-k\tau} + e^{-2k\tau}) \cdot e^{-k\tau}$
	$D \cdot (1 + e^{-k\tau} + e^{-2k\tau})$	$D \cdot (e^{-k\tau} + e^{-2k\tau} + e^{-3k\tau})$

More generally,

$$Ab_{\max,n} = D \cdot (1 + e^{-k\tau} + e^{-2k\tau} + e^{-3k\tau} + \cdots + e^{-(n-1)k\tau}) \tag{D.5}$$

The expressions contain a geometric series. Let R represent the geometric series:

$$R = 1 + e^{-k\tau} + e^{-2k\tau} + e^{-3k\tau} + \cdots + e^{-(n-1)k\tau} \tag{D.6}$$

Thus,

$$Ab_{\max,n} = D \cdot R \tag{D.7}$$

Multiply R by $e^{-k\tau}$:

$$R \cdot e^{-k\tau} = e^{-k\tau} + e^{-2k\tau} + e^{-3k\tau} + \cdots + e^{-nk\tau} \tag{D.8}$$

Subtracting equation (D.8) from equation (D.6) gives us

$$R - R \cdot e^{-k\tau} = 1 - e^{-nk\tau}$$
$$R = \frac{1-e^{-nk\tau}}{1-e^{-k\tau}} \tag{D.9}$$

Recall from equation (D.7) that $Ab_{\max,n} = D \cdot R$:

$$Ab_{\max,n} = D \cdot \frac{1 - e^{-nk\tau}}{1 - e^{-k\tau}} \tag{D.10}$$

As $Cp = Ab/Vd$,

$$Cp_{\max,n} = \frac{D \cdot (1 - e^{-nk\tau})}{Vd \cdot \left(1 - e^{-k\tau}\right)} \tag{D.11}$$

A trough concentration ($Cp_{\min,n}$) occurs when the time after the dose, $t = \tau$ and is given by ($Cp_{\min,n} = Cp_{\max,n} \cdot e^{-k\tau}$):

$$Cp_{\min,n} = \frac{D \cdot (1 - e^{-nk\tau})}{Vd \cdot \left(1 - e^{-k\tau}\right)} \cdot e^{-k\tau} \tag{D.12}$$

The plasma concentration at anytime, t after a dose (Cp_n) during a dosing interval, is given by ($Cp_{,n} = Cp_{\max,n} \cdot e^{-kt}$)

$$Cp_n = \frac{D \cdot (1 - e^{-nk\tau})}{Vd \cdot \left(1 - e^{-k\tau}\right)} \cdot e^{-kt} \tag{D.13}$$

Including the salt factor and bioavailability as potential modifiers of the dose, we obtain

$$Cp_n = \frac{S \cdot F \cdot D \cdot (1 - e^{-nk\tau})}{Vd \cdot \left(1 - e^{-k\tau}\right)} \cdot e^{-kt} \tag{D.14}$$

In summary:

1. The basic equation for the plasma concentration at any time during therapy with multiple intravenous bolus injections is given by equation (D.14):

$$Cp_n = \frac{S \cdot F \cdot D \cdot (1 - e^{-nk\tau})}{Vd \cdot \left(1 - e^{-k\tau}\right)} \cdot e^{-kt}$$

2. Peak plasma concentrations occur at the time a dose is given ($t = 0$):

$$Cp_{\max,n} = \frac{S \cdot F \cdot D \cdot (1 - e^{-nk\tau})}{Vd \cdot \left(1 - e^{-k\tau}\right)} \tag{D.15}$$

3. Trough concentrations occur just before the next dose is given, when $t = T$:

$$Cp_{\min,n} = \frac{S \cdot F \cdot D \cdot (1 - e^{-nk\tau})}{Vd \cdot (1 - e^{-k\tau})} \cdot e^{-k\tau} \tag{D.16}$$

D.3   STEADY-STATE EQUATIONS

The equations for steady-state plasma concentrations simplify somewhat. These equations are derived in Chapter 12 but are summarized here. During therapy, n increases with each successive dose. As steady state is approached:

1. $nk\tau$ gets large.
2. $e^{-nk\tau}$ decreases and tends to zero.
3. $(1 - e^{-nk\tau})$ becomes equal to 1 and disappears from equation (D.14).

$$Cp_{ss} = \frac{S \cdot F \cdot D}{Vd \cdot \left(1 - e^{-k\tau}\right)} \cdot e^{-kt} \tag{D.17}$$

The peak plasma concentration at steady state:

$$Cp_{\max,ss} = \frac{S \cdot F \cdot D}{Vd \cdot \left(1 - e^{-k\tau}\right)} \tag{D.18}$$

The trough plasma concentration at steady state:

$$Cp_{\min,ss} = \frac{S \cdot F \cdot D}{Vd \cdot \left(1 - e^{-k\tau}\right)} \cdot e^{-k\tau} \tag{D.19}$$

APPENDIX E

ENZYME KINETICS: MICHAELIS–MENTEN EQUATION AND MODELS FOR INHIBITORS AND INDUCERS OF DRUG METABOLISM

Sara E. Rosenbaum and Roberta S. King

E.1 KINETICS OF DRUG METABOLISM: THE MICHAELIS–MENTEN MODEL

E.1.1 Overview

The Michaelis–Menten model is the most common approach used to model the kinetics of enzymatic metabolism, and it is the basis of the approach used to derive mathematical expressions for the effects of inhibitors and inducers of drug-metabolizing enzymes. An understanding of the Michaelis–Menten model and its associated parameters of Vmax and Km is important to fully understand the models used to describe altered enzyme activity.

This appendix begins with a brief description of the derivation of the Michaelis–Menten equation and is followed by a presentation of the approaches used to model the effects of modifiers of the drug-metabolizing enzymes. Detailed derivations of the Michaelis–Menten equation and some of other equations found in this appendix may be found in enzyme kinetics textbooks [1, 2]. The value of the Michaelis–Menten equation (and model it is based on) is that it allows enzymatic reactions to be expressed mathematically using only experimentally measurable or controllable parameters. However, the model is valid only under specific experimental conditions that conform to assumptions utilized in the mathematical derivations. These assumptions and experimental conditions will be emphasized in this text.

Traditionally, the Michaelis–Menten model is described using the letter "S" to indicate Substrate, "P" to indicate Product, and "E" to indicate Enzyme. When applied specifically to drug-metabolism enzymatic processes, it is useful to replace "S" with "D" for Drug, and to replace "P" with "M" for Metabolite. Thus, the processes involved in metabolism of a drug are shown below:

$$D + E \underset{k_2}{\overset{k^1}{\rightleftharpoons}} ED \underset{k_{\text{cat}}}{\rightarrow} M + E \tag{E.1}$$

Free drug, D, binds to the free enzyme, E, at the site of metabolism (e.g., hepatocyte and enterocyte) with a forward rate constant of k_1, to produce a drug-enzyme complex, ED. This is a reversible process and the rate constant for the backward process is labeled as k_2, which represents dissociation of the ED complex to yield the unchanged drug and enzyme. Subsequently, a second forward reaction can occur resulting in the enzyme-mediated chemical modification of the drug to form the metabolite (M) with rate constant of k_{cat}, indicating rate of catalysis.

E.1.2 Assumptions for Validity of Michaelis–Menten Model

The Michaelis–Menten model equation is valid under specific experimental conditions that conform to assumptions utilized in the mathematical derivations. One necessary assumption is that the conversion of metabolite M back to unchanged drug D does not occur, and thus the Michaelis–Menten model is only valid under experimental conditions where the reverse catalytic reaction does not substantially occur. These conditions occur during the early stage of the reaction when the concentration of metabolite M is essentially zero. This is referred to as **initial-rate** (also called **initial velocity**) **conditions.** Experimentally, initial-rate conditions are sufficiently maintained by ensuring that no more than approximately 10% of total drug is converted to metabolite during the time of the experimental assay. Under these conditions, product formation is linear with time of incubation.

Another assumption is that the enzyme reaction occurs under **steady-state conditions**. Steady-state conditions require that the concentration of the *ED* complex once formed remains steady, meaning its rate of formation equals its rate of decomposition, and [*ED*] does not change with time during the experimental assay. Experimentally, steady-state conditions occur when the total enzyme concentration [E_t] is much lower (at least 1000-fold lower) than the initial drug concentration [*D*]. These are described as "catalytic" concentrations of enzyme.

E.1.3 *Km* and *Vmax*

It is helpful now to define the two parameters, *Km* and *Vmax*, which are the cornerstones for the Michaelis–Menten model. The Michaelis constant (*Km*) is always defined as the combination of rate constants involved in the formation and decomposition of the *ED* complex. In our model shown in equation E.1, the rate of formation (k_1) and decomposition ($k_2 + k_{cat}$) of the *ED* complex results in

$$Km = \frac{(k_2 + k_{cat})}{k_1} \tag{E.2}$$

Maximum velocity (*Vmax*) is defined as the maximum possible rate of metabolism, which only occurs when all the enzyme (E_t) is being used in the catalytic process k_{cat}. *Vmax* is a function of the total concentration of enzyme multiplied by the rate constant for the catalytic process k_{cat}:

$$V\max = [E_t] * k_{cat} \tag{E.3}$$

The Michaelis–Menten equation uses the defined parameters, *Km* and *Vmax*, to mathematically relate the experimentally determined rate of product formation (*V*) during an enzyme assay to the experimentally controlled total drug concentration in the assay. And because *Vmax* is mathematically dependent on the total concentration of enzyme present [E_t], the enzyme concentration added to the system must also be experimentally controlled. According to the Michaelis–Menten model, the rate of metabolism (*V*) is given by:

$$V = \frac{[D] * V\max}{[D] + Km} \tag{E.4}$$

E.1.4 Derivation of the Michaelis–Menten Equation

In order to fully understand the necessity of the initial-rate and steady-state conditions, it is helpful to see the full derivation of the Michaelis–Menten equation. The derivation of the Michaelis–Menten equation starts with definition of the rate of metabolism (*V*), which can be experimentally determined by measurement of the amount of metabolite formed during the time of the experimental assay,

$$V = \frac{dM}{dt} \tag{E.5}$$

Under the necessary initial-rate and steady-state experimental conditions, this rate will be linear and equal to the rate at which ED turns into E + M, which is equal to $k_{cat} * [ED]$. Thus,

$$V = \frac{dM}{dt} = k_{cat} * [ED] \qquad \text{(E.6)}$$

However, we do not experimentally know $[ED]$ or k_{cat} so we need to solve for $[ED]$ and k_{cat} in terms of other knowable or defined quantities.

Remember V_{max} was defined as $V_{max} = [E_t] * k_{cat}$ (E.3), thus, we can substitute for k_{cat}:

$$V = k_{cat} * [ED] = \frac{V_{max}}{[E_t]} * [ED] \qquad \text{(E.7)}$$

To solve for $[ED]$, remember from our assumptions of steady state that the rate of ED formation (rate constant, k_1) equals the rate of ED dissolution (overall rate constants, $k_2 + k_{cat}$), and thus,

Rate of Formation of ED = Rate of Breakdown of ED

$$[E] * [D] * k_1 = [ED] * (k_2 + k_{cat}) \qquad \text{(E.8)}$$

Rearranging results in:

$$\frac{[E] * [D]}{[ED]} = \frac{(k_2 + k_{cat})}{k_1} \qquad \text{(E.9)}$$

And remember Km was defined in equation (E.2) as

$$Km = \frac{(k_2 + k_{cat})}{k_1}$$

Thus,

$$\frac{[E] * [D]}{[ED]} = Km \qquad \text{(E.10)}$$

which rearranges to

$$[ED] = \frac{[E] * [D]}{Km} \qquad \text{(E.11)}$$

Next, we need to use the initial-rate assumption. The free enzyme concentration $[E]$ and enzyme-drug complex concentration $[ED]$ cannot be exactly determined, but it is known that the total enzyme concentration ($[E_t]$) added to the experimental system must be equal to the free enzyme concentration plus the concentration of the drug-enzyme complex,

$$[E_t] = [E] + [ED] \qquad \text{(E.12)}$$

which rearranges to

$$[E] = [E_t] - [ED] \tag{E.13}$$

Similarly, the free drug concentration $[D]$ cannot be exactly determined, but because of the assumption that $[E_t]$ is much lower (at least 1000-fold lower) than the initial drug concentration, $[ED]$ will be insignificantly small relative to $[D]$. Thus, we can use the initial drug concentration $[D]$ without adjusting for conversion to ED or metabolite.

Now that we have knowable quantities for $[E]$, $[ED]$, and $[D]$, substituting for $[E]$ as given in equation (E.13) into (E.11) yields:

$$[ED] = \frac{\left([E_t] - [ED]\right) * [D]}{Km} \tag{E.14}$$

Rearrangement yields:

$$Km\,[ED] = [E_t] * [D] - [ED] * [D] \tag{E.15}$$

Add $[ED] * [D]$ to both sides of equation (E.15) which yields:

$$Km\,[ED] + [ED] * [D] = [E_t] * [D] \tag{E.16}$$

Rearrangement yields

$$[ED] = \frac{[E_t] * [D]}{(Km + [D])} \tag{E.17}$$

Finally, $[ED]$ from equation (E.17) is substituted into equation (E.7):

$$V = \frac{V\max}{[E_t]} * \frac{[E_t] * [D]}{(Km + [D])} \tag{E.18}$$

$[E_t]$ divides out, resulting in the traditional Michaelis–Menten equation,

$$V = \frac{V\max * [D]}{(Km + [D])} \tag{E.4}$$

E.1.5 Summary, Practical Considerations, and Interpretations

The Michaelis–Menten equation shown above is useful because it links measurable quantities (drug concentration and rate of metabolite formation) to the drug-specific parameters (Vmax and Km). This enables the parameters of the model to be determined from *in vitro* experiments where the rate of metabolism is determined at different drug concentrations.

The following practical considerations must be in place for proper Michaelis–Menten enzyme assay design and conduct:

1. User controls the total volume of the experimental assay.
2. User controls the total amount (and concentration) of Drug added to the assay.

3. User controls the total amount (and concentration) of Enzyme added to the assay.

4. Preliminary range-finding experiments are needed to determine proper combinations of [D], [E], and time so that steady state and initial-rate conditions are maintained.

5. User measures the total amount of Metabolite formed per period of time, which is the rate of metabolite formation (under steady state and initial-rate conditions).

The following interpretations and conclusions can be drawn from properly conducted Michaelis–Menten enzyme assays:

1. The *Km* is constant for a given enzyme and substrate pair, no matter the enzyme source. Thus, two different enzyme sources resulting in equal calculated *Km* (for otherwise equivalent assay conditions) provide evidence supporting the conclusion that the same enzyme catalyzes the reaction in both sources.

2. *Km* is *not* a true indication of binding affinity of drug for the enzyme. *Km* includes not only drug binding affinity, but also the catalytic step. Thus, *only* when k_{cat} is much smaller than k_2, is *Km* truly a reflection of drug binding affinity (K_d). Under these conditions, no catalysis would occur and no product would be formed. However, for practical considerations, the *relative Km* can be compared across a series of chemically similar drugs for which the rate of catalysis is expected to be approximately equal.

3. Relative efficiency of a single enzyme catalyzing metabolism of two different drugs can be compared using the relative measure of *Vmax/Km* (called intrinsic clearance, discussed in Section E.1.6).

4. When different enzyme samples are compared under otherwise equivalent assay conditions, the rate of product formation (*v*) is dependent on the amount of enzyme present. Thus, higher product formation (activity) provides evidence that supports the conclusion that more enzyme is present in the higher activity sample (i.e., different expression levels of active protein).

E.1.6   Relationship Between Intrinsic Clearance and the Michaelis–Menten Parameters

In clinical pharmacokinetics, the primary pharmacokinetic parameter for elimination (metabolism and renal) is a drug's clearance. The relationship between clearance and the Michaelis–Menten parameters will now be presented.

Metabolism is driven by the free (unbound) drug concentration at enzyme site, [D], which has units on the molar scale.

As discussed in Chapter 5, the therapeutic concentrations of most drugs display linear metabolism because their therapeutic concentrations in the body and at the enzyme site are much less than their *Km*. As a result, the denominator in equation (E.4) can be simplified: because $Km>>>[D]$, $Km +[D] \approx Km$:

$$V = \frac{[D] * V\,max}{Km}$$

(E.19)

The rate of metabolism can also be expressed in terms of intrinsic clearance, which is the constant of proportionality between the rate of metabolism and the free drug concentration at the enzyme site (see Chapter 5)

$$V = Cl_{int} * [D]$$

(E.20)

where Cl_{int} is the fundamental or intrinsic clearance of the unbound drug at the enzyme site. Thus,

$$Cl_{int} = \frac{V\max}{Km} \tag{E.21}$$

Perpetrators of metabolism-based drug–drug interactions (DDIs) produce their effects by altering a drug's Vmax and/or Km, which then results in changes in intrinsic clearance:

$$Cl_{int}^{P} = \frac{V\max^{P}}{Km^{P}} \tag{E.22}$$

where the superscript P indicates parameter values in the presence of a perpetrator.

Changes in intrinsic clearance are then translated into changes in hepatic clearance and/or hepatic bioavailability. The ratio of a drug's intrinsic clearance in the absence and presence of a modifier of the drug-metabolizing enzymes is commonly used to assess the impact of the modifier on a single pathway. This ratio is known as "R." Dividing equation (E.21) by equation (E.22)

$$R = \frac{Cl_{int}}{Cl_{int}^{P}} = \frac{V\max}{Km} * \frac{Km^{P}}{V\max^{P}} \tag{E.23}$$

E.2   EFFECT OF PERPETRATORS OF DDI ON ENZYME KINETICS AND INTRINSIC CLEARANCE

E.2.1   Reversible Inhibition

E.2.1.1   Mathematical Model for the Effect of Reversible Inhibitors on Enzyme Kinetics

A reversible inhibitor competes with the substrate for the enzyme. It has no effect on the total concentration of enzyme in the system nor on the drug-enzyme complex. A representation of the action of an inhibitor is shown in Figure E.1. The inhibitor binds to the enzyme to produce an inhibitor-enzyme complex ([IE]). This is a reversible process with forward and backward rate constants of $k_{1,i}$ and $k_{2,i}$ respectively. The dissociation constant of the inhibitor (K_i, where $K_i = k_{2,i}/k_{1,i}$) is a reciprocal measure of the inhibitor's affinity for the

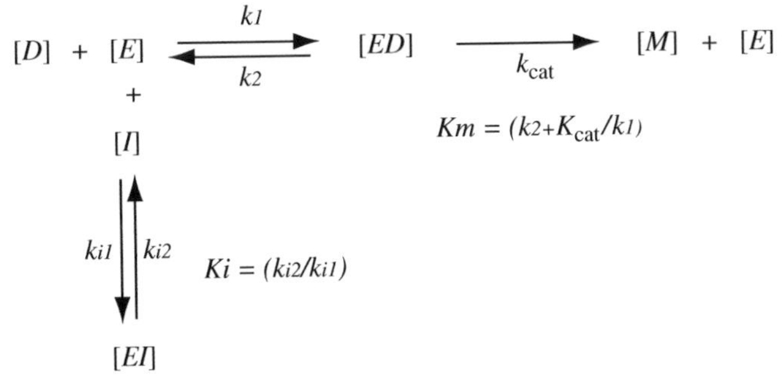

$$[D] + [E] \underset{k_2}{\overset{k_1}{\rightleftharpoons}} [ED] \xrightarrow{k_{cat}} [M] + [E]$$

$$+$$

$$[I] \qquad Km = (k_2 + K_{cat}/k_1)$$

$$ki_1 \updownarrow ki_2 \quad Ki = (ki_2/ki_1)$$

$$[EI]$$

FIGURE E.1   Both the victim drug [D] and the inhibitor [I] bind to and compete for the enzyme [E]. The inhibitor's dissociation constant (Ki) is an inverse measure of the inhibitor's affinity. The inhibitor produces an apparent increase (reduced affinity) in the victim drug's Km.

enzyme. This is a key parameter for the inhibitor. The smaller the value of K_i, the greater is the inhibitor's affinity for the enzyme, and the more potent the inhibitor. For example, the K_i values for ketoconazole and fluconazole have been reported to be 0.006 and 3.4 μM, respectively, for CYP3A4 [3], demonstrating that ketoconazole is the more potent inhibitor.

The equation used to describe the effect of reversible interactions on enzyme kinetics was first proposed by Rowland and Matin [4]. The equation for the total concentration of enzyme presented in the Michaelis–Menten derivation (E.12) must now be modified to reflect that some of the enzyme is taken up to form the inhibitor-enzyme complex. Thus, in the presence of a competitive inhibitor, the concentration of enzyme available for metabolism of the drug will be lower. The equation expressing the effect of a reversible inhibitor on the metabolism of a victim drug will be derived:

As always, the rate of metabolism is given by:

$$V = [ED] * k_{cat} \text{ and } V\text{max} = [E_t] * k_{cat} \tag{E.24}$$

Thus,

$$k_{cat} = \frac{V\text{max}}{E_t} \tag{E.25}$$

and

$$V = [ED] * \frac{V\text{max}}{E_t} \tag{E.26}$$

(a) Probing an expression for [ED], which cannot be measured, it was previously shown in equation (E.11):

$$[ED] = \frac{[E] * [D]}{Km} \tag{E.27}$$

(b) Probing an expression for E_t. In the presence of an inhibitor, the total enzyme concentration (E_t) will be:

$$[E_t] = [ED] + [E] + [EI] \tag{E.28}$$

An expression for [EI] can be obtained using the law of mass action:

$$[EI] = \frac{[E] * [I]}{K_i} \tag{E.29}$$

where, $K_i = k_{2,i}/k_{1,i}$

An expression for [ED] was given above [equation (E.27)].

Substituting the expressions for [ED] and [EI] into the equation for the total enzyme concentration (E.28)

$$[E_t] = \frac{[E] * [D]}{Km} + [E] + \frac{[E] * [I]}{Ki} \tag{E.30}$$

$$[E_t] = [E]\left(1 + \frac{[D]}{Km} + \frac{[I]}{Ki}\right) \tag{E.31}$$

Substituting the expressions for $[ED]$ given in equation (E.29) and E_t given in equation (E.31) into equation (E.26)

$$V = \frac{V\max * [D]}{Km\left(1 + \dfrac{[D]}{Km} + \dfrac{[I]}{Ki}\right)} \qquad (E.32)$$

Rearranging

$$V = \frac{V\max * [D]}{[D] + Km(1 + [I]/K_i)} \qquad (E.33)$$

Comparing the equation for the rate of the enzymatic process in the absence (equation E.4) and presence (equation E.33) of the inhibitor, it can be seen that the inhibitor produces an apparent increase in the victim drug's Km value. Let Km^l be the apparent Km of the victim drug in the presence of the inhibitor and:

$$Km^l == Km\left(1 + \frac{[I]}{K_i}\right) \qquad (E.34)$$

E.2.1.2 IC50 of Reversible Inhibitors

The IC50 of a reversible inhibitor is the inhibitor concentration that reduces the rate of a victim drug's metabolism by half. Its value and relationship to K_i can be confusing because the value of the IC50 depends on the concentration of the victim drug. With increasing concentrations of the victim, more of the victim binds to the enzyme and a larger amount of an inhibitor is required to displace it to inhibit metabolism by a certain extent, for example, 50%.

By definition, when the rate of metabolism of a victim drug is reduced by 50% (at any drug concentration), the inhibitor concentration is defined as the IC50.

As shown in equation E.33, in the presence of an inhibitor

$$V = \frac{V\max * [D]}{[D] + Km(1 + [I]/K_i)}$$

When $[I] = IC50$ and the rate is half that in the absence of the inhibitor.

$$V = \frac{V\max * [D]}{[D] + Km(1 + [IC50]/K_i)} \qquad (E.35)$$

Half the normal (in the absence of the inhibitor) rate of metabolism can also be expressed:

$$V = \frac{V\max * [D]}{([D] + Km)} * \frac{1}{2} \qquad (E.36)$$

Equating equations (E.35) and (E.36)

$$\frac{V\max * [D]}{([D] + Km) * 2} = \frac{V\max * [D]}{[D] + Km(1 + [IC50]/K_i)}$$

Rearranging

$$K_i = \frac{IC50}{\left(1 + \dfrac{[D]}{Km}\right)} \tag{E.37}$$

Experimentally, it can be difficult and time-consuming to measure the K_i of an inhibitor. The estimation of an IC50 is more straightforward and is often measured as an alternative to the K_i. From the relationship between the K_i and IC50 shown in equation (E.37), it can be demonstrated that:

- If the IC50 is measured when the concentration of the victim drug is equal to its Km, the IC50 is equal to $2*K_i$ and the K_i can be estimated by dividing the IC50 by 2.
- If the concentration of the victim drug is much lower than its Km ($D \ll Km$), the rate of metabolism will be in the first-order range and the value of the IC50 will be approximately equal to the Ki. For example, let the concentration of the victim drug equal 10% its Km, calculating the Ki from equation (E.37):

$$K_i = \frac{IC50}{\left(1 + \dfrac{[D]}{Km}\right)} = \frac{IC50}{\left(1 + \dfrac{[0.1Km]}{Km}\right)} = IC50 * 0.91$$

The IC50 is often used as an alternative to the K_i to assess possible DDIs for transporters [5].

E.2.1.3 *Ratio of the Intrinsic Clearance of a Victim Drug in the Absence and Presence of a Reversible Inhibition*

Recall R (equation E.23), the ratio of a victim drug's intrinsic clearance in the absence and presence of a perpetrator, is used to assess the impact of altered metabolism on a single pathway (equation E.23). For reversible inhibitors, the ratio is referred to as R_1 and is given by:

$$R_1 = \frac{Cl_{int}}{Cl_{int}^I} = \left(1 + \frac{[I]}{Ki}\right) \tag{E.38}$$

The larger the value of R, the greater the magnitude of the predicted DDI. Equation (E.38) demonstrates that the magnitude of change in intrinsic clearance brought about by a reversible inhibitor is dependent on both the inhibitor's potency (K_i) and $[I]$, its unbound concentration at the enzyme site. The ratio $[I]/K_i$ can be used to predict the extent of effect produced by reversible inhibitors. The larger the ratio, the greater is the effect on intrinsic clearance of the pathway affected. Note when the inhibitor concentration, $[I]$, is equal to K_i, there is 50% reduction in intrinsic clearance.

E.2.2   Time-Dependent Inhibition

E.2.2.1 *Mathematical Model for the Effect of TDI on Enzyme Kinetics*
The underlying mechanism of time-dependent inhibition is much more complex and varied than that of competitive inhibition [6,7], and a detailed discussion of this type of inhibition is beyond the scope of this book. Although multiple mechanisms may result in time-dependent inhibition (TDI), one of the most common causes results from the formation of metabolic intermediates (MIs) that bind very strongly, often irreversibly to the enzyme and destroy its activity. The inhibition increases over time as increasing amounts of MI are formed.

$$[I] + [E] \underset{k2}{\overset{k1}{\rightleftharpoons}} [EI] \xrightarrow{k_{cat}} [P] + [E]$$

$$\Big\downarrow k_{inact}$$

$$[E.MI]$$

FIGURE E.2   The interaction of a time-dependent inhibitor with an enzyme. The inhibitor $[I]$ binds to the enzyme $[E]$ to form an inhibitor-enzyme complex (k_1 and k_2 are the rate constants for the forward and backward processes, respectively). The inhibitor-enzyme complex could dissociate to release the drug and the enzyme, undergo catalytic metabolism to form a product $[P]$, or the inhibitor's metabolic intermediate could bind to the enzyme and destroy its activity. The first-order rate constants for the catalytic and inactivation processes are k_{cat} and k_{inact}, respectively.

Recovery from the inhibition requires the synthesis of new enzyme, and thus may persist long after the inhibitor has been fully eliminated from the body. The inhibition produced by TDI is parameterized *in vitro* by two parameters: the inhibitor's potency, K_I, which is defined as the concentration of the TDI required for half-maximal inhibition; and a measure of the destructive power of the MI, k_{inact}, which is defined as the maximal rate constant of inactivation. These parameters are discussed in more detail below.

Figure E.2 shows the interaction of a TDI with an enzyme. The kinetics and associated equations for TDI have been described in the literature [8, 9]. The inhibitor ($[I]$) binds to the enzyme ($[E]$) (rate constant k_I) to form the enzyme-inhibitor complex ($[EI]$) from which three outcomes are possible. First, the inhibitor can dissociate to yield the unchanged enzyme (rate constant k_2). Second, a productive catalytic metabolism can yield a metabolite or a product (P) (rate constant, k_{cat}). Finally, the inhibitor's MI can bind tightly and irreversibly to the enzyme, destroying it and abolishing its activity.

The inhibitor potency K_I and k_{inact} are complex functions of several rate constants (e.g., k_1, k_2, and k_{cat}) [7]. However, several simplifying assumptions can be made in order to develop an expression for k_{inact} and K_I and allow the role of k_{inact} and K_I in controlling inhibition to be better understood [9]. The derivation assumes, first that the initial binding of the inhibitor to the enzyme is fast and that an equilibrium is rapidly achieved. Second, it is assumed that the productive enzymatic pathway and the enzymatic pathway leading to inactivation of the enzyme are very rapid, and nonrate limiting [9]. Under these conditions, K_I represents the dissociation constant for the inhibitor and k_{inact} the rate constant for the formation of the inactive form of the enzyme. The rate of inactivation is assumed to be a first-order process driven by the concentration of the enzyme-inhibitor complex and the first-order rate constant for the process, k_{inact}.

Normally, when a TDI is absent, the enzyme concentration is constant and at steady state. Like all endogenous proteins, the enzyme undergoes a natural turn over process in the body. Usually, the rate of synthesis of an endogenous protein is assumed to be a zero-order process (rate, k_{syn}) and the rate of enzyme degradation assumed to be first order (rate constant k_{degrad}) (see Chapter 20), (Figure E.3).

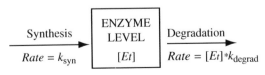

FIGURE E.3   Enzyme turnover. The enzyme is produced by a zero-order process (rate $= k_{syn}$). The degradation of the enzyme follows first-order kinetics with a rate constant of k_{degrad}.

Under normal steady-state conditions, the enzyme concentration $[E_t]$ in the absence of inhibitors is given by

$$\text{Rate of synthesis} = \text{Rate of degradation}$$

$$k_{\text{syn}} = [E_t] * k_{\text{degrad}} \tag{E.39}$$

$$[Et] = \frac{k_{\text{syn}}}{k_{\text{degrad}}}$$

Rearranging

$$k_{\text{syn}} = k_{\text{degrad}} * [Et] \tag{E.40}$$

In the presence of the TDI, there is additional loss of the enzyme through inactivation by the MI. (Figure E.3).

Thus, the rate of inactivation can be expressed as:

$$\text{The Rate of Inactivation} = -\frac{d\left[E_t^I\right]}{dt} = k_{\text{inact}} * [EI] \tag{E.41}$$

where E_t^I is the total enzyme concentration in the presence of the inhibitor. An expression for $[EI]$, which cannot be measured, will now be probed. Under the simplifications and assumptions made above, according to the law of mass action:

$$[EI] * K_I = [E] * [I] \tag{E.42}$$

where K_I is the dissociation constant (k_2/k_1) for the enzyme-inhibitor complex $[EI]$, and $[E]$ is the concentration of free enzyme.

The free enzyme concentration at any time is equal to the total enzyme concentration minus the concentration of the complex. Thus,

$$[E] = \left[E_t^I\right] - [EI] \tag{E.43}$$

Substituting for $[E]$ in equation (E.42)

$$[EI] * K_I = \left(\left[E_t^I\right] - [EI]\right) * [I] \tag{E.44}$$

Solving for EI

$$[EI] = \frac{\left[E_t^I\right] * [I]}{K_I + [I]} \tag{E.45}$$

Substituting the expression for $[EI]$ given above into equation (E.41), the inactivation rate of the enzyme is expressed as:

$$-\frac{d\left[E_t^I\right]}{dt} = k_{\text{inact}} * \frac{\left[E_t^I\right] * [I]}{K_I + [I]} \tag{E.46}$$

Rearranging

$$-\frac{d\left[E_t^I\right]}{dt} = \left[E_t^I\right] * \frac{k_{\text{inact}} * [I]}{K_I + [I]} \tag{E.47}$$

Let,

$$k_{\text{obs}} = \frac{k_{\text{inact}} * [I]}{K_I + [I]} \tag{E.48}$$

Substituting k_{obs} into equation (E.47)

$$-\frac{d\left[E_t^I\right]}{dt} = \left[E_t^I\right] * k_{\text{obs}} \tag{E.49}$$

It can be seen from equation (E.49) that the rate of inactivation can now be viewed as an apparent first-order process driven by the total enzyme concentration and an apparent first-order rate constant of k_{obs}, which is dependent on the inhibitor concentration, K_I and k_{inact} (Figure E.4). Further, it can be seen in Figure E.4 that when $[I]$ is very high $k_{\text{obs}} = k_{\text{inact}}$. Also note from equation (E.48), it can be seen that when $[I] = K_I$, k_{obs} is equal to half k_{inact}. **Thus, k_{inact} and K_I can be defined as the maximal inactivation rate constant and the inhibitor concentration causing half-maximal inactivation, respectively.**

The model for the action of the inhibitor on the enzyme concentration can now be viewed more simply (Figure E.5) in which the enzyme is subject to two first-order destruction pathways: degradation (rate constant k_{degrad}) and inactivation (rate constant k_{obs}).

In addition to the assumptions noted above, this derivation also assumes that k_{syn} and k_{degrad} are not affected by the inhibitor, there is no competitive inhibition, and that the function of the enzyme molecules not inactivated remains unchanged by the inhibitor [6]. When the assumptions or simplifications used to derive these formula do not hold, other rate constants for the enzymatic processes will also control K_I and k_{inact} but even under those circumstances, K_I will represent the concentration of the inhibitor that results in 50% the maximal rate of inactivation. Thus, in TDI or mechanism-based inhibition, K_I is defined as the inhibitor concentration that produces 50% maximum inhibition and k_{inact} is referred

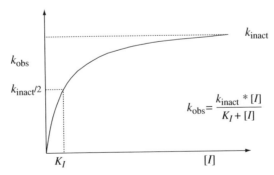

FIGURE E.4   Relationship between k_{obs} and $[I]$. The value of k_{obs} increases with increases in the inhibitor concentration, $[I]$. At high concentrations, k_{obs} becomes equal to k_{inact}, the maximal inactivation rate constant. Note when the inactivation is half maximal, the inhibitor concentration is equal to K_I. Thus, K_I is defined as the inhibitor concentration that produces half maximal inhibition.

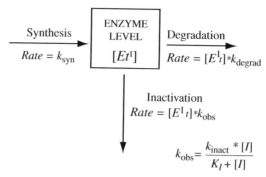

FIGURE E.5 Inactivation viewed as an apparent first-order process driven by the total enzyme concentration and k_{obs}. See the text and Figures E.2 and E.3 for definitions of the symbols.

to as the constant producing the maximal rate of inactivation. Note, for drugs that are both reversible and mechanism-based inhibitors, there is no correlation between the values of K_i and K_I [10].

Recovery of enzyme activity after TDI is dependent on the synthesis of new enzyme, which is controlled by the first-order degradation constant (k_{degrad}) (see Chapter 20, Section 20.3.2) and will typically take about four k_{degrad} half-lives. Thus, the duration of action of a TDI is controlled by a physiological parameter, the degradation rate constant of the affected enzyme.

E.2.2.2   Understanding the Parameters of TDI through Simulation: http://web.uri.edu/pharmacy/research/rosenbaum/sims

Go to model 13, Time-Dependent Enzyme Inhibition simulation model: DDI 1 Time Dependent Enzyme Inhibition (http://web.uri.edu/pharmacy/research/rosenbaum/sims/Model13).

The model is based on the TDI of CYP3A4. The normal steady-state enzyme concentration of CYP3A4 was set to 5 μmol per liver (Assuming 70 pmol/mg microsomal protein [11]; 40 mg microsomal protein/g liver and a liver weight of 1648 g provides a value of 4.6 μmol, which was rounded to 5), and k_{degrad} to 0.0192 h^{-1} (see [3]). To maintain that steady amount of 3A4, with a k_{degrad} of 0.0192 h^{-1}, the k_{syn} must be 5*0.0192 = 0.096 μmol. h^{-1}. The inhibitor's concentration is in units of K_I, which is set to 1 μM. The k_{inact} of the inhibitor is initially set to 2 h^{-1}.

Perform a simulation with the default values ([I] = 1 unit of K_I).

1. *Observe how the total enzyme concentration decreases in a monoexponential manner over time.*

2. *The rate constant for the first order fall in the enzyme concentration is k_{obs}, which is shown in the display window. Notice how it compares to k_{inact}, which is also displayed. Recall, from equation (E.48)*

$$k_{obs} = \frac{k_{inact} * [I]}{K_I + [I]}$$

Note that in this simulation, [I] = K_I and $k_{obs} = (k_{inact}/2)$.

3. *Increase the inhibitor concentration [I]. Note as it increases the enzyme concentration falls more steeply, which reflects the increase in k_{obs}. Note how k_{obs} is approaching k_{inact}. When [I] becomes very large relative to K_I, k_{obs} becomes equal to k_{inact}.*

4. *Use different values of K_I. Observe how the inhibition becomes less as K_I increases.*

5. *Go to the Recovery page. Turn on the short-term exposure button, which removes the inhibitor from the system at time = 1 day. Thus, at 1 day, [I] will become equal to zero. Perform a simulation. Note the enzyme level returns to normal at around 8 days. The time for the system to recover from the enzyme is determined by the first-order degradation rate constant for the enzyme (see Chapter 17). It will take about $4*k_{degrad}$ half-lives to restore the system to about 90% of its normal values. For the default setting of k_{degrad} (0.0192 h^{-1} or 0.461 days), the enzyme level is about 90% of its original value 6 days after the inhibitor was removed. Adjust k_{degrad} and note how it affects the time to recover from the inhibitor.*

E.2.2.3 Ratio of the Intrinsic Clearance of a Victim Drug in the Absence and Presence of a TDI

TDI inhibitors reduce the amount of enzyme. Thus, they reduce $Vmax$ but do not affect Km.

The ratio of $Vmax$ in the absence and presence of the inhibitor is given by the ratio of the total enzyme in the absence and presence of the inhibitor:

$$\frac{V\max}{V\max^I} = \frac{[E_t]}{[E_t^I]} \tag{E.50}$$

From equation (E.39)

$$[Et] = \frac{k_{syn}}{k_{degrad}} \tag{E.51}$$

In the presence of the TDI, there is additional loss of enzyme through degradation and:

$$[E_t^I] = \frac{k_{syn}}{k_{degrad} + k_{obs}} \tag{E.52}$$

Thus, from equations (E.51) and (E.52)

$$\frac{[E_t]}{[E_t^I]} = \frac{k_{degrad}}{k_{degrad} + k_{obs}} \tag{E.53}$$

$$\frac{V\max}{V\max^I} = \frac{[E_t]}{[E_t^I]} = \frac{k_{degrad} + k_{obs}}{k_{degrad}} \tag{E.54}$$

The impact of the inhibition is assessed by calculating the ratio (R) of intrinsic clearance in the absence and presence of the inhibition of the affected pathway. For TDI, the ratio is referred to as R_2. Recall equation (E.23),

$$R = \frac{Cl_{int}}{Cl_{int}^I} = \frac{V\max}{Km} * \frac{Km^I}{V\max^I}$$

The value of *Km* is not altered by TDI and substituting in for the *V*max ratio given in equation (E.54):

$$R_2 = \frac{Cl_{\text{int}}}{Cl_{\text{int}}^I} = \frac{V\max}{V\max^I} = \frac{k_{\text{degrad}} + k_{\text{obs}}}{k_{\text{degrad}}} \tag{E.55}$$

Substituting in for k_{obs} as given in equation (E.48)

$$R_2 = \frac{Cl_{\text{int}}}{Cl_{\text{int}}^I} = \frac{k_{\text{degrad}} + \dfrac{k_{\text{inact}} * [I]}{K_I + [I]}}{k_{\text{degrad}}} \tag{E.56}$$

E.2.3 Enzyme Induction

E.2.3.1 *Model for Effect of Induction on Enzyme Kinetics*

Inducers of drug metabolism do not bind to the enzyme itself, nor do they interfere with the binding of the drug to the enzyme. Instead, they affect the regulation of the gene encoding the enzyme and increase production of the enzyme. This results in higher enzyme concentrations. Although inducers can activate a number of transcription factors, the pregnane-X receptor is most commonly the target for inducers of drug metabolism enzymes and drug transporters.

The model for the effect of inducers on the amount of enzyme assumes that steady-state enzyme levels have been achieved in the presence of the inducer. A simple $E_{\max}$ model (Chapter 19) is used to incorporate the effect of the inducer on enzyme synthesis.

In the presence of the inducer:

$$k_{\text{syn}}^{Ind} = k_{\text{syn}} + k_{\text{syn}} * \frac{E_{\max} * [I]}{EC50 + [I]}$$

where k_{syn}^{Ind} is the zero-order rate of enzyme synthesis in the presence of the inducer, $E_{\max}$ is the maximum fold induction the inducer can produce, EC50 is the inducer concentration that produces 50% maximum induction, and $[I]$ is the concentration of the inducer.

At steady state, the total enzyme concentration in the presence of the inducer $[E_t^{Ind}]$ is now expressed as:

$$[E_t^{Ind}] = Et * \left(1 + \frac{E_{\max} * [I]}{EC50 + [I]} \right) \tag{E.57}$$

E.2.3.2 *Ratio of the Intrinsic Clearance of a Victim Drug in the Absence and Presence of an Inducer*

The value of the ratio (R) of a drug's intrinsic clearance in the absence and presence of an inducer is known as R_3. Recall from equation (E.23) generally R is expressed as:

$$R = \frac{Cl_{\text{int}}}{Cl_{\text{int}}^P} = \frac{V\max}{Km} * \frac{Km^P}{V\max^P}$$

where the superscript P indicates a value on the presence of a perpetrator. Inducers affect Vmax. As discussed above, inducers do not alter Km, but only Vmax. Thus:

$$R_3 = \frac{Cl_{int}}{Cl_{int}^{Ind}} = \frac{V\max}{V\max^{Ind}} \tag{E.58}$$

where Cl_{int}^{Ind} and Vmax^{Ind} are the drug's intrinsic clearance and Vmax in the presence of an inducer.

As shown in the previous section (equation E.50).

$$\frac{V\max}{V\max^{Ind}} = \frac{[E_t]}{\left[E_t^{Ind}\right]}$$

Substituting in for $[E_t]$ as given in equation (E.57)

$$\frac{[E_t]}{\left[E_t^{Ind}\right]} = \frac{[E_t]}{[E_t] * \left(1 + \dfrac{E_{\max} * [I]}{EC50 + [I]}\right)} = \frac{1}{1 + \dfrac{E_{\max} * [I]}{EC50 + [I]}}$$

$$\frac{Vmax}{V\max^{Ind}} = \frac{1}{1 + \dfrac{E_{\max} * [I]}{EC50 + [I]}}$$

Thus, substituting into equation (E.58)

$$R_3 = \frac{Cl_{int}}{Cl_{int}^{Ind}} = \frac{1}{1 + \dfrac{E_{\max} * [I]}{EC50 + [I]}} \tag{E.59}$$

E.2.3.3 Understanding Induction through Simulation:
http://web.uri.edu/pharmacy/research/rosenbaum/sims
Open the model 14, Enzyme Induction model: DDI 2 Enzyme Induction (http://web.uri.edu/ pharmacy/research/rosenbaum/sims/Model14), which is based on the induction of CYP3A. The steady-state enzyme concentration of CYP3A4 is set to 5 µmol per liver (see Section E2.2.2). The units of concentration are EC50 and the $E_{\max}$ is set to 20-fold increase from normal, which is around the maximum fold increase reported for potent inducers, such as rifampin; [I] = 1 unit of EC50.

(a) *Perform a simulation in the absence of induction. Turn the inducer switch on and set [I] to 50 EC50 units. Notice that maximum induction is observed ($E_t \approx 5 + 5*20 = 105$ µM).*

(b) *Set [I] to 1 unit of EC50. Note that there is 50% maximum induction.*

(c) *Set [I] to 0.1 units of EC50. Note that with this inducer, even at a very low inducer concentration, the amount of enzyme has more than doubled.*

(d) *Reset [I] to 50 units of EC50, turn on the Recovery button and perform a simulation. The inducer will be withdrawn at time = 1 day. Note that it takes around 6–7 days for the enzyme system to recover. As noted above for TDI, recovery is a function of the degradation rate constant for the enzyme (0.0192 h^{-1} in this model). It will take about four degradation half-lives ($4*36$ h = 144 h = 6 days) to get to 95% recovery.*

REFERENCES

1. Segel, I. (1975) *Enzyme Kinetics. Behavior and Analysis of Rapid Equilibrium and Steady State Enzyme Systems*, John Wiley & Sons, New York.

2. Nagar, S., Argikar, U., and Tweedie, D (Eds.) (2014) *Enzyme Kinetics in Drug Metabolism. Fundamentals and Applications*, Springer.

3. Fahmi, O. A., Hurst, S., Plowchalk, D., Cook, J., Guo, F., Youdim, K., Dickins, M., Phipps, A., Darekar, A., Hyland, R., and Obach, R. S. (2009) Comparison of different algorithms for predicting clinical drug-drug interactions, based on the use of CYP3A4 in vitro data: predictions of compounds as precipitants of interaction. *Drug Metab Dispos, 37*, 1658–1666.

4. Rowland, M., and Matin, S. (1973) Kinetics of drug-drug interactions. *J Pharmacokinet Biopharm, 1*, 553–567.

5. Giacomini, K. M., Huang, S. M., Tweedie, D. J., Benet, L. Z., Brouwer, K. L., Chu, X., Dahlin, A., Evers, R., Fischer, V., Hillgren, K. M., Hoffmaster, K. A., Ishikawa, T., Keppler, D., Kim, R. B., Lee, C. A., Niemi, M., Polli, J. W., Sugiyama, Y., Swaan, P. W., Ware, J. A., Wright, S. H., Yee, S. W., Zamek-Gliszczynski, M. J., and Zhang, L. (2010) Membrane transporters in drug development. *Nat Rev Drug Discov, 9*, 215–236.

6. Venkatakrishnan, K., Obach, R. S., and Rostami-Hodjegan, A. (2007) Mechanism-based inactivation of human cytochrome P450 enzymes: strategies for diagnosis and drug-drug interaction risk assessment. *Xenobiotica, 37*, 1225–1256.

7. Monhutsky, M. H., and Hall, S. D. (2014) Irreversible enzyme inhibition kinetics and drug-drug interactions, in *Enzyme Kinetics in Drug Metabolism* (Nager, S., Argikat, U. A., and Tweedie D. J, Eds.), pp. 57–61, Humana Press, New York.

8. Silverman, R. B. (1988) *Mechanism-Based Enzyme Inactivation: Chemistry and Enzymology*, CRC Press, Boca Raton, FL.

9. Mayhew, B. S., Jones, D. R., and Hall, S. D. (2000) An in vitro model for predicting in vivo inhibition of cytochrome P450 3A4 by metabolic intermediate complex formation, *Drug Metab Dispos, 28*, 1031–1037.

10. Zhou, S., Yung Chan, S., Cher Goh, B., Chan, E., Duan, W., Huang, M., and McLeod, H. L. (2005) Mechanism-based inhibition of cytochrome P450 3A4 by therapeutic drugs. *Clin Pharmacokinet, 44*, 279–304.

11. Wolbold, R., Klein, K., Burk, O., Nussler, A. K., Neuhaus, P., Eichelbaum, M., Schwab, M., and Zanger, U. M. (2003) Sex is a major determinant of CYP3A4 expression in human liver. *Hepatology (Baltimore, Md.), 38*, 978–988.

APPENDIX F

SUMMARY OF THE PROPERTIES OF THE FICTITIOUS DRUGS USED IN THE TEXT

SARA E. ROSENBAUM

Lipoamide Lipoamide is a novel antipyretic drug that is believed to work by reducing the synthesis of cytokines. It appears to be safe in both children and adults. At concentrations above 300 µg/L, there is an increased incidence of fairly minor concentration-related side effects, including nausea and diarrhea. Lipoamide is available in both an IV formulation and an oral tablet.

Nosolatol Nosolatol is a β_1-adrenergic antagonist selective for receptors located in the heart and vascular smooth muscle. However, like all selective β_1 agents, at high doses (>300 mg/day for nosolatol), it loses its selectivity and can block β_2-adrenergic receptors, with undesirable results. Nosolatol shows no inherent α-activity. Like many other agents in this class, nosolatol has been found to be beneficial in treating hypertension, chronic stable angina, heart failure, and myocardial prophylaxis. Nosolatol is available in both an IV formulation and an oral tablet.

Disolvprazole A member of the proton pump inhibitor family of drugs, disolvprazole is an irreversible inhibitor of H^+, K^+-pumps in the parietal cells of the gastric mucosa and it shows many of the same characteristics as other drugs in this class. Disolvprazole has shown similar efficacy in ulcer-healing rates as other drugs in this class and is effective in the elimination of *Helicobacter pylori* when used at the doses recommended. Disolvprazole is available in both an IV formulation and an oral tablet.

Detailed information on the physicochemical and pharmacokinetic properties of these drugs is provided in Table F.1.

TABLE F.1 Physiochemical and Pharmacokinetic Properties of Lipoamide, Nosolatol, and Disolvprazole

	Lipoamide	Nosolatol	Disolvprazole
Physicochemical properties			
Acid/base	Base	Acid	Base
MW	396	365	221
Log P	3.2	2.1	0.2
Log $D_{6.0}$	3	1.8	−2.8
Highest dose strength (mg)	150	250	50
Solubility: pH 1–7.5	High: 1 g/L	Low: 0.5 g/L	High: 5 g/L
Fraction of oral dose recovered as metabolites in humans	99.00%	99.00%	0.05–0.03
Pharmacokinetics			
Cl (L/h)	62	12.6	12
Vd (L/kg)	6	3	0.5
k (h^{-1})	0.15	0.06	0.34
$t_{1/2}$	4.70	11.6	2.02
k_a (h^{-1}) (fasting)	4	2	2
fe	<0.01	<0.01	~0.98
fu	0.05	0.6	>0.95
Main enzyme involved in its metabolism	CYP2C9	CYP3A4	None
Substrate for intestinal uptake transporter	None known	None known	OATP1A2
Substrate for intestinal efflux transporter	None known	P-gp	None known
F_a	1	1	0.5
F_g	1	0.7	1
F_h	0.21	1	1
F	0.21	0.7	0.5
Substrate for renal transporter	No	No	OAT
Cp/Cb	1	1	1
Pharmacodynamics			
Target Cp_{ss}	50 µg/L	1.2 mg/L	400 µg/L
Other PD information	Indirect effect model I	E_{max} = 30 ± 3.2 bpm EC$_{50}$ 75 ± 15 µg/L	See Section 20.7.1.1

APPENDIX G

COMPUTER SIMULATION MODELS

SARA E. ROSENBAUM

All the computer simulation models were created using Stella 9.1.3 or 10.1.2 (isee Systems, Lebanon, NH; http://www.iseesystems.com/). The models were published on the Web as isee NetSim files using Simulate (Forio, San Francisco, CA). All the underlying models can be downloaded as Stella or Runtime files. The model interfaces are not downloadable.

A complete list of the models can be found at the following link:

http://web.uri.edu/pharmacy/research/rosenbaum/sims

Basic Pharmacokinetics and Pharmacodynamics: An Integrated Textbook and Computer Simulations,
Second Edition. Edited by Sara E. Rosenbaum.
© 2017 John Wiley & Sons, Inc. Published 2017 by John Wiley & Sons, Inc.

GLOSSARY OF TERMS

A, B	Intercepts of exponential terms in a two-compartment model
A1	Amount of drug in the central compartment
Aa	Amount of drug in the arterial blood
Ab	Amount of drug in the body
$Ab_{max,n}$	Maximum amount of drug in the body after the nth dose
$Ab_{min.n}$	Minimum amount of drug in the body after the nth dose
ADME	Absorption distribution metabolism and excretion
Ae	Amount of drug eliminated
A_{GI}	Amount of drug in the gastrointestinal tract
α	Hybrid rate constant for distribution or intrinsic activity or slope representing how a disease status changes over time
Ap	Amount of drug in the plasma
At	Amount of drug in the tissue(s)
Au	Amount of drug in the urine
Au^{∞}	Amount of drug excreted in urine by infinity
AUC	Area under the plasma concentration–time curve
AUC^p	The area under the curve in the presence of a perpetrator
AUCR	The ratio of the AUC in the presence and absence of a perpetrator
AUMC	Area under the first moment-time curve
Av	Amount of drug in the venous blood
β	Hybrid rate constant for elimination
BCRP	Breast cancer resistance protein
BP	Blood:plasma concentration ratio of a drug
BSEP	Bile salt export pump
BW	Body weight
Ca	Drug concentration in arterial blood

Basic Pharmacokinetics and Pharmacodynamics: An Integrated Textbook and Computer Simulations,
Second Edition. Edited by Sara E. Rosenbaum.
© 2017 John Wiley & Sons, Inc. Published 2017 by John Wiley & Sons, Inc.

Cb	Drug concentration in blood
Ce	Concentration of drug in the effect compartment or the concentration at the site of action
C_{EC}	Concentration in extracellular space
Ch_u	Unbound drug concentration in the hepatocyte
C_{IC}	Concentration in intracellular space
Cl	Clearance
$Cl_{intact,t}$	Transporter intrinsic clearance
Clb_h	Hepatic blood clearance
Cl_{efflux}	Intrinsic clearance of efflux transporter
Cl_h	Hepatic clearance (based on plasma)
$Cl_{h,b}$	Blood hepatic clearance
Cl^I	Clearance in the presence of an inhibitor
Cl_{int}	Intrinsic hepatic clearance
Cl_{intg}	Intestinal intrinsic clearance
Cl^I_{int}	Intrinsic clearance in the presence of an inhibitor
Cl^{Ind}_{int}	Intrinsic clearance in the presence of an inducer
Cl^P_{int}	Intrinsic clearance in the presence of a perpetrator
Clr	Renal clearance
Cl_{uptake}	Intrinsic clearance of uptake transporter
Cm	Concentration of metabolite
$Cm50$	Steady-state concentration of the metabolite that produces 50% maximum tolerance
$Cmax$	Maximum observed plasma concentration
$Cmax_{hi,u}$	Maximal unbound hepatic inlet concentration
Cp	Plasma concentration
$Cp_{av,ss}$	Average steady-state plasma concentration
Cp_{max}	Peak plasma concentration
Cp_{min}	Trough plasma concentration
Cp_n	Plasma concentration during the nth dosing interval
Cp_{ss}	Steady-state plasma concentration
Cp_u	Concentration of unbound drug concentration in the plasma
Cp_{ut}	Unbound concentration in the venous plasma
Ct	Tissue concentration
CT	Concentration of a hypothetical tolerance drug in an additional compartment
Ct_u	Unbound tissue concentration of the drug
Cv	Drug concentration in venous blood
Cv_{ut}	Unbound drug concentration in venous blood
Cvt	Drug in the venous blood emerging from a tissue
D	Distribution coefficient (lipophilicity); diffusion coefficient (Noyes–Whitney)
D	Dose administered
DDI	Drug–drug interaction
D_L	Loading dose
D_M	Maintenance dose
ε	Intrinsic efficacy, efficacy per unit receptor
e	Efficacy, efficiency with which an agonist generates a stimulus in a tissue
E	Extraction ratio
E	Drug effect
E	Free enzyme

E_0	Baseline effect
Ec	Vasoconstriction effects
EC50	Concentration of drug that produces half its maximum response
Ed	Vasodilation effects
Eg	Fraction extracted in the intestine (1-Fg)
E_t^{Ind}	Total enzyme in the presence of an inducer
E_t^I	Total enzyme in the presence of a TDI
Em	System's maximum response
E_{max}	Drug's maximum response
EP	Erythrocyte:plasma concentration ratio
Et	Effect of a drug at time t
E_t	Total enzyme concentration
Et	Total amount of enzyme
F	Bioavailability factor (fraction of the dose absorbed)
F_a	Fraction of the dose that is absorbed into GI membrane
fe	Fraction of the dose excreted unchanged
F_g	Intestinal bioavailability
Fg^p	Intestinal bioavailability in the presence of a perpetrator
F_h	Hepatic bioavailability
fm	Fractional contribution of a specific pathway of metabolism to the overall AUC
fu	Fraction of the drug in the plasma that is unbound
fu_b	Fraction of drug unbound in blood
fu_{IC}	Fraction of drug free in intracellular space
fu_t	Fraction of the drug in the tissues that is unbound
GFR	Glomerular filtration rate
GI	Gastrointestinal
GIT	Gastrointestinal tract
Ht	Hematocrit
I	Inhibitory effect
I	Inhibitor concentration at enzyme site
IC50	Drug concentration that produces 50% inhibition
ICTT	Intercompartmental transit time
Ig	Intestinal perpetrator concentration
Ih	Perpetrator concentration at site of action in the liver
I_{max}	A drug's maximum inhibitory effect
I_{max}	maximum observed plasma concentration of a perpetrator
$I_{max,u}$	maximum observed unbound plasma concentration of a perpetrator
$I_{u,hi,max}$	maximum unbound concentration in the portal vein or maximum unbound hepatic inlet concentration
$Jmax_t$	Maximum rate of transport
k	Overall elimination rate constant
$k10$	Elimination rate constant in a two-compartment model
$k12$	Rate constant for distribution between the first and second compartments
k_{1e}	First-order rate constants for distribution into the effect compartment
k1m	Rate constant for formation of tolerance mediator
$k21$	Rate constant for redistribution between the second and first compartments
ka	First-order rate constant for absorption
k_{cat}	The rate constant for the productive enzyme pathway
k_{circ}	First-order rate constant for the loss of neutrophils

kd	First-order rate constant for distribution to a tissue
Kd	Dissociation constant, reciprocal measure of affinity. Drug concentration that results in 50% receptor occupancy
k_{degrad}	First-order degradation rate constant of an enzyme
k_{e0}	Rate constant for removal of drug from the effect compartment
KF	Kill factor
K_I	TDI inhibitor concentration that produces 50% maximum inactivation
K_i	Dissociation constant for an inhibitor.
k_{in}	Zero-order rate constant for the formation of a physiological response variable
k_{inact}	Maximum first-order inactivation constant for a TDI or mechanism-based enzyme inhibitor
k_{irr}	Second-order rate constant for the irreversible destruction of a response variable
km	First-order rate constant for the elimination of a drug by metabolism
Km	Michaelis–Menten constant
Km^I	Michaelis–Menten constant in the presence of an inhibitor
k_{m0}	Rate constant for the destruction of tolerance mediator
Km^P	A drug's Km in the presence of a perpetrator
Km_t	Michaelis–Menten constant for a transporter
k_{obs}	The constant of proportionality between the rate of inactivation of an enzyme and the total enzyme concentration
k_{off}	Rate constant for the disassociation of a drug with its receptor
k_{on}	Rate constant for the interaction of a drug with its receptor
k_{out}	First-order rate constant for the degradation of a physiological response variable, R
k_p	First-order rate constant for production
k_{prog}	First-order rate constant for disease progression
k_{prol}	Rate constant for the proliferation of neutrophils from the stem cell pool
Kp_t	Tissue to plasma partition coefficient
kr	First-order rate constant for the elimination of a drug by renal excretion
k_{syn}	Zero-order rate constant for the production of an enzyme
k_{tr}	First-order rate constant for progression between compartments
LogD	Log diffusion coefficient
LogP	Log partition coefficient
MATE	Multidrug and toxin extrusion protein
MEC	Minimum effective concentration
MRP	Multidrug resistance-associated protein
MRT	Mean residence time
MTC	Maximum tolerated concentration
MTT	Mean transit time
n	Power function
N_o	Baseline neutrophil count
N_t	Number of neutrophils at time t
OAT	Organic anion transporter
OATP	Organic anion transporting polypeptide
OCT	Organic cation transporter
P	Partition coefficient
P-gp	Permeability glycoprotein
PS_t	Permeability surface area product
Q	Tissue blood flow

Q_{ent}	Blood flow to the enterocytes
Q_g	Blood flow to the enterocytes
r	Accumulation ratio
R	Concentration of a physiological factor or the response variable
R	Ratio of intrinsic clearance in the absence and presence of the perpetrator
R_0	Baseline concentration of the physiological response variable
RC	Concentration of the drug receptor complex
RC_{E50}	Concentration of the drug receptor complex that produces 50% the system's maximum effect
R_I	Reversible inhibitor
R_m	Maximum response achieved at a given dose in an indirect effect model
R_{max}	Maximum achievable response of the drug in an indirect effect model
R_T	Total concentration of receptors
S	Salt factor; stimulatory effect
S_0	Status of the disease at time zero
SC50	Drug concentration that results in 50% of the maximum stimulatory action of the drug
$S_i(t)$	Weibull function value at a given time t
S_{max}	Maximum stimulatory effect of a drug
S_{SS}	Terminal disease status of a progressive disease
St	Status of the disease at time t
t	Time or time after a dose
τ	Transduction ratio or dosing interval or intercompartmental transit time
τ	Dosing interval
t_0	Absorption lag time
$t_{1/2}$	Half-life
TDI	Time-dependent inhibitor
T_{MAX}	Time of maximum observed plasma concentration
T_{Rm}	Time of maximum response
v	Rate of an enzymatic process
V1	Volume of the central compartment
V2	Volume of the peripheral compartment
Va	Volume of the arterial blood
Vd	Volume of distribution
Vd_β	Volume of distribution during the elimination phase
Vd_{ss}	Volume of distribution at steady state
Ve	Volume of the erythrocytes
V_{max}	Maximum rate of an enzymatic process
$Vmax^I$	A drug's $Vmax$ in the presence of an inhibitor
$Vmax^{Ind}$	A drug's $Vmax$ in the presence of an inducer
$V_{max}{}^P$	A drug's $Vmax$ in the presence of a perpetrator
Vp	Volume of plasma
Vt	Volume of tissue or volume outside the plasma into which a drug distributes
Vv	Volume of the venous blood
V_β	Volume of distribution in the postdistribution phase
WE	Weibull function parameter

INDEX

Note: Page numbers followed by f refer to figures; page numbers followed by t refer to tables; page numbers followed by s refer to simulations; page numbers followed by p refer to problems; and page numbers followed by e refer to examples.

Basic Pharmacokinetics and Pharmacodynamics: An Integrated Textbook and Computer Simulations,
Second Edition. Edited by Sara E. Rosenbaum.
© 2017 John Wiley & Sons, Inc. Published 2017 by John Wiley & Sons, Inc.